The
CANCER
SURVIVOR'S
BIBLE

Everything that everyone should know about cancer
How to recover from cancer
How to protect yourself from damaging treatments

Jonathan Chamberlain

Long Island
Press

I dedicate this book to the memory of Bernadette, Sau-fong—
for whom the information came too late.

A CIP catalogue record for this book is available from the British Library.

Published by Long Island Press

ISBN 978-1-908712-09-7

www.fightingcancer.com

Disclaimer

I am not a doctor. The information in this book is for educational purposes only. None of the treatments in this book are recommended for any particular person with any particular cancer. You, and you alone, bear the responsibility for any decisions you make in relation to any cancer treatment you may choose, be it orthodox or alternative. The best decisions are based on the best understanding of the facts.

Foreword 2012 Edition

This book—The Cancer Survivor's Bible—is the final stage of an 18 year journey that started the day my wife was, very belatedly, diagnosed with cancer.

This news was so shocking and unexpected, and we were so uninformed and unprepared, that neither Bernadette nor I had any thought but to go along with what the doctor recommended. Fifteen months later Bernadette was dead and the year that we battled her illness was one of great pain and suffering. She died not just from the cancer but also from the appalling impacts of her treatment. There is no doubt that she was extremely unlucky. She would have been better off doing absolutely nothing.

I would like to say that, on learning of her cancer, I immediately went to the bookshop and to the local cancer support group's resource library and set out to find out what I could. But I didn't. It took me a couple of weeks to take those important steps. What I discovered as I read book after book was that there was a great deal we could do or might have done. But these options were such a radical departure from our world view that we simply didn't take them on in time.

Part of the problem was the variety of books and, more important, the variance of world-view that they expressed. One book would promote the curative value of a particular therapy while other books would pour scorn on the idea. Trying to get a grip, a coherent understanding of the situation, was difficult. And to make things worse, the different ways in which we were approaching the disease was tearing apart our marriage.

I read book after book, looking for that book that would wrap its arm around my shoulder and say: 'Look Jonathan, this is the way it is'. What I needed was a sane, personal, intelligent, critical—and above all bluntly honest - book that could lead me through the contending beliefs; that could put both sides of the case and point out the limitations of any arguments there might be. But I never found this voice so I set out to provide this voice for others.

My first attempt was a book called *Fighting Cancer: A Survival Guide* which was picked up by a major British publisher, Hodder Headline. They put out two editions and then let it go out of print. I was then approached by a French publisher to produce a new edition and his criticisms of the first book led me into doing further research and re-organising what information I had. The end result of this process was the book *Cancer: The Complete Recovery Guide*, which I published in 2008.

Now, just because you have written the 'complete' guide to cancer doesn't mean that you stop learning about new approaches, new perspectives and above all new facts. So I set up a blog site at www.cancerfighter.wordpress.com where I could archive this new information that was coming in week after week and at the same time make it available to others.

Then along came Kindle and other ebook readers. I felt the book was too long to be uploaded as a single volume into Kindle so I had the idea that I could kill two birds with one stone. I could update the book by inserting all the new material that had come my way and at the same time break the book into eight short, easy to read volumes. This I did and the result is my *Cancer: The Complete Recovery Guide Series, Books 1-8* (see www.cancerfighter.wordpress.com for details).

But having done this, I felt something was lacking. I had turned a one-stop source of information into a fragmented series of books. I wanted to recreate the wholeness of the enterprise, to give people like myself, who wanted to buy a single volume that had all the information needed within one set of covers, the book they wanted. So this is what I have done—and so as not to create more interference with my other books (for I had in the meantime produced a short book called, *Cancer Recovery Guide: 15 alternative and complementary strategies for restoring health*), I have decided to call this book *The Cancer Survivor's Bible*.

This book is not about taking sides. It is not about telling you what you should do. Rather, this book aims to present all the information available to me, that I consider relevant to decisions about getting well again, in a reasonable and fair manner. The decisions you eventually make must be your own decisions. You and I will make different decisions because we are different people, we have different life experiences, different cancers to deal with, different amounts of money to throw at the problem, different personalities, different attitudes and all the rest of it. There is no single set of decisions that will be right for everybody—and we need to respect these differences. And we need to recognise that there is a place for surgery just as there is a place for vitamin C. But whatever decisions we do make for ourselves, we should make sure those decisions are based on as clear and as full an understanding of the facts as is possible. That is where this book comes in.

Please read this book thoughtfully. It is there to serve you in the situation you find yourself in. I have tried to write clearly and accessibly so that you can read this book quickly—so that you have time not just to read the book but also to reflect on it and then hopefully to use this information to change your response to your cancer.

This has been my journey. You too are on a journey of discovery. I wish you the best of luck on that journey and I hope it leads you to a place of safety.

Jonathan Chamberlain
Brighton 2012

Testimonials for Cancer, the Complete Recovery Guide

'From the depth of my tired (at the moment) heart, I thank you for being YOU—for turning the light on the dark corner, where people wanted to keep cancer; for turning your personal, in part tragic experience, into a dignified triumph of life, for yourself and other people. Your book has become as important to me as my deceased mother's letters. Such clarity and honesty in your writing that I keep it on my bedside table.'—*Victoria McLaurin, Cancer survivor*

'This book helps to put things in perspective and was invaluable to me in making my decisions about follow-up treatment …. The author does not advocate either the 'orthodox' or 'alternative' route, but suggests the reader should decide on the treatment—or combination of approaches—that are right for themselves. Please, absorb the vast amount of information within this book and make the right choices—knowing you now have so much more information at your fingertips than the doctors will ever tell you.'—*Lucy W. (Amazon review)*

'Since I was diagnosed with the dreaded C disease, I have read many books on and around the subject, and when I read this one, I wish now I had not wasted any money on the rest. The info here is virtually all you need to know.'—*Funland Addict (Amazon review)*

'This book gives hope …. It explains clearly the arguments for and against a multitude of treatments …. I wish I'd read this book before I was diagnosed. My doctor and the cancer charities didn't tell me any of this.'—*D Bushell*

'A very well written book, beautifully organised and easy to read and understand.'—*June Black, cancer survivor*

'Being someone diagnosed as a terminal cancer patient, I have scoured the 'net and read many books. This is the best. And it gives hope too …. Get this book; read it; be inspired by it.'—*Ian Clements, cancer survivor*

'I now can recommend your book to the people in my support group, as the book to read. You have covered just about everything that I have read, and it took me over twenty books and innumerable downloads to do it. Thanks again, and no I'm not going to give your hard work away! The book is more precious than gold!'—*Richard Thompson*

'I work with cancer patients and have found this book incredibly helpful to them (and me and my work colleagues). Very well laid out, well written.'—*S Lumley (Amazon review)*

Further testimonials can be found at the end of this book.

Acknowledgments

The original version of this book was *Fighting Cancer: A Survival Guide*. I would like to thank Brian Stratford for introducing me to Pam Dix who, in turn, agreed to be my agent and for finding me my first publisher, Hodder Headline. Without Pam's enthusiasm the book might very well have died an early death.

I also owe a profound debt to Vicky Parker who supplied detailed comments on the chapter on radiation and whose commentary enabled me to avoid many errors. Vicky was one of the leading activists of RAGE—an organisation founded by and for victims of radiation treatment. Sadly, this organization has ceased its activities, as the radiation victims were physically unable to maintain their work.

In writing this book I have also been very fortunate in having the library resources of the Hong Kong Cancer Fund. Without access to these books it is unlikely I would have been able to start work on this project.

I wish also to acknowledge the invaluable help of Edith Segall, Annette Crisswell, Gary Oden, Hazel Thornton, Charles Ha, Alan and Martha Cheng, Louise Aylward, Chris Teo, Dr Alan Greenberg, Jack Gontier, editor of the French edition, whose input has resulted in this new edition of the book being very much better than its predecessors; Leonard Rosenbaum, who combined editorial savvy with unbridled enthusiasm and support for this book; and to Dr Shamim Daya and her staff at the Wholistic Health Centre in London, for reviewing this book and educating me in some of the latest testing modalities; to Pete Spurrier for facilitating the publication of the 2008 edition and Margit Whitton, whose critical support on the home front was very much appreciated.

I would also like to acknowledge the input of the people whose stories appear in Section 8: *Survivors' Stories: They did it. You can too!*, who had the courage to follow the alternative route, solely or partly in their own cancer journey, and who have shared their stories in books or in emails to me personally—in particular, Ian Clements and Nuro Weidemann whose input and involvement went beyond simply telling their story. Thanks are also due to those contributors to various health Yahoogroups who provided many much needed discussion and information that has moulded my own understanding.

Finally, serendipity led me to Andie Davidson who has played an important editorial, design (and sometimes even educational) role in guiding this latest incarnation of the *Complete Recovery Guides* and *The Cancer Survivor's Bible* to press.

To them all, I would like to say thank you.

Contents

Cancer? What Now?

Make sure the first steps in your cancer journey are going in the right direction

In this section, I describe the basic facts about cancer, the two ways cancer can be visualized and the four sensible strategies for responding to your cancer. But the first step in your cancer journey is to become aware of and to evaluate your own attitudes to health, healing, doctors and so on. By becoming aware you will be more in control and therefore more able to take a long view as to how you—you in particular—wish to respond to your cancer. I then provide you with resources that will help you take the next step in your cancer journey.

And of course, a natural strategy that cures cancer is very likely to be a strategy which, put in place ahead of time, might very well help you avoid that cancer in the first place.

About this Section

In this section, I describe the basic facts about cancer, the two ways cancer can be visualized and the four sensible strategies for responding to your cancer. But the first step in your cancer journey is to become aware of and to evaluate your own attitudes to health, healing, doctors and so on. By becoming aware you will be more in control and therefore more able to take a long view as to how you—you in particular—wish to respond to your cancer. I then provide you with resources that will help you take the next step in your cancer journey.

And of course, a natural strategy that cures cancer is very likely to be a strategy which, put in place ahead of time, might very well help you avoid that cancer in the first place.

When you have read this book you will know more about cancer than you ever thought possible: the two ways of conceptualizing cancer, the causes, the diagnostic tests, the problems with the orthodox treatments and the enormous range of alternative approaches that there are. You will also learn about the business of cancer and cancer research.

However, I know from experience that it is no good simply hoping that the information you will read in this book will help you. You come to this book with a world view and a whole bag full of prejudices. These have been formed by your reading, the newspapers, television. And almost all your prejudices, thoughts and ideas about cancer are almost certainly wrong. But it may be that my telling you this has merely served to make you defensive: How do you know that what I know is wrong? Who are you to …? etc.

Let's just say that I've been there. Goethe put it succinctly: 'The half-known hinders knowing. Since all our knowing is only half, our knowing always hinders our knowing.' In short, what we think we know gets in the way of our learning something new.

I am not a Guru; I am a Tour Guide

This book was written to provide you with quick—but at the same time sufficiently detailed—overviews of the facts, the arguments and the evidence supporting them. If you want someone to tell you what to do, then you have come to the wrong place. My job is to give you sufficient information for you to make your own decisions. Your decisions will very likely be different from my decisions—but that doesn't mean we shouldn't respect each other's opinions. That is why I have written this book in a reasonable and fair-minded way. There are lots of books that vilify the alternative approaches and many more books that vilify the conventional approaches. What you need is a reasonable voice that can weave a rational path through the controversies. That is what I have attempted to provide. Let me put this as clearly as I can. This is the book I wish I had had when my wife was first diagnosed with cancer. If we had had this information we would certainly have made different decisions to the ones we did make—and we would have been saved a great deal of pain.

Together, it is my hope, this book will provide you with the confidence to make decisions that suit you and will, I hope, lead to you becoming well again—possibly without having to undergo damaging treatments—or, if you decide to undergo these treatments, you will have learnt ways in which you can help limit the damage.

In this brief foreword, I'm going to suppose that you fall into one of three groups of people and I'd like to say something to each of you.

1. You have just recently discovered that you have cancer

You are, I imagine, suddenly very scared. Life that seemed so firmly based has now become very precarious. You have to a certain extent closed yourself off from the world. You are locked inside your own head. Your fears are echoing around the empty chambers of your mind. You are trying to strengthen your grip on things by saying to yourself: 'I will do whatever is necessary to get through this thing!' You know that it is going to be fearfully damaging and painful. But you're going to do it. Yes, you are! And you will ignore all obstacles in the way. You are going to grit your teeth and … STOP!

Yes, please stop this line of thinking. I am going to tell you two things. One will scare you a little more and one, I hope, will reassure you.

The scare

The minute you heard that you had cancer, your cancer almost certainly started to become just a little more aggressive. The problem is stress and anxiety. The biochemistry of these emotional states is actually provoking the tumour to grow faster. Your doctor probably didn't tell you that—he thought it would just make matters worse. And perhaps it would make matters worse if I left it there. But by knowing this fact you can now start working to change this stress to a state of relaxation, even calm acceptance perhaps: Meditate, swim, go for long walks, book yourself an aromatherapy massage, take up singing, listen to Javanese gamelan music or the hypnotic Indian dulcimer (santoor) music of Shiv Kumar Sharma.

Yes, go and do it now. This will, hopefully, have the reverse effect of slowing the growth of the tumour. Also, get the amino acid supplement L-theanine. This is widely available on the Internet and is a proven, quick acting and totally safe anxiety eliminator. Take up yoga and/or meditation. Go and watch a funny film.

The reassurance

Cancer can be beaten—there are dozens of 'cures' in this book. I have put the word 'cure' in inverted commas because it is a contentious word but I do believe that many of these 'cures'—either alone or in conjunction with others—can lead to a real, long term state of being cancer-free. It's true that none are 100 per cent certain but several have extremely good track records –and you will be relieved to know that most of them are pain-free. If one therapy—or one combination of therapies—doesn't work, you can move on to another. There is time.

Also I would like you to tell yourself the following message. Say to yourself these important words:

I am not going to do anything until I have read this book. I want any decision I make to be truly informed. I want to know something more about cancer. I will spend the next few days reading. Maybe I will get a copy for a close friend to read at the same time so that I can talk about it. Then I will be in control. Above all I am not going to undertake a treatment just because the doctor or my wife, husband or mother says that's what I should do.

Read also the personal stories in Section 8: *Cancer Survivors' Stories.* These people cured themselves of their cancers—you can too. Good luck.

Get access to the Internet

If you do not have access to the Internet—for whatever reason—then find someone who does. Or go down to the library and find out how you can learn. This is a vital resource for many of the products recommended in this book.

2. You have undergone cancer treatment but now you want to learn more about the options just in case it returns

When you first got cancer you probably went along with what your doctors advised. Why wouldn't you? The doctors have 'science' on their side. (Again I have used inverted commas because science too is a word that is often misused. Doctors claim that they have science on their side—but in fact most authorities accept that 80 per cent of what doctors do is not in fact strongly supported by science—and there is a great deal of science supporting many of the alternative options.) Well, now maybe you are prepared to reconsider that position. I hope so. The problem is that there are large areas of health-related information and expertise that doctors know nothing about—certainly they are not taught about them during their medical studies: diet, supplements, herbs, electromagnetic interventions and a great deal more. In many places—the USA, for example—doctors are in fact forbidden by their medical boards from discussing these subjects. If they insist on doing so they can find themselves struck off the medical register. So if there is any value in these areas you will not learn about them from your doctor —which is a great pity.

Also, if you are wise you will already have come to understand that you can't treat cancer as a disease that you can 'cure' and then forget about. Your cancer hasn't come from Mars. Cancer is the result of a natural process that is almost certainly connected with the way you choose to live your life. If you don't change your way of life then you can probably expect the cancer to return at some stage. But what do you need to do to avoid this happening?

I liken cancer to the war in Afghanistan. Dropping powerful bombs that destroy remote villages will not win the war. Force alone cannot be successful. We need to understand the causes of the problem too and deal with those. I hope this book will help you find answers that you can happily incorporate into your life. Good luck.

3. You Are Helping Someone Who Has Cancer

You have a very difficult job. You want to help but you're not sure how. As someone who has been in this position let me tell you some of the conclusions I have come to.

a) Not everyone wants information

Recently I met Peter. On our first meeting he told me that he had liver cancer. It had been treated but had returned. 'Well, this is your lucky day,' I said to him. 'I happen to know what you can do.' But Peter waved me away. 'Oh don't tell me anything. I just have to live with it as long as I can.' 'Really,' I assured him. 'I know something you can do. It's cheap and people say it has a 90 per cent chance of working.' 'No,' he said. 'I don't want to know.' So I smiled and we talked about something else. Over the next three years I continued to see Peter on summer afternoons. He was a large and very jovial man who liked to gather around him old age pensioners who he entertained with his bizarre stories— like how he became a besotted Marlene Dietrich fan. But last summer he wasn't there, nor this one. So, perhaps the cancer finally got him but … he was happy. He lived his life on his own terms.

The truth is denial does have some survival value—it stops people getting overstressed (and stress exacerbates cancer) and if that's how he wanted to deal with it, fine. I just had to accept it.

And, it is true, the older you are the less sense it makes to do anything for any cancer you might have. And if you don't want to do anything, you probably also don't want to think obsessively about it either.

b) You may disagree about what to do

This is particularly difficult if you are living with someone who is making decisions that you think are wrong. Perhaps they want to do chemo and radiation while you think the Budwig approach (see Section 4: *Cancer: Detox and Diet*) is best. Or they want to see a spiritual healer while you think surgery is the only sensible thing to do. Well, here is what you have to do: say your piece—once, twice or even three times—and then shut up. The person who has cancer is the person whose decision counts. I can tell you this is not an easy thing to do. But it is important because …

c) Your relationship is vital

The person you are caring for is utterly vulnerable. Your relationship may be one of the things that is making the present bearable. Do everything you can to nurture it. This is not a time for you to impose your feelings on the relationship. Instead, it is a time for you to listen and to quietly be of help. Again this is often not easy but I assure you it is important. If you feel frustrated take your frustrations elsewhere.

d) Is your relationship part of the problem?

This is a hard question to ask and an even harder one to answer. If there are problems between you and the person you are caring for then this is the time to confront them. Nagging emotional obstacles can hinder healing. Healing the emotions can release very profound energies. Perhaps counselling—for both of you—would be beneficial.

e) Take care of yourself

You are not perfect. You can't do everything. There will come a time when you, yourself, will need the support of others. From time to time you will need to put your own needs first. Give yourself treats. Pamper yourself too. Nurture yourself.

Good luck
Jonathan Chamberlain
Brighton, July 2011

'Fast decisions are usually bad decisions.'

Vincent Gammill,
Center for the Study of Natural Oncology (CSNO),
Solana Beach, California

Your cancer took a long time getting to where it is today. Unless it is highly aggressive, another month or so won't make much of a difference in terms of making the cancer worse—but the time spent researching your options will certainly improve the decisions you will make.

This is the truth: There are literally dozens of options that have a very good chance of stopping your cancer in its track—within weeks or months. Tumours will disappear and you will feel healthy.

It is also true that no one option will work 100 per cent of the time in 100 per cent of cancers. So it's best to do a number of options together simultaneously and be constantly prepared to modify your regime in the light of new information.

People who are open to new ideas will tend to have better outcomes.

Introduction

This section is designed to help you formulate your own strategy for treating your cancer—one that is right for you in your situation. And then it tells you where to find information resources relevant to your own healing or treatment journey. Here is an overview of what you will find in this section:

Part One: Knowing Your Enemy: the basic facts of cancer

Here you will learn some of the basic concepts that will help you understand what your doctor is talking about.

Part Two: Knowing Yourself: what kind of cancer patient are you?

Here you will be given a questionnaire designed to help you become aware of your own attitudes. Why are your attitudes important? Because they inform, or get in the way of, your ability to make the right decisions. But attitudes aren't permanent. They can be changed. The more you are aware of your attitudes—and what the other possible attitudes are—you can either confirm yourself in the attitudes you hold or begin a process of negotiation with yourself so that you open yourself up to change.

Part Three: The four sensible strategies

Here I discuss the four sensible strategies for dealing with your cancer. Your job is to think about these strategies and decide which of them makes most sense to you. It is for you to decide which makes most sense for you in your situation.

Part Four: Resources

Here you will be given details of some information resources that will help inform you further of the options available—of which there are an enormous variety!

The idea is to quickly load you with some key concepts and then direct your path so that you can speedily reach a level of understanding that will allow you to affect the course of your treatment.

Part One
Understanding the Enemy
some basic facts about cancer

Preamble

Some interesting statistics

The incidence of cancer is rising inexorably as the following statistics show (unless otherwise stated, these figures are from Ralph Moss's excellent book *The Cancer Syndrome*—reprinted as *The Cancer Industry*, 1982).

Early 1800s: One in 50

1900: One in 27

1920: One in 20

1930: One in 12

1940: One in nine

1950: One in seven

1960: 'According to present government statistics, one out of every six persons in our population will die of cancer. It will not be long before the entire population will have to decide whether we will all die of cancer or change fundamentally all our living and nutritional conditions.' (Max Gerson (1958) author of *A Cancer Therapy*)

1980: 'If the present trend continues, at least one in four of us will contract cancer. One in five will die of the disease.'

1993:   'Cancer may be the most feared disease of our time. It is second only to heart disease as a leading cause of cancer in the United States, and it is estimated that one in every three Americans will develop cancer at some point in their lives.' Geoffrey Cooper (1993) author of The Cancer Book.

2000:   'More than 1 million people in the United States were diagnosed with cancer in 1990. Cancer (in the USA) … claims more than 500,000 lives every year. Basing its estimates on statistics, the American Cancer Society … predicts that by the year 2000, about 1 out of every 2 people will develop the disease.' (Dr I William Lane and Linda Comac (1992)—authors of Sharks Don't Get Cancer)

2002:   'Today, one of every two men and one of every three women in the United States alone will confront cancer over the course of their lives.' (Andrew von Eschenbach MD, Director of the National Cancer Institute—preface to Everyone's Guide to Cancer Therapy, 2002)

I hope those figures got your attention because they certainly got mine. Decade after decade cancer incidence has risen inexorably. However, some have suggested that in 2004–6 these figures may have peaked, others have pointed out that the post-war baby boomer generation are just beginning to hit the age when cancer incidence rises markedly so the apparent flattening out of the curve may be a very temporary phenomenon. For some these figures are merely impersonal abstractions that have little immediate personal relevance. But there are those whose experience of cancer's seemingly insistent onward march is more traumatic.

'Cancer, and cancer, and cancer. My mother, my father, my wife. I wonder who is next in the queue?'
C S Lewis

Cancer is now the cause of a third of all deaths in Western industrialised countries—up from about 20 per cent not much more than a decade ago. And it is not just because people are living longer—actually they—we—aren't! The life expectancy of a 45 year old person hasn't changed significantly in the last 100 years. In 1870, the 45-year-old person could expect to live to the age of 70 to 75. Now, he or she can expect to live to somewhere between 75 and 80. If average life expectancy appears to have increased by great leaps in that time it is because there are fewer diseases decimating children—and fewer women are dying in childbirth. Several thousand years ago writers of the Old Testament were able to estimate a normal life expectancy of 'three score years and ten' (70 years). So the argument that there's more cancer because people are living longer is not a very good one. The fact is, overall cancer incidence is increasing at every age level. In 2000, for example, more women of 40 had breast cancer than they did in 1950. Cancer incidence is rising at approximately one per cent a year.

Until recently, cancer was almost a taboo word. Fortunately, it has now come out of the closet. It is no longer seen to be an automatic death sentence. The good news is the fact that people with cancer are, according to statistics, living longer and that 40–50 per cent of people diagnosed with cancer do not die of the disease. The bad news is that the statistics cannot be trusted, for reasons that will be explained later in this section.

The fact is, more and more people are developing cancer. While death rates for most cancers have not changed in decades, some have declined (often for reasons unknown), while some are increasing at an enormous rate: lung cancer being the prime example. With the possible exception of breast cancer (where there may—I stress 'may', for reasons unknown—have been a slight improvement in survival rates in recent years), the so-called 'orthodox' methods of treating cancer—surgery, radiation and chemotherapy—have not had a clear impact on death rates. Many people have therefore taken the view that alternative ways of treating cancer hold out more hope. These alternative ways include dietary regimes, the taking of vitamin and herbal supplements—and a host of other approaches from copper coils to magnetic beds, from acidophilus to visualisation—details of which you will find in this book

The problem for the patient is that doctors, generally speaking, are very hostile to these alternative approaches. It is not excessive to describe the present state of affairs as a war of ideas. Anyone wishing to make reasoned decisions in this battlefield needs to understand where the battle lines are drawn. I have discussed these issues in Section 3: *Cancer: Research and Politics.*

Can we avoid getting cancer?

For those of us who do not (yet?) have cancer, two questions pose themselves:

- Is there any way that we can reduce our chances of getting cancer?
- If we do get cancer, what is the best way to making sure that we are among the 40–50 per cent who do not die from the disease within five years—perhaps even one of the 25–30 per cent who does not die of the disease at all?

How to improve your chances of not getting cancer

The quick answer is to stop smoking—one in two smokers dies from a smoking related disease—and to reduce dietary fat to not more than 30 per cent of total calories (but note that very low fat diets are also associated with some cancer risks—a median fat diet is optimal), eat more fibre, take more exercise, avoid burnt or barbecued foods, avoid drinking alcohol in liver damaging quantities. Alcohol in reasonable quantities does not appear to be measurably carcinogenic on its own but evidence suggests that it can speed the passage of other carcinogens into the cells. For heavy drinking heavy smokers, this is bad news. You should also avoid chemical pollutants and excessive radiation.

But cancer prevention is not simply about avoiding cancer-causing substances. A more pro-active regime will involve increasing exposure to the sun (for the vitamin D), changing one's diet to one that includes lots of apples, oranges, carrots, cabbage and other dark green vegetables—preferably organic (pesticides have been linked to breast cancer). It may also involve taking vitamin and herbal supplements.

You are going to have to change the way you live to maximise your chances of living a longer cancer-free life. That's your responsibility, no-one else's.

Being prepared for cancer

Let's look back at the statistics. These demonstrate beyond a shadow of doubt that something very frightening is happening. It is not exploding as fast as AIDS, maybe, but the cancer spectre is much larger and affects many more people. And dying of cancer is a painful, debilitating, traumatic and traumatising experience. To give you an indication of how great the problem is, imagine eight fully-loaded jumbo 747s crashing every day with no survivors: That is the number of people dying of cancer every day in North America and Western Europe combined. That's right. Eight jumbo jets today, another eight tomorrow, eight more the day after that and so on. Or perhaps there is a more potent image. Imagine an event of the magnitude of the 9/11 incident in New York. Imagine that many people dying every day. Now double that. That's close to what is happening globally with cancer.

For myself, confronted with my wife's newly diagnosed illness, I discovered I knew nothing at all about cancer. Cancer was just a word. I talked to my friends, supposedly bright, literate, and highly-educated. None of them knew anything worth a damn about cancer or its treatments. Here is a disease that is going to kill one in two of us within the foreseeable future and we knew nothing about it. We weren't doing anything about it either. We had simply blinkered ourselves to reality. We didn't do it consciously but we were doing it. We were heading like lambs to the slaughter.

If the situation is that bad why isn't everyone panicking?

I think part of the reason is that it is all happening so slowly. There is an experiment that went as follows. A number of frogs were put into a shallow pan containing scalding hot water. Without exception they immediately leapt out. A number of other frogs were placed in a similar pan containing water at room temperature. This water was ever so gradually heated. The water heated up but the frogs didn't move. They all eventually died of heat shock.

The moral of this experiment is that when something is gradual, it slips under our genetically primed warning systems that are geared to protect us against sudden or gross changes in our environment. We become habituated. The slow creeping increase in cancer and heart disease has slipped through more or less unannounced. Oh yes, there have been stories in the press. But the sense of urgency is entirely missing. We may be able to perceive it intellectually. But we are not emotionally alerted. Our fight or flight systems are not switched on. There's no adrenalin. There's no panic. We continue to live as we have always lived.

One of the purposes of this book is to trigger a little adrenalin.

You have the choice of being or not being a victim

Let me state this bluntly: If you don't inform yourself about cancer, you will significantly increase your chances of being a victim. Why do I say this? Because when confronted with a diagnosis of cancer, you may make choices that you will possibly regret later. You need to be informed that there is a medical war out there. There are major disagreements as to how cancer should be treated. You need to know what the issues are. You need to understand what is happening in the world of cancer, what the arguments are, what the options are. You need to read this while your mind is clear and unworried. Imagine the doctor were to tell you today that you had cancer. How would you react? What decisions would you make? Remember, it is your decision. You, and you alone, are responsible for making whatever treatment decisions that are made—not your doctor.

Here is the opinion of a qualified doctor, Dr Eugene D Robin:

> 'The doctor's opinion is not infallible … you, the patient, have the highest stake in the decision—the most to gain and the most to lose. You, the patient, are the one to decide what constitutes a happy and productive life. Don't let your doctor, however well intentioned, usurp this right.'

Dr Eugene Robin is saying here that if you don't want an operation because you don't want to live with the consequences of the operation then it is your right not to have the operation. To make any decision, you need to understand the range of options that are available. We can define a victim as someone to whom damaging things are done without him or her having any say in the matter. A non-victim is someone who makes the decisions about what is done, who takes responsibility.

What is the right decision?

And what are the right choices? The right choice is simply the choice each patient makes for him-or-herself based on the best information at hand, and based on each person's own personal situation and world view.

Over the last 15 years in which I have been giving advice through my website, it has become very clear to me that there cannot be one set of right answers that cover all situations. Not only are the specific situations unique to themselves—but so too are the people who find themselves faced with cancer. Some are fearful, others are aggressive; some want to take control, others want control to be taken away from them—still others just don't want to know. I have therefore summarised the options that people can take as follows:

1. Follow the orthodox regime only. Do what the doctor advises. Avoid anything unorthodox.
2. Follow a regime of a combination of alternative therapies only. Do not consider any of the orthodox regimes.
3. Follow doctor's orders first and if that doesn't work then try the alternative route later.

4. Follow the alternative approaches first and if they don't succeed, fall back on the orthodox treatments
5. Combine orthodox and alternative therapies together from the start.
6. Do nothing.

It is possible to make out a sensible case for each one of these options—even the last one. I have explained the arguments later in this section.

How do we decide? It is ultimately a decision-making problem. For some, the decision will be made on essentially emotional grounds. Others will want to base their decisions on hard evidence. Some people will insist that there must be proof that a treatment works before they will do it. Others will accept that there are many types of evidence and that low quality evidence (a friend of a friend told me …) need not necessarily be rejected out of hand. In this case, a risk-benefit analysis may be more appropriate. If the risk is low and the potential benefit high then this might be an adequate reason for choosing a course of action.

Each person facing a diagnosis of cancer needs to consider the options coolly. Read this book, then keep it on your shelf so that when you, or a member of your family, or a friend, or a colleague, or a neighbour, gets cancer—as they assuredly will—then you will have immediate access to advice.

And the decision to follow an alternative path need not be a lonely one. There are doctors who support the complementary/ alternative point of view—not many, it's true, but there are some.

Basic Facts

What is cancer?

Doctors and other health professionals usually give one of two answers. One answer is that cancer is not one disease, but a general name for a group of over two hundred (possibly two thousand) diseases all of which are characterised by rapid and irregular cell growth. Another characteristic is the spread of the disease from one site to another (a process called metastasis). That, in brief, is the first answer. The other answer is that cancer is really a disease of the whole body, one of the symptoms of which is rapid and irregular cell growth in one or more sites.

At first sight there doesn't appear to be much difference between these two answers. But there is a crucial difference. Is the area of rapidly dividing cells the disease itself or only a symptom of the disease? Is it one disease or two hundred or more? Dr Salomon, a French oncologist at the National Center for Scientific Research, stated the matter in the following words: 'The notion that cancer is a localized disease which tends to spread and become general may be opposed by the idea that cancer is a general disease which results in a local tumor.'

It is very important that we answer this question correctly. How we define the disease affects how we treat the disease. So we must ask ourselves: is the tumour the disease, or is it a symptom of the disease? Do we concentrate on attacking the tumour or do we try to heal the body?

Orthodox modern western medicine considers the cancerous tumour to be the disease itself. How or why it arose they have no idea (or if they do have an idea, they don't find it an important question). But the tumour having arisen, it must be attacked. It must be surgically removed. Or it must be irradiated. Or it must be killed with highly toxic chemicals. Or it must be defeated with the aid of some sort of immunological vaccine. Or some combination of these.

So-called 'alternative' medicine, on the other hand, posits that the tumour-symptom will disappear once the root cause disappears. And the root cause, they say, is the fact that the body as a whole has been poisoned and is not getting the right kind of nutritional and/or natural support.

To put it another way, there are those who believe that cancer cells have something wrong with them, that they are deviant cells and because they are deviant they must be destroyed. The other view is that cancer cells are essentially normal cells forced to live in and accommodate themselves to an abnormal tissue environment. The problem is not the cells per se, but the surrounding environment.

Who is right?

We are so used to right-wrong polarities that it seems easy to ask this question. But potential patients—and we are all potential patients—must be very wary of taking a 100 per cent position. Perhaps we need to embrace the question with both hands and suggest that there may be an element of right on both sides.

It is certainly true that some people have been diagnosed with cancer, have undergone surgery with or without radiation and chemotherapy and have gone on to live long and happy lives. This was true of my own mother who had breast cancer, and who had no further problem with cancer after having had surgery and radiation treatment. It is also true that what appears to work for one type of cancer will not work for another—and therefore it makes sense to talk of different types of tumour. So, on these grounds, we have to accept that the orthodox medical approach has some merit.

It is also undoubtedly true that some people have utterly rejected these therapies and have cured themselves of cancer by doing no more than drinking or taking a particular substance, or even by simply mentally rejecting the cancer. One case is that of Dr Benjamin Spock, the 'world's best known paediatrician' who in his early eighties was reportedly diagnosed as having a bone cancer in his spine. Being so old he had no desire to undertake any burdensome treatment. He knew in any case that cancers grow slowly in elderly people. He decided therefore simply to refuse to believe he had the cancer. A few years later tests showed that he no longer did have any cancer.

What often happens in cases like this is that sceptics call into question the original diagnosis of cancer. How can we know that he really did have cancer? They ask. But they don't call into question the cases that respond to their orthodox treatments.

So the answer we choose for ourselves to the question 'What is cancer?' depends on the model—or paradigm—of medicine that we choose to follow. What is important is that we know there is a question and that there is no simple black and white answer.

Complementary or alternative?

Often there is confusion over these two terms—and they are often bracketed together as Complementary and Alternative Medicine (CAM). However, the distinction is a useful one. Alternative approaches are non-conventional ways that directly aim to attack the tumour or heal the body. Complementary approaches, on the other hand, tend to be designed to lessen the impact of conventional treatments. Sometimes the same approach—taking a good quality vitamin C, for example—could be done as a curative approach (in which case it would be an alternative therapy) or it could be taken alongside chemotherapy (in which case it would be used as a complementary therapy). Doctors are warming towards 'complementary' approaches (because the tide of opinion is strongly in that direction) but are very hostile to 'alternative' approaches.

Cancer cells versus normal cells

One point that does need to be made clear is that cancer cells were once normal cells that have become abnormal. This change can be reversed. It is possible to turn a cancer cell back into a normal cell. This fact has enormous implications as we shall see.

At a metabolic level there is a key difference between normal and cancer cells as to how they get their energy. The normal cell generates its energy needs using oxygen generated by mitochondria, which are rod-like structures within the cell. These mitochondria are also responsible for controlling cell death. In a cancer cell the mitochondria are de-activated and the cell, unable to get its energy in the normal way, is forced to use a whole-cell energy-production process that requires a large amount of sugar. This process has been likened to fermentation and it requires a low-oxygen environment. That is the first difference. Actually, it is better to describe this process in the reverse way: the low-oxygen environment forces the cell to get its energy in another way and in order to achieve this, the mitochondria are de-activated. The cause of the cancer is the low oxygenation of the surrounding tissues.

The second difference between normal and cancer cells is that the cancer cells cannot die because the cell death-controlling mechanism—which is also controlled by the mitochondria—has been switched off. The cells become immortal. They keep dividing and dividing until they take over the system.

Basic cancer terms

A *tumour* is a growth that contains both normal and abnormal cells. The abnormal cells divide faster than the normal cells. The rate of division varies. Some tumours grow very slowly while others are more aggressive. Tumours are not always cancerous. The classic division is between tumours that are benign and those that are malignant.

A **benign tumour** generally has limited growth potential and does not destroy normal cells while they are growing. It does not metastasize, (another way of saying: 'spread to other parts of the body') and remains localised in one site. It grows in an orderly fashion and does not produce serious side effects unless it is pressing against an organ like the brain in a limited space.

By contrast, a **malignant tumour** will keep on growing relentlessly and is capable of sending particles away from the main tumour which can then travel to distant parts of the body to develop other tumours. This process is called **metastasis**. Frighteningly, this can happen many years later.

About 90 per cent of cancers are **solid** cancers and ten per cent **liquid** cancers such as the various leukaemias and lymphomas. Tumours are classified according to the type of tissue involved:

Carcinomas: The most common form of cancer, arising, unsurprisingly, in the tissue that divides most often: the surface cells of organs or the cells that form the linings of the body and its organs: e.g. skin, lung, intestinal, uterine and breast cancers.

Sarcomas: These arise in the muscle and connective tissue. They attack bone, and muscle.

Myelomas: These attack the blood plasma cells in the bone marrow.

Lymphomas: Lymph is a water-like fluid that bathes and cleanses all the cells of the body. It originates in small bean-sized nodes and glands. Lymphomas attack these lymph organs.

Leukaemia: Cancer of the blood forming tissue and blood cells characterised by the over-production of white blood cells.

Cancers are also classed according to the stage of their development.

> **Stage 1:** small tumour with no signs of spread
> **Stage 2:** some local spreading has occurred
> **Stage 3:** more widespread local metastasis is detected
> **Stage 4:** the cancer has spread to different sites

> You may also hear the following terms:

In situ cancer: This is a cancer that has not spread to surrounding tissues.

Invasive cancer: This is a cancer that has spread to surrounding tissues. Note that this term is not used with mesothelioma, leukaemia and lymphoma as these diseases are by their very nature invasive and widespread throughout the body.

It is also very important that patients understand the words that doctors use to describe the success of treatment and to understand what they mean by these words. Here are the key words and their real meaning.

Response rate
This indicates the number of patients for whom the cancer shrank more than 50 per cent after treatment. But tumours that have shrunk can quickly return. This measure is meaningless for patients. There is no connection at all between response rate and survival.

1-3-5-10 year survival rate
This means what it says. This is the per centage of the patients who were treated who have survived for the period indicated. Short- and medium-term survival rates are highly suspect, as they are skewed

by improvements in diagnosis. If cancers are found earlier the survival rates will apparently go up without any actual improvement in treatment.

Disease-free survival

This is the measure of how long the patient survives without any signs of the tumour. Length of life may not be increased in any way even with increased disease free survival. The tumour, when it returns, may grow with aggressive speed.

Regression/Partial Remission

The tumour has grown smaller. Again this is meaningless, though it may give rise to some short-term hope.

Complete remission

Complete disappearance of cancer tumours for a significant period.

Cure

Doctors rarely use this word. If a doctor uses this word, ask what is meant by it. It may mean no more than five-year survival.

What are the symptoms of cancer?

The development of most tumours usually goes unnoticed. They are painless and do not have an obvious negative impact on health. Generally speaking, only tumours that are located on the surface of the body are likely to be detected by chance or by means of precautionary examination. Deeply located tumours such as tumours of the brain, stomach, intestines, kidneys or lungs are hardly ever discovered early. So, unfortunately, it is rare for any symptoms to become evident before a cancer has reached a fairly advanced stage. The American Cancer Society issues the following warning signs:

- unusual bleeding or discharge from any orifice
- a solid lump
- a sore that doesn't heal
- changes in bowel or bladder habits
- persistent hoarseness or coughing
- indigestion or difficulty in swallowing
- any change in a wart or mole.

Another symptom is sudden unexplained weight loss.

Cancer doesn't necessarily kill

It is not inevitable that a cancer left untreated will proceed to a terminal stage—some cancers grow very slowly (e.g. most prostate cancers) and some simply disappear of their own accord or remain in a stable state. This is sometimes associated with some deep seated change in the emotional life of the patient, but may be associated with what doctors would call placebo cures, or dietary changes that are assumed to have no therapeutic effect. Or it may simply be because that is their natural progression.

Other patients appear to be able to live in a static, symbiotic relationship with their cancer—the tumour growing neither bigger nor smaller. One woman with breast lumps describes how they tended to harden when she was stressed and so acted as a warning signal. They would then soften when she was more at ease with herself.

Then there is the fact that some cancers are known not to be fatal. Professor Michael Baum of King's College Hospital, London estimates that thirty per cent of all breast cancers are self-limiting— i.e. they need no treatment at all.

Cancer and pain

Cancer is generally painless—but if you feel pain, don't accept your doctor's opinion that it can't be cancer. If a tumour presses against a nerve or other healthy tissue it may indeed cause pain, and cancer does cause pain when it reaches a terminal stage. This pain is extreme and it is managed—if that is the word—usually with morphine. This is when the tumour takes over the body's energy generating system for the purpose of its own energy requirements that the patient feels pain. This is the pain of the body's own tissues dying, a state known as cachexia.

There are other ways of managing pain apart from morphine, and anyone suffering chronic pain should investigate the books generally available on the subject. (I also deal with this subject in Section 2: *Cancer Diagnosis and Conventional Treatments*).

What causes cancer?

This is the question everyone wants an answer to and which the experts duck to avoid. The truth is that there is no one generally accepted answer. However, there is an answer that is widely accepted among those who favour the alternative approaches. In their view, the cause of cancer—and indeed the cause of all diseases—is a low oxygen environment within the body's tissues. Many things can cause this low-oxygen environment, ranging from saturated fats and toxic chemicals to nanobacteria that cause calcification at a cellular level. This low-oxygen environment forces cells to get their energy through a fermentation process which creates an environment suited to agents of disease. Otto Warburg, a Nobel-prize winning scientist explains the situation with extreme clarity:

'Cancer, above all other diseases, has countless secondary causes, but there is only one prime cause. ... The prime cause of cancer is the replacement of the normal oxygen respiration of body cells by an anaerobic cell respiration.'

Having said this, some people fear that a search for single causes obscures the reality of cancer and at the same time leads to too much focus on research to discover single intervention 'cures'. Instead, they suggest, we should talk about contributing factors. The following is a list of the leading contributory factors.

Smoking

We all know that smoking causes lung cancer. This is true but can never be 'proved'. The evidence is statistical: smokers die of lung cancer in much larger numbers than non-smokers. It is also historical: before smoking became a wide-spread habit lung cancer was an extremely rare disease.

Dietary fats and sugars

Not all fats or sugars are unhealthy. The baddies are the saturated and hydrogenated fats and the refined sugars. Although a high intake of fats is implicated in a number of cancers—very low fat diets are also implicated in some forms of cancer. A median fat diet should be attained—but as we shall see in Section 4: *Cancer: Detox and Diet*, the oils and fats you take in should be mainly vegetable oils. Omega 3 oils are very important for fighting cancers while omega 6 oils tend to promote inflammation, and by implication cancer. However, there are those who argue that omega 6 oils also have a positive role to play in the fight against cancer.

Sugar in the form of glucose is very directly correlated with tumour growth as it supplies the fuel tumours need for their anaerobic metabolism—as well as stimulating the release of cancer promoting hormones. While simple sugars should be avoided, fruits and vegetables, grains and legumes, which are complex carbohydrates, are important cancer fighters and are very definitely OK. Also OK is the natural sweetener, Stevia. Aspartame on the other hand is possibly not good—it is considered to be carcinogenic by some, though most studies, according to the FDA, appear to show it is safe. It has, among other things, been fingered as a trigger for brain cancers, the incidence of which is rising. It is best to avoid it to be on the safe side.

In general, foods that are low on the glycaemic index (which is a measure of sugar content of food) are preferred and are healthier than those that are high on the index.

There are also good sugars—known as glyco-nutrients—which play an important role in fighting cancer. Blackstrap molasses also has a claim to be a good food despite its sweetness.

Dietary fibre

Low fibre diets are strongly correlated with high incidences of cancer of the colon and rectum.

Obesity

Body size, large waist measurements and high body mass index (BMI) are correlated with an up to 500 per cent increase in the risk of developing myeloid leukaemia, a malignant disease of the white blood cells, from which more than 9,000 people die each year in the US alone.

It has been suggested that obesity may significantly impair immune function and that the chronic hyper-insulinaemia (the persistent elevation of insulin levels in the blood) that commonly accompanies obesity may be associated with increased levels of insulin-like growth factor (IGF-1), which is also present in dairy products. This has been shown to increase the rate of cell division and has been linked to the development of a number of cancers.

Nitrites in processed foods

Pickled, smoked and cured foods are associated with stomach cancer. They contain large amounts of nitrites which can be easily converted to a class of highly potent carcinogenic chemicals called nitrosamines. Vitamin C is known to interfere with the formation of these compounds.

Burnt and chargrilled foods

Foods that are burnt, especially barbecued foods have been found to be carcinogenic.

Pharmaceutical drugs

The following is a Reuters news release dated January 23, 2006 (Reuters Health):

> 'Two prescription eczema drugs, pimecrolimus and tacrolimus, will now carry a black box warning about the possible risk of skin cancer, lymphoma and other cancers. Novartis AG's Elidel (pimecrolimus) and Astellas Pharma Inc.'s Protopic (tacrolimus) issued the warning 10 months after the Food and Drug Administration first called for them. FDA officials said that while a clear link between the drugs and cancer risk had not been found, there have been enough cancer reports to warrant the change. A total of 78 cases were reported for both products as of October 2005, they said.'

This is just one example of standard pharmaceutical drugs possibly causing cancer. It is known, for example, that even anti-cancer chemotherapy drugs are implicated in long-term cancer risks. One study has found that women who have combined radiation and chemotherapy for their breast cancer have 28 times higher than normal incidence of leukaemia.

Stress and reduced immunity

Stress is a well-known precursor of illness, particularly cancer. Stress is known to result in a lowered immune response. If the lowered immunity is allowed to remain for any length of time then the chances of serious illness occurring rise sharply.

However, the connection between cancer incidence and lowered immune systems is not absolutely proven. For example, people with AIDS, whose immune systems have completely collapsed do not have a higher incidence of most cancers. They do have a higher incidence of Karposi's sarcoma, an otherwise rare cancer, lymphomas and cancers of the anal/genital area which are known to have a viral cause.

Stress causes release of corticosteroids, which can have the effect of making any existing cancer more aggressive and invasive. This may mean that simply receiving a diagnosis of cancer will make a cancer worse. The herb gingko biloba has demonstrated an ability to interfere with this process. Conversely, relaxation and release from stress, especially emotional conflicts (anger, the desire for revenge etc.), have been notable parts of many healing stories. Many survivors have stressed that their healing seemed to start with a fit of crying despair or from a sincere act of forgiveness. (Read Section 7: *Cancer: Energy, Mind and Emotions* for further details.)

Anxiety attacks can be eliminated or reduced with the help of the amino acid L-theanine. Other useful natural interventions include: lavender essential oil, evening primrose oil, valerian herb, St John's Wort, and Bach's Rescue Remedy. If anxiety attacks are acute and continuing it may be useful to have thyroid functioning checked. If this is a concern—and even if it isn't—increased iodine intake should be considered.

Viruses and microbes

As many as one-third of cancers are believed to be caused by viruses of one sort or another. One minority view is that all cancers are caused by microbes that can change shape so that sometimes they appear to be viruses and at other times appear to be bacteria.

Campylobacter pylori, recently discovered to be the cause of stomach ulcers, has also been implicated as a cause of colon cancer. Cervical cancers are now known to be caused by human papilloma virus (HPV) and a vaccination has now been developed which, hopefully, will eliminate the virus. More recently, researchers at Tulane Medical School have identified a virus that is present in 90 per cent of breast cancer cases, known as human mammary tumour virus (HMTV). This appears to be present in the blood of 15 per cent of otherwise healthy women and men. A vaccination for breast cancer could very well be the next big development.

Fungal infections

There is increasing and very much belated recognition that fungal infections may be a major cause of cancer. A number of doctors have noted that in the case of Leukaemia, the co-presence of a severe fungal infection is extremely common. Intriguingly, treatment with an anti-fungal drug has also been associated with a number of remissions from cancer. Patrick Quillan, in his book, *Beating Cancer with Nutrition*, quotes the story of a well-known oil magnate, 'Doc' Pennington, who was diagnosed with advanced colon cancer in 1972. He persuaded his doctor to prescribe Griseofulvin, an anti-fungal drug, and three months later his cancer had disappeared. He went on to live another 22 years, dying aged 92 in 1994. He founded the Pennington Biomedical Centre to study the link between yeast, nutrition and cancer. Research that he funded has shown the Griseofulvin causes cell death in cancer cells in test tubes.

An Italian doctor, Dr Tullio Simoncini, bases his radical approach on this assumption that cancer is caused by fungus (specifically Candida albicans) and treats his patients, with seeming success, with five per cent solution of sodium bicarbonate injected close to the site of the tumour. For more detailed discussion of his treatment go to www.curenaturalicancro.com.

In 1999 Meinolf Karthaus, MD, reported that he had seen three children with leukaemia suddenly go into remission upon receiving a triple antifungal drug cocktail for their 'secondary' fungal infections. This was echoed by the experience of another doctor, Dr Doug A Kaufman:

> '[A] young lady phoned into my syndicated radio talk show. Her three-year-old daughter was diagnosed last year with leukaemia. She believes antifungal drugs and natural immune system therapy has been responsible for saving her daughter's life. She is now telling others with cancer about her daughter's case. After hearing her story, a friend of hers with bone cancer asked her doctor for a prescriptive antifungal drug. To her delight, this medication, meant to eradicate fungus, was also eradicating her cancer. ... When she could no longer get the antifungal medication, the cancer immediately grew back.'
> (reported by Dr Mark Sircus in an email 2007)

Chronic viral and bacterial infections and chronic inflammation (especially of the gums)

The body's normal response to inflammation is to flood the area with stem cells and various growth factors to aid healing. Where the inflammation, for whatever reason, persists (perhaps because an irritant persists or because of low immune function) then these growth factors transform the stem cells into malignant cells.

Bacterial and viral infections that cause inflammation that is not speedily resolved, can result in cancer. The teeth, for example, have long been seen as a potential source of such problems and some doctors in the past have recommended removal of infected teeth—or teeth with root canals—for this reason. The other side of the coin is that anti-inflammatory drugs and herbs will tend to be useful in the fight against cancer. Note, however, that pregnancy and cancer are closely related in metabolic terms, and anything that is effective against cancer is likely to lead to a miscarriage of a foetus.

Free radicals

Free radicals are highly reactive molecular fragments that are hungry for oxygen. If left uncontrolled they would quickly destroy every living creature as they scavenge for oxygen in the cell walls—so damaging the cells. They cause mutations to the cell's DNA and this can result in cancer. Very little, if anything, is mentioned about them in orthodox medical cancer books. One reason for this is that the main orthodox anti-cancer weapons create free radicals and the best known means of controlling or minimising their effects are through the use of anti-oxidant vitamins (vitamins A, C and E). Since the use of vitamins has been very generally vilified by proponents of orthodox medicine, the whole area of free radicals was for many years an intellectual 'no go' area in some scientific circles.

It should be noted that there are situations in which free radicals are beneficial—such as when the body is fighting acute bacterial infections.

Trauma

Another cause of cancer appears to be physical or emotional trauma. This is why some people disapprove of mammograms, which require the breasts to be squeezed and therefore traumatised. Some studies have indicated that breast cancer is more common among women who have annual checks than among women who don't.

Toxic chemicals

There are now around 30,000 chemicals in everyday use. The safety of these chemicals on their own has only been established in a rough and ready way. However, what happens when any of these chemicals combines with one or more of the other chemicals? It is impossible to test all the possible combinations. We are living guinea pigs in an enormous experiment.

Rough and ready estimates for safe levels of these compounds assume a simple linear reality in which higher doses always lead to worse results. But the truth is infinitely more complex. Sometimes an organism may be unaffected by relatively high doses but seriously disrupted by low level doses. Also, organisms are not static. At various stages in their life cycle they may be extremely vulnerable to extremely slight biochemical aspects of their environment. It is believed that hormone disruption during the foetal stage is the main cause of testicular cancer and falling sperm counts.

And of course many chemicals do not break down easily. Every one of us is carrying chemical residues in our fat layers. Various studies have found that the average person is carrying residues of 40 or more potentially toxic chemicals—and that even animals in remote habitats (polar bears and arctic seals) are polluted chemically in the same way. What effects are all these chemicals having? Who knows?

It is well known that sudden exposure to large doses of any pollutant for a limited period of time is unlikely to lead to cancer. But even low doses of a pollutant over a long period of time may result in cancerous growths as the tissue attempts to adapt to the change in its environment. New carpets that have been treated with a variety of chemicals have been implicated as a cancer cause. There are studies that show long-term exposure to vehicle exhaust is a definite risk factor. Benzene and vinyl chloride are known to be dangerous to chemical workers. These occupational carcinogens are now found in drinking water!

Almost every pesticide used today is recognised by one or more regulatory agencies in Europe or America as being disruptive to our endocrine system—which controls and regulates every gland and every hormone in the body.

Plastic containers release dioxins, a family of chemicals that are known to be carcinogenic, into the fats of the food it contains—especially when microwaved. This also applies to the plastic wrap used to cover foods that are being microwaved. Also, dioxins are released into water when plastic bottles are put in the freezer

Electromagnetic fields (EMFs)

Electro-magnetic fields have also been implicated as a major cause of cancer. This link has never been proved—but evidence is mounting, and in 2011 the World Health Organisation reclassified EM fields as a Class 2b possible carcinogen. One study conducted by the University of North Carolina School of Public Health found that children of mothers who slept under electric blankets developed 250 per cent more brain tumours, 70 per cent more leukaemias, and 30 per cent more cancers than those who didn't.

One of the earliest reports on the dangers of EMFs appeared in the *Journal of Occupational Medicine* in 1985. This article reported that deaths in Maryland from various cancers were up to three times higher among electricians, electrical engineers and linesmen than any other occupation. Since World War II, we have filled the air with electromagnetic waves. They beam down on our houses through telephone wires, television satellite dishes, AM and FM radio receivers. Add to this pagers, cell phones , CB radios and other radios. Add to this the overhead power lines, and we see how dependent we are on EMF-producing equipment. Dr Robert Becker, a world expert in this field is in no doubt:

> *'At this time the scientific evidence is absolutely conclusive: 60 cycle magnetic fields cause human cancer cells to permanently increase their rate of growth by as much as 1,600 per cent and to develop more malignant characteristics.'*

It's not just cancer. EM fields have now been linked with suicides, nervous system disorders, sexual dysfunction, reproductive hazards, abnormal foetal development and heart disease. Mobile (cell) phones are also being investigated as possible causes of brain cancer.

The new vogue for digital phones has also increased the threat of harmful frequencies in the home—the base units in particular are at fault. These frequencies can be detected with an electro-smog detector. For further details see www.electrosmog.org.uk and www.lessemf.com. There is growing concern that mobile phone use will precipitate an epidemic of brain cancers.

Oestrogen (US: estrogen)

Excessive oestrogen in the body is a cancer causing factor—as are the intermediary metabolites of oestrogen created as oestrogen is broken down in order to be eliminated from the body (a metabolite is the chemical produced in the body as it breaks down a primary chemical either to make use of it or to process it into a form where it can be eliminated from the body). If there are problems relating to this process so that these metabolites cannot be further broken down then they can remain in the body and are potentially even more carcinogenic than the original oestrogen. This is particularly so if we have a high sodium/low magnesium and high glucose levels in the tissues. The combined effect is to cause havoc in normal cells and potentially making them malignant.

This is not just a concern for women. Unfortunately there are a lot of oestrogen-mimicking chemicals in our environment—the chief of which is bisphenol A, a chemical used in plastics and food packaging. Bisphenol A has been shown to have biological effects at levels 200,000 times lower than the presumed safety level. The lubricants on condoms are also oestrogen mimics.

One of the side effects of excessive oestrogen is an increase in body weight. The large size of many Americans may reflect their oestrogen levels as much as their food intake.

Over-exposure to the sun's rays

It has recently become a mantra that the sun's rays are bad for us—certainly it is true that one or two relatively benign forms of skin cancer are associated with over-exposure to the sun. However, the association of over-exposure to sunlight and malignant melanoma is not so clear. Melanomas are often found in parts of the body least exposed to the sun—and the difference between melanoma rates in Florida and New York is not enormous. Scandinavian research, however, suggests that there is a connection between melanoma and broadcast frequency radio waves.

But, more importantly, there is strong evidence that sunlight is good for us—and that people who spend a large part of their lives outdoors under the hot sun have significantly lower incidences of most cancers. Most of the vitamin D in our bodies comes from exposure to sunlight—and vitamin D is increasingly being recognised as very powerful medicine. (See Section 7: *Cancer: Energy, Mind and Emotions* for a detailed discussion of this contentious subject.)

Genes and oncogenes

Some genes appear to provoke the onset of cancer. Such genes are referred to as oncogenes. In some cases these oncogenes are triggered by a genetic predisposition. The result is that there are families with high incidences of certain cancers. However, it has been estimated that this genetic cause accounts for fewer than five per cent of cancers. And genes only trigger events in the body if they are activated. Diet can prevent a gene from being activated.

Alcohol

There appears to be, in excessive quantities, and in association with other pollutants, a measurable tendency for alcohol to exacerbate a cancer risk in cases of cancers of the lips, tongue and other areas in the mouth and throat. Against this, it is now generally accepted that alcohol in smaller quantities has a beneficial effect on health—more so for men than women. The divisive question is this: at what level of intake does alcohol cease to be beneficial? And alcohol's benefits relate not to cancer but to heart disease. So it is possible that a slight cancer risk is outweighed by greater heart disease benefits.

Certainly, rural Greeks who like to drink a glass of red wine with their meals have one of the highest life expectancies in the world. But French men, who are not abstemious, have one of the world's highest cancer rates for men (fifth)—more than double that of French women who have a far lower incidence (35th).

Bras

Many women wear poorly-fitting bras. In fact, some experts have suggested that as many as 85 per cent of women are wearing the wrong size bra. This is not just a problem of fashion or even comfort. Bras cause breast cancer according to a Harvard University study. (Hsieh C C, Trichopoulos D, *European Journal of Cancer,* 27:131-5, 1991)

It's not the fabric of the bras, it seems, but the fact that they constrict lymphatic drainage and, at the same time, have a negative impact on melatonin secretion. The results were that: women who wore their bras 24 hours per day had a three out of four chance of developing breast cancer; wearing for more than 12 hours a day resulted in a one in seven risk, while wearing a bra for less than 12 hours a day brought the risk down to one in 152—very close to the risk factor for women who never wore bras (one in 168). A number of other studies have supported this conclusion. Go to (www.breathing.com/articles/ brassieres.htm) for a more detailed discussion on this.

Metal-underwired bras, because of their dimensions, are also thought to act as re-radiating antennae for radio-frequencies (see electromagnetic fields, above).

Miscellaneous

Almost every day it seems that some new cancer cause is announced. Some fear chemicals in shampoos, others talcum powder. The latter certainly does seem to worth avoiding, especially near female genital areas. It has been likened to asbestos. Similarly, fears have been expressed about aluminium and parabens in underarm deodorants—especially in relation to breast cancer. Fingers have also been pointed vociferously at the mercury laden dental amalgams that dentists have used for fillings and also at root canals, and indeed any form of gum disease (which also has serious impacts on heart health). Some people are so convinced of these threats that they have all their fillings replaced with non-toxic materials. However, the process of doing this replacement, unless with the greatest care and awareness, is likely to release large amounts of heavy metals into the bloodstream.

How should we respond to these threats?

The problem each of us faces is what to do in the face of these suggested threats. Should we maintain a very high level of scrutiny on every product we buy or should we just shrug our shoulders and carry on regardless, taking the view that life cannot be lived entirely without risk?

There is a well-known controversy dating back to two French scientists—Louis Pasteur, with his germ theory and Claude Bernard with his biological terrain theory. The question is do you focus your attention on the germ or the terrain of the body. Here is a useful summary of the issue:

'The germ—or microbian—theory of disease was popularized by Louis Pasteur (1822-1895), the inventor of pasteurization. This theory says that there are fixed, external germs (or microbes) which invade the body and cause a variety of separate, definable diseases. In order to get well, you need to identify and then kill whatever germ made you sick. The tools generally employed are drugs, surgery, radiation and chemotherapy. Prevention includes the use of vaccines as well as drugs, which—theoretically at least—work by keeping germs at bay.

'Just prior to the time that Pasteur began promoting the "monomorphic" germ theory, a contemporary by the name of Claude Bernard (1813-1878) was developing the theory that the body's ability to heal was dependent on its general condition or internal environment. Thus disease occurred only when the terrain or internal environment of the body became favorable to disease.

'An extremely brilliant contemporary of Claude Bernard's was Antoine Bechamp (1816-1908). Bechamp had degrees in physics, chemistry and biology. In addition he was a medical doctor and a university professor. Bechamp built upon and extended Bernard's idea, developing his own theory of health and disease which revolved around the concept of "pleomorphism".

'Through meticulous research and in contrast to Pasteur's subsequent, misinformed promotion of "monomorphic" or single-formed, fixed state microbes (or germs), Bechamp had discovered tiny organisms (or microorganisms) he called "microzyma" which were "pleomorphic" or "many-formed" (pleo = many and morph = form). Interestingly, these microzyma were found to be present in all things whether living or dead, and they persist even when the host has died. Many were impervious to heat as well.

'Bechamp's microzyma, including specific bacteria, could take on a number of forms during the host's life cycle and these forms depended (as Bernard contended) primarily on the chemistry of their environment, or the biological terrain, or to put it a third way, the condition of the host. In other words there is no single cause of disease. Instead disease results when microzyma change form, function and toxicity according to the terrain of the host. Bad bacteria, viruses and fungi are merely the forms assumed by the microzymas when there is a condition or terrain that favors disease and these 'bad' microzyma themselves give off toxic byproducts, further contributing to a weakened terrain.' (thehealthyadvantage.com)

My own view is that we should not be too obsessive in trying to avoid these contributory factors—a healthy body can withstand all manner of assaults. Our key focus should be on strengthening the health of our bodies. Nevertheless, it is worth knowing the dangers so that we can make responsible decisions. No point in breathing in asbestos if you can avoid it, to take one obvious example.

Causes don't always lead to results

Some people argue that carcinogenic substances cannot adequately explain the cause of cancer because in most cases of exposure to a carcinogen, there are some, usually a minority, who will get cancer—the others won't. That suggests that the physical and mental health of the person exposed to the carcinogen is a key factor. There is no doubt that the terrain of the body has a key say in whether the seeds of cancer will be able to take root and thrive.

For us, the key question that arises from this is whether we are going to spend our lives examining the external world checking it obsessively for things to avoid—pesticides, chemicals in shampoos and so on—the so-called defensive shopping syndrome—or whether it is enough to focus on our own physical, mental and spiritual health. This is the crux of a scientific schism that split 19th century France and which has had repercussions ever since. Are the causes of disease, the alien germs and environmental poisons that attack us or is it the weakened soil of our bodies. Is it the toxin or is it the terrain? Where do we place the emphasis? If poor soil causes diseased plants, can we cure the plants by just looking at the plant, or must we treat the ailments of the plant by focussing on the soil?

A sensible strategy, it seems to me, is to minimise as far as possible the chemical impacts on the body while at the same time not being too over-concerned about occasional lapses. At the same time, we need to make sure that the food we eat, the supplements we take and the daily habits we follow are adequate to maintain good health. *Mens sana in corpore sano*: a healthy mind in a healthy body. This is the prescription for happiness and longevity.

Incidence of cancer

Epidemiological studies show that cancer incidence varies greatly from country to country, being low in the developing world and increasingly high in the west. It also varies widely from province to province within China. How can we explain these variations?

'The difference is far too big to be explained by genes. We have to take a look at diet, at excess calories. It may be that diet is linked in a very complicated way.' (Dr Gordon McVie, scientific director of the Cancer Research Campaign in *The Independent*, 25 March 1994)

This kind of research reveals that 70–90 per cent of cancers relate to lifestyle and environmental factors, while only three to five per cent is gene-related. Such research is clearly valuable because prevention is better than cure. You can't change your genes but you can change your diet and other aspects of your environment. And changes in the diet can change the way genes operate.

There is of course genetic involvement in all cancers—but this is simply because any change in a cell involves the genes at some level. What we are talking about here is specific genes which, if activated, will control and direct the cancer causing process.

Cancer statistics

If you want to look on the bright side of things it is possible to conjure up figures that show that there has been significant progress in the battle against cancer. The National Cancer Institute publishes a chart of five-year Relative Survival Rates. These figures show clear improvement. But statistics are only meaningful when they are accurate. One source if inaccuracy is exposed by the following personal testimony: 'my husband recently died of pancreatic cancer and he was listed as death by heart attack because he was in the end stages of his cancer and his heart gave out. Statistics can be whatever the people keeping the results want them to be.' (quoted by Ralph Moss in his newsletter 1 February 2007)

Another problem is that five-year survival rates, while seeming to represent increased survival may actually only measure improvements in diagnosis.

Incidence statistics for cancer depends upon accurate diagnosis. Improved screening programmes tend to raise incidence figures because they lead to the detection of many 'early cancers' which are either not cancers, or they find cancers that would resolve themselves without treatment, or they find cancers earlier than they would otherwise. Even with no improvement in treatment, these will have a major impact on official survival figures, as we can see from the following example. Take two identical twins aged 65 both of whom have prostate cancer. One, Man A, is diagnosed as having prostate cancer and starts treatment. The other, Man B, also has prostate cancer but this is not diagnosed till he is 70. Let us imagine that Man B's cancer is now too advanced and so no treatment is given. Now, it is possible that Man A's treatment has no effect and does not help to extend Man A's life. Both men die of their prostate cancer at the age of 72. However, for the statistician, Man A was diagnosed early, received treatment and lived seven years. Man B however, was diagnosed late and only lived two years. Early diagnosis appears to have allowed Man A to have live three and a half times longer than Man B. So, the statistics appear to demonstrate huge benefits for early diagnosis— but in fact these huge benefits are in this case entirely illusory.

It may be that the apparent slight improvement in prognosis for women with breast cancer is not a result of improved chemotherapy but may, rather, be a result of improvements in diagnosis and the consequent impact on survival statistics. Or, of course, it may also be due to the fact that women are much more aware of the range of alternative therapies and are taking more vitamins etc., while at the same time not discussing this with their doctors.

Another problem with statistics

Statistics also don't tell us what any individual's likelihood of recovery will be. If we discover that we have a cancer for which there is a fifty per cent chance that we will die within five years, some people will become very depressed, while others will interpret this to mean that there is a fifty per cent chance that they will live longer than five years. Both are correct, but the second patient has the better prognosis.

Imagine a group where half the people died before six months and the other half lived ten years. The doctors would say you have only a fifty per cent chance of living for six months! A much gloomier picture than we would get from saying, equally correctly, you have a fifty per cent chance of living ten years.

Even if the five-year survival rate is only ten per cent the positive patient will see that ten per cent of the population survive somehow. Statistics demonstrate this clearly. How do these people do it? This question cannot be answered yet for the simple reason that very little research is done on survival. But clearly they are doing something different.

It is also important to know what is meant when you read that the average life expectancy for a particular form of treatment is five years, say. Most people think that this means you add up all the life spans of a particular group and divide by the number in the group. But that is unlikely to be the case. Almost certainly, it is the point at which half of the group being measured died. So fifty per cent of any group will live longer than the average life expectancy—and how long they live is not factored into the figures at all. The Harvard biologist, Stephen Jay Gould wrote an essay on the subject that is a must-read. You can find it at Steve Dunn's website at www.cancerguide.org/ median_not_msg.html

Relative benefit versus absolute benefit

Every so often the newspapers erupt with news of a new wonder drug. The result is cancer patients become desperate to get their hands on this new drug that, according to the newspapers, will give them a 30 per cent, or 50 per cent, or 70 per cent better chance of being cured. Sadly, these people are victims of innumerate newspaper reporters who are doing little more than rewriting press releases issued by the pharmaceutical companies. It's not that the drug companies are lying. They are telling a sort of truth—but it is a highly inaccurate truth, as you will see.

Let us imagine that out of a group of 100 women with stage 4 cancer, ninety eight are expected to die of their disease within five years. These women are given a drug (drug X) and after five years it is found that only 96 died. In this case there is a *relative benefit* of 100 per cent (four people survived instead of the expected two). The newspapers will carry headlines saying that drug X doubles your chances of living for five years; they may even say it doubles their chances of being cured.

But we can see that in fact only two of the group of 100 women actually benefited. There is, in this case, an *absolute benefit* of two per cent. This is not a figure that will sell many newspapers.

Herceptin is the current new wonder drug that is prompting people to re-mortgage their houses and take on massive debt. It actually has an absolute benefit of only 0.6 per cent (one-year survival) and 5.5 per cent (one-year disease free status). So the benefits are marginal at best and have to be set against the possibility (2–3 per cent) of heart damage (cardiotoxicity in doctor-speak).

So add the terms 'relative benefit' and 'absolute benefit' to your vocabulary and you are less likely to be taken in by drug company propaganda or newspaper headlines.

Cures for cancer?

The word 'cure' carries with it a lot of implicit baggage that it is worth looking at more closely. First of all, to talk of cures implies a situation where there is a clear-cut opposition between a state of health and a state of illness. You either have cancer or you don't have it—as though cancer is a thing in itself separate from the body in which the cancer is present and that it is there or, preferably, not there. If it was there before and now no longer is there then you say there has been a cure.

But how real is this image? Are there not intermediate stages between not having a cancer and having one? And similarly, if you get rid of a cancer tumour but make no change to the bodily environment that produced the cancer tumour, how long is the state of not having a tumour going to last? What causes a cancer to appear in the first place? What is being done to correct this situation? If these two questions are not addressed, as they usually aren't under an orthodox clinical setting, then to talk of cures, even in the absence of a tumour for an extended period of time is probably inappropriate. Doctors use a five-year term as their definition of a successful outcome—a permanent state of being cancer free. But cancer may, and often does, recur after this period. There is nothing sacred about this five year period. It is in fact an arbitrary cut off—useful for pragmatic reasons but otherwise meaningless.

Some cancers are fast growing others are slow growing. Some stop of their own accord. Others stop after some form of treatment and others still resist all forms of treatment.

The hard reality is that between 1930 and 1990, in the USA, for men, only two cancers have actually declined in incidence: stomach cancer has dropped from 38 to seven per 100,000 men and liver cancer has dropped by 50–65 per cent, and now only kills about five per 100,000 men per annum.

For women there have been significant improvements in cancer of the uterus, stomach, liver and some improvement in colon and rectal cancer.

The problem for orthodox medicine is that none of these improvements are recent; and for many cancers there has been either no change at all, or a slow but steady increase in death rates. Prostate deaths have nearly doubled—as have deaths from cancer of the pancreas and leukaemia. And lung cancer deaths have just gone through the roof. One possible exception is with breast cancer. There does appear to have been a recent improvement in death rate figures. The problem is there has not been any change in treatment to account for this improvement. Could it be that more and more women are following alternative treatments that are having an impact?

But there is another way to look at the subject. Cancers are never cured—even when they appear to have gone. The potential for cancer is always there lurking in the microscopic depths of the body. Hazel Thornton who was diagnosed in 1991 with breast cancer wrote this to me:

'Whilst I believe that attitude is crucially important in coming to terms with a life threatening disease so that one may live one's life fruitfully and in tranquillity, I cannot accept that one can say at any given moment that one has 'beaten' the illness …. I hope that I am in a state of truce with my body's inefficiencies, rather than waging war with it.' (personal communication, December 1995)

This book was written to help you make your decision as to what you should do should you get cancer, or if you already have cancer. I have surveyed the orthodox anti-cancer weapons with a critical eye and I have listed the alternative approaches—of which there a great many. But the final act must be yours, and yours alone. You must look through the options provided and make the choices that seem most sensible to you. Your choices will be different from my choices. But we are different and we must respect those differences. This is one of the most difficult things to do when you and a loved one take divergent views as to what to do. I have been through this and know the damage it can do to couples. So I have one word of advice. It is for the person with cancer to make the final decisions about what therapies to follow, and those who are in a supporting role should support these decisions as far as they can—putting the need to give loving support over all other considerations.

Introduction

The first thing that has to be said is this: We are all different. We have different cancers; we have different perceptions of how the world is; we have different social responsibilities; we have different budgets; different personalities; different lifestyles, and we are of different ages. Each of these factors will impact any decision we make in relation to our cancers.

This book is based on the principle that *you* are in charge and that *you* should make any treatment decisions that are made. Obviously it is much better to make decisions that are based on a broad understanding of the whole situation. There is a very famous saying (in China) attributed to the military strategist Sun Tzu that contains a very powerful idea:

Know yourself
Know your enemy
One hundred fights
One hundred victories

Note that the first step on the path to victory is to 'know yourself'. So, what kind of cancer patient are you? On the next few pages is a quick questionnaire. Circle the letter of the answer that most closely approximates to the views you hold.

Jonathan's cancer attitudes questionnaire

Question 1

A   Doctors know what's best for cancer. They have had years of training. Everything they do is scientifically tested. If doctors don't do something, there is a good reason for this. Therefore it makes sense for me to put myself in the hands of the experts and do exactly what they tell me to do—no more, no less.

B   Doctors can generally be trusted to do the right thing—but they often ignore the side-effects of their treatments and patients need to protect themselves. So I will do what the doctors recommend but I will also do what I feel might improve my situation—but I won't necessarily tell the doctors in case they disapprove.

C   Patients have a duty to consider all options—conventional and alternative—whether or not their doctor approves. Holistic approaches may work and I have a responsibility to myself and to my family to explore this area to see if these approaches might work for me. If I consider any holistic approaches to be better than the conventional approaches I will certainly choose to do them.

D   The conventional approaches to cancer are painful, damaging and do not respect the body. For me, cancer cannot be treated simply by attacking the tumours with force. This ignores the question: What caused the tumours to arise in the first place? I believe in healing through natural means to bring the body back to a state of health—and when the body is healthy the tumours will go away on their own. By following a route that respects my body, I fully expect to get well again.

I agree with opinion: ☐ A   ☐ B   ☐ C   ☐ D

Jonathan's cancer attitudes questionnaire

Question 2

A   For me a cure means simply that the tumour is gone. I just want to get rid of the tumour and return to my old way of life. If that means I have to suffer some pain, so be it. You just have to grit your teeth and get on with it.

B   Getting rid of a cancer tumour is essential—but it is likely that the course of treatment will be damaging so I need to do other things—vitamins and herbs—to protect myself and hopefully to reduce the pain.

C   Getting rid of a cancer tumour may or may not be sensible, but it makes sense to ask where the cancer tumour comes from. If we don't change the context of cancer how can we be sure the cancer won't return? So we need to address this issue—and that probably will mean some change to my diet and might involve taking a number of supplements.

D   Getting rid of a tumour by some violent means cannot be called a 'cure'. Violent therapies weaken the body and harm our long term health—which cannot be sensible. The important thing is to return the body to a state of vibrant good health. To get rid of a cancer and to prevent the cancer returning I need to change my whole life: my diet, habits, attitudes— perhaps I even need to do emotional counselling.

I agree with opinion: ☐ A   ☐ B   ☐ C   ☐ D

Jonathan's cancer attitudes questionnaire

Question 3

A   Cancer is a hard nut to crack so you have to hit it with a heavy hammer. For most cancers, chemotherapy is an essential part of any potentially successful treatment plan. You just have to grit your teeth and get on with it.

B   While I am resigned to the fact that chemotherapy will almost certainly be prescribed for my cancer—I will do everything I can to minimise its effects—perhaps with acupuncture, supplements and herbs.

C   I will only do chemotherapy if I am totally convinced that it has significant benefits—by which I mean at least a 30 per cent absolute benefit or better. I believe that for most cancers there are far better therapies—both mainstream and alternative.

D   Chemotherapy is never justified. It is far too damaging and it has virtually no proven benefit whatsoever. Often it makes cancers more aggressive. Even when there is a benefit, the long term damage is horrendous. It can damage you for life. I am not prepared to live with the pain and damage that radiation and chemotherapy causes.

I agree with opinion: ☐ A   ☐ B   ☐ C   ☐ D

Jonathan's cancer attitudes questionnaire

Question 4

A   It is complete nonsense to think that a simple thing like diet can cure something as serious and life threatening as cancer. If diet was curative doctors would tell us to go on a diet. But they don't, so clearly diets don't work. I believe in eating well to keep up my strength.

B   It makes sense not to eat too many fried or fatty foods and you should try to eat some fruit every day. You should try to eat a balanced meal including meat, dairy, cereals and fruit and veg.

C   For someone with cancer, I believe that it is important to eat lots of vegetables and fruit but little, if any, meat or dairy. But I would also take lots of vitamin and mineral supplements as I don't think diet alone is sufficient. Whether or not that would be sufficient to cure the cancer I couldn't say, but it is certainly a step in the right direction.

D   Diet is the foundation of health. In fact our whole health is entirely dependent on what we eat. If we have cancer that is a sign that there is something wrong with our diet. Cancer cannot continue to exist in a truly healthy bodily environment. The only way to return our bodies to vibrant health is through diet. It follows that the right kind of diet can be curative.

I agree with opinion: ☐ A   ☐ B   ☐ C   ☐ D

Jonathan's cancer attitudes questionnaire

Question 5

A Herbs were fine in the Middle Ages when there were no scientifically demonstrated pharmaceutical medicines. Now that we have drugs we can throw away the herbs. Drugs have been rationally tested, herbs haven't. Drugs are strong, herbs aren't. I can't see any reason why anyone would choose to take herbs to try to cure something as powerful as cancer.

B It's important to take the drugs that the doctor prescribes but often these have side-effects. These side-effects can often be effectively treated with herbs. So, in those circumstances, it makes sense to take herbs to minimise the impact of the drugs.

C I believe some herbs can have a very powerful effect and I can see that a herb or a herbal mixture might be able to cure cancer. At the moment there is no agreement as to what are the best herbs so I would have to do some research. I would be very happy to take herbs for my cancer as part of a general anti-cancer therapy. However, I wouldn't just rely on a single herbal remedy.

D Herbs are natural. Drugs are artificial. Herbs contain many complex chemicals that work together in a synergistic way. Drugs are toxic concentrations of a single chemical. Herbs support the health, drugs damage the body. Obviously herbs are far superior to drugs.

I agree with opinion: ☐ A   ☐ B   ☐ C   ☐ D

So what kind of person are you?

On the basis of your answers, does the result indicate that you are mainly an A, B, C or D type person?

   If it's not clear (i.e. your answers are scattered across all the letters then convert your answers to a numerical value (A=1, B=2, C=3, D=4).

Score 5-8 points   Read Profile A
Score 9-12 points   Read Profile B
Score 13-17 points   Read Profile C
17+ points   Read Profile D

Profile A

You are a very conservative person. You believe that the structures of society are good and you do not wish to interfere with them in any way. You will not allow yourself to entertain any criticism of doctors—indeed you believe absolutely that what doctors tell you is absolutely true, and that anyone who disagrees must be wrong. Doctors, in your opinion, have only one goal and that is to help you get better and they will always seek to give you the right treatment.

You are also very attached to your own habits of life—mental and behavioural. You do not like change. You are certainly not prepared to change what you eat.

You are prepared to put up with pain—even extreme pain—as long as this seems to be required.

You take the view that science is concerned to find the truth by strictly rational procedures and that anything that has not been through the process of rigorous scientific testing is not worth considering.

Profile B

You are fairly conservative in character. You believe that doctors know best but you also understand that you need to defend yourself. Doctors can be too focused on the objective aspect of a problem—but may not pay enough attention to the emotional and subjective—especially when it comes to pain.

You feel that the doctor is the one with authority and you don't feel confident enough to go against the decisions he or she is making on your behalf. However, you are also prepared to listen to friends and to consider other approaches.

You are happy to do anything—and you may even lie to the doctor if you think she or he will disapprove. You accept that you will have to make some changes to your way of life—especially when it comes to taking vitamins and other supplements and even, possibly, changing your diet.

Profile C

You are a very practical, no-nonsense person and you trust yourself to make decisions—but you want to know all the facts first. You have proper respect for doctors but you know very well that they are only human too and are subject to professional pressures that you are unlikely to be aware of. You understand that a surgeon will always think in terms of surgery—because that's his job. So you want to know how likely any recommended treatments are to result in a cure.

However you are not committed to mainstream treatments. If a herb or a diet makes more sense you will go that route. In fact you will try anything that you believe to be based on good reasoning or evidence, that does not carry with it much in the way of risk, and which does not cost an excessive amount.

Essentially, you want to have the big picture before you make your decisions.

Profile D

You have almost certainly been involved in so-called 'alternative' or 'new age' circles over many years and this has shaped your attitudes. You already believe very strongly that the basis of good health is a diet founded in organic, natural principles. You are also aware that good health has an energetic, even spiritual, basis. For you, cancer is not a localised disease—but a disease of the whole body. And what affects the body also affects the mind.

The idea of attacking the body and causing it damage and pain in the name of medicine is repugnant to you. You know in your heart that there must be a better way, a way that is natural, a way that respects the body.

As with any illness you will want to start the healing process by cleansing the body, and eliminating any harmful factors in the environment (such as work stress, friends with negative attitudes, and so on).

Comment

I hope you found that exercise helpful and that you have read the other profiles for comparison—and possibly even reconsidered your answers to the questions in order to change your profile to one you think more exactly describes you. Let me now tell you something of my story so that you can see where I am coming from.

In 1994 my wife, Bernadette, was diagnosed with cancer and although I took a very proactive approach to reading up on the subject, we were basically Profile A people and went along with what the doctors suggested. Back then there was less public acknowledgement that there were other options. However, my reading quickly led me to the view that we were going down the wrong path. Unfortunately, my wife wasn't interested in doing any reading so she remained a devout Profile A, while I skittered across the range until I was somewhere between C and D. Obviously this caused a great deal of tension at home.

If we had had a book like this one, that pointed out why we were having such stressful disagreements, things might have been better. That is why all books you read should be thoroughly shared with those who are closest to you.

The person who has the cancer is the one who must make the final decision—and everyone else needs to accept that fact. That doesn't mean you can't revisit and re-evaluate the situation from time to time but I do urge you not to lock yourself into a mental framework that cannot be changed in the light of new information or as events unfold.

My wife died very quickly (15 months after diagnosis, despite—or possibly (indeed almost certainly) because of—surgery, radiation and chemotherapy) and I was left not knowing how I would confront any new cancer that I might have. Clearly the route we had taken with my wife had not worked. But if I was going to reject that route I needed to have reasons to do so and other options that seemed better. As I had a fifty per cent likelihood of getting cancer (the same as everyone else) it seemed to me sensible to continue my reading until I reached a point where I felt I had a strategy that I would follow myself. I needed in fact a global picture of cancer because, without that, I couldn't be sure that any strategy that I might formulate would be valid. Eventually, I did reach a point where I felt I had a handle on the whole thing—and I wanted to share that understanding and so I wrote my first cancer book.

Now, to fully understand my situation I need to go back to 1986, eight years before my wife's cancer was diagnosed. It was in February of this year that my daughter Stevie was born. She was a beautiful little baby but she had Down's Syndrome and a heart condition that needed to be corrected. During the heart operation, which she had at the age of six months, something caused her to have a brief moment of oxygen shortage—just a few minutes—but it was to cause brain damage that left her profoundly disabled, epileptic and blind. She lived another eight years before dying of the pneumonia that was inevitable in a girl who could barely move.

Why am I telling you this story? Because Stevie transformed my life. She was the single best thing ever to happen to me. She made me aware of the power of love and sharing, and also of the value and power of being proactive and taking responsibility for myself. Because of her, I was to found two charities. I could barely support my family but there I was going out and founding charities. One of those charities—the Hong Kong Down Syndrome Association—is now, 24 years later, a major Hong Kong charity and the other charity helped to set up a parent resource centre in Guangzhou, China (The Yang Ai Parent Resource Centre) and establish an annual conference to which people come from many distant parts of China.

It gives me an extraordinary sense of pride to know that I have helped to benefit, however slightly, the welfare of developmentally disabled children throughout China, and helped establish a blueprint for the decades to come. Don't get me wrong. I didn't do all of this alone. Many people were involved in both these charities—but neither of these charities would have happened without me doing something, and having certain thoughts. And that only happened because I was awakened to the possibility, and indeed the necessity, of these things happening as a result of my experience with Stevie. She seeded in me the love and she empowered me to go out and to help others.

I have written the story of my life with Stevie and Bernadette in my memoir: *Wordjazz for Stevie*. ('Maybe the most moving story you will ever read.'—*Sunday Telegraph*)

The reason I am writing this book, and the other cancer books that I have written, and why I am maintaining an archive of more recently acquired cancer information at www.cancerfighter.wordpress.com (and also my Facebook group: Cancer Recovery) is that I believe I have some information that might help you—and because of Stevie, I am impelled to offer it to you.

Another point I want to make here is that when Bernadette was diagnosed with cancer, I was already an Olympic-level athlete (because of my experiences with Stevie) in terms of being proactive and taking responsibility—and yet events sped away from me so fast I was never able to catch up and influence them one iota. I hope I can help you get the information you need to avoid Bernadette's fate in time to influence the decisions you make.

Part Three
The Four Sensible Strategies

Introduction

Cancer is everywhere. It is, as one newspaper headline recently put it, the new normal. ('Cancer is the new normal', *The Guardian*, 15 January 2011). It is in all our lives. You may or may not have already been diagnosed with cancer—indeed, you might at this very minute be suffering from the shock of a recent diagnosis—but there is no doubt that cancer is going to visit you. It is going to come knocking on your door. Whether or not that cancer is going to be your cancer or your wife's, husband's, lover's, brother's, sister's, mother's, father's, son's, or your daughter's, it is coming and it will affect you.

If we take a statistical cross-section of the situation right now, then we can say that approximately 45 per cent of all adults over the age of 18 will get cancer (rather more than the 'one in three' mantra that we have been hearing for the last decade and more). But this is a static photograph. It is averaging out all the probabilities for people of all ages. But a dynamic photograph is going to show that the vast majority of those 18 year olds alive today are going to grow into 70 and 80 year olds, and in the intervening 50–60 years cancer incidence in all probability will have risen markedly overall—just as it has done over the last 50 years and is generally expected to continue doing. So it is reasonable to argue that a dynamic whole-life cancer probability of an 18 year old today is likely to be closer to 70–80 per cent.

A very scary thought. So the next step in the search for a life free of cancer is to consider what strategy you want to take—what is your perception of the solution?

We will now look at what I call the four sensible strategies for dealing with cancer. When I say sensible I don't mean to suggest that I agree with them, merely that it is possible to argue reasonably in favour of them. And since we are all different, we are going to be attracted to different strategies. The important thing is to respect these differences.

Strategy 1: Do what your doctor advises

This is the strategy that most people follow by default. Why would they not? The doctors know best. They have had years of training and experience. And they have science on their side. Surely it's a no-brainer.

It's obvious that cancer is a killer so you have to try to get rid of it or kill it in some way (surgery, radiation, chemotherapy etc.) and doctors have some very, very powerful tools at their fingertips that enable them to do just that—in theory. They are also, usually, hostile to alternative therapies—calling them (derisively) 'unproven'—so it's best to keep in the doctor's good books by not doing anything that the doctor might disagree with.

Many people will certainly be attracted to this view of the solution because it takes them off the hook. They don't have to think about their situation. Many people lack the education and more importantly the confidence to think they could make better decisions than a doctor could. After all, they will say to themselves, he or she, (the doctor), knows everything and I (the patient) know nothing.

If you choose to follow this strategy, then all you have to do is what the doctor recommends up to the financial limits of whatever health system or insurance package you have. If things work out, great! If they don't, well, that's just bad luck and it is just the way the cookie crumbles and everyone did their best.

We can see that Strategy 1 will appeal to people who fit the Profile A of the last chapter.

Even if you are strongly attracted to this argument, I would like to suggest that you read on.

Strategy 2: Ignore what your doctors advise. Don't do any of the conventional treatments. Instead only do the alternatives.

This may seem crazy to you (if you are a Profile A person) or so obvious that it doesn't need explaining (if you are a Profile D person) but, whatever your profile, it is a perfectly sensible approach. Let me spell out the reasons as to why someone would take this approach in slightly more detail.

There are both positive and negative arguments. The positive arguments look at the benefits of following the strategy while the negative arguments focus on the benefits of avoiding strategy 1. I will deal with these negative arguments first.

■ **The first part of the negative argument is this: the conventional treatments have not proven as effective as we would hope.**

The facts appear to be that 50–60 per cent of all cancers are effectively treated by conventional means—that is to say that 50–60 per cent of cancer patients live at least five years having received conventional treatments. Unfortunately this leaves 40–50 per cent of cancer patients who don't.

Of the conventional treatments, surgery is far and away the most effective. It is estimated that 90–95 per cent of cancer patients who recover after conventional treatments do so directly as a result of surgery.

It is also known that chemotherapy—although widely used (about 75 per cent of all cancer patients in the USA are treated with chemo)—only has a proven benefit for about six per cent of all cancers—and in those cancers, perhaps only 50 per cent become cancer free in the long term. So we can see that many people—indeed the vast majority of people who undergo chemotherapy do not gain any benefit from doing so.

Radiation, bizarrely, has not been much studied on its own by means of a double-blind clinical trial, though it would be easy to do so. It isn't studied in this way because its effectiveness is assumed. And, so the doctors argue, since it is effective, it would be unethical to deprive cancer patients of it. Some statistical studies do appear to show some limited benefits—for example, one study by Yale School of Medicine doctors (published in the *Journal of the National Cancer Institute*, 17 May 2006) shows an absolute benefit of four per cent over five years among women over 70 years of age with breast cancer. If you think that an absolute benefit of four per cent over five years is worth the risk of lymphoedema (one of the more common side effects of radiation treatment—see Section 2: *Cancer Diagnosis and Conventional Treatments* for further discussion), that's your decision. This result is usually quoted as being a 70 per cent improved chance of survival—because there was a 70 per cent relative benefit. But relative benefits are misleading—only absolute benefits should be taken into account.

Another study ('Radiation Benefits Women with Small Cancers After Lumpectomy' by M F X Gnant and others, *San Antonio Breast Cancer Symposium*, December 8, 2005, Abstract 8) followed several thousand women of all ages, and found that after ten years there appeared to be a two per cent absolute benefit (or a 60+ per cent relative benefit) among those who had received the radiation over ten years.

We have already discussed the issue of relative versus absolute benefit. My own personal view is that I would not be swayed by any proposed treatment that carried with it the threat of serious side effects unless there was an absolute benefit of 20–30 per cent at the very least. You, very likely, will take a different assessment of what you think is a reasonable benefit. Remember that any claim less than three per cent could be caused by statistical or experimental error.

■ The second part of the negative argument is that conventional treatments can be very painful and damaging to long-term health.

I have written at length about the pros and cons of surgery, chemo and radiation in Section 2: *Cancer Diagnosis and Conventional Treatments*. Here I will simply note that while it is hard to argue against a lumpectomy in the case of breast cancer, the removal of a significant section of the colon could mean you are permanently beset by problems associated with poor digestion and a requirement to be close to a toilet at all times. Since diet and absorption of nutrients through the gut is vital for long-term health you could be setting yourself up for a life that requires very careful management.

Although not all chemotherapy is excruciatingly painful, some is. Here is a description written by someone who has undergone a very painful chemotherapy regime: 'I lost 50 per cent of my body fat and looked like a scarecrow. I lost my hair, my skin looked a whitish-green-grey color, I could not keep any food down, I totally lost my appetite, my immune system was non-existent, I became anaemic, and I almost died.' (Carol Patterson, author of *Cure Yourself of Cancer*).

People have been so damaged by radiation that they have lost important bodily functions.

In one study, breast cancer patients treated with combined chemotherapy and radiation were later found to have 28 times more leukaemia than the general population.

■ The third part of the negative argument is that conventional methods can make cancers more aggressive

It is known that surgery can have the inadvertent effect of promoting cancer growth. In addition, radiation and chemotherapy while seeming to make tumours shrink, often (usually?) end up making the tumours faster growing. In the end there is little benefit in terms of increased life span.

■ The fourth part of the negative argument is that conventional treatment targets the wrong thing.

Broadly speaking, the objective of conventional treatment is to kill or remove the tumour. Conventional doctors do not address in any way the question of what has caused the tumour to grow. It may be that they subscribe to the 'evil cell' hypothesis, i.e. that cancer cells are simply deviant in some lethal way—and that it is just randomly our bad luck if they happen to be in our body. Since it is known that no more than five per cent of cancers are genetic, this does not seem to be a reasonable cause for most cancers—something else is at work.

If we do not address the cause of the tumour, reason suggests that a new tumour will likely appear. More likely, there will be a continual production line of tumours until the cause is identified and corrected—or until the host dies.

Those then are the negative arguments for not choosing the conventional treatments. But what about the positive arguments in favour of doing alternative therapies?

The positive arguments in favour of choosing alternative therapies

■ The first part of the positive argument: tumours are not the disease

Firstly there is the argument that cancer should not be seen simply as an issue of tumours. It is best to see the tumours not as the disease but as symptoms of the disease. After all, we don't cut off the itchy red spots when we have measles. We understand the spots are just symptoms that will disappear once the disease state has left the body. Why do we think that tumours are different?

Some, (but not all) alternative methods address this question by arguing that cancer is really the result of dietary deficiencies and that if these deficiencies can be corrected then the body can be returned to a state of good health. They point to the analogous situation 100 years ago when millions of Indonesians suffered terribly from the disease of beriberi, many of them dying the most wretched deaths. Health authorities attempted to treat this disease with drugs to no avail. Eventually it was discovered that the problem was caused by thiamine deficiency (vitamin B1). So here was a case where a simple change of diet or addition of a supplement proved to be infinitely more powerful than the most powerful of drugs.

That is just one instance of an approach that might be defined as alternative—in that it revolves around diet—that proved to be very effective.

There is an enormous range of alternative viewpoints and approaches, and they are certainly not all in agreement. However, mostly they would agree with the following:

1.   Cancer cells can be persuaded to kill themselves by returning the body to a state of alkalinity and high tissue oxygenation. This can be done through diet and supplements.
2.   There are natural ways of alerting the immune system to the presence of cancer cells and getting this immune system to help eliminate the cells from the body.
3.   There are ways of engaging the mind, the emotions and the body's living energy system in such a way that vital health is promoted and that these can be useful anti-cancer weapons.

■ The second part of the positive argument: anecdotal successes

The argument is this: an increasing number of people have followed alternative approaches, and they seem to have been cured.

Beata Bishop, for example, was in her late forties working for the BBC when she discovered she had untreatable stage 4 melanoma. This was in the early 1980s. She is alive and well today (2011) because she threw herself into the Gerson diet, a regime she continues to follow rigorously thirty years later. She has written about her own cancer journey in her book, *A Time to Heal*. This book was originally published with the heading, *My Triumph Over Cancer*, a title that Beata abhorred. I personally had the pleasure of interviewing her and you can see our discussion at www.conscious.tv/lifestories.html (under 'healing'). You can see from this interview that she was doing very well on whatever regime she was on. The Gerson diet is routinely vilified by conventional doctors but she is living proof that, for some, this is a potential anti-cancer approach that has worked.

Felicity Corbin-Wheeler is a fervent Christian, and so when she was discovered to have untreatable pancreatic cancer—a diagnosis that few people survive—she turned to prayer and seeds, in particular the extract of bitter almonds known as laetrile. She is today alive and cancer free. She wrote her story up in the book, *God's Healing Word*.

Elonna McKibben had an untreatable cancer on her spinal cord that has left her wheelchair bound—yet she too is now cancer free having experimented with a chemical called CanCell. If you want to read her story, go to her website at www.elonnamckibben.com.

These three people are high profile. They have written books or have websites telling their stories. These and other cases demonstrate that 'terminal' cancers needn't be fatal. So, for those attracted to these approaches, there is some support that they can be successful.

I have described many more stories in Section 8: *Cancer: Survivors' Stories—They did it. You can too.* (also available as a free pdf from www.fightingcancer.com)

■ The third part of the positive argument: scientific evidence

Normally, the dispute between conventional and alternative approaches is phrased as being a dispute between science, on the one hand, and airy-fairy thinking or quackery on the other. This is extremely unfair.

In the first place we should note that there is very little proof supporting the use of surgery and radiation, and chemotherapy (while certainly proven in some cases) has actually been disproven for the vast majority of the cases in which it is still used as a standard treatment. I discuss all these questions in relation to 'proof' and 'evidence' in Section 3: *Cancer Research and Politics*. Here I will just say that there is a great deal of laboratory research supporting many of the so-called alternative approaches. Indeed it is possible to argue that there is more science on the alternative side of the argument than on the conventional. The problem is that conventional medicine is very tied into patentable medicines—because that is where the money is and that is what doctors have been trained in.

Evidence-based medicine?

Conventional medicine makes a great point of stating that it is evidence-based. But how much evidential support for it is there? You would imagine a great deal. But is this in fact the case?

The *British Medical Journal* has an offshoot publication, *BMJ Clinical Evidence*, whose mission is to provide physicians and patients with the best available evidence, garnered wherever possible from randomized, controlled clinical trials (RCTs), which are considered to be the most reliable and rigorous standard for measuring treatment effectiveness. The journal describes itself as 'the international source of the best available evidence for effective health care'.

'What proportion of commonly-used treatments are supported by good evidence, what proportion should not be used or used only with caution, and how big are the gaps in our knowledge?' asks the publication's website (BMJ, 2007).

Of around 2,500 treatments so far reviewed by the journal's distinguished team of advisors, peer reviewers, experts, information specialists and statisticians, only 13 per cent have been found definitely beneficial. A further 23 per cent are rated as likely to be beneficial; eight per cent can be classified as a trade-off between benefits and harms; six per cent as clearly unlikely to be beneficial; four per cent are likely to be ineffective or harmful, and a whopping 46 per cent—almost half of all treatments reviewed—are rated as being of unknown effectiveness. That's the word from the horse's mouth.

But what about all the research that is published in the medical journals? Dr Marcia Angell, author of *The Truth About the Drug Companies: How They Deceive Us and What to Do About It*, issued this statement after leaving *The New England Journal of Medicine* as Editor in Chief: 'It is simply no longer possible to believe much of the clinical research that is published'. Why not? Because it is manipulated by the pharmaceutical companies who pay for it. Often the supposed author of an article has nothing to do with the research discussed in it. This is a problem that has also been admitted by the editors of *The Lancet* who believe that as many as half the articles they publish suffer from some form or other of deceitful practices.

But surely new drugs are better than the ones they replace? According to Iain Chalmers of the *British Medical Journal*, there is evidence that 'new treatments are as likely to be worse as they are to be better' than the current treatments. Amazing, isn't it?

Conclusion

While it is true that alternative approaches cannot demonstrate their effectiveness through large-scale research studies—for the simple reason that these research studies have not been done (and why haven't they?), it is also true that they generally have sensible rationales and there is often empirical evidence—in the form of personal experiences—and laboratory research to support their use. The danger, though, is that their effectiveness may be exaggerated, or that results from laboratory experiments do not translate into effectiveness in real life.

Strategy 3: Mix and Match

The first strategy was to do only what the doctor recommended. The second strategy was to do anything and everything except what the doctor recommended. Now we come to Strategy Three. You may take the view that while there is a lot that seems to be interesting and potentially valuable in the alternative point of view—diet, herbs, supplements, emotional and spiritual support, energy healing etc.—you are not entirely comfortable with the idea of rejecting the conventional methods. You therefore propose to do both.

There are three ways of mixing and matching:

i)   Do conventional treatments first and then, if that doesn't work, do the alternatives.

This is the strategy that many people follow by default. First time round, they do everything that the doctor recommends. However, very often, when a cancer returns, patients take the view that having experienced the effects of the conventional approaches and finding that they have been unsuccessful, they now feel free to turn to the alternatives. By this time too, they are often less prepared to take on board their doctors' professional biases against the alternative approaches.

ii)   Do the alternatives first and if they don't work, fall back on the conventional

Unless a cancer is highly aggressive then you have time to make decisions. Cancers have generally been growing for several years before they are detected. A few months experimenting with the alternatives may not make much difference. And it could mean you will amaze everyone by curing yourself through nutritional means.

iii)   Do the conventional and alternative approaches in parallel right from the start.

There is increasing evidence that this is already what many people are doing—particularly women with breast cancer. Often the alternative approaches are being used to soften the impact of the conventional treatments—so-called complementary therapies—but very often cancer fighters are using non-conventional therapies to attack their cancers directly. A 2005, Canadian study into the use of alternatives by women with breast cancer found that 80 per cent of them were using alternatives alongside conventional treatments. Cristiane Spadacio, a cancer researcher studying this phenomenon commented:, '… there has been an exponential growth in interest in—and use of—complementary and alternative medicine (CAM), especially in developed western countries …. Studies show that the number of patients who use some form of alternative therapy after the diagnosis of cancer is high … [and they experience] high levels of satisfaction with alternative therapies.'

So there you are. Mix and match the conventional and alternative whichever way you like. It is interesting to note that doctors are finding that breast cancer patients are living longer now than they were twenty years ago. It is often assumed that this is because of developments in conventional treatment. However, since there haven't been any real developments, it is much more likely to be because more and more breast cancer patients are doing CAM on the side.

It has also been noted that cancer survivability in the UK lags behind that in France and German, for example, two countries with a stronger tradition of herbal medicine. Is there a connection?

Strategy 4: Do nothing for your cancer

Our final strategic option is to do nothing at all for your cancer. This may surprise you, but it is a perfectly reasonable strategy. The older you are the stronger this argument becomes. If you're 80 years old, who can say how many years you have left? You may not wish to risk the damage and pain of conventional approaches on the one hand while, at the same time, you are probably happy with your habits and way of life and may not wish to change these for some disruptive alternative program—after all there's no guarantee that that will work either.

You might take heart from the fact that the older you are the slower the cancer tends to grow.

Also, a medical statistician, Dr Hardin Jones, once calculated that on average you are likely to live four times longer by doing nothing than if you do something (by which he meant something conventional). Dr Hardin Jones of the Department of Medical Physics at the University of California studied the question of how effective various treatments were in terms of the future life expectancy of the patients undergoing them. This was his controversial conclusion:

'My studies have proven conclusively that untreated cancer patients actually live up to four times longer than treated individuals. For a typical type of cancer, people who refused treatment lived for an average of twelve and a half years. Those who accepted surgery and other kinds of treatment lived an average of only three years.'

Recently, I was giving a talk to a Rotary Club and one of the audience told me this story: his mother had been diagnosed at the age of 87 with breast cancer. The doctors had told her what they proposed to do but she declined their services saying she was old enough and she had to die of something, so she would do nothing. His mother had continued her life as before and eventually died—aged 100!

Also, if you are a man diagnosed with prostate cancer, a strategy of 'wait and see' is often recommended—largely because most people with prostate cancer do not die of their disease and the consequences of surgical and radiological intervention—impotence, urinary incontinence—generally impact very negatively on quality of life.

And intriguingly, some people have ignored their cancers and their cancers have simply disappeared on their own.

People who are extremely anxious may prefer just to forget they have cancer. It is easier for them to cope psychologically. Obviously this is not a rational decision but denial sometimes does work.

Which strategy is for you?

So, you have read the four options. Which one of these strategies makes sense for you? The choice is yours. All we do know is that there is no 100 per cent 'cure' that will work for everyone. We are all different: our cancers are different (even two men with prostate cancers will, most likely, have different types of cancer cell), our situations are different, our characters are different. There is no one single right answer, only the answer you feel is right for you.

Decision making: the voice of authority versus a risk-benefit analysis

How can we make decisions in the face of cancer? One way is by means of authority. We find someone who we consider to have authority in this area and we ask them what decisions we should make—and then we do that. We are happy to let the pilot fly the plane because he is an expert and we are not. But would we be happy to let bankers run the economy? I am assuming not. Why not? After all they too are experts.

Another way we can arrive at a decision is by way of proof. We see what action has been proven to be effective by means of careful scientific studies. In the case of medicine, proof consists of finding something to be true or false by submitting it to a large scale double blind clinical trial. For a full discussion of what this involves see Section 3: *Cancer: Research and Politics.*

A third way of making decisions it to use a risk-benefit analysis (or even a risk-cost-benefit analysis). If a therapy seems potentially interesting, then it is reasonable to say to yourself: the potential benefit of doing this is that I will be cured. That would be a big plus. Are there any negatives that I need to put alongside this big plus? What are the costs? Drawbacks? Potential damage?

I think this is a very useful tool for making decisions.

Let's look at the suggestion that we should take megadoses (doses of 3–40+ grams a day) of vitamin C, according to a risk benefit analysis.

Potential benefits:
Cure the cancer, slow down the growth of cancer, relieve pain, extend life.

Potential risks:
Side effects? The only negative side effect associated with vitamin C is that it causes diarrhoea when you take in too much. This can be solved by reducing intake. Some forms of vitamin C are less effective than others.
Effectiveness? It may not be effective.

Impact? Because it is an important nutrient for the body it will have impacts—to avoid any possibility that these impacts will be negative, dosage needs to be increased and decreased gradually.

Potential costs:

Vitamin C is cheap. Note that when I talk of vitamin C I am *not* talking about the fizzy orange pills you can buy in the supermarket or chemist. See Section 6: *Cancer: Vitamins and Other Supplements* for a full discussion of vitamin C.

We see from this analysis that vitamin C might have enormous benefits while the risks of using it are small and the cost issue is negligible. So we can reasonably apply Pascal's famous conclusion and take megadoses of vitamin C (a megadose is usually defined as a dose measured in grams rather than milligrams).

Pascal's conclusion

Blaise Pascal, a French mathematician and philosopher, believed that even though God's existence might be 99.99 per cent unlikely, we would be foolish not to believe in him. Why? Because if he doesn't exist it makes no difference whether we believe or not; but if God exists then our belief or non-belief might be the difference between going to Heaven or not.

Applying this theorem to vitamin C, we can argue thus: If taking 20, 30 or 40 grams a day of vitamin C doesn't work it makes no difference whether we take it or not, but if it does work then the only way to benefit is by taking it. There is no obvious danger involved and the cost of exploring this option is not excessive. So the sensible thing is to take it.

Part Four
Resources

Different Journeys

Hopefully you are more self-aware now than before you started to read this book. You are more aware also of the strategies that you might wish to take and what your rationale is. It is now time to look at the next steps on your cancer journey:

Step 1

If you want to find out more about mainstream approaches for your own cancer, then go to www.cancer.gov/cancertopics/pdq. This is an information resource for both doctors and patients (and there is no reason at all why patients should not read the information provided to doctors). This is the most up-to-date information available anywhere and it is updated regularly.

Step 2

If you want to find out what the alternative therapies are—and if you want to get an overview of the arguments, the history, the issues, the strategies and the options—then you will want to read this book in detail, particularly sections 4 to 7, which cover diet, herbs, vitamins and a wide range of other therapies. You may also wish to read the short companion volume: *Cancer Recovery Guide: 15 alternative and complementary strategies for restoring health*.

Step 3

If you want a guru to tell you what to do in terms of alternative therapies, then these books may be helpful:

Cancer Free, Bill Henderson
Beating Cancer with Nutrition, Patrick Quillin
Healing the Gerson Way, Charlotte Gerson

Step 4

If you would like some personal testimonies of people who have chosen the alternative route I would highly recommend the following:

Cancer Cause and Cure, Percy Weston
> *Percy was an Australian farmer whose cancer story is fascinating in pinpointing a cause of his own cancer. Diagnosed as terminal in his late 30s, he went on to live to the age of 100, free from cancer, heart disease and the arthritis that had plagued him when young.*

A Time to Heal, Beata Bishop
> *Beata was diagnosed with stage 4 melanoma in the 1980s, as a woman in the prime of life. As I write this (2011), she is alive and well, and still working—although she is well past the normal retirement age of 60.*

Cancer Battle Plan, Ann Frahm
> *Ann had suffered through surgery, radiation, chemo and even a bone marrow transplant when she was told that all these treatments had failed and she had at most weeks to live. Five weeks later she declared herself cancer free having turned to a nutritional therapy. She lived another ten years.*

Step 5

If you need some background on the politics of the major cancer institutions and how the major pharmaceutical companies have infiltrated the profession I would recommend the following books:

The Cancer Industry, Ralph Moss
> *This is a book that everyone should read. It is a view of the 'Cancer Industry' from the inside of Sloan Kettering—a major cancer research centre.*

The Emperor of All Maladies by Siddhartha Mukherjee
> *This is an excellent history of the development of conventional cancer treatments.*

Step 6

There are other books not directly related to cancer that are nevertheless valuable in teaching useful lessons

Health at the Crossroads, Dean Black
> *Now out of print, this slim book packs a big punch*

Anatomy of an Illness, Norman Cousins
> *Empowering book on how Cousins took himself out of the hands of his doctors and using common sense healed himself from an acutely debilitating metabolic disease.*

Quantum Healing, Deepak Chopra
> *A very readable attempt to bring some serious scientific backbone in support of an esoteric understanding of what health means and how it might be achieved.*

Confessions of a Medical Heretic, Robert Mendelsohn MD
> *The often amusing ruminations of a doctor on the defects of conventional medicine.*

You Can Fight For Your Life, Lawrence LeShan
> *A psychologist's approach to helping cancer patients.*

On The Take: How Medicine's Complicity With Big Business Can Endanger Your Health , Jerome P Kassirer MD
> *Kassirer's credits include Adjunct Professor of Medicine at Yale University and Editor-in-Chief of the New England Journal of Medicine. This is a man right at the heart of the 'Medical Establishment' and he is disgusted with the very negative impact of the pharmaceutical industry on the medical profession and, more importantly, our health.*

The China Study, T Colin Campbell
> *This is the most persuasive book on why diets with low animal protein are healthy and those with a high animal protein component are not. Campbell is a leading US nutritional scientist. Since his conclusions, based on the largest nutritional survey ever done, conflict with what he calls 'The Status Quo', meaning vested interests in the food industry, and the collusion of scientists in maintaining that status quo, he is interesting too on political in-fighting in the world of the scientific establishment.*

There are many other useful books but this is a good selection to start off with.

Now what?

Reading this section has, I hope, helped you to refine your views on cancer and how you wish to proceed. You know where to go to, so go there. Start reading and follow the path that your heart tells you is the right path—the path that is right for you.

If you feel you are tempted to do something either in addition to or instead of the conventional treatments then I will start you on the way with these four suggestions:

1.   Eat a plant-based diet.
     See Section 4: Cancer: Detox and Diet for the rationale and for details of which foods are most recommended.

2. Take increasing amounts of vitamin C.
    See Section 6: Cancer: Vitamins and Other Supplements for details of what type of vitamin C is best, and which should be avoided.
3. Do exercise.
    See Section 7: Cancer: Energy, Mind and Emotions for a full explanation of why this is beneficial
4. Take a herbal formula such as Essiac.
    See Section 5: Cancer: Herbs and Botanicals for a full range of options.

These suggestions are provided simply as a platform for a wider-ranging approach, something you can activate right now while you settle down to the business of informing yourself of all the other options you may want to do. I wish you the very best of luck.

Cancer: Diagnosis and Conventional Treatments

The pros and cons of cancer tests, surgery, radiation and chemotherapy

In this section I look in detail at the pros and cons of the conventional treatments for cancer, with particular emphasis on surgery, radiation and chemotherapy. I also discuss the other mainstream options from the use of lasers to smart drugs. No-one should opt for these treatments without a full understanding of the limitations and dangers associated with these treatments. However, since most people will assume that this is the only way to go, I have an extensive section on ways in which you can protect yourself. This section also takes a detailed look at issues relating to diagnostic tests—and suggests a number of tests that your doctors will not mention. We also look at the particular issue of lymphoedema—a common consequence of conventional treatment.

Cancer Testing

'I have no difficulty in dating the origin of my own doubts about the conventional assessment of the work of doctors. They began when I went to a London hospital as a medical student after several years of graduate research in the Department of Biochemistry at McGill, and Human Anatomy at Oxford. There were two things that struck me, almost at once. One was the absence of any real interest among clinical teachers in the origin of disease, apart from its pathological and clinical manifestations; the other was that whether the prescribed treatment was of any value to the patient was often hardly noticed, particularly in internal medicine .... Indeed there seemed to be an inverse relationship between the interest of a disease to the doctor and the usefulness of its treatment to the patient.'

Professor Thomas McKeown
Professor of Social Medicine, University of Birmingham
(*The Role of Medicine*, 1979)

The first step in any approach to cancer—as with any disease—is diagnosis. Initial suspicions of cancer may arise from a regular health check-up or, more likely, as the result of noticing some bodily changes.

There are a number of ways in which these suspicions can be confirmed or ruled out. However, there are also a number of dangers associated with testing, and you should be aware of these dangers before proceeding.

First let's look at the kind of tests that are available.

Blood tests

Most blood tests are non-specific—that is, they can indicate the presence of a health problem but not clearly specify the exact cause. The blood test may show, for example, that you are anaemic, but there are many possible reasons, including cancer, for why you might be anaemic.

There are also a number of specific blood tests that look for chemical markers produced by specific cancers. For example, breast, lung and bowel tumours produce a protein called carcino-embryonic antigen (CEA). If a very high CEA level is found, then a tumour is assumed to be present until proved otherwise. Cancers of the prostate, testicles and ovaries also produce known chemical markers that can be tested for.

Markers	Cancer
CEA	Colon, Rectum, Lung, Breast, Pancreas
CA-125	Ovaries, Uterus
CA 15-3	Breast
C 19-9	Colon, Pancreas, Stomach, Liver
PSA	Prostate
PAP	Prostate

Blood tests can also directly indicate blood-related cancers. The presence of blood in the stool, for example, may itself be an indicator of cancer. Sometimes, blood in the stool is not obvious and thus has to be tested for. This test is known as the 'faecal occult blood test' ('occult' in medical matters—and particularly in relation to cancer—means 'hidden', not clearly visible).

Imaging techniques

Doctors have access to a number of imaging techniques that help them to see into the body: X-rays, CT scans, MRI scans, ultrasound, PET scans and so on. While these may be helpful in determining the presence and location of cancer tumours, none is 100 per cent effective. Most of these imaging techniques provide ill-defined results—as one doctor describes it: they show that 'something is taking up space'. The PET scan is significantly more likely to pick up metastases than other types of scan, but still picks up on average less than 90 per cent of metastatic lymph nodes. Even so, neither the PET scan nor any of the others can distinguish between cancer and benign lumps. Also, with a number of these scans, a problem for the patient is the extent of exposure to radiation. One new technology, Electron Beam Tomography, uses very low doses of radiation.

Endoscopy

In addition, there are a number of ways of achieving direct visual access to parts of the body with specially constructed telescopes. The general name for these kinds of tests is endoscopy—which is Latin for 'looking at the insides'. Specific terms relate to the part of the body they are looking at: colonoscopy takes a look at the colon, bronchoscopy looks at the lungs, and so on. In all cases, this involves feeding a fibre optic tube with a camera at the other end into the body, usually through the nearest major orifice.

Cytology (biopsies)

Finally, there are the cytological tests which study cells that have been removed from the body. Cells are usually obtained by cutting them out of the body. With *excisional biopsies* the tumour, or lump, is removed in its entirety. This is best. Alternatively, an *incisional biopsy* may be performed. This involves the cutting out of part of the tumour/lump or, in the case of *needle biopsies*, the removal of cells from the interior of a tumour/lump using a needle. Lymph nodes surrounding a tumour may also be removed at this stage for analysis, to see whether there has been any spread.

Problems with tests

False results

The first problem associated with any test is that of reliability. The perfect test would be one where a positive result would always mean 'yes' and a negative result would always mean 'no'. Unfortunately, by this standard, almost all tests are unreliable.

The first risk of any test is the so-called 'false positive' result. That is, the test indicates the presence of cancer when in fact there is no cancer. The problem for people with false positives is that they may undergo cancer treatment: surgery, radiation and chemotherapy, unnecessarily. They may suffer permanently from this treatment, and they may even die from it.

The opposite problem is the 'false negative,' where the patient gets a negative result when in fact cancer does exist.

These are not rare problems. Almost every test has a failure rate, and sometimes this can be as high as 20–30 per cent. It is always therefore worth asking what the reliability rate of any test is—and it is worth getting re-tested if you have any concerns. For example, if you have worrying symptoms but the test comes back negative, it is probably worth repeating the test.

Safety

Another problem relates to the safety of the test. For example, some tests require the inspection or removal of tissue in an operating theatre—all such tests have what professionals refer to as a morbidity factor—a possibility of causing permanent injury. Incisional biopsies particularly should be avoided where possible, for two reasons. One is the high risk of releasing cancer cells into the bloodstream. The second reason is that the tumour can be provoked into becoming aggressive when it may previously have been slow-growing. Dr Vincent Gammill has reported: 'I have seen lesions that have been quiescent for years become aggressively malignant and apparently metastatic after a biopsy.' However, he dismisses the suggestion that exposure to oxygen can cause a cancer to become more malignant.

But excisional biopsies, and indeed surgical removal of a tumour, may also raise other safety issues. There is the curious fact that a primary tumour is known to be able to inhibit the growth of distant, microscopic metastases by releasing two substances, angiostatin and endostatin, into the bloodstream. These prevent the growth of the blood supply (known as angiogenesis) that the metastases need to develop into full-blown tumours. Once the primary tumour has been removed, so too has this constraint on growth. The result of surgical removal of one tumour therefore has a catastrophic impact on the body by stimulating the unrestrained growth of these metastases. The surgery itself requires that the body initiate healing activities that also have the unfortunate side effect of helping to stimulate the growth of cancer tumours. This caution against surgical removal of a tumour applies particularly to cases of node positive breast cancer in premenopausal women, where the estrogen-rich environment also promotes the dissemination of cancerous cells.

Long-term impacts

Some aspects of biopsies can have long term—even permanent—impacts. The main culprit is the case of lymph node excision. I have discussed this in more detail at the end of this section. The key point to make though is that some procedures do have serious impacts and you would be wise to consider the matter very carefully before doing anything that does have the potential to cause long-term harm.

Usefulness of the test

Again, a test should be done only if it is likely to lead to a treatment. There is no point in discovering that something exists for which there is no known treatment. This is well illustrated by the following personal story. I know a man whose chest X-ray indicated that there was a possibility something was seriously wrong with his lungs. 'These shadows could be old tubercular scars, in which case there's no problem, or it could mean lung cancer,' the doctor told him. 'If it's cancer, it has spread throughout your lungs and I can only give you a few weeks or months to live. The only way I'll know for sure is by going in and having a look.' Amazingly, my friend opted for a visual inspection and the result was painful and expensive surgery that showed there was no problem. I had to laugh when I heard this. 'Why didn't you just wait to see if you were still alive in six months' time?' I asked.

This was a stark case, and my initial reaction was perhaps unhelpful. Faced with the same situation now, I would probably recommend that a second opinion might be useful—and not just a second opinion by another surgeon. It might in this circumstance be more valuable to find a doctor who was not dismissive of alternative approaches, who would know about other tests that might cast light on the situation. An advanced cancer stamps its signature on the body in many ways. We don't necessarily have to open up the rib cage for a visual inspection of the lungs to determine whether advanced lung cancer exists.

The reporting of tests

Finally, another problem with tests—one that is rarely mentioned—is the reporting of the results. Often this is done by a nurse to the patient over the phone. 'The results are negative,' my wife was told. She died, in part, because she accepted this information over the phone. If she had seen the test report she would have seen that there was a comment that indicated something was not 100 per cent right. She would have had a retest. So do ask for a copy of the test results 'for your files'. A good doctor will welcome this as a sign that you are willing to take responsibility for your own health and well-being. A doctor who refuses needs to be removed from your environment.

The lymph node excision issue: lymph node excision and oedema

Lymph node excision is a common feature of many biopsy procedures and will accompany most tumour surgery as well. The claimed object is to see if there are cancer cells in the lymph nodes (selected because they are close to the lump or tumour) which, if there are, would indicate that the cancer has spread. However, there has recently been a large-scale study that casts doubt on the value of cutting out lymph nodes (a procedure known as lymphadenectomy).

The trial, organised American College of Surgeons Oncology Group, published in *The Journal of the American Medical Association* (Feb 2011), was conducted at 115 medical centres and included 891 women. The median age was in the mid-50s, and the participants were followed for a median of 6.3 years. After an initial node biopsy, women were randomly assigned to have ten or more additional nodes removed or to leave the nodes alone. There was no difference in survival or recurrence between the two groups. According to the authors of the study Dr Grant Walter Carlson and Dr William C Wood, the study 'definitively showed that axillary lymph node dissection is not beneficial …. Survival was independent of lymph node status.'

One of the authors of the study goes on to say: 'This is such a radical change in thought that it's been hard for many people to get their heads around it.'

The author of an editorial accompanying the study, Dr Grant W Carlson, said: 'I have a feeling we've been doing a lot of harm (by routinely taking out many nodes).'

One of the findings supporting this view is that women in the study who had nodes taken out were far more likely to have complications (70 per cent versus 25 per cent). These complications included infections, abnormal sensations and fluid collecting in the armpit, and lymphoedema.

Dr Armando E. Giuliano, the lead author of the study and the chief of surgical oncology at the John Wayne Cancer Institute at St John's Health Center in Santa Monica, California, reported that the standard practice of lymph node removal has been so ingrained that 'some prominent institutions wouldn't even take part in (the study).'

Long-term impact

The removal of lymph nodes will make you very susceptible to oedema (US: edema). This is the very painful swelling of a limb as a result of lymph being unable to drain away. It is a problem that for most people cannot be completely corrected, only ameliorated with the aid of pressure bandages or by using one or other of a variety of manual lymphatic drainage procedures. One school of lymphatic drainage, the Dr Vodder School of North America, is specifically recommended. There is a worldwide list of qualified practitioners at their main site, www.vodderschool.com. There are also a number of lymph drainage remedies that are claimed to be effective. A homeopath can advise if this is a problem—or do a web search for 'lymph drainage remedies'. See also www.jovipak.com for various lymphoedema products. Other suggestions can be found under 'Lymphoedema relief' on page 136.

A closer look at some specific tests

The Pap smear

This is the most common test for cervical cell analysis. Cells have to be removed through a surgical procedure that involves scraping and brushing the inside of the cervix to obtain cells for analysis. The removed cells are put on slides, stained with dyes and examined with a microscope. The cytologist will look for the characteristic appearance of malignant or pre-malignant cells. A pathologist should also examine the slides and either diagnose cancer or report a strong suspicion of cancer. According to conservative doctors, all women who are 18 or older or sexually active should have a Pap smear test every year or every three years after three normal yearly exams. Other doctors disagree vehemently with this suggestion, saying for instance that it is not 'based on any acceptable clinical trial of the risks versus benefits of Pap smear' (Eugene D. Robin, 1984). The Pap smear is one of the most widely used of all cancer tests, and in Dr Robin's view the dependency on the test is dangerous. The reason? It has a very high rate of false results.

How are these false results possible? Highly qualified specialists study the slides and the cancerous cells have a 'characteristic shape', so how is it possible for mistakes to happen?

First of all, Pap smears require interpretation. Different doctors examining the same specimen under the microscope will vary widely in their opinions. In one study, quoted by Dr Robin, ten experts disagreed about the presence or absence of cancer cells in about 40 per cent of the specimens.

One reason for the confusion is a non-cancerous state called dysplasia, which occurs in the cells of the cervix and may be difficult or impossible to distinguish from CIS—carcinoma in situ—a form of cancer or pre-cancer where the cells remain localized; CIS does not necessarily become invasive cervical cancer (ICC). Abnormal cells can also appear in the Pap smear as a result of fungal infections, changes in the metabolic state of the subject, or for other reasons. As Dr Robin remarks, 'The possibility of finding in the Pap smear abnormal non-cancerous cells that can be mistaken for cancer is substantial.' In the case of the Pap smear, the number of false positives and false negatives amount to over 30 per cent of all test results.

A more recent test, known as liquid-based cytology (LBC), has demonstrated no meaningful improvement in reliability, according a report in *The Lancet*, January 2006.

The mammogram

The mammogram, in which breasts are X-rayed, has also been severely criticized for squeezing and bruising breast tissue—and in that way actually promotes the problem that it is supposed to be testing for. Physical trauma is considered to be one possible cause of cancer, and if there is cancer present it may also act to make the tumour more aggressive. Cancer incidence has been shown in some surveys to be higher among women who have annual checkups than among those who have never had a mammogram. The only group of women for whom regular mammograms have been shown to have any value is in the over 65, and then the degree of benefit is considered to be marginal.

Professor Michael Baum, a leading British cancer researcher, is horrified at the extent to which mammograms are promoted, without any evidence that they are beneficial, and despite a great deal of evidence that they pick up a great many non-invasive tumours which are then dealt with unnecessarily by radical surgery. (*Journal of the National Cancer Institute*, Vol. 96, No. 20, 1490–1491, October 20, 2004)

Cornelia J Baines, MD, deputy director of the Canadian National Breast Screening Study, writes: 'an unacknowledged harm [of mammography] is that for up to 11 years after the initiation of breast cancer screening in women aged 40–49 years, screened women face a higher death rate from breast cancer than unscreened control women, although that is contrary to what one would expect .... 'Shouldn't women aged 40–49 years know that, three years after screening starts, their chance of death from breast cancer is more than double that for unscreened control women? Shouldn't they be informed that it will take 16 years after they start screening to reduce their chance of death from breast cancer by a mere nine per cent?'

For a fuller account of what should perhaps be referred to as 'the mammography scandal' go to www.rense.com/general64/mam.htm.

Scintimammography

This is a new form of mammography which you may prefer to undergo as it does not involve bruising of breast tissue. Essentially it involves the injection of a slightly radioactive chemical—usually into a vein in the foot. The patient undergoing this procedure is then required to lie still while a gamma camera takes photos. Ask your cancer centre for details. This is not suitable for pregnant or breast-feeding women.

Tests for prostate cancer

The presence of prostate cancer is determined in the first place by a test known as the PSA (prostate-specific antigen) test. However, some men have been diagnosed with prostate cancer and yet have a normal low PSA reading, while others who have a high PSA reading have been found not to have the disease.

The simple fact is that most men, as they grow older, get prostate cancer. That's the bad news. The good news is that this form of cancer is usually very slow growing and not aggressively metastatic. You can live a long time with a cancer of this type and not even know it. So, the question is: who cares? There is no point in testing for something that is almost certainly present. Unfortunately, a very small number of cases of prostate cancer are aggressively metastatic.

The PSA is not the only way of testing for prostate cancer. Other tests include ultrasound and 'manual palpation'—this involves feeling the prostate to see if it is enlarged, asymmetrical, or nodular.

Summary

If you are asked to undergo any form of testing, make sure you understand:

- the risks that the test may involve
- the reliability of the results
- the likely treatment you may require if the test shows you have cancer. If you do not wish to have the proposed treatment you may prefer not to undergo the test.

Alternative Testing Procedures

I first thought of calling this section 'Alternative Diagnostics', but the word 'diagnosis' tends to be reserved for the identification of specific diseases or illnesses. Most alternative tests do not diagnose disease conditions, but rather they analyze aspects of the body's biochemistry to determine if everything is as it should be. We diagnose herpes, for example, but test to evaluate the pH of the body's tissues.

Just as the orthodox doctor relies on information derived from blood and urine tests, X-rays and CAT scans, so too practitioners of alternative medicine rely on information gained from an array of testing procedures and equipment. We will look at some of these procedures that are useful for the person who has cancer.

Bloodwork

'Bloodwork' is the American slang word for blood tests. Regular blood tests have a strong role to play in an overall anti-cancer strategy.

If we go back to the very definition of cancer, you will remember that there are two opposing views. The first is the view that the tumour represents the disease. Once you have rid the body of that object, then the cancer can be considered cured. Opposed to this is the view that the tumour is only a symptom of the disease. The cause of the cancer is an unhealthy body. Eliminating the symptom will do nothing in the long run. It may delay the inevitable for a while but the ill-health of the body will eventually provoke new cancer tumours. In this view, only by returning the whole body to a state of health can cancer be truly cured.

The relevance of this to blood tests is that instead of doing tests simply to detect the chemical markers for various cancers, we need to do tests that will measure the overall health of the body's ecology—the terrain in which the disease arises. This is the area where it is good to have the co-operation of a friendly doctor who will agree to carry out these tests while you experiment with the diets, supplements, herbs and other alternative strategies listed in the following chapters.

There are a number of tests that should be done regularly to keep track of the body's basic health. In this way, you can see clearly if what you are doing is working. However, remember that all tests suffer from the problems of false negative and false positive results so, if there are anomalous results, get re-tested. It is also a good idea to use two tests that may test the same thing in different ways so that you build in a degree of redundancy. This will help you see more clearly where the problems may lie—in the body or in specific test results. So what blood tests will measure the basic health of the body?

Blood sedimentation rate test

The erythrocyte sedimentation rate (ESR) test, which in medical jargon is known as the 'sed rate', measures the speed at which red blood cells settle at the bottom of a glass tube. The speed of sedimentation reflects the concentration of certain proteins in the blood.

This is a screening test for overall health. It is not specific to any one illness. A slow rate of sedimentation is good. Speedy sedimentation may be caused by infection, inflammation and the presence of cancer.

Complete blood count

This test will determine the quantity of red and white blood cells—which in turn will provide useful information on the general health of the body.

AMAS

AMAS (anti-malignin antibody screen) test is able to detect cancers well in advance of other signs and symptoms, and months before other conventional medical tests can detect it. However, it remains the preserve of a single laboratory, Oncolab, which developed the test, and has not gained wide acceptance. You may therefore have to bring this test to the attention of your doctor. See www.oncolabinc.com for more details. You should also note that it appears to produce a relatively high number of false negatives—so don't assume a 'no cancer' result means what it says 100 per cent of the time. Get a re-test in three months' time just to be sure.

DR-70

The DR-70 is a simple blood test that screens for 13 different cancers all at the same time. Clinical studies have been conducted all over the world, and the results showed that it detected cancers of the lung, colon, stomach, liver, pancreas, rectum, ovaries, oesophagus, cervix, uterus, thyroid, breast and even malignant lymphoma. The test is simple, non-invasive, and costs around $100. It is highly 'sensitive' in that it will detect most cancers (so the risk of false negatives is low) and 'selective' in that it will not say cancer is present when it isn't (so the risk of false positives is low). However, a positive result will not tell you which form of cancer you have—only that there is a high probability that you have one of the thirteen.

C-reactive protein test

The liver produces C-reactive protein in response to acute inflammation. The presence of this protein is therefore a good sign that there is acute inflammation. Since inflammation is strongly associated with cancer (and heart disease and arthritis) it is good to be able to detect the extent of inflammation in the body—even if this test does not tell us where the inflammation is or what is causing it.

CEA (carcino-embryonic antigen) test

This is a back-up test that measures inflammation. Although low scores cannot be taken as evidence that there is no cancer in the system, and high scores cannot definitively point to which cancer is present, if you already know where a tumour is, a high score will generally indicate that inflammation is present. Note that pregnancy will also cause high levels of CEA.

Liver tests

The liver is a key organ. If the liver is unhealthy, the whole physical system suffers. It is therefore vital that the liver be returned to good health as quickly as possible. This is something that most detoxification regimes do not fully recognize. It is no good attempting to flush toxins out if the liver, whose job is to deal with these toxins, is unable to deal with them. There are a number of tests that look at various liver functions. The following tests are usually undertaken in tandem and are known by the initials of the enzyme markers they relate to: GGT, AST, ALT, ALP and LD. The levels of bilirubin are also tested for. Taken together these provide a detailed picture of liver health. GGT, in particular, is an extremely sensitive test. When cancer develops, the liver finds itself forced to work harder and harder to try and maintain normal functioning. GGT is the test that reveals overactive liver action.

Other tests

Interleukin 6

This is a measure of angiogenesis activity. Angiogenesis is the process by which a cancer tumour creates a blood supply to support its growth. The IL6 tests for activity in this area. By itself, it should not be taken as an indicator of cancerous activity simply because it can give false readings. However, when used in conjunction with other tests, it is a very good indicator that something is going wrong. If cancer is present and active, it will inevitably be growing its own life support and IL6 levels will become elevated. It is important to get this marker into the normal range. If you can do this, you will win the fight against cancer. If you can't, your cancer wins.

Biological terrain assessment (BTA)

There has long been a dispute between the supporters of Louis Pasteur—who argue that diseases are caused by viruses, bacteria and so on—and the supporters of Pasteur's rival, Claude Bernard, who argued that the terrain in which the viruses are found is the real cause of disease. According to this view, the viruses could not flourish in a cellular terrain that was healthy. The diseased terrain allows the agents of disease to operate. Pasteur is often quoted on his death bed as having admitted that his rival was correct: 'The germ is nothing, the terrain is everything.'

Taking the logic of this one step further, it follows that a sick terrain will lead inevitably to ill health and that a plant is only as healthy as the soil it grows in. And so, we can conclude, in order to cure the unhealthy plant, it is more effective to fix the soil than to treat the plant itself.

This idea that disease may first be detected in the cellular terrain has led to the development of BTA. BTA does a computerised analysis of blood, urine and saliva looking at three specific features: the pH of the cellular environment; the degree of oxidative stress and mineral concentration levels.

Obviously, results of this test will not diagnose any specific disease, but they will reveal areas of the body's ecology that can be improved by means of diet, supplementation or other intervention. Generally speaking this is not a test that your doctor will carry out. An Internet search will be needed to find a therapist near you who offers this type of analysis.

Digital infrared thermal imaging (DITI)

This is a non-invasive scanning technique that measures changes in the surface temperature of skin. It converts the infrared radiation that is emitted from the skin into visual images that look like a Technicolor weather map. This visual image is called a thermo-gram. The body is usually symmetrical in its functioning, so any asymmetrical patterns that appear on the thermo-gram demonstrate areas of concern.

The value of this to a person scanning for cancer is that a hot spot can be detected long before a cancer tumour has grown to the size where it can be picked up by standard scanning equipment. The precancerous activity shows up hot because it is developing its own blood supply—a process referred to as neo-vascularisation.

A DITI thermogram provides a visual picture of what's going on in the body rather than being a precise diagnostic technique—but for the purpose of acting as an early warning system for cancers close to the skin surface it is an excellent tool. For deeply-rooted cancers it is less useful.

This is a technology that is developing fast both in complexity and in popularity. It is entirely non-invasive and does not traumatize tissue—unlike the standard mammogram.

At present, it is still viewed with suspicion by mainstream diagnostic centres—though this is likely to change rapidly in the coming years. One reason for this suspicion is simply that the technology detects precancerous changes far earlier than they can be dealt with surgically. You can't take out a lump before a lump has formed.

It is also a testing procedure with an excellent record of accuracy. Only nine per cent of test results are false (either false positive or false negative) according to research at the Pasteur Institute in

France. It can clearly distinguish between cancer (which is hot) and fibroadenoma cysts (which are cold). In this way it eliminates 80 per cent of the false positives that result from mammography.

For more detailed information and to view some example thermograms go to: www.healthybreasts.info.

That is the positive spin on thermograms. However, some critics have pointed out that it does not pick up more deep-seated tumours—so an all clear is not in any way conclusive. Also, an asymmetrical heat pattern can have a number of causes, and does not necessarily indicate a precancerous situation. Finally some slow-growing cancers do not show up on thermograms. The DITI should therefore be viewed as only one test among several.

Bio-resonance testing

Bio-resonance testing (also known as autonomic response testing) is one umbrella name for a number of different practices which measure bio-feedback, usually using some form of equipment: applied kinesiology, EAV (electro-acupuncture according to Voll), electrodermal screening, contact reflex analysis, Omura O-Ring test, QXCI, VEGA and others. Here I will look at the first two. You should understand that, although I will be describing them favourably, on their own terms, this technology and these techniques are on the ideological fringes of what is on offer to the cancer patient and are certainly not proven in any way.

Applied kinesiology

Most cancer patients see their problem in the following way: I have cancer. I want to get rid of it. I wish I knew of some way of just eliminating the cancer—I just want it to go away so I can get on with the life I was leading before it came along.

The problem with this way of thinking is that, almost certainly, it was precisely the way of life you were leading that gave rise to the cancer in the first place. Something, possibly major, maybe very minor, happened that eventually led to the cancer forming in your body. If that is the case then just getting rid of the cancer isn't going to work. If the conditions remain unchanged the cancer is almost certain to return. This is one of the problems that orthodox medicine signally fails to recognize. They—the oncologists—are focusing all their attention on making the tumour go away so that you can get on with your life. Sadly, they are unable in the majority of cases to do even that—but that's another issue.

This may be very annoying, but it is a fact that those cancer patients who survive, generally come to terms with. They need to know what it is that's going wrong in their body. Once they know that, they can correct it. Now, the exciting possibility is that once they have got rid of the causes of the cancer, the cancer itself might go away.

Dr Max Gerson explained his own realization of this truth in these words: 'I gradually came to the basic conclusion that, in a body with normal metabolism, cancer cannot develop. The normalization of the damaged metabolism is therefore the essential aim of any therapy.'

This is one of two basic assumptions underlying applied kinesiology. The second assumption is that the body knows what is wrong with it and will tell you if you ask the right questions in the right way.

Applied kinesiology, therefore, is a system of evaluating the body's weaknesses and strengths using the body itself as a sounding board. The basic idea is that the body is wise. It responds to contact with any item in one of three ways. If the body needs a substance, it will show this by strengthening the muscles. If it finds the substance detrimental in some way, it will weaken the muscles and if it is neutral to it, there is no response. The applied kinesiologist therefore approaches the diagnostic problems posed by a patient by taking a muscle group (e.g., an arm or a leg) and exerting a little pressure against it while the patient resists the pressure. Then substances that will reveal the inner workings of the body are placed in contact with the body and the effect on the muscle is tested—does the muscle remain strong or does it weaken?

Having personally undergone an applied kinesiological evaluation, I can tell you that the muscle responses appear to be consistent and repeatable. Indeed, if it didn't work, it is unlikely that it would become widely accepted as a health promoting approach—but it has. A large number of otherwise orthodox doctors have also trained in kinesiology. The founder of the approach, George Goodheart Jr, is still alive today and was the first chiropractor to serve on the US Olympic medical committee. Nevertheless, it is fair to say that it has not conclusively proven its claims and that a number of clinical trials have been done and the results have tended to be negative.

But what makes applied kinesiology potentially such a powerful and important weapon is that it may be able to reveal very subtle biochemical problems immediately—there's no waiting for days or weeks to get lab results—and without the necessity for invasive procedures. Indeed, if it is not a sham, the analysis is at levels of precision way beyond what most orthodox doctors will do, or indeed can do using orthodox means. Perhaps it is this potential that seduces us to ignore or question the negative results of clinical trials. It is not my desire to undermine the idea of applied kinesiology—but I do wish to point out that it is one of the most contentious areas of alternative medical practice.

To help you understand applied kinesiology a little better, I will give an example. The body is a system in which every cell is both manufacturing and breaking down numerous hormones, neurotransmitters and other biochemical molecules necessary for the body to function. To take a specific example, the amino acid tyrosine that is extracted from food is transformed in the body first into L-dopa, which in turn is transformed into dopamine, which is transformed into noradrenalin, and that is then transformed into adrenalin. Once each of the chemicals in this chain is no longer needed there is a three-stage process by which the chemical is changed to make it capable of being eliminated in the urine. That is just one of thousands of cycles that the body does seemingly effortlessly all the time. However, each of these transformations requires other substances to be present—vitamins, minerals and so on. If these other chemicals are not present then the result is that one of the intermediate products cannot be broken down for elimination and so it remains in the body—usually in the fatty tissue—such as the breasts for example. The problem is that these intermediate products are toxic and have the potential to cause precancerous changes, among other things. So, the lack of a vitamin or a mineral can have very serious consequences. The point needs to be made here that a serious result may have an apparently minor cause. One boy losing his balance on a trampoline may simply bounce on the sprung surface and think it's funny while another boy, falling on the same trampoline, might crack his neck against the steel rim and be paralyzed for life. Same cause different results.

Unfortunately, the orthodox doctor ignores this level of biochemistry completely. One way, potentially, of finding out what is needed is to undergo an applied kinesiological evaluation.

The applied kinesiologist also understands that each body is unique. For him it is not sufficient to say, for example, that magnesium is required. In my own case, further testing showed that the common supplement magnesium citrate would be of no value to me. For me, magnesium chloride and magnesium oxide were the preferred salts. For you, the answer would be different.

Depending on what the applied kinesiologist discovers, you might be directed to nutritional supplements or osteopathic manipulation or other forms of therapy. A list of trained applied kinesiologists can be found at www.icak.com.

EAV (electro-acupuncture according to Voll)

Hans Larson, editor of *International Health News*, puts the matter succinctly: 'Imagine if you could go to your doctor, sit for an hour in a comfortable chair where you are hooked up to some highly sophisticated electronic equipment, and then receive a detailed assessment of your health status. Sounds farfetched? Perhaps, but thousands of progressive practitioners around the world are already providing this service.'

The machine Larson describes is an EAV machine which measures the electrical impulses found in acupuncture points and other locations. It is able, very quickly, to tell the therapist about the patient's toxic metal loads, the health of the organs (particularly liver function), the presence of any inflammation, fungi, food intolerances, and mineral deficiencies.

It was developed initially in the 1950s by a German doctor Dr Reinhold Voll while studying the electrical properties of acupuncture points.

With this machine, the patient holds a brass bar and a probe is then placed on a suitable acupuncture point. A wide range of subtle frequencies are then fed into the patient's body and the body's responses to these are noted by the computer that is hooked up to the machine. The result is a global health analysis in well under an hour.

What this means is that the complex of energy patterns in the body reveals the health or otherwise of every component and process in the body. The EAV machine measures these energy patterns.

But EAV is not just an assessment tool for diagnosis. Actually diagnosis is not the right word for what it does. EAV cannot tell you that you have cancer or diabetes or TB. What it can tell you is the specific problems facing specific parts of the body. Together all the information might add up to a probability of a particular disease, but the EAV practitioner cannot definitively draw that conclusion.

EAV is also a means of providing treatment. If a disharmony is detected, the practitioner can reverse the procedure, using the EAV machine to create homeopathic-strength vibrational remedies which will help to reverse the energetic imbalance and so correct the original health problem. This is, in fact, a form of energy medicine and not a form of chemical medicine. The results are at levels of sensitivity far exceeding what is possible in any other way. Because of this, the results cannot be checked to assess whether the results are true or false. Using the modality therefore becomes an act of faith. Both applied kinesiology and EAV are challenging modalities—challenging to our sense of the world. However, the proof of the pudding is whether or not they work—and, in the absence of clear proof or disproof, each person needs to decide that for him- or herself.

Live blood and dried blood analysis

These are two techniques for looking at the blood using different types of high-resolution microscope. Dried blood analysis uses a light field microscope while live blood analysis uses what is called a dark field microscope. In both cases, using only a small amount of blood—a single drop of live blood from the patient's finger—the therapist can see the vital components of the cell clearly. These can be viewed on a video monitor. The blood analysis provides information about the condition of the red cell membranes, the activity levels of white blood cells and the quantity and quality of various blood plasma elements.

Both tests allow even very early signs of ill health to be picked up. It is possible to see free radical damage, vitamin deficiencies, hormonal imbalances, digestive problems, the degree of toxicity, pH and mineral imbalances, as well as the extent of parasite, fungus and yeast infestation. These provide information relevant to immune system function and nutritional status.

These blood tests are good basic screening tools that provide information that can help the therapist target more specific tests. When abnormalities or deficiencies are detected in the blood the therapist will seek to provide treatments, the aim of which will be to bring the blood quality back to that associated with normal good health. While a live blood test cannot make a definitive diagnosis of cancer, it provides important information about the basic biological terrain of the patient's body, and is therefore a useful and relatively cheap clinical tool.

Hair analysis

Hair is a highly metabolically active tissue and an analysis of hair will normally reveal significant details concerning the nutritional and endocrine status of a patient well before these abnormalities will be found using standard blood tests. It will often also disclose information that cannot be easily determined from more conventional diagnostic tests.

Hair analysis simply involves cutting off some hair—a small clump is required—from the scalp, and sending it to a laboratory where it will be tested for mineral and toxic metal content.

This is an analytical tool that tends to be frowned on by doctors but is used by forensic scientists as a matter of course. American law enforcement agencies have used hair analyses for decades, considering them conclusive as evidence in crime investigations and for drug testing. Death by poisoning can be determined conclusively only by means of a hair analysis. A three-inch strand of hair will contain a record of chemical exposure over the previous six months (hair grows at an average rate of half an inch a month).

The purpose of a hair analysis is to determine whether metal and mineral contents indicate an overload which may impact on our health. Once identified, detoxification can be done through herb and vitamin supplementation or dietary changes.

Saliva and urine hormone analysis

For many health investigations, it is necessary to determine the levels of a range of hormones in the body, and their ratios. Normally, in mainstream clinical settings, this is done using blood tests, but in fact the hormone fractions (unbound fractions) present in saliva and urine provide a better picture of what is happening hormonally in the body than those found in blood (bound fractions). Saliva and urine tests can therefore provide useful information about the biochemical functioning of the body.

The Navarro urine test

The Navarro test looks at the amount of the hormone, hCG (human chorionic gonadotrophin), there is in your urine. The higher the Navarro score, the more likely it is that you have cancer.

People use this test for two purposes. The first is to see if there is any sign of cancer. The test is so sensitive that it can, they claim, detect cancers up to two years before they become visible by other diagnostic means.

The second reason people use this test is to determine if their alternative anti-cancer therapy is working. For this purpose, people have a series of tests every one or two months—a six week interval is common—and check to see if the Navarro scores are heading in the right direction. If the scores are dropping, then it indicates that the regime is being successful.

The Navarro test is administered by the Navarro clinic in the Philippines. For full details of how to operate the test go to their website at www.navarromedicalclinic.com/index.php

The test costs $55 a time.

Note that pregnancy also raises HCG in the urine so you should not do this test if you are pregnant.

Dr Emil K Schandl's cancer profile tests

Dr Emil K Schandl is a clinical biochemist and oncobiologist based in Hollywood, Florida. He has developed a series of seven blood tests which he calls the Cancer Profile. He claims they can detect with remarkable accuracy the earliest presence of cancer of any test—as much as ten or twelve years before they are detectable by other means. Among the tests is an HCG test. The panel of blood tests is said to have about a 93 per cent accuracy in stating whether a person has cancer or not.

The CA Profile is not site- or organ- specific, however, it will detect metabolic changes leading to or indicating cancer. hCG hormone, PHI enzyme, GGTP enzyme, CEA, TSH, and DHEA-S are the components. The actual, supersensitive cancer markers are hCG (sensitivity 0.3mIU/ml), PHI and CEA. The other three are peripherally related to malignancies: GGTP monitors the liver and biliary systems, TSH measures low or high thyroid activity, DHEA-S is the adrenal 'anti-stress, pro-immunity, longevity' hormone. Low thyroid and/or adrenal activity is a predisposing factor in cancer. The PHI enzyme regulates the anaerobic metabolism associated with cancer cells (normal cells are aerobic in their metabolism, but it is also the *autocrine motility factor,* the factor that aids the spread of malignant metastases.

While each of the blood tests has varying levels of predictive accuracy, the cumulative accuracy claimed is very high. According to Schandl's website: 'The CA Profile was positive in 92 per cent of established breast cancer patients, 97 per cent of lung cancer patients, and 93 per cent of colon cancer patients. Statistical studies done on 571 patients with cancers of all sites resulted in 89.8 per cent positives. Our current statistics indicate that 68 per cent of 'healthy' American women and 56 per cent of 'healthy' American men present with elevated tumour markers. They may be in the process of developing cancer. Note, it may take 10–12 years to diagnose.'

It costs about $300 to get all seven tests. For further information contact American Metabolic Testing Laboratories—http://caprofile.net.

A standard pregnancy test

Both pregnancy and cancer increase the levels of the hormone, human chorionic gonadotrophin (hCG). If you know you're not pregnant and the pregnancy test tells you that you are, then you have problems. This is a cheap way of assessing yourself—though you may, if you're a man, get funny looks from the pharmacist.

Ian Clements' overall health status tests

Ian Clements is a cancer survivor whose story appears in Section 8: *Cancer Survivors' Stories.* He has a very deep understanding of the situation facing someone who is battling cancer—and its potential to return. He makes a point of testing himself regularly to see how his cancer markers are doing—but crucially, he also tests his overall health status too. He has devised a shorthand assessment and feels that if the results of three specific tests are good then so is his overall health. The three tests are as follows:

'I assess my wellness by measuring my levels of vitamin D3, homocysteine, and Essential Fatty Acids (EFAs). These are simple tests that your doctor should be prepared to arrange. Vitamin D3 levels should be high (not just normal)—above 200mmol/l; Homocysteine levels should be low, and as for the essential fatty acids I am aiming for an AA/EPA ratio of 1.5.'

Rather than repeat the further explanation of these tests, which Ian explains in his story, I will simply direct you to his story on page 499.

Surgery

Historical background

To put cancer surgery into some kind of perspective, it is worth looking at its history. Surgery was known to the ancients but was expressly condemned in the case of cancer. Hippocrates' famous comment was: 'It is better not to apply any treatment in cases of occult [i.e., hidden] cancer; for, if treated, the patients die quickly; but if not treated, they hold out for a long time.' This is a conclusion supported by some contemporary medical statisticians. One researcher, Dr Hardin Jones, professor of Medical Physics, calculated that cancer patients are on balance likely to live four times longer if they do nothing for their cancer than if they do something. This conclusion has never been decisively challenged in the four decades since he made this claim.

In Europe, medical practitioners between the twelfth and nineteenth centuries repudiated the use of any kind of surgery, leaving it to barbers to perform. Without asepsis or anaesthetics, it was cruel and generally unsuccessful. The great doctor Paracelsus (1493–1541) said, 'It should be forbidden and severely punished to remove cancer by cutting, burning, cautery and other fiendish tortures. It is from nature that the disease arises and from nature comes the cure.'

So doctors six hundred years ago were able to talk of curing cancer. It was also their combined experience of the disease that surgery was the wrong approach. Now it is considered the standard approach—and natural cures are considered beyond the pale. Clearly something has happened to medical thinking on the way.

It was only with the discovery of asepsis and anaesthetics that surgery, against much opposition, became accepted. It became accepted as a necessity during the Napoleonic wars—because men needed treatment for their battle wounds. Since then, surgical procedures and technology have improved by leaps and bounds. There is no doubt that for cases of severe physical trauma—resulting from war, traffic accident, or any other cause—surgery is essential if many victims are to survive. But cancer is not a severe physical trauma that needs to be corrected. It matters not what great advances have been made in the area of surgery; the question of its appropriateness in the case of cancer remains contentious, and no amount of technological improvement can change that, because the problem relates almost entirely to the nature of cancer rather than to the nature of surgery.

The dangers of surgery

The simple fact is that surgery is dangerous and results in deaths. What is the combined death rate from all forms of surgery? Recent investigations in Britain suggest that the average surgeon has a patient mortality rate of between two and seven per cent. This is measurably greater among those who have had the least experience. It is therefore better to go to a big hospital than a small local one. It is better not to be in hospital when medical students graduate and relieve their more experienced superiors. A specialist is always better than a general surgeon. Make sure any doctor doing surgery on you is a specialist. Insist on it.

Then there is the simple fact that surgery requires hospitalization—and hospitals are very unhealthy places to be. Apart from very real problems of dying directly from negligent treatment, drug overdoses, and so on, there is the increasing danger of hospital-acquired infection or, as doctors call it, nosocomial infection.

One of the most serious forms of infections that arises from a stay in hospital is MRSA (methicillin-resistant Staphylococcus aureus), which is a bacterial infection resistant to the antibiotic methicillin. Staphylococcus aureus is a common bacterium found on the skin of healthy people. If 'staph' gets into the body, it can cause anything from a minor infection such as boils or pimples to more serious infections such as pneumonia or blood infections.

MRSA usually infects hospital patients who are elderly or very ill; specifically, you may be at more risk if you are a regular or long-term user of antibiotics or you are immunosuppressed. Cancer patients fall right into the heart of this most vulnerable sector.

Symptoms of infection can range from red and inflamed areas around wound sites, fever, lethargy, and headache. MRSA can also cause urinary tract infections, pneumonia, toxic shock syndrome, and even death.

Within hours of admission to hospital, colonies of hospital strains of bacteria develop in the patient's skin, respiratory tract, and genitor-urinary tract. These are caused by such actions as intubation, urine catheterization and so on or by the administration of drugs that lower the immune response. Also there are the risks posed by neighbouring patients, poor ventilation systems, contaminated water systems, and above all inadequate sterilization procedures in the operating theatre and surrounding environment. Ironically, intensive care units are the place you are most likely to be infected.

How frequent are nosocomial infections? Official figures estimate occurrence at 5 per cent of all acute care hospitalizations which in the USA alone, means more than 2 million cases per year, resulting, according to one calculation to added medical costs of over US$2 billion.

Mortality/morbidity: nosocomial infections are estimated to more than double the mortality and morbidity risks of any admitted patient. The official figures suggest that they cause about 20,000 deaths a year in the USA. It is also accepted that the real figure is very likely much higher, as the following statement which appeared in the *Journal of the American Medical Association* shows.

'Over a million patients are injured in US hospitals each year, and approximately 280,000 die annually as a result of these injuries. Therefore, the iatrogenic death rate dwarfs the annual automobile accident mortality rate of 45,000 and accounts for more deaths than all other accidents combined.' (*JAMA*. 1995 Jul 5, 274(1):29–34)

The word 'iatrogenic' means 'caused by doctors'. Deaths from nosocomial infections are always understated as this is rarely the reason given on death certificates, and only death certificate causes are counted for official purposes. If you have cancer but die of MRSA, the cause of death is still likely to appear as cancer.

Other common nosocomial infections are vancomycin-resistant enterococcus (VRE), pseudomonas, candidiasis, legionella, respiratory syncytial virus, thrush, Clostridium difficile and necrotising fasciitis, the increasingly common flesh-eating, bacteria which is associated directly with surgical procedures. If you want to scare yourself, do a Google search for 'nosocomial infection' on the Internet.

Since it is the most vulnerable who are most affected, it makes sense to take action to strengthen the immune system before going into hospital if that is unavoidable.

Some hospitals are recognizing the threat and are housing cancer patients in hotels where there is much less likelihood of infection.

'Localised' versus 'radical' surgery

Against this background we can now take a hard look at cancer surgery. Surgery can be categorized as localized surgery when it aims simply to remove the tumour and nothing else. It is called 'radical surgery' when parts of the affected or neighbouring organs or lymph glands are also removed.

Localized surgery

The argument for simple localized surgery to extract a tumour only—with only the minimum of surrounding tissue (e.g., a lumpectomy, in the case of breast cancer)—appears to make a degree of sense. As long as metastasis has not occurred, the tumour is small enough to be removed, and the tumour is accessible, the chances, most surgeons say, are reasonably good that surgery will, on its own, be quite sufficient.

'Early stage tumours (e.g., carcinomas in situ) that have not yet invaded surrounding normal tissue can be completely removed and are virtually 100 per cent curable.' (Cooper, *The Cancer Book*, 1993)

This is comforting, but unfortunately neglects an important point. Cancer tumours are highly individualistic. Just because a tumour is small does not mean it hasn't metastasized; just because it is big does not mean it is going to metastasize. And, in any case, most tumours are relatively far advanced by the time they are detected—even though they may appear small to the naked eye. So, it is not at all obvious before an operation which tumours are best treated by localized surgery and which are not.

Added to this is the question of surgical competence on the part of the surgeon. One American study suggests that even when a tumour appears to be singular and operable, in only 50 per cent of cases is the entire tumour removed. In half the cases some cancerous cells are left to rebuild the tumour. In other cases the cancer tumour may be inadvertently cut, releasing cancerous cells into the bloodstream. The result? A cancer that spreads much more quickly. When this happens—and it undoubtedly does happen—the result is that surgery not only does not cure, it hastens death—just as Hippocrates observed.

As we have already noted, this caution applies even to diagnostic, incisional biopsies. The more aggressive the malignancy, the more dangerous the procedure is, and the more it must be avoided. In cases of testicular cancer, one of the most aggressive of all cancers, biopsies absolutely must not be performed.

It has also recently become apparent that a primary tumour in one site, in addition to seeding metastases to other sites, has the ability to control these metastases in such a way as to prevent them from growing. It does this by secreting two substances, angiostatin and endostatin, that inhibit the development of a blood supply. Once the primary tumour is removed, the means of control is also removed, and the result is that each metastasis quickly blossoms into a full-grown tumour of its own. A patient who has had one tumour successfully removed is therefore quickly inundated with numerous other tumours. This is another argument against proceeding automatically with surgery.

Radical surgery

While some argument can be made in favour of localized surgery, the same cannot be said of radical surgery. Radical surgery is a desperate—and very likely vain—attempt to remove a cancer that has spread by cutting out all the tissue surrounding a tumour—or trying to locate and remove all the metastases of a tumour. With any major surgery of this kind the mortality risk must necessarily be greater. And for the patient the pain and suffering is greater—and for no good purpose. Patients may not only be seriously disfigured, lacking in basic bodily functions, and seriously weakened but, on top of that, they may have their remaining life-span reduced. The quality of that life will also be substantially impaired.

Dr Hardin Jones, professor of Medical Physics at the University of California, studied the effectiveness of standard cancer therapies. It was his opinion—based on statistical analysis—that there was no relationship between the intensity of treatment and survival rates. Radical surgery, in short, does not improve one's statistical chances of full recovery. He is on record as saying: 'radical surgery does more harm than good'.

To conclude: For most cancer patients, the stated need for radical surgery will be for the reason that the tumour is known to have metastasized—or is strongly assumed to have done so. Once a tumour has metastasized, there is no knowing where the secondary tumours will appear. The tissue closest to the tumour will not necessarily be the tissue first affected by a new metastasis. The cancer cells will have been borne by the bloodstream to areas of the body far from the original site. Breast tumour cells may grow in lung tissue or in the bone—nevertheless it remains a breast cancer cell identifiable as such under the microscope. Once a tumour is suspected of metastasizing, surgery ceases to be an option that makes very much sense: what is the surgeon going to cut out? When will the surgeon finish cutting?

Modern approaches to surgery

As with any skill dependent on technology, there will continually be developments. In surgery, the use of lasers, computer-controlled radiation surgery and tissue-freezing techniques are areas where a lot of new work is being done. Some of these techniques, such as the CyberKnife, are described later—and they certainly are a big step forward for the simple reason that they allow surgery to be done non-invasively and on an outpatient basis.

But, to repeat what I have said earlier, the problem is really not so much with the surgical procedures as with the nature of cancer. It therefore matters very little what the new developments are. These do not alter the basic question: is surgery the right thing to do?

The problem for the cancer patient is not just the problem of asking the right questions. There is the additional problem of who you ask—who you expect the answers to come from. A surgeon's job is to cut out cancer tumours. A cancer surgeon who believes that surgery is not an appropriate form of treatment would be arguing himself out of a job—and surgeons, like everyone else, have mortgages and children to put through school. Therefore, when we ask the surgeon: Is surgery the right thing to do? The surgeon, almost certainly, unless he considers you already too far gone, will say 'Yes, of course.' That's his job. What else can he say?

Mastectomy: a special case

The most common form of radical cancer surgery is mastectomy, the amputation of the breast. Any mastectomy could be termed 'radical surgery', as it involves removing tissue surrounding a tumour, but confusingly, there is a particular kind of procedure known as a 'radical mastectomy'.

Around the turn of the century, William Halsted of Johns Hopkins Hospital in Baltimore developed the radical mastectomy. His procedure involved removing the entire breast, removing the two underlying main chest wall muscles leading to the shoulder and removal of all the lymph nodes in the armpit. Ewan Cameron and Linus Pauling comment:

> *This was an extensive and very mutilating procedure, leaving the woman not only without a breast but also with a deep depression where the underlying muscles had been removed, an ugly scar, and almost always a permanent brawny swelling of the arm because of the surgical interference with the lymphatic drainage.'*

What Cameron and Pauling don't say is that this swelling—oedema—is extremely painful and debilitating in its own right. In fact, it is a potentially permanent effect of any surgery that involves removal of lymph nodes. It needs to be repeated that this is a very painful condition that cannot be corrected.

After the Second World War, Scottish surgeons started to do a simplified mastectomy, removing the breast but not the underlying muscles or the lymphatic nodes. This was accompanied by radiation. The results appeared to be better than the Halsted procedure. In the 1950s, Finnish doctors developed the lumpectomy—and claimed even better results than with the mastectomy. This seems to have been supported by later studies.

Statisticians looking at the whole picture, comparing different cohorts of women with breast cancer choosing different treatments, have found that there is no difference at all in the death rate of women who have had mastectomies and women who have had no treatment at all. 'There is no evidence that mastectomy affects survival. If women knew that they would probably refuse surgery' (Dr L. Cunningham, *The Lancet*, 1980).

Despite this, until the 1970s or 80s, American surgeons still tended to do radical mastectomies, while European surgeons tended to do 'simple' mastectomies or lumpectomies. The reason for American surgeons' preference for the radical mastectomy appears to be a combination of income—they earned more for doing more—and fear of litigation; you can't be sued for doing the maximum possible.

The current trend even in America is away from the Halsted procedure to lumpectomies or 'resections'—the cutting away of part of the breast. However, the Halsted procedure—or a modified, less-disfiguring version—may still be advised where there is significant spread. In such a case the patient might prefer not to undergo any surgery whatever, as there is no proof that extensive surgery in breast cancer has any impact on survival.

Amazingly, of those women who survive long-term after a mastectomy, 5–10 per cent will later find a cancerous nodule on the mastectomy scar.

Despite this, in America, large numbers of mastectomies are performed as a preventative measure. Many women volunteer to have their breasts removed in order to avoid breast cancer. Figures from one New York hospital showed that such so-called 'prophylactic mastectomies' accounted for 20 per cent of the total!

Ewan Cameron and Linus Pauling, who were by no means opposed to surgery as a first line of attack against cancer, had this to say: 'The observations from Halsted on seem to be showing that the less that is done for breast cancer patients, the better their chances of survival. The damage done to the body by surgical or radiotherapeutic intervention may be greater than the benefit resulting from partial control of the disease. This trend has led many thoughtful surgeons to question seriously whether they should treat breast cancer patients at all—whether these patients might not better be left alone. The question is a serious one, demanding an answer.' (Cameron and Pauling, *Cancer & Vitamin C*, 1979).

The conclusions we draw from the case of mastectomy will almost certainly be valid for any other surgery that may be proposed. While there may or may not be some argument for limited localized surgery, there is very little if any support at all for radical surgery.

Not all doctors approve of surgery

Medicine is an arena of contending ideologies. One of these ideologies is the surgeon's creed that the best thing to do with a tumour is to cut it out. This belief has become so dominant that it is now almost unquestioned within the temples of modern medicine, but there have been many doctors along the way who have disagreed.

A hundred years ago, homeopathic doctor Compton Burnett, a scathing critic of surgery for cancer, remarked: 'Surgeons may think the cutting out and cutting off processes "curing"; I think them a last refuge of helplessness.'

He was not alone. Dr Robert Bell, a senior staff member of the Glasgow Hospital for Women, agreed. In 1906, he wrote the following:

'I had been taught that this (surgery) was the only method by which malignant disease could be successfully treated, and, at the time, believed this to be true. But failure after failure following each other, without a single break, inclined me to alter my opinion. The disease invariably recurred with renewed virulence, suffering was intensified, and the life of the patient shortened.' He went on to say: 'That cancer is a curable disease … if rational dietetic and therapeutic measures are adopted and rigidly adhered to, there can be no doubt whatever.'

It is not just doctors of a century ago who criticise surgery. Professor Michael Baum, a leading and very orthodox cancer specialist, published a report (*European Journal of Cancer*, March 2005) in which he argued that surgery—whether to take out a lump or remove a breast—could enable breast cancer to spread more quickly, especially in young patients whose cancer isn't advanced.

Baum's argument is that the body's response to surgery creates circumstances that help to stimulate the growth of tumours. For example, surgery creates a wound. The wound healing process requires angiogenesis, the formation of new blood vessels, and these help to feed the tumours. Surgery also stimulates the production of growth factors as part of the postoperative wound healing process which in turn can promote tumour growth. 'A likely trigger for "kick-starting" the growth of micro-metastases could be the act of surgery itself,' he wrote.

Another way in which primary cancer tumours control metastasis is by releasing an angiogenesis inhibitor, angiostatin. When you remove the primary tumour—or irradiate it—the result is to stimulate the growth of metastases.

In short, surgery should not be an automatic knee-jerk response to cancer. Sadly, the desire to 'get rid of the damn thing' will in many cases propel patients unhesitatingly and unswervingly towards surgery. There is also the desire to eliminate this deadly 'poison' from the body. I would urge anyone contemplating surgery to re-read this section and meditate on the potential consequences of this act.

How far do you want to go? putting limits on surgery

However, in a particular circumstance there may be very good reasons why cancer surgery is an attractive, or at least the preferred, option. Whether or not any major organ is removed is a matter for patients, not the doctors, to decide—although they will try to convince you otherwise. Every patient has the right to say that a procedure may or may not be done on his or her body. This decision should be made in writing, and if possible it should be witnessed.

Patients undergoing any form of surgery should therefore be very clear in their own minds as to how far they are willing to go. If a woman with suspected breast cancer, for example, is willing to have a lumpectomy but not a radical mastectomy, it is for that woman to write this down on the permission form before she signs it. Unfortunately, the legal protections for patients are not as strong as they should be. Doctors are allowed a great deal of leeway as to what they can do in the operating theatre, so it is best to get legal advice.

Surviving surgery

The first step to ensure you survive an operation is to go into the operation with the most positive of thoughts. In your case, everything is going to work out fine. Positive thinking works. It helps to boost the immune system. Spend as much time as you can watching funny films and laughing your head off.

Another effective action is to take very large doses of vitamins C, and E starting a week or two before the operation and continuing for a month or so after. Similarly, acidophilus and other friendly bacteria should be taken in capsule form. Large doses of magnesium (1g/day) are also highly recommended. Afterwards, you should also smear undiluted lavender essential oil on all the scars to aid healing. Lavender oil is a marvellous healing agent. The enzyme serrapeptase should also be taken after the operation, as it is a powerful anti-inflammatory and pain reliever.

Another precaution that you can take, especially if surgery is not scheduled for a number of weeks, is to build up a supply of your own blood to be used if necessary. This is to prevent the admittedly low possibility of catching hepatitis or HIV from infected blood. The estimated risk of HIV infection in the States is 1 in 225,000, while the risk of hepatitis is 1 in 6,000. Blood transfusion from other donors can also cause problems when there is a reaction to the foreign blood platelets and/or white blood cells—these may cause hives or fevers. The risk of one or other of these is apparently in the region of 1 in 15–20.

Finally, many testimonials relating to the Quantronic Resonance System testify to its value in helping people recover from surgery (see Section 7: *Cancer: Energy, Mind and Emotions*).

Radiotherapy

X-rays were discovered in 1895 by Wilhelm Konrad Roentgen and nowadays are largely restricted within the public domain to medical use—either diagnostic or therapeutic.

Diagnostic radiation uses very low doses—but even these low doses have been associated with a number of dangers, the two key ones being its potential for causing cancer and the possibility that it might cause genetic damage that may not reveal itself for generations. Since diagnostic radiation is used in mammograms, women who have regular check-ups for breast cancer may actually be exposing themselves to a higher risk than those who choose not to have a check-up.

Therapeutic radiation uses high-energy ionizing radiation to attack and kill cancer cells. But even therapeutic X-rays have been implicated as a cause of cancer! Medical history contains many murky corners, and the following is a well-known case. In the 1940s and 50s it was common to irradiate the thyroid glands of children who were believed to have a particular thyroid condition. Many of these babies later developed cancer of the thyroid as adults. It was only when this connection was made that irradiation of children's thyroids was stopped. Subsequently it was discovered that the initial thyroid condition itself did not exist and had never existed—it had been a figment of the medical imagination. Bizarre but true!

Delivery of therapeutic radiation

Therapeutic radiation is given in the form of ionizing radiation. The process of ionization is very destructive to the DNA of all living tissue cells, but normal healthy cells are better able to repair the resulting DNA damage than are cancer cells. That is the theory. However, in practice many types of cancer cells are highly resistant to being destroyed by radiation. How they defend against the radiation is not yet known.

Radiation is normally given as external beam therapy in which a beam of high-energy rays is directed at the tumour. With the latest machines, the beam is rotated around the patient so that it irradiates the tumour from many different directions and so does not continuously pass through the same healthy tissues. Each patient undergoing radiation will have been individually assessed, and a total dose will be calculated. This total dose will then be divided into fractions, and each treatment will deliver one of these fractions until the total dose has been delivered. Once a tissue has been irradiated in this way it can never be radiated again.

Brachytherapy

In addition to external beam therapy, radiation can be delivered internally. The use of sealed radioactive sources in the form of rods or small wires that are surgically inserted into a tumour to produce a highly localized dose is called brachytherapy. For cancers of the uterus and cervix, a machine called the Selectron will be placed in the vagina. Another way of delivering radiation internally is to give it in a form that will be selectively taken up by the target tissue. For example, radioactive iodine may be swallowed to treat cancer of the thyroid.

Another form of brachytherapy is the GliaSite radiation therapy system which is a balloon catheter device for the delivery of radioactive liquid to the brain. The liquid is inserted into the surgical cavity after the tumour has been removed. This way, high doses of radiation can be delivered locally at the tumour site and its surroundings. Currently, Iotrex (iodine-125) is used as the liquid radiation source; however the company plans to market a proprietary isotope cesium-131 (Cs-131). With brain tumours, as one report states: 'Typically, surgeons remove most of the tumour followed by treatment of the surrounding areas with radiation therapy. However, brain tumours often recur shortly following the surgery.' Apparently there is some improvement in preventing recurrence of the tumour with this technique—but I would be very interested in figures for absolute benefits along with some understanding of the potential long-term side effects of introducing radioactive substances to the brain. To put this another way, how many of us would choose to live next to Fukushima or Chernobyl power stations. Anyone agreeing to undergo any form of brachytherapy must understand that any negative consequences can never be corrected.

The problem of locating the tumour

One of the problems faced by radiologists using older radiation machines is that of determining the exact spot where the tumour is. This has led to the development of a number of machines that combine a means of visualizing the exact location of the tumour. With three-dimensional conformal radiation therapy, the patient first undergoes a CT scan while lying in the treatment position. These scans are transferred to a computer, and the doctor can then plan a treatment that will allow the avoidance of organs that are more vulnerable to radiation damage—as the machine delivering the radiation rotates around the body. It is important to remember that these machines work with a virtual image of the tumour and surrounding tissues. If there is any change in real life this will not be taken into account. This issue has led to the development of a true image guided machine which has a CT scanner integrated with the treatment machine. This ability to correct for small movements means there are fewer set up errors—and consequently the likelihood of damage is decreased. Nevertheless, damage cannot be eliminated.

This is admitted by the UK's Health Protection Agency whose website says this: 'For a cure, sufficiently high doses must be delivered to kill all the living cells within the tumour and this will inevitably cause some damage to surrounding healthy tissues.'

The CyberKnife or Gamma Knife is a form of radiation technology that uses a beam of radiation to perform excisional surgery guided by a CT scanner.

Radiation therapy for cancer patients: the official version

The US National Cancer Institute publishes a booklet entitled *Radiation Therapy and You*, where we are assured that radiation is an effective means of treating cancer.

> *'High doses of radiation can kill cells or keep them from growing and dividing …. Although some normal cells are affected by radiation, most normal cells appear to recover more fully from the effects of radiation than do cancer cells. Doctors carefully limit the intensity of the treatments and the area being treated so that the cancer will be affected more than normal tissue.*

> *'Radiation therapy is an effective way to treat many kinds of cancer in almost any part of the body. Half of all people with cancer are treated with radiation, and the number of cancer patients who have been cured is rising every day. For many patients, radiation is the only kind of treatment needed. Thousands of people are free of cancer after having radiation treatments alone or in combination with surgery, chemotherapy or biological therapy.'*

On the question of risks, the brochure advises us that there are a number of side effects. But we are assured that 'Your doctor will not advise you to have any treatment unless the benefits—control of the disease and relief from symptoms—are greater than the known risks. Although it will be many years before scientists know all the possible risks of radiation therapy, they now know it can control cancer.'

The problem here is that the doctor assumes the terminal risk of malignant cancer is 100 per cent. Therefore any amount of radiation risk, by this standard, would be acceptable.

Also, we are informed that 'it will be many years before scientists know all the possible risks of radiation therapy.' Medical use of radiation therapy has been in existence for almost a century, yet the full extent of the risks is still not known. This is worrying. It suggests that no one has looked very carefully at the consequences of radiation. This does not sit well with orthodox medicine's claim to be 'scientific' or 'evidence-based'.

What about the side effects?

Side effects, the National Cancer Institute brochure goes on to inform us, may be negligible, or they may be serious—but does not go on to elucidate how serious. The British Medical Association *Complete Family Health Encyclopaedia* is also reassuring: '…normal cells suffer little or no long-term damage (from radiation). [However,] Radiotherapy may produce unpleasant side-effects, including fatigue, nausea and vomiting (for which anti-emetic drugs may be prescribed) and loss of hair from irradiated areas. Rarely there may be reddening and blistering of the skin.'

This is as much as the average cancer patient is told about radiation and its consequences. Certainly it is very reassuring—especially as the encyclopaedia goes on to say, 'Radiotherapy cures most cancers of the larynx or skin. The cure rate for other types of cancer varies depending on how early the treatment is begun, but the cure rate can be 80 per cent or higher.'

So what's the problem? Eighty per cent cure rate sounds good and a cure is worth a bit of pain. However, these contrasts with the 33 per cent or the 40 per cent or the 50 per cent that various other experts say are being cured. The cancers where radiation is supposed to be particularly successful are cancers of the cervix, testicles, prostate, lymphosarcoma and Hodgkin's disease.

Other views

Radiation is not without its detractors. Dr Hardin Jones, a medical statistician, makes caustic comments on radiation: 'Most of the time it makes not the slightest difference whether the machine is turned on or not.' Another biostatistician, Dr Irwin Bross, was quoted in 1979 as saying, 'For the situations in which most radiotherapy is given, the chances of curing the patient by radiotherapy are probably about as good as the chances of curing him by laetrile ... because the chances of curing any patient in advanced stages of cancer are very poor, regardless of the method employed.'

Hang on! On the one side, we have a claim of a very-high success rate, and on the other side we have a claim, made by people whose job it is to look at the actual numbers, that its success rate is close to zero. We need a third opinion.

Dr Lucien Israel is a highly regarded French oncologist. In his opinion, radiation should be used in the early stages of Hodgkin's disease (he quotes a five year survival of 80 per cent) but he is quite blunt in admitting that radiation is not a proven form of treatment: '... apart from Hodgkin's disease and lymphosarcoma, there is much disagreement as to its effectiveness—indeed there have been no conclusive trials—and many physicians prefer surgery, despite the mutilation it entails, because it has the advantage of making a clean sweep—total sterilization by radiation often remains problematical.'—note the comment about surgery causing mutilation!

This is a less than ringing endorsement. Neither does research support the view that radiation is successful in extending people's lives. This question was studied by The National Surgical Adjuvant Breast Project, who, in 1970, summarized their findings in these words: 'From the data available it would seem that the use of post-operative irradiation has provided no discernible advantage to patients so treated in terms of increasing the proportion who were free of disease for as long as five years' (Fisher B et al., 'Postoperative Radiotherapy in the Treatment of Breast Cancer; Results of the NSAPP Clinical Trial', *Annals of Surgery*, 172, No.4, Oct. 1970). Although this study was conducted over 40 years ago, there has been no major change in standard radiation therapy since that time and no change in cancer's response to radiation. The findings then remain valid today. It is unknown whether new radiation technologies would make a difference.

Dr Richard Evans of the Texas Cancer Center, a leading American cancer clinic—on his website at www.texascancercenter.com—says this of radiation in relation to breast cancer: 'Radiation can reduce local recurrence with some patients, but it does not increase survival.' And in the case of prostate cancer, he says: 'Physicians at Stanford (University Medical Center) no longer recommend radiation for patients with curable prostate cancer.' Clearly Dr Evans is not convinced of the value of radiation.

Let us restate the situation. Radiation has been around for a very long time. It has been used medically against cancer for well over half a century and it is still not able to present a clear case that it is of curative value. In some cases, it is true, lung cancer being one, radiation does appear to extend life expectancy by a short time but generally, even here, it is used not to cure but to shrink the tumours and so hopefully extend the life of the patient. Radiation is good at shrinking many different kinds of tumour. The problem, unfortunately, is that when these tumours grow again, they grow more quickly and are more malignant. In exchange for the pain of radiation, some cancer patients may gain a limited period of life. This may seem to some to be worthwhile.

Non-response to radiation

Not all cancers respond well to radiation. Many cancers indeed are highly resistant to radiation. Also, any cancer that has already metastasized cannot be successfully treated with radiation—because radiation focuses a beam of ionizing radiation at a single spot or area in the body. It is most successful when used to slow down or reduce the size of aggressive tumours—and then its success may be, as we have seen, very short term. Some tumours—of skin, tongue and lips—respond very slowly to radiation treatment, but in these cases the radiation often appears to have comparatively good long-term results—at the expense however of the salivary and other glands in the mouth and neck. 'Dry mouth' is an extremely unpleasant and permanent condition. The taste buds are also severely damaged so that food that was once enjoyed can become inedible. In other cases, a tumour may appear to melt away only to return with greater force.

Radio resistance, as this effect is called, is a major problem and it has led some doctors to consider giving radiation in small daily doses rather than at intervals of days or even weeks. In this way the cells are given less time to repair themselves. Early evidence suggests that anyone deciding to take radiation should have many sessions with small doses of radiation on a daily basis rather than fewer sessions of larger doses at longer intervals. However, pressure on radiotherapy services often makes this impossible. This is a case of health service administration procedures impeding possible beneficial medical practice.

It is possible to conclude the discussion so far by saying that radiation, as a curative approach to cancer, has not proven itself in any way, it has not even demonstrated much in the way of medium-term benefits for most cancers. As a short-term method for making tumours appear to go away it seems to be more successful—but at a potentially serious cost.

Dangers

However, we need to note that there are a number of very serious dangers associated with radiation.

Radiation can itself cause cancer

Diagnostic radiation is known to be associated with cancer: First, it is known that radiologists as a profession have a higher than average likelihood of getting cancer. Frequency of radiation also increases vulnerability to cancer. A large scale study of 700,000 children compared children of mothers who had received pelvic X-rays during pregnancy with the children of mothers who had not been X-rayed. Cancer mortality was 40 per cent higher among the children with X-rayed mothers (reference: figure quoted in *Death by Medicine*, Gary Null et al. 2003, www.garynull.com—MacMahon B, 'Prenatal X-ray Exposure and Childhood Cancer', *Journal of the National Cancer Institute* 28 [1962]: 1173).

Dr John Gofman, in his book *Preventing Breast Cancer* (CNR Books, USA, 1996) argues that X-rays are very likely responsible for over 50 per cent, and possibly even 75 per cent, of all breast cancer cases. Dr Gofman was Professor Emeritus of Molecular and Cell Biology at the University of California at Berkeley, so we should take his views seriously.

Radiation makes tumours more aggressive

One problem is that many cancers treated by radiotherapy, with apparent success, return—some more quickly than others, and when they do so they are unstoppably aggressive. American Senator Hubert Humphrey's bladder cancer returned three years after being irradiated. No further treatment was able to slow the progress of the disease. In my wife's case, her cervical tumour disappeared after combined radiation and chemotherapy. However, within three months of stopping chemotherapy, five months after completing the radiation treatment, a tumour five inches long was suddenly found to be wrapped around one of her ureters. She was given three months to live, and she in fact died almost exactly three months later. By that time the cancer had spread widely in the pelvic area.

This effect—of making a tumour more aggressive—should be kept firmly in mind by those patients for whom radiation therapy is advised.

Radiation makes tumours impervious to new treatment

Mice that have been irradiated do not respond at all to substances that have a beneficial effect on the cancers of non-irradiated mice. This is an important point to bear in mind for any patient interested in working with alternative approaches.

Radiation can cause severe injury

One of the worst consequences of radiation is the injury it can cause. Injury, unfortunately, is not a random, rare and unforeseeable consequence of radiation treatment. It is an inevitable consequence. The fundamental fact is that radiation damage to normal tissues is a necessary and inevitable part of radiotherapy and this is clearly understood by all radiotherapists, but by very few patients. The reasons for this is as follows. One of the problems with radiation, according to Dr Lucien Israel, is that each time a tumour is irradiated, 37 per cent of the tumour cells are not affected at all. The next time, 37 per cent of this 37 per cent is not affected—and so it goes on. Unless surrounding tissue is also attacked, it is impossible to eliminate all the malignant cells by radiation alone. From this we can see that radiotherapy can never succeed on its own if it is aimed only at the tumour.

If radiation is used to affect the surrounding tissue, then the likelihood of success increases dramatically. In fact, one can say that the success of radiation as a therapeutic tool rises in exact proportion to the amount of damage caused to surrounding tissues. Some damage will be discovered very quickly. Other damage may not appear for ten or twenty years—and may then not be attributed to the radiation treatment.

'Radiation can cause...loss of function of the irradiated tissues. The different organs vary in their vulnerability to this sort of complication. The liver, kidneys and lungs are particularly fragile; the muscles are also susceptible' (Israel, *Conquering Cancer*, 1976).

This damage may be very mild, or it may be permanently incapacitating or even life threatening. The fairly recent use of radiation and chemotherapy together has resulted in higher numbers of patients suffering from radiation-induced problems. Some doctors have established a grading for radiation damage:

Grade I: Minor symptoms that require no treatment.

Grade II: Minor symptoms that can be managed by simple outpatient methods.

Grade III: More severe symptoms. May have to be admitted for diagnostic procedures or minor surgery.

Grade IV: Prolonged hospitalization and major surgical intervention necessary.

Grade V: Fatal complications.

What this list tells us clearly is that some patients die from their radiation treatment and that for all patients suffering grade II, grade III and grade IV damage, pain—even extreme pain—and serious discomfort are the norm.

Radiation can cause problems five or ten years into the future

Radiation damages healthy tissue—but this damage may not show up for months or even years. There are cases of radiation recipients suffering haemorrhages as blood vessels rupture. It is also well established that radiation to the chest area—particularly on the left side—creates a high likelihood of heart disease. Heart attacks are two and a half times more likely in irradiated groups compared with the general population. The problem is that when these effects occur it is not immediately clear that they have been caused by radiation. However, long-term comparisons of radiated and non-radiated groups of patients have established a clear picture that there are significant long-term risks—so great that they cancel out any presumed immediate benefit.

But what exactly is the risk?

As we have seen, this is a difficult question to answer because there is so much variation in therapeutic procedure from one hospital to another. But doctors have begun to state a figure of five per cent. Five per cent of patients undergoing radiation suffer some kind of serious complication. But this figure does not appear to have any basis in fact. One critic, Vicky Parker, believes that it actually represents a theoretical level of morbidity that would be professionally and ethically acceptable. Medical textbooks say that a morbidity rate of ten per cent is 'ethically unacceptable'.

One group which strongly suspects that the figure of five per cent is a gross under-estimate is RAGE (Radiotherapy Action Group Exposure), a patients' rights group that, while it was active, advocated on behalf of people suffering from radiation damage and that organized mutual support groups in the UK for radiation-damaged patients (Sadly, the group is no longer active, as leading members have become too incapacitated to carry on their work). Their private estimate is that more than ten per cent of all people receiving radiotherapy are permanently damaged as a result. This figure will certainly be higher for women who have radiotherapy for cervical cancers, because of the number of organs so close together in the pelvic area that can also be irradiated. In their case, one would suspect a very high morbidity rate.

It is also becoming clear that some people are more sensitive to radiation than others. Different studies indicate that between ten per cent and 40 per cent of women may be highly sensitive to radiation—and so will react more seriously to 'normal' radiation doses. But the patient's own sensitivity to radiation is not taken into account when designing a course of radiotherapy treatment. The result of being overly sensitive to radiation is the increased likelihood of injury. Just how seriously debilitating some of these side effects and after effects are can be seen from the following examples. These are the words of one member of RAGE:

> 'I had my (internal radiation) in 1989. By 1992 I had lost my bladder, womb, ovaries and half my vagina. I had lost my career and my self-respect. I also almost lost my family, my mind and my sense of humour. "At least you don't have cancer", my urologist cheerfully informed me. No, I thought, I don't have a lot of things, like a sex life, or healthy kidneys. Is this the price for not having cancer? I wouldn't have minded so much but they insisted I didn't have cancer in the first place. Just a few suspicious cells which could turn cancerous if left untreated ….' (Kath Ridgard, quoted in the Rage National Newsletter, Summer 1994)

A very common effect of radiation is that it damages or kills the glands. This is a very important consequence for patients receiving radiation in the area of the neck or head, as the salivary glands will be destroyed. The consequence is a complete inability to produce saliva. Destruction of the neck glands and muscles also impacts on the ability to swallow. My brother-in-law lived with this condition for five years and it was distressing to watch him masticate his food. In the end he died because a lump of food went down the wrong way and blocked off his air passages. He choked to death.

In 1989, Ryan Werthwein, a ten-year-old American boy was diagnosed with a highly malignant brain tumour. He underwent radiation treatment, which proved to be ineffective. 'The radiation burnt out most of Ryan's pituitary gland, stunted his growth, and hurt his mental functioning, We were never told about radiation's possible long-term effects.' (Ryan's mother, Sharon Werthwein, quoted in Options, Richard Walters, 1993)

Radiation of any of the hollow organs: intestine, bladder, ureters, uterus, fallopian tubes and so on will have the inevitable effect of damaging the mucous membranes which secrete the moisturising substances that protect the inside surfaces of these organs. Note that this damage becomes far more certain when radiation is combined with chemotherapy, because chemotherapeutic agents are designed to attack cells that divide and multiply rapidly—such as the cells of the mucous membrane.

One form of damage is adhesion: where the sides of any tube stick together, another problem is that the cells lining the inside of the intestine can become fibrous, tough and rigid. When this happens in the intestine, blockage occurs, requiring urgent surgery to bypass the problem. The destruction of the organ linings is usually followed by erosion making perforations inevitable. This allows the contents of one organ to leak into another.

Damage to the lymph system is another common consequence of radiation. This results in extremely painful lymphatic swellings, called oedema—which vary in intensity and duration and which can be permanent.

Blood vessels are also vulnerable and haemorrhaging can also result—even as long as ten years or more later. Patients receiving radiation for brain tumours are therefore at risk of strokes.

Damage can also occur to the ureters, the tubes linking the kidneys and the bladder, so that they become blocked. Sometimes a straw like device, called a stent, is forced up to maintain the flow of urine. The problem is known as stenosis, or narrowing. Where stenting doesn't work, and where both ureters are affected, renal failure becomes a distinct possibility.

Radiation also can weaken tissues so that they fail at a later date. Intestines can rupture, for example:

> 'Eighteen months after the radiotherapy, I started having violent abdominal pains followed by vomiting …. Eventually … I was in absolute agony. The pain was indescribable. I began to vomit faecal matter and was rushed into hospital. On arrival the surgeon warned me that I needed life-saving surgery … when I came round from the anaesthetic the surgeon (informed) me that … the radiotherapy had burned my intestines resulting in the perforation, causing the bowel contents to leak into the peritoneal cavity resulting in peritonitis. The reason now, looking back, that I put up with the pain and vomiting … was because apart from being advised that there would be only some slight side effects during treatment, I was given no warning about long term side-effects …. Had I been forewarned it would have saved me a great deal of both physical and emotional trauma.'
>
> ('Mandy' quoted in the RAGE National newsletter, Summer 1994)

Mandy and Kath were victims of an iatrogenic episode resulting from experimental use of a new way of delivering radiation in a number of hospitals in Manchester, and elsewhere in England, using one or both of two new machines: the curiously named Hex 2 and the Selectron. (Iatrogenesis is the term applied to diseases or harmful consequences that are directly caused by doctors or by standard medical practice.)

The Selectron, which is still very much in use, is a way of giving radiation internally. In this particular case relatively high doses were given to the women. There was an economic basis for this decision. The bigger the dose, the fewer the number of sessions needed and so the greater the number of patients that can be treated within a given time span. Radiation machines are expensive. The budgets of radiotherapy units are huge. The problem with such high costs is that there will be continual pressures to find savings. The result was tragic: some 300 women were condemned to a life such as this:

'My life is totally controlled by my condition. I'll never have sex, never marry and have kids, never work again. I'm luckier than some though—some of the women are housebound or bedridden. I can go out when I feel better, though I have to carry morphine syrup with me everywhere …. The colostomy bag and my urostomy bag have burst when I've been out, so that's a constant worry, and I have to use incontinence pads all the time. I can't start the day until about 2pm and I tire very quickly. There's always something: vomiting, bleeding. I'm always back in hospital before my three-monthly appointment comes round …. I've been in the operating theatre over two dozen times. Doctors say "but at least you're still alive". But this is no life. It's a nightmare.'

(Vicky Parker, one of the founders of RAGE)

No official figures have emerged from this disastrous episode—funds are rarely provided to investigate possible iatrogenic episodes—but one unofficial estimate is that nearly sixty per cent of the women receiving this treatment up to 1982 subsequently suffered horrific damage to internal organs. Many are believed to have died. The hospitals in question have never offered apologies or explanations or in any other way accepted responsibility.

It is possible to argue that this is the sort of episode that one might expect from a monolithic state medical system, such as the NHS in Britain, and that it is most unlikely to occur in a freer, more competitive medical environment. However, even this episode would not have blipped on the radar if some very brave women had not organized themselves into an activist group. It is to honour the memory of these women that I dedicate this chapter. It may be that this was an exceptional episode, exceptional in the concentrated devastation that was caused. How common are such cases? Very likely they are not common at all. I certainly hope not. But I fear that they are more common than they should be. The truth is we shall never know.

Radiotherapy textbooks state very clearly that radiotherapy is an inexact science in which procedures are decided upon in an 'empirical manner' (i.e., if it works, it works, and if it doesn't, then tinker with it until it does work). There is very wide variance in practice between one centre and another. And it cannot be restated too often: fewer problems are associated with smaller fractions given frequently, than larger fractions given at longer intervals.

Women undergoing radiation for breast cancers are also at risk. Radiation can damage the brachial plexus, a nerve tissue in a sensitive area which can be heavily irradiated in an attempt to kill a breast tumour. More than 1,000 women are known by RAGE to have suffered injuries in the brachial plexus. Some have lost the use of a hand or an arm, some suffer intractable pain, and a few have even had to have their arms amputated. This problem affects approximately one per cent of all women irradiated for breast cancers—but this is only one of fifteen or more possible types of damage that can result from breast radiation.

Oedema (US: edema) of the lymph gland is another common result of radiation and the result is painful swollen limbs. This is an intractable problem that requires very careful management. Radiation of the neck, head or throat will almost certainly result in the destruction of all the salivary glands. The result is a very dry mouth and an inability to taste many foods. Very probably it will also result in the eventual loss of the teeth.

Finally, a number of less-well-known effects:

- If you have received radiation and you subsequently require surgery in that same area, complications are very likely to result as the body's healing powers will have been very negatively affected.
- Secondly, irradiation of the brain can lead to dementia or loss of the ability to maintain one's balance. The British politician, Mo Mowlam, died as a result of head injury caused by a fall. This happened eight years after receiving radiation treatment for a brain tumour which left her unable to control her balance.

If it's so dangerous why is it used?

One reason why such a dangerous form of treatment as radiotherapy is allowed to be used is that doctors assume that all cancers will inevitably lead to death. Professor Karol Sikora explains the general case thus: 'For some forms (of cancer), such as cervical cancer, it is the only hope of cure and without it thousands of women would have died.' But what this neglects to say is that cervical cancer is, generally speaking, a very slow growing cancer. Certainly women with this particular cancer in the early stages can afford to spend some time examining alternatives to radiation.

Another argument is economic. Large sums of money have been invested in some very expensive equipment, and in training people to use the equipment. How would the medical authorities justify a decision to stop using these machines? Unfortunately it is like a juggernaut. Once it has been set in motion, it becomes almost impossible to stop.

But perhaps I am wrong. Perhaps radiation makes sense as a key component in the war against cancer. That is for each reader to judge. I will leave the last word to John Cairns, a professor at Harvard University School of Public Health:

'The majority of cancers cannot be cured by radiation because the dose of X-rays required to kill all the cancer cells would also kill the patient.' (*Scientific American*, November 1985)

This contrasts markedly with the views of the US National Cancer Institute quoted at the beginning of this chapter: 'For many patients, radiation is the only kind of treatment needed.'

New developments

As with any other area of technology, there is a constant development of new machines that can do new procedures based on new assumptions. These are always tested empirically, that is to say they are tested out on patients—just as the Hex 2 and the Selectron were. It is a fair bet that almost every cancer patient that undergoes any form of treatment will, knowingly or otherwise, be part of an experimental study.

Having said all that, the move towards a reduced use of radiation has recently been reported: this is the use of a microbeam which fires a beam of helium ions just a thousandth of a millimetre wide, one at a time, at individual cancer cells. Apparently the cells that are killed send out 'suicide signals' which cause nearby cells to die as well. This is known as the 'bystander effect'. This is certainly a move in the right direction but there is, of course, no evidence as yet that it is effective, let alone safe. What will the side effects be? What damage might it cause? These are reasonable questions for each person discussing treatment options with an oncologist to ask.

Proton therapy

Another development is proton therapy. The use of a proton accelerator to direct a stream of protons at hard-to-get-at tumours appears to have long lasting impact with minimal side effects. It is particularly used against prostate cancer tumours.

The key difference between proton therapy and standard radiation therapy is that X-rays affect everything in their path right through the body along the line they travel. Protons can be so focused that they do not affect anything in front of the target and come to a stop just beyond the target. There are testimonials to the effect that even many years later virtually no negative side effects have been experienced.

Most centres offering this therapy are in the USA but this may change with time. For more information, go to www.prostateproton.com.

Neutron therapy

This makes use of heavier neutrons, rather than lighter protons, and appears to have better effects against larger solid tumours. It is used mainly for prostate and salivary gland tumours.

However, side effects can be more serious: 'Neutrons deposit greater amounts of energy in all tissues through which they pass—not just the tumour cells. Hence, they generally give rise to more severe side effects than conventional radiotherapy. There is a much more severe mucositis reaction (sore mouth and throat) that may make it difficult for the patient to swallow. While any form of radiotherapy to the head and neck can cause xerostomia (dryness of the mouth).' (www.rare-cancer.org)

Gamma Knife surgery: radiation used as a surgical tool

Developed in 1968 by Swedish professors Lars Leksell and Borge Larsson, the gamma knife is a highly advanced instrument used mainly to remove brain tumours. Without making any incision, it uses a concentrated radiation dose from Cobalt-60 sources. A total of 201 beams of radiation intersect to form a powerful tool focused on a targeted area of abnormal tissue within the brain. Clinics using this technology claim that the Gamma Knife is so precise that it damages and destroys the unhealthy tissue while sparing adjacent normal, healthy tissue. The success rate of the gamma knife, according to its advocates, is unprecedented. More than 41,000 patients have had Gamma Knife radio-surgery with no mortality and minimal morbidity reported.

The risk of surgical complications is greatly reduced because the procedure is performed without having to make an incision. Therefore, Gamma Knife radio-surgery is virtually painless. Patients routinely use only a local anaesthetic along with a mild sedative to help them lie still during the procedure. Patients can undergo the procedure and go home in the evening.

A variation of this technology is called the CyberKnife. This system uses a miniature radiation machine and a robotic arm that moves around the patient's head while delivering small doses of radiation from hundreds of directions. During treatment a computer analyzes hundreds of brain images and adjusts for slight movements by the patient. This makes it possible to deliver the treatment without using a frame to hold the patient's head still. Only the tumour receives the high doses of radiation and healthy tissue is spared.

Given the apparently clear benefits of this approach, it is odd that it isn't used more widely for all tumours.

Another form of remote surgery is high intensity focused ultrasound (HIFU). It has been used successfully in Japan for several years and is particularly used for the treatment of prostate cancer.

Total body irradiation

This is used only in relation to bone marrow transplantation. Some human studies were done to see if it had curative potential on patients with Ewing's sarcoma. The results were negative and this use has been discontinued 'outside of clinical trials' says one source. I do hope no-one reading this book will ever consider undergoing any form of clinical trial involving radiation procedures.

Postscript

As this book was going to press, the news of Kara Kennedy's death was announced. Kara Kennedy was the daughter of Senator Edward Kennedy. She died shortly after a workout at her gym: Here is the report as published in the *Daily Mail* (UK):

> 'On Tuesday, a cardiologist and Kara Kennedy's brother Patrick said her death may have been caused by an aggressive cancer treatment she received in 2002. Dr Sharonne N. Hayes, a cardiologist and founder of the Women's Heart Clinic at the Mayo Institute, told ABC: "Depending upon where the lung cancer was, her heart could have taken a direct hit." When she was diagnosed with the cancer, Mrs Kennedy was told it was inoperable but her father found a surgeon who was able to treat it by removing part of her right lung. She then received chemotherapy and radiation. Her brother, former Rhode Island Rep. Patrick Kennedy, 44, said the gruelling treatments had left his sister physically weakened. Dr Hayes told ABC that cancer patients who have aggressive chemotherapy and radiation, particularly in the chest, are at risk of heart problems . She said: "The heart muscle can be weakened. This is probably widely under-appreciated. People are so fearful of cancer, but in order to save people from cancer, other organs are put at risk—the heart, in particular."'

Chemotherapy

According to the National Cancer Institute, chemotherapy drugs can produce cures in about 15 per cent of cancer cases. According to less enthusiastic experts, the figure is really three per cent. In fact, it is hard to see where the 15 per cent figure can possibly come from, as only about five per cent of the various types of cancer respond to chemotherapy to the extent that it can be called curative. But in none of these cases is it 100 per cent effective. Against this, it has been estimated that 75 per cent of cancer patients are given chemotherapy. This is not a very good success rate, especially as we know which five per cent of cancer types respond well to chemo. Given the negative impacts of chemotherapy it is very possible to argue that chemotherapy kills more patients than it cures, and injures very many more.

What does chemotherapy involve?

Chemotherapy simply means that chemical substances are used to treat a medical problem. Taking aspirin for a headache is a relatively innocuous form of chemotherapy (though 750 people a year die in the US from aspirin abuse!). But, as applied to cancer treatments, chemotherapy involves the use of very powerful chemical substances.

Over 100 different drugs can be used either alone or in combination. These drugs are used because they are poisonous. They kill cells. They kill normal cells in the same way that they do cancer cells because, to this date, it has not been possible to develop a totally cancer-specific chemotherapeutic agent.

Chemotherapy drugs act generally by killing DNA or the DNA synthesizing process. Those that focus on the synthesizing process will attack all fast-dividing cells, including the cells that line the intestinal tract, blood-forming cells and hair cells. The result is that anyone taking one of these agents will suffer some degree of nausea, infection and hair loss. The resulting infections are themselves potentially life threatening. It is not uncommon for people undergoing chemotherapy to develop pneumonia, for example—some dying as a result. Liver and kidney damage along with bone marrow suppression are the most widespread damage from chemotherapy.

Different agents have different effects. For example, Adriamycin (doxorubicin) is very damaging to the heart—serious cardiac damage occurs in over 20 per cent of those taking it. This is one of a group of chemotherapy agents—the anthracyclines (epirubicin and idarubicin are others in this family of drugs)—that have been used almost as a default, against breast cancer in particular. Recent research shows that it has benefit (but 'benefit' does not mean anything as wonderful as cure. It could mean something as little as a month or two increase in life expectancy)—for only a small per centage of breast cancer patients (eight per cent is one quoted figure, two per cent is another). Its nickname in some quarters is 'red death'.

Another example: A small per centage of those taking interferon will suffer psychotic breakdowns. In addition to these side effects, some, if not the majority, of chemotherapeutic agents are themselves carcinogenic (i.e., they will cause cancer themselves in a number of cases).

If anyone should doubt the reality of the seriousness of the side effects, let them consider this. According to Dr Gerald Dermer, in some drug trials as many as 20 per cent of cancer patients died not from the disease but from the chemotherapy—which he referred to as 'toxic deaths'.

There appear to be a large number of deaths associated particularly with an intense form of therapy known as high-dose chemotherapy. Often the dose given is so lethal that it kills the bone marrow. This requires that patients undergo a further procedure known as autologous bone marrow transplantation, in which some of their bone marrow is taken out before the chemotherapy treatments and cultivated. At the end of the chemotherapy treatments this marrow is then transplanted back into the patient. This is an expensive, high tech but gruelling treatment which appears to have some short-term benefit in increasing disease free periods but long-term benefits in terms of substantially increased survival has not been clearly demonstrated for most cancers.

As with radiation, side effects are to be expected from chemotherapy, because damage to the body is inevitable. One study reported that between 1965 and 1969 the one-year survival rate for colon cancer was 68 per cent but that this fell to 65 per cent over the next two years, 1970–71, the reason being that it was now being treated more vigorously with chemotherapy.

The successes of chemotherapy

However, some cancers have shown a very positive response to chemotherapy. It has been shown to be very effective in the treatment of the following cancers: Burkitt's lymphoma, Hodgkin's disease, acute lymphocytic leukaemia, choriocarcinoma, embryonal testicular cancer, Ewing's sarcoma, lymphosarcoma, retinoblastoma, rhabdomyosarcoma, and Wilms' tumour. Unfortunately, together, these account for only about five per cent of all cancer cases. There also appears to be a small sub-group of breast cancer cases who might benefit. In his January 2007 newsletter, Ralph Moss says 'Current research indicates that the most commonly used breast cancer chemotherapy regimen almost certainly provides no benefit whatever to 92 per cent of patients. A test is now being developed to identify the eight per cent of women who have the greatest chance of benefiting from chemotherapy.' But even so the absolute benefit is not great (between seven and 11 per cent). Against this benefit has to be set the substantial risk of permanent damage caused by the chemotherapy drugs.

The cancers that respond best to chemo are penile and testicular cancer and the fast-growing lymphomas and the leukaemias. In the case of non-Hodgkin's lymphoma, low-grade (slow growing) tumours are incurable by any regime but medium- and high-grade tumours have a good response to chemotherapy, and cure rates are estimated at 50–80 per cent. The form of leukaemia affecting most children is the form that responds best to chemotherapy. When leukaemia affects adults, it tends to be a form that is less responsive—though a five-year survival rate of 50 per cent is still claimed.

Unfortunately, chemotherapy will almost certainly cause serious side effects to children. Toxicity effects have been described as 'horrendous'—in one study 61 per cent suffered seizures. Strokes and other 'acute mental status changes' are high-frequency effects. It also causes immune system collapse, and children often have to spend months at a time in germ-free zones.

Its long-term effects are also serious. According to the largest study ever done on cancer survivors who have entered adulthood, only about one in three remain healthy. 'Thirty years after their diagnosis, 40 per cent of survivors have a serious health problem, and a third have multiple problems, including stroke, heart disease and kidney failure. It is now clear that damage to the organ systems of children caused by chemotherapy and radiation therapy may not become clinically evident for many years,' said the research team, led by Kevin Oeffinger of the Memorial Sloan-Kettering Cancer Center in New York.

The survivors were 54 times more likely to have required a major joint replacement, 15 times more likely to have congestive heart failure or develop a second malignant tumour, ten times more likely to have heart disease, and nine times more likely to have suffered a stroke or kidney failure.

While it may appear that treating leukaemia with chemotherapy, horrible though it is, is the only way to deal with the problem, there are some who argue strongly that the fatal aspect of leukaemia is in fact a form of scurvy. This view is forcefully put by Dr Irwin Stone, a long-time vitamin C advocate, as follows:

> 'Leukemia is not a single disease but a combination of a neoplastic blood disease and severe biochemical scurvy. The scurvy can be relieved by massive daily dosing with ascorbic acid or sodium ascorbate. The secret is to employ 25 to 100 grams (25,000 to 100,000 milligrams) or more of ascorbate per day (spaced into four or five doses), given orally or intravenously or in a combination of both. Relief of the ascorbutic burden will give the patient a fighting chance for his body to battle with the neoplastic process. It may be found that without the severe biochemical scurvy, leukemia may be a relatively benign, non-fatal condition.' (www.whale.to/cancer/stone.html)

Finally, it is worth quoting a Reuter's report:

> 'Experts estimate that at least 25 per cent of chemotherapy patients are affected by symptoms of confusion, so-called "chemo brain", and a recent study by the University of Minnesota reported an 82 per cent rate, the statement said. "People with 'chemo brain' often can't focus, remember things or multi-task the way they did before chemotherapy."

> 'Prof. Silverman who led the study said: "Our study demonstrates for the first time that patients suffering from these cognitive symptoms have specific alterations in brain metabolism."' (CNN, Reuters, October 5, 2006)

To put it simply, chemotherapy has a life-long impact on your ability to think straight.

Chemotherapy: long-term effects

In addition to 'chemo brain', chemotherapy, even when successful, can have a number of serious long-term effects: heart damage being one—leaving you short of breath and in greater danger of a heart attack. This is a particular danger with Adriamycin and Herceptin. Some people find that they are left with permanent shakes or other signs of nerve damage: numbness or tingling or burning sensations—signs of what doctors call peripheral neuropathy. Osteoporosis is another long-term effect as is the possibility of damage to liver, kidneys, and bladder. Increased risk of a new cancer is also an issue.

The failure of chemotherapy

Even such a cancer research establishment figure as Harvard Medical School's Geoffrey Cooper has had to admit the poor prognosis for the chemotherapy treatment of most cancers: 'Unfortunately, curative chemotherapy for most common adult malignancies (e.g., breast, colon and lung carcinomas) remains elusive,' he says in his book (*The Cancer Book*, 1993). 'Chemotherapy of metastatic disease usually fails …. Advances in chemotherapy have led to successes against a few malignancies, but not against the majority of common cancers.'

One estimate is that 75 per cent of cancer patients are prescribed chemotherapy (a figure that needs to be put against the recognized benefit to only five per cent of all cancer patients—it is probably fair to say that more people are killed by chemotherapy than are cured by it). In many cases, doctors will point to its evident effects on chemical markers indicating the presence of cancer. But these effects are almost always too temporary. This must be a very frustrating experience for oncologists, but it is certainly no reason for them to persevere in this futile exercise—yet persevere they do.

The case of breast cancer

In the last decade, there has been an intensive focus on breast cancer and every week a new advance is announced in the press suggesting that some major improvement has been developed. It is very easy to find on the Internet websites that say things like 'Chemotherapy is effective against cancer cells because the drugs love to interfere with rapidly dividing cells' (www.breastcancer.org).

Uncritical statements of this sort are common on websites operated by cancer charities, cancer clinics and other sites wedded to the orthodox view. They give the patient who has been diagnosed with breast cancer an unrealistic view of the likelihood that chemotherapy will be effective in relation to their disease. However, this seductively rosy view is contradicted by other, less propagandistic sources:

> *'In women with metastatic breast cancer, chemotherapy is usually given with palliative rather than curative intent. Cure (meaning that the cancer goes away completely and never comes back) is an unlikely*

outcome for women with metastatic breast cancer …. Cure is possible, but uncommon in women with metastatic breast cancer …. Despite the disappointing cure rate, treatment most likely prolongs survival in women with metastatic breast cancer ….' (www.patients.uptodate.com)

This statement is very much at odds with other statements suggesting that, today, the woman diagnosed with breast cancer can expect to live another 20 years. Where does the truth lie? What does appear to be clear is that the form of chemotherapy known as high-dose chemotherapy is completely ineffective.

Two cancer researchers from Addenbrooke's Hospital, Cambridge, UK, Astrid Mayer and Helena Earl, published a paper in November 2000 (quoted in www.breast-cancer-research.com) in which they reported: 'Four trials of high-dose chemotherapy with stem cell support in breast cancer in the adjuvant and metastatic settings have shown no long-term disease-free or overall survival gain.'

Later in the same paper, these same researchers refer to: 'the resounding failure of conventional high-dose chemotherapy approaches in breast cancer.'

Certainly, the early approaches to chemotherapy in the case of breast cancer were not effective. As long ago as 1975, the British medical journal *The Lancet* reported on a study that compared the effect on cancer patients of chemotherapy versus no treatment at all. Those having no treatment at all had a better life expectancy and better quality of life.

So, has there been a chemotherapeutic revolution since then? The answer is no. As I write, a great deal of publicity has been given to a drug called Herceptin. Some cancer patients are reported as choosing to sell their houses to pay for this very expensive drug. The press is claiming that it improves survival by 50 per cent. Yet the truth is rather different. First, Herceptin is potentially of use to only the 20–30 per cent of breast cancer patients who have an aggressive form of the disease characterised by the overproduction of a protein called HER-2. In fact, Herceptin is an antibody to this protein and is used in addition to other chemotherapy regimes. According to the Genentech website, clinical trials demonstrated the following. With the addition of Herceptin to first-line chemotherapy, there was a significant improvement in median survival (the point at which half the group have died) to 25.1 months versus 20.3 months in the control group. The median time to disease progression was increased to 7.2 months in women treated with chemotherapy plus Herceptin, compared with 4.5 months in women treated with chemotherapy alone.

These results relate to women whose breast cancer has already metastasized and so does not apply to most breast cancer cases. But these figures clearly demonstrate the low expectations that anyone undergoing chemotherapy should have with regard to the effectiveness of the treatment.

A recent analysis of the benefits of chemotherapy was conducted by three senior Australian oncologists: Associate Professor Graeme Morgan, Professor Robyn Ward and Dr Michael Barton, was published in the journal *Clinical Oncology*. [Morgan G, Ward R, Barton M, 'The contribution of cytotoxic chemotherapy to 5-year survival in adult malignancies', *Clin. Oncol. (R. Coll. Radiol.)* 2004;16(8):549–60—This reference is for you to give to your doctor.]

They did a meta-analysis of *all* clinical trials of chemotherapy drugs for *all* the major cancers affecting adults that reported positive results for five-year survival conducted in Australia and the USA 1990–2004. Their conclusion was that chemotherapy for the major cancers—breast, lung, colon, rectum, etc.—was responsible for increased survival in 2.1 per cent of cases overall. For breast cancer, the figure was 1.5 per cent. Of all the cancers studied, only testicular cancer and Hodgkin's disease showed significant benefit from chemotherapy.

An Australian study into the use of chemotherapy in Australia in 1998 came up with the following data: Out of the total of 10,661 women who were newly-diagnosed with breast cancer, 4,638 women were considered eligible for chemotherapy. Of these 4,638 women, only 164 (3.5 per cent) actually gained some survival benefit from chemotherapy. As the authors point out, the use of newer chemotherapy regimens including the taxanes and anthracyclines for breast cancer may raise survival by an estimated additional one per cent—but this is achieved at the expense of an increased risk of cardiac toxicity and nerve damage.

But the general public is not told of any doubts about chemotherapy as a cancer treatment. On the contrary, they (we!) are fed an almost weekly diet of reports announcing the success of new treatments.

Ralph Moss has reported on this problem in his excellent newsletter, 'Cancer Decisions' (www.cancerdecisions.com):

> 'When physicians reporting the results of a major clinical trial announce a 23 per cent improvement in survival for lung cancer patients taking a new drug, it would be hard to see this as anything less than a breakthrough. But examine this claim a little more closely and you will discover that the 23 per cent improvement in survival actually translates into patients living for 12.5 months, rather than 10.2 months. Furthermore, a significant proportion—4.5 per cent—of patients receiving the new wonder drug can be expected to die as a direct result of the treatment itself, a mortality rate which, according to one of the lead researchers involved, is "well within accepted limits."'

So re-mortgaging your house to buy the latest wonder drug would not appear to be a very sensible decision.

The problem of 'chemo brain'

It is only fairly recently that this problem of chemo brain has become discussed. The following description is an edited down version from The American Cancer Society site:

> 'For years cancer survivors have worried about, joked about, and been frustrated with the mental cloudiness they sometimes notice before, during, and after chemotherapy. This mental fog is commonly called 'chemo brain.' Doctors have known for years that radiation treatment to the brain could cause problems with thinking and memory. Recently, they have found that chemo is linked to some of the same kinds of problems. Though the brain usually recovers over time, the sometimes vague yet distressing mental changes cancer patients notice are real, not imagined. They might last a short time, or they might go on for years. These changes can make people unable to go back to their school, work, or social activities, or make it so that it takes a lot of mental effort to do so. They affect everyday life for many people, and more research is needed to help prevent and cope with them.

'Here are just a few examples of what patients call chemo brain:

- forgetting things that they usually have no trouble recalling (memory lapses)
- trouble concentrating (they can't focus on what they're doing, have a short attention span, may "space out")
- trouble remembering details like names, dates, and sometimes larger events
- trouble multi-tasking, like answering the phone while cooking, without losing track of one task (they are less able to do more than one thing at a time)
- taking longer to finish things (disorganized, slower thinking and processing)
- trouble remembering common words (unable to find the right words to finish a sentence)

'Doctors and researchers call chemo brain "mild cognitive impairment". There is a wide range of estimates of how many people get chemo brain. One expert noted that, among people who get chemo, between 15 per cent and 70 per cent have brain symptoms.

'Imaging tests have shown that in some patients, the parts of the brain that deal with memory, planning, putting thoughts into action, monitoring thought processes and behaviour, and inhibition are smaller after chemotherapy.

'Pictures of the brain have shown lower resting brain activity of breast cancer survivors treated with chemo when compared with those who were not treated with chemo. These changes were still seen on scans of some women five to ten years after treatment stopped. And during memory testing, these women had to call on and use larger areas of their brains than women who had not gotten chemo.

'In people with brain problems, tests of memory usually show the person is slow to learn new things, and they take longer to recall what they know. Response or reaction times slow down; attention and concentration often suffer. Most often, tests find that the person with chemo brain has more trouble in using recalled information (executive function), and in using language. The causes of chemo brain are still being studied, and at this time there is no known way to prevent it.'

So why is chemotherapy still so commonly prescribed?

The simple fact is: chemotherapy is big business. The chemotherapy business is worth literally billions of dollars to the pharmaceutical companies.

Then there is the cancer research industry. The major proportion of the money donated to cancer research goes to the search for chemotherapeutic drugs. It's a lucrative business for the institutes engaged in cancer research.

It's also a lucrative business for private oncologists. There have been accusations that patients have been put on ineffective low doses for long periods of time just to ensure the patient keeps coming back. No one wants to kill the goose that lays the golden egg.

This may seem like a cheap and unsupported accusation against respectable, hard-working doctors. Yet doctors have not been shy in stating publicly that it is better for a patient to be kept uselessly on a regime of chemotherapy rather than allow them to explore the unorthodox avenues.

Dr Charles Moertel of the prestigious Mayo Clinic investigated the value of one of the most common of chemotherapy agents, 5-FU, in combination with other chemotherapy agents, and found that only about 15–20 per cent of patients with gastro-intestinal cancers had any form of response and that for most of them these responses were only partial and transient. 'There is no solid evidence that treatment with (5-FU and related compounds) contributes to the overall survival of patients with gastrointestinal cancer regardless of the stage of the disease at which they are applied.' (Moertel, 1978, quoted by Pauling 1986). Moertel also, according to Pauling, came to the same conclusion with regard to the effect of 5-FU in combination with other chemotherapeutic agents for a variety of cancers from the throat to the rectum.

It would seem to follow that 5-FU and related chemotherapeutic agents were contraindicated for these cancers. But Moertel goes on to say: 'By no means, however, should these conclusions imply that these efforts should be abandoned. Patients with advanced gastrointestinal cancer and their families have a compelling need for a basis of hope. If such hope is not offered, they will quickly seek it from the hands of quacks and charlatans.' (Moertel, 1978, quoted by Pauling 1986) He is here urging doctors to continue to offer expensive, debilitating and pointless chemotherapy treatment to stop them investigating the alternatives. You will have to make up your own mind how that makes you feel.

In 1994, *Everyone's Guide to Cancer Therapy*, the official version of orthodox cancer medicine as seen fit for the un-medically-qualified member of the general public, mentions the use of 5-FU with the following cancers: anal, bile duct, bladder, breast, cervical, colorectal, oesophageal, gall bladder, gastrointestinal tract, head and neck, liver, ovarian, pancreatic, penile, small intestine, stomach, uterine, vaginal, and vulvar. To be fair, it doesn't always recommend its use. For example, in the case of bile-duct cancer it says, 'Studies have not shown that chemotherapy can prolong survival, but the standard drugs used (mitomycin-C or 5-fluorouracil) may cause tumours to shrink and help about 25 per cent of patients … however, patients may not be better off after chemotherapy. The treatment has side effects and the tumour ultimately re-grows.' (Dollinger et al., 1994)

This means that, in the opinion of the best-informed doctors, a number of chemotherapy drugs, which are used sufficiently often so that they can be referred to as 'the standard drugs used', don't work. They certainly don't do what patients want them to do, which is to help them live significantly longer to justify the pain of undergoing the treatment.

The 2002 edition of the same book continues to refer to the use of 5-FU as an investigational drug in relation to colon cancer. The message seems to be: it hasn't worked so we must try harder to make it work.

It is extremely worrying that the medical profession seems so wedded to chemotherapy that they would rather use a useless chemotherapeutic than contemplate looking at alternative therapies.

How is it that this situation is allowed to continue? One reason is the baleful influence of the pharmaceutical companies who benefit from maintenance of the current situation. They are making huge profits, and it is reasonable to expect that they, like the tobacco industry, will do everything they can to defend themselves. They do this in a number of ways: combining political muscle with the power of the dollar. Politically, they have ensured that they are well represented on the executive committees of the National Cancer Institute (NCI) and the major cancer research centres in the USA—the Mayo Clinic and Sloan-Kettering, for example—as any analysis of membership of these committees will demonstrate. National cancer policy in the USA is largely in the hands of representatives of the drug industry. According to former NCI director, Samuel Broder, the NCI has become 'what amounts to a governmental pharmaceutical company'. Broder should know because, on leaving the National Cancer Institute in 1995, he went to work for IVAX Pharmaceuticals. In doing so he was following a well-worn track. This aspect of cancer, the politics and operations of the pharmaceutical industry and the major cancer charities, is further discussed in Section 3: *Cancer: Research and Politics*.

If you don't believe me then maybe you will believe Jerome Kassirer MD, former editor-in-chief of the *New England Journal of Medicine* (one of the biggies)—he wrote a book on the subject, *On The Take: How Medicine's Complicity With Big Business Can Endanger Your Health.*

Improved chemotherapy success rates?

Roaming the Internet, one comes across a myriad articles discussing chemotherapy and its success or otherwise in treating cancer. One that caught my eye suggested that chemotherapy success rates had been substantially boosted by some new approach. Naturally I read further, wondering what had had this boosting effect. It turned out that that the new technique involved giving chemo to fewer patients!

That's right.

In fact I could make a suggestion that would boost chemo's success rates exponentially from its current level of about 3–6 per cent to 50–60 per cent overnight. Just give chemo to say the 5–10 per cent of cancer patients who might possibly benefit. Simple. This is just another example of how scientists play with statistics.

But why doesn't chemotherapy work?

The main problem is resistance. Chemotherapy is often quite successful at first. After its use, the tumour shrinks and there is a decline in the chemical markers in the blood. These markers are indications of the cancers presence and degree of activity. But then, even though the drugs are still being given, there is a relapse and the cancer starts to grow again.

Resistance is not only very common; it is the normal result. This has led doctors to use two or more chemotherapy agents together in combination. The problem is that once resistance to one drug combination occurs, there is an increased likelihood that there will be resistance to other combinations.

The main problem is that most tumours contain a small per centage, approximately two per cent, of cells that are resistant to multiple drugs. These are known, naturally enough, as multiple drug-resistant (MDR) cells. Since a tumour mass is composed of both normal and cancerous cells, most of which are vulnerable to chemotherapy, the first result of chemotherapy is a very much reduced tumour. Chemotherapy therefore can be said to have put the tumour into remission. The response will be good. Everyone will be happy. But the problem is that the MDR cells will now start to replicate themselves and the tumour will regrow. This time, however, the tumour is composed entirely of MDR cells. It is both more aggressive, because of the higher concentration of cancer cells in the tumour, and totally resistant to chemotherapy.

So, in the majority of cases, the end result of using chemotherapeutic drugs is to make cancer cells more cancerous. This is recognized by the experts. In 1985 a prominent cancer researcher named Robert T Schimke publicly announced the problem in a lecture he gave at the National Institutes of Health. The problem, he explained, is that cancer cells resist chemotherapy and that resistance mimics the very processes of cancer itself. As a result, chemotherapy tends to make cancer worse.

Insulin potentiation therapy and low-dose chemotherapy

It may be that, despite the discussion above, some cancer patients may still feel it is worth exploring the chemotherapy route. If so, they should perhaps consider insulin potentiation therapy (IPT). In this therapy, a small dose of insulin is injected, causing a state of low-blood sugar, which leads to hypoglycaemic symptoms of light-headedness and weakness. At this stage, very-low doses of chemotherapy are administered. The cells, thinking they are going to get food, become more absorbent to the chemotherapy. In this way, low doses have an enhanced impact. In fact, they are capable of very substantially enhancing the effect of chemotherapy. This approach has been in use for over 75 years, and many patients claim to have been cured in this way, with no painful or harmful side effects whatsoever.

So, why isn't the IPT approach used all the time? Ask your oncologist.

For more information on Insulin Potentiation Therapy, go to www.iptq.com and www.getipt.com/location.htm.

Chemotherapy as 'palliative' treatment

To be fair to doctors, in the majority of cases, chemotherapy is not expected to be curative. It is recommended as a palliative treatment. Here is the World Health Organisation's definition of this term:

Palliative care is an approach that improves the quality of life of patients and their families facing the problem associated with life-threatening illness, through the prevention and relief of suffering by means of early identification and impeccable assessment and treatment of pain and other problems, physical, psychosocial and spiritual. Palliative care:

- provides relief from pain and other distressing symptoms
- affirms life and regards dying as a normal process
- intends neither to hasten or postpone death
- integrates the psychological and spiritual aspects of patient care
- offers a support system to help patients live as actively as possible until death
- offers a support system to help the family cope during the patients illness and in their own bereavement
- uses a team approach to address the needs of patients and their families, including bereavement counselling, if indicated
- will enhance quality of life, and may also positively influence the course of illness
- is applicable early in the course of illness, in conjunction with other therapies that are intended to prolong life, such as chemotherapy or radiation therapy, and includes those investigations needed to better understand and manage distressing clinical complications.'

When deciding to accept or reject chemotherapy—or indeed radiation—as a form of 'palliative care', each person has to decide whether the pain of the treatment is worth the benefits in terms of pain relief afterwards and or extended life span.

Chemotherapy as a 'last throw of the dice'

Chemotherapy does have one thing going for it, and it may be possible to harness this effect in an interesting way. Ian Clements, whose story I tell in Section 8: *Cancer Survivors' Stories,* owes his life in the first instance to a decision to undergo chemotherapy for his bladder cancer, despite three oncologists saying it would not be curative. A fourth oncologist gave it a five per cent chance of working and since Ian was in a hospice and expected to die within days, he decided to go for it. He said he was able to cope with the pain of the chemo because he was feeling so bad anyway. Nevertheless, it was not an easy decision and he was effectively bed-bound for six months after.

What is it that chemo does? It shrinks tumours. It's quite good at this. But there is a time limit and inevitably, in the majority of cases, the cancer comes screaming back more aggressively. But, if you put in place a rigorous complementary programme of diet and supplements then maybe there is hope. Ian is still alive today and, crossed fingers, cancer free. But to this day it is a battle that he never believes he has entirely won and he keeps a close eye on his health status. Do read his story.

A non-toxic non-conventional chemotherapy regime? Amyloxine

This is a non-toxic chemotherapy drug that is currently going through the drug trials hoopla. Originally developed for use with HIV patients, it was discovered to be extremely effective against arthritis and cancer (as well as chronic fatigue, multiple sclerosis and 'all forms of metabolic dysfunctions'). To quote from the information sheet of the clinic offering this treatment: 'Amyloxine was designed to control metastasis, penetrate tumour cells, and inactivate protoplasm that goes into the cells and feeds the tumour cells. When the nutritional protoplasm is eliminated the cancer cells starve to death …. Amyloxine was used in 212 breast cancer patients over a two-year period with a 92 per cent remission rate.' While this is impressive, it would be worth talking to them further about what that remission rate is now that they claim to have treated several thousand cancer patients.

Currently this treatment is only offered at one clinic, Life Force Hospitals, located in Nuevo Laredo, Mexico (just across the US border from Laredo). It is not cheap at US$12,000 to $18,000. For further information call 1-888-205-3262 or go to their website at www.lifeforcehospitals.com.

Looking at some web forums, I have found some positive views on Amyloxine. Here is one: 'I received Amyloxine in Dec.[2008] and I feel wonderful. Although I have melanoma I found out about Dr Truitt because of a woman with ovarian cancer who had received all that they could do for her at MD Anderson. She received Amyloxine and changed to a plant-based diet and is doing great six years. later. I myself and two others that I know personally have chosen Amyloxine and severe restriction of animal products in our diet and we are doing very well. Please don't be afraid of going to Mexico. There are sooo many success stories!'

And another testimonial: 'My dad was told there was nothing that could help him from US doctors so he went to Dr Truitt and had his treatment. US doctors are amazed at his results. He was diagnosed w/ stage IV prostate and stage IV bone cancer and now when he sees the US doctors they tell him his bones are in better shape now than when he was diagnosed.'

Conclusion

On examining this evidence, I can come to no other conclusion than that chemotherapy is a dangerous and desperate approach to the treatment of any cancer except for the treatment of a few cancers where its benefits have been well established.

Sadly, the oncologist, talking privately face to face with the patient, who recommends chemotherapy, as a wise precaution perhaps, will always carry a lot of weight. But do oncologists with cancer themselves opt for chemotherapy? No they don't.

In 1986, researchers at McGill University Medical Center in Montreal approached 118 doctors who routinely recommended patients for clinical trials involving chemotherapeutic agents and asked them to imagine that if they had cancer, which of six chemotherapy treatment plans they would choose for themselves. Only 79 replied and of these, 58 said they would choose none. The reasons they gave were the ineffectiveness of chemotherapy and the unacceptably high degree of toxicity.

Not all doctors have been silent

Here are some statements that some very knowledgeable scientists and doctors have made about chemotherapy.

'If I contracted cancer I would never go to a standard treatment centre. Cancer victims who live far from such centres have a chance.'—Professor George Mathé, French cancer specialist, 1989.

'Success of most chemotherapies is appalling …. There is no scientific evidence or its ability to extend in any appreciable way the lives of patients suffering from the most common organic cancer ….'—Dr Uhlrich Abel, Stuttgart, 1990. Dr Abel's conclusion was drawn at the end of the most comprehensive evaluation of chemotherapy ever undertaken by a single doctor.

'Aside from certain rare cancers, it is not possible to detect any sudden changes in the death rates for any of the major cancers that could be credited to chemotherapy. Whether any of the common cancers can be cured by chemotherapy has yet to be established.' John Cairns, professor of Microbiology at Harvard University, Scientific American, Nov. 1985

'Most cancer patients in this country die of chemotherapy. Chemotherapy does not eliminate breast, colon, or lung cancers. This fact has been documented for over a decade, yet doctors still use chemotherapy for these tumours,' Allen Levin, MD—The Healing of Cancer, 1990

'We have a multi-billion dollar industry that is killing people, right and left, just for financial gain. Their idea of research is to see whether two doses of this poison is better than three doses of that poison.' Glen Warner, MD, oncologist

'As a chemist trained to interpret data, it is incomprehensible to me that physicians can ignore the clear evidence that chemotherapy does much, much more harm than good.'—Alan Nixon, PhD, Past President, American Chemical Society

'I wouldn't have chemotherapy and radiation because I'm not interested in therapies that cripple the immune system, and, in my opinion, virtually ensure failure for the majority of cancer patients.'—Julian Whitaker, MD

'Patients who underwent chemo were 14 times more likely to develop leukemia and six times more likely to develop cancers of the bones, joints, and soft tissues than those patients who did not undergo chemotherapy' (NCI Journal 87:10).'—John Diamond MD

'My studies have proven conclusively that untreated cancer victims actually live up to four times longer than treated individuals. For a typical type of cancer, people who refused treatment lived for an average of twelve and a half years. Those who accepted surgery and other kinds of treatment lived an average of only three years'—Dr Hardin Jones, Dept. of Medical Physics, University of California, 1969

Final comment

I was once asked by a woman who was preparing for chemotherapy to comment on whether vitamin C supplements would interfere with the chemotherapy. I suggested to her that a better way of looking at the situation was to ask whether the chemotherapy would interfere with the vitamin C.

Childhood Cancers: Late Effects of Chemotherapy and Radiotherapy

The following is an edited summary of the information to be found at the American Cancer Society website (www.cancer.org).

Brain

Children who are most likely to have late effects in the brain are those with brain tumours or with acute lymphocytic leukaemia (ALL), but children with other cancers may be affected as well. Treatments that can affect the brain include surgery, radiation therapy, and chemotherapy.

The learning problems, often called *cognitive impairments*, usually show up within a few years of treatment. They may be seen as:

- lower IQ scores, which can vary depending on how intense the treatment is
- lower academic achievement test scores
- problems in memory and attention
- poor hand-eye coordination
- slowed development over time
- behaviour problems.

Non-verbal skills like maths are more likely to be affected than language skills like reading or spelling, but nearly any area of brain development can be affected.

Other late effects that may show up, depending on the type of treatment used, include things like seizures and headaches. Treatments that affect the brain can also lead to other effects in the body. For example, radiation therapy can also affect the pituitary gland, which is found at the base of the brain. Symptoms of pituitary problems can include fatigue, listlessness, poor appetite, cold intolerance, and constipation, which may point to low levels of certain hormones. Other problems can include delayed growth and/or sexual maturation, which are described below.

Eyesight

Cancer treatment can affect vision in a number of ways, and is more likely if the tumour was in or near the eye. Vision problems after treatment are most common with retinoblastomas, which are childhood cancers that start in the back of the eye. In many cases, the vision in the eye has already been destroyed by the tumour at the time of diagnosis. Surgery may be needed to remove the affected eye. If this is done, an artificial eye is inserted to take the place of the eyeball.

Radiation therapy to the eye can sometimes damage inner parts of the eye, which can lead to vision problems. Radiation in the area of the eye can also sometimes cause cataracts (clouding of the lens of the eye) over time. Radiation treatment to the bones near the eye may also slow bone growth, which can change the shape of the child's face as it grows.

Certain chemo drugs can be toxic to the eye and may lead to problems like blurred vision, double vision, and glaucoma. Many times, these effects go away over time.

Children who have had a stem cell transplant may be at higher risk for some eye problems if they develop chronic graft-versus-host-disease. This is a condition in which the new immune system attacks cells in the eye.

Other late effects on the eye may include:

- dry eye
- watery eye
- eye irritation (feels like something is in the eye)
- discoloured sclera (white part of the eye may be a different colour)
- poor vision
- light sensitivity
- poor night vision
- tumours on the eyelid
- drooping eyelid.

Hearing

Certain chemo drugs and antibiotics may cause hearing impairment (especially with high-pitched sounds). Radiation given to the brain or ear can also lead to hearing loss, as can surgery in these areas. This risk may be increased in children who are young at the time of treatment. Other late effects may include:

- ringing in the ears (tinnitus)
- trouble hearing words when background noise levels are high
- dizziness
- hard, crusty earwax.

Growth and development

Slowed growth during childhood cancer treatment is a common problem. A certain amount of catch-up growth may occur after treatment, but in some children, short stature (height) is permanent.

Many of the late effects on growth and development are linked to radiation therapy. Radiation has a direct effect on the growth of bones that are in the area that is being treated (see 'Muscle and bone', below).

Radiation (and sometimes surgery) in the head and neck area can also affect overall growth and development in the body. Treating this area can damage the pituitary gland, which is the main gland of the endocrine system.

The endocrine system is a group of glands that help regulate many important body functions, including growth, metabolism, puberty, and responses to stress. Endocrine glands include the pituitary, thyroid, adrenals, testicles (in boys), and ovaries (in girls). These glands work by releasing hormones into the bloodstream, which can then affect cells throughout the body. For example, the pituitary releases growth hormone, which stimulates body growth in children. Hormones from the ovaries and testicles affect sexual maturation and fertility.

The hormone changes that result from damage to endocrine glands such as the pituitary can slow the child's growth, and may affect bones, height, and full maturity. Again, very young children are most likely to be affected. The slowing of growth is usually seen within five years of treatment.

Treatment with growth hormone may reverse some of these effects if the pituitary gland is damaged. But growth hormone treatment has its own risks. The choice to use growth hormone replacement should be made with your child's doctor, and you should fully discuss its possible side effects.

Thyroid

The thyroid gland, found at the base of the neck, is an important part of the endocrine system. Hormones from the thyroid affect growth and development in children, as well as help regulate the body's metabolism.

Thyroid function may be affected by radiation therapy or surgery in the head and neck area, or by total body irradiation, which may be used as part of a stem cell transplant. Treatments may damage the thyroid directly, or they may damage the pituitary, which in turn affects thyroid function.

Low thyroid function (hypothyroidism) occurs when the thyroid no longer makes enough thyroid hormone. It can cause extreme tiredness, dry skin, unexplained weight gain, constipation, slowed bone growth, and thinning hair. Thyroid hormone replacement can be given in the form of daily pills, if needed.

An overactive thyroid (hyperthyroidism), is less likely, but it can happen. Signs of this include nervousness, weight loss, trouble sleeping, diarrhoea, and enlarged thyroid gland (goitre). If treatment is needed, radiation or surgery may be used to lower thyroid hormone levels.

Regular thyroid blood tests can help detect these problems early, often before symptoms appear. Testing may be needed for more than ten years after radiation treatment. In fact, thyroid problems have been found more than 20 years after treatment.

Muscle and bone

Radiation treatment can have serious effects on the proper growth of bone and muscle in young people. Very young children have a lot of growing to do, and radiation can slow the growth of any given area. Bones, soft tissue, muscle, and blood vessels are very sensitive to radiation during times of rapid growth. Young children and children going through a growth spurt at puberty are at great risk for late effects.

Along with stunted bone growth, other late effects related to bone and muscle can include:

- unequal growth of body parts (the treated side doesn't grow the same way as the untreated side)
- bone pain
- joint stiffness
- gait changes (changes in the way the child walks)
- weak bones that can break easily (osteoporosis)
- decreased calcium in the bones.

Surgery for some types of childhood cancers can have obvious effects on muscle and bone growth in certain parts of the body. This is most likely with cancers that start in bones (such as osteosarcomas or Ewing tumours) or muscles (such as rhabdomyosarcomas).

Some problems in bone growth can be due to damage to the endocrine system (see 'Growth and development', above).

Sexual development and fertility

Males

Both radiation therapy and chemo can reduce sperm production and may also affect sexual development. In general, the cells in the testicles that make sperm are more likely to be damaged by cancer treatments than are the cells that make hormones. The effects may be short-term or permanent, depending on the intensity of the treatment.

Sex hormone levels in the body are also influenced by the pituitary gland, so radiation therapy to the head area can affect these as well. Treatments that affect sperm production can alter the patient's ability to father children. For some, this may be only temporary, but for others it may be long lasting or even permanent. It is important to think about this before starting cancer treatment in the older child. For boys who have gone through puberty, sperm banking (collecting and freezing sperm samples) may be an option that can allow them to father children later in life. Infertility is less of a risk in young males who are treated before puberty.

The effects of treatments that alter testosterone levels can include failure to complete puberty, delayed or accelerated puberty, decreased sexual desire, and impotence (being unable to get and keep an erection).

Females

The ovaries can be affected by both chemotherapy and radiation therapy. The degree of problems mostly depends on the intensity of treatment and the girl's age and stage of puberty at the time of treatment. Girls who have not yet been through puberty are less affected. Radiation treatment to the abdomen or pelvis can directly damage the ovaries. Radiation to the head can also affect the pituitary gland, which in turn can interfere with the hormones needed for the ovaries to work as they should. In girls who are already menstruating, this can cause a stoppage of menstrual periods, which may be temporary or more long lasting. Girls who get treatments that affect the ovaries are at risk for early or delayed puberty and start of menstruation, irregular menstrual periods, early menopause, and reduced fertility, as well as other health problems. Doctors may recommend hormone replacement therapy to help with some of these issues if they remain after cancer treatment.

The uterus can be affected, too, especially if radiation is given to the abdomen. Late affects can include a uterus that is smaller than normal or which may not stretch as it should. This can increase the risk of miscarriage, low birth-weight babies, and premature birth.

Reproduction

Studies continue to look at the possible risk of congenital (present at birth) abnormalities in the children of cancer survivors. Most studies thus far have not shown a link, but treatments given today may use different drugs or doses not yet proven safe to future offspring.

Heart/cardiovascular system

Heart disease can be a serious late effect of certain cancer treatments. The actual damage to the heart may occur during treatment, but the effects may not show up until many years, or even decades later. A class of chemotherapy drugs called *anthracyclines*, which are used to treat many childhood cancers, can damage the heart muscle or affect its rhythm.

Radiation therapy to the chest or spine, or in the form of total body irradiation can also damage the heart muscle or cause problems with its rhythm. Radiation can also damage the heart valves or the blood vessels (coronary arteries) that supply the heart muscle with oxygen.

Most people who receive these treatments do *not* develop significant heart problems. This is especially true in children being treated today, as modern approaches have reduced treatment doses and lowered the risk. Problems are more likely in people who received more intensive treatment, but doctors can't always predict who will or won't have problems.

Lungs

Certain cancer treatments can affect the lungs.

Lung problems can occur in children who have had radiation therapy to the chest or total body irradiation. The risk of problems depends on the dose of radiation, the proportion of the lungs that is irradiated, and the age of the patient. The use of certain chemotherapy drugs at the time of radiation may also increase the risk. Possible late effects include:

- decreased lung volume (lungs can't hold as much air)
- shortness of breath, which may be worse with exercise
- chronic (ongoing) dry cough
- lung tissue that becomes scarred and thickened (called pulmonary fibrosis), which may limit the lungs' ability to expand
- inflamed lung tissue, which can cause trouble breathing (called pneumonitis)
- increased risk of lung infections
- increased risk for lung cancer later in life.

Certain chemo drugs, such as bleomycin, may also cause lung problems, especially fibrosis and pneumonitis. The risk of problems increases with higher drug doses.

Some people who receive these treatments may have no noticeable symptoms, but for others, problems may start as soon as within the first or second year after treatment.

Teeth

Chemotherapy or radiation therapy in an area that involves the teeth and jaw can lead to late effects, mostly in children who are treated before the age of five. But older children may have problems too. Late effects of these treatments can include:

- small teeth
- missing teeth or delayed tooth development
- tooth enamel is not normal (teeth may be discoloured or not have a normal shape)
- increased risk of cavities
- roots of teeth are shorter than they should be, which can lead to early loss of teeth.

Radiation in the area around the mouth can also affect the salivary glands, which can lead to decreased saliva and dry mouth. This can cause tooth decay and gum disease.

Second cancers

Childhood cancer survivors have a small increase in risk of developing a second cancer during their lifetime. As childhood cancer survivors live longer into adulthood, they are also at higher risk of developing other cancers usually seen in adults, such as prostate, breast, or colon cancer. As these children grow up and age, things like genetics, diet, activity level, overall health, body weight, exposure to viruses, and environmental exposures all play a part in their cancer risk.

That is the end of the American Cancer Society information. Not everyone is in agreement about the 'small increase in risk' of developing a new cancer. John Diamond MD (not to be confused with John Diamond the British journalist who died of cancer) writes:

'A study of over 10,000 patients shows clearly that chemo's supposedly strong track record with Hodgkin's disease (lymphoma) is actually a lie. Patients who underwent chemo were 14 times more likely to develop leukemia and six times more likely to develop cancers of the bones, joints, and soft tissues than those patients who did not undergo chemotherapy (NCI Journal 87:10).'

And in 1996 (March 21) the New England Journal of Medicine reported that children who are successfully treated for Hodgkin's disease are 18 times more likely later to develop secondary malignant tumours. Girls face a 35 per cent chance of developing breast cancer by the time they are 40—which is 75 times greater than the average. The risk of leukaemia increased markedly four years after the ending of successful treatment, and reached a plateau after 14 years, but the risk of developing solid tumours remained high and approached 30 per cent at 30 years.

Other Treatments

Laser therapy

This involves focusing a beam of high-intensity light at tumour cells. The use of laser is restricted at present to treating precancerous states and small tumours. It works by vaporizing tissue at very high temperatures. The result of laser treatment can be a hole or ulcer. The problem with laser treatment is that it can be used against only the portion of a tumour showing on the surface. But tumours are like icebergs. For cervical precancerous conditions it is claimed to be very effective—but the jury is still out as to whether or not it can be effective as more than palliative care.

In Germany, a technique called laser-induced interstitial thermo-therapy (LITT) has shown itself to be successful against liver metastases. In a study of 232 women with breast cancer who had a total of 578 liver metastases, six months after LITT treatment fewer than five per cent of them showed tumour progression, and no new tumours had developed.

Photodynamic therapy (PDT)

Can cancer be killed by a death ray? In his book *Light: Medicine of the Future*, Jacob Liberman reported that over 3,000 people with a variety of malignant tumours had been treated with a method known as photodynamic therapy, and that the results had been very exciting: 'Although they had been treated previously with surgery, chemotherapy, radiation, immunetherapy or a combination of these, their tumours responded positively to the light treatment 70 per cent or 80 per cent of the time, after only one treatment.'

This therapy is based on two facts. The first is that there is a family of substances known as porphyrins which, when injected into the body, are selectively taken up by cancer cells—but not by most normal cells. The interesting thing about porphyrins is that they are light sensitive to a high degree. They are not toxic in the dark but are highly toxic when exposed to light.

The second fact is that when the cancer cells have taken up the porphyrins they will fluoresce under ultraviolet light. This allows their position to be ascertained with a high degree of accuracy if they are not too deeply embedded in tissue.

Using these two facts, cancer patients are injected with porphyrins and then, once the sites of the cancer cells have been located, a red light, tuned to a wavelength of 630 nanometres, is delivered, using an argon pumped-dye laser, directly to the treatment site using a fibre-optic tube no thicker than a hair.

'Within hours of the light treatment, the cancer cells begin to die, leaving most normal tissues unharmed. Even in tissues that are just partially cancerous, only the cancerous portion of the tissue will die. Since specific photosensitive dyes are combined with highly tuned laser light, the treatment is extremely precise.' (Liberman, 1991)

One problem with this therapy is the fact that the liver, kidneys and spleen also retain porphyrins. For this reason a gap of 24 to72 hours between injecting the porphyrins and turning on the red light. This time lapse allows the normal tissues to clear out the porphyrins. The second problem is that patients undergoing this treatment suffer from increased skin sensitivity to sunlight, which may result in intense skin irritation for 4 to 6 weeks after.

A combination of photodynamic therapy and hypothermia is offered under the name LIESH therapy (light-induced enhanced selective hyperthermia) by Lase Medical Institute in Jacksonville, Arkansas. For further details go to www.lasemedinc.com. Using a non-drug method—they use nano-particles instead—they claim to be able to attack large tumours with '100 per cent effectiveness'. However, this therapy is most suitable for cancers on or near the surface of the skin.

For more information about Photodynamic Therapy go to www.killingcancer.co.uk. More and more people are urging the use of this approach as it is effective and does not damage the body.

Hyperthermia

This refers to the raising of the temperature of the body to about 108°F (42°C)—and sometimes higher—by various means. The whole body may be heated or localized heating can be achieved using microwaves. There is some disagreement as to its usefulness. At present, heating treatments are generally limited to one-hour sessions, but it appears that longer sessions have achieved some exciting results—the longer the better. This is, in fact, a therapy that has crossed the orthodox-alternative divide and is recommended by both. Since the high heat interferes with the cell's ability to repair itself after radiation treatments, it is now being used along with radiation, and it appears that immediate response rates nearly double as a result.

One study showed that radiation on its own had a 31–37 per cent response rate, while radiation with heat treatment had a response rate of 63–71per cent. Response rates, however, as we have seen, mean little on their own. Nevertheless, some studies claim long-term benefits. This suggests that, if radiation is to be chosen as the form of treatment, the best way of conducting it would be to have very small fractions of radiation every day with long-term hyperthermia treatment in between.

Hyperthermia may be used regionally, in a part of the body only, using microwaves, or may involve the whole body. In the case of liver cancer, this method is being used, apparently, with some success in those cases, the majority, where surgery cannot be undertaken because of the cancer's spread. The side effects of hyperthermia are minimal.

Radio-frequency ablation (Rfa)

This technique involves the use of a high-frequency electric current to heat tumours and kill them. It was at first used to provide palliative relief to terminal patients, particularly those with liver cancer. However, its effects were so positive that it is now being considered as a replacement of both surgery and radiation.

The Life Extension Foundation website (www.lef.org) describes the advantages of the therapy: 'Because of its therapeutic value and cost effectiveness, along with its non-invasive, low-risk profile, RFA has the attention of both physicians and patients. The National Institutes of Health consider RFA the most predictable, safest, and simplest method for thermal ablation in bone, liver, kidney, prostate, breast, and brain cancers.'

In this therapy an MRI scanner is used to pinpoint the location of the tumour and a titanium electrode is then inserted into it. The radio-frequencies transmitted through the electrode to the tumour can in a matter of 10–12 minutes kill a sphere of 1–2 inches. In the case of a large tumour the electrode is moved to a number of sites in the tumour until the whole tumour is killed. Radio frequency thermal ablation is another way of inducing highly localized increases in temperature. For more information about radio frequency thermal ablation, visit www.cancerablation.com.

Hormones

Hormone treatment is often recommended with breast and prostate cancers.

Hormones for breast cancer

Hormone therapy is designed to inhibit oestrogen and progesterone which, in some cases of breast cancer, are having the effect of promoting cancer cell growth. In some cases, doctors will prescribe drugs to turn off the production of hormones from the ovaries—alternatively they will recommend the surgical removal of the ovaries to achieve the same result. If diagnosis shows that the cancer cells have oestrogen or progesterone receptors, it means that growth of the cancer tumour will be stimulated by these hormones. If a cancer is found to have these receptors, hormone therapy is recommended as part of the treatment plan.

Unfortunately, although the theory may be sound, the practice is less than perfect. Tamoxifen is the best known hormone treatment for breast cancer. Sherrill Sellman, a health writer, has investigated the subject intensively, and I recommend that you read her article in full. It can be read at www.all-natural.com/tamox.html. She concludes that Tamoxifen has shown a very marginal benefit—but only for post-menopausal women—but that it comes with such serious side effects (risk of blood clots, endometrial cancer, uterine sarcoma and fibroids) that it should almost certainly be avoided. More recently two similar drugs appear to have better results with reduced negative impacts: raloxifene and anastrozole (Arimidex). However, the list of side effects for these two drugs still makes for sober reading:

Side effects of raloxifene:

More common: Bloody or cloudy urine; chest pain; difficult, burning, or painful urination; fever; frequent urge to urinate; infection, including body aches or pain, congestion in throat, cough, dryness or soreness of throat, and loss of voice; runny nose; leg cramping; skin rash; swelling of hands, ankles, or feet; vaginal itching.

Less common: Abdominal pain (severe); aching body pains; congestion in lungs; decreased vision or other changes in vision; diarrhoea; difficulty in breathing; hoarseness; loss of appetite; nausea; trouble in swallowing; weakness.

Rare: Coughing blood; headache or migraine headache; loss of or change in speech, coordination, or vision; pain or numbness in chest, arm, or leg; shortness of breath (unexplained).

Side effects of Arimidex

More common: Abdominal pain, accidental injury, anxiety, arthritis, back pain, bone pain, breast pain, cataracts, chest pain, constipation, cough, depression, diarrhoea, dizziness, dry mouth, flu-like symptoms, fractures, headache, heart disease, high blood pressure or cholesterol, hot flashes, infection, insomnia, joint disease or pain, loss of appetite, nausea, osteoporosis, pain, pelvic pain and stiffness, 'pins and needles', rash, shortness of breath, sore throat, stomach and intestinal upset, sweating, swelling of arms and legs, urinary tract infection, vaginal discharge or inflammation, vomiting, weakness, weight gain.

Less common or rare: Blood clots, bronchitis, confusion, drowsiness, feeling of illness, fever, hair thinning, heart attack, increased appetite, itching, muscle pain, nasal or sinus inflammation, neck pain, nervousness, severe blisters in the mouth or other mucous membranes, sluggishness, stroke, temporary tumour growth, tense muscles, vaginal bleeding, vaginal dryness, weight loss.

It is important to note that the older you are the more likely it is that you will suffer the side effects.

Hormones for prostate cancer

Hormones cannot cure prostate cancer but they can slow the growth. The idea behind the treatment is that the male hormone, testosterone, helps prostate cancer cells to thrive. Removing this hormone slows the rate of growth. One way in which this can be done is through surgical castration. Another way is through oral hormone pills that feminize the patient.

The side effects of this therapy are severe: besides breast development there is deep-vein thrombosis (blood clotting). In fact the side effects of all such drugs should be read with care. Those for hydrocortisone, one of the hormone drugs used includes raised blood pressure, heart trouble, mood changes, blood clots, thinning of the bone leading to increases in fractures, bruising, changes in vision and acne. Loss of sexual interest (libido) too will almost certainly happen.

Currently, hundreds of thousands of men (around 600,000) are being treated with androgen deprivation therapy, ADT, as this treatment is called.

University of Michigan Medical School researchers recently examined data from 107,859 prostate cancer patients aged 67 and older. According to their analysis, men treated with ADT had a 30 to 40 per cent higher risk of colorectal cancer than men who didn't receive the treatment. The risk increased the longer the men received the therapy. ADT is also associated with structural bone decay.

So not a good idea it would seem. And, in fact, this therapy seems to run counter to common sense. The idea that high testosterone levels are associated with prostate cancer growth runs counter to the fact that men with the highest testosterone levels (teenagers and young men) have the lowest prostate cancer incidences. In fact it is now known that there is no connection at all between testosterone levels and prostate cancer incidence.

Cryotherapy

Cryotherapy, also called cryosurgery, cryoablation or targeted cryoablation therapy, is a minimally invasive treatment that uses extreme cold (liquid nitrogen or argon gas) to freeze and destroy cancer cells. Mostly it is used on surface tumours but image guidance techniques (MRI, ultrasound etc.) are used to deliver these freezing substances to tumours located inside the body. Normally it will take at least two treatments to treat any tumour.

According to one source (drugs.com) the impacts of this therapy are such that: 'You may have discomfort, burning, or pain during and right after your skin cryosurgery. Your treated skin may become red and swollen. It may bleed, or get an infection. You may get a fever. If cryosurgery was done to treat a lesion on your face, you may get a headache after the procedure. The treated skin may take longer than expected to heal, and you may get a scar. A new lesion may grow in the same area. Your nerves may get hurt and your skin may grow numb (lose feeling). Skin cryosurgery may also cause your treated skin to get lighter or darker, or to lose hair. If your body cannot handle cold, your blood pressure may decrease, and you may pass out.'

Another problem is that healing takes a long time. While some sources say that healing will result in six weeks for small and 14 weeks for larger wounds, I personally have met someone who treated himself with liquid nitrogen and years later he still had a small wound that refused to heal.

Biological therapies

The idea behind biological therapies is that the immune system can be activated to target cancer cells—and if these defences can be activated, the cancer tumour would be destroyed by the body's own immune system. Sometimes this happens spontaneously.

In 1986 Molly O'Connor, a five-month-old baby, was diagnosed with a neural blastoma which had already spread to the liver. The cancer tumour swelled up and distended the stomach. The specialists, however, detected certain signs (not explained) that were positive and decided not to proceed with chemotherapy. Instead they observed her. At a certain point the cancer stopped growing and retreated of its own accord. She is still alive to this day. This was a case of spontaneous remission. Somehow the immune system kicked in and once it had done so the cancer tumour retreated and finally disappeared.

In order to replicate this process, a large number of biological substances, extracted from tumour and immune cells, have been investigated: interleukins, interferons, tumour necrosis factor, prostaglandin and others. All of these substances have been trailed on cancer patients. Some have very minor side effects, some cause flu-like symptoms and some, such as interleukin-2, has severe and life-threatening effects. To date, this approach has not been particularly successful.

Vaccination

Vaccination is another form of biological therapy. Cancer vaccines are different from other prophylactic vaccines in that they are not preventive. Rather, cancer vaccines are therapeutic—they are used to treat the disease rather than prevent it.

One pioneer in this field is Dr Donald Morton, Director of the John Wayne Cancer Institute. He has used the standard BCG vaccination with some success against malignant melanoma—four of the first seven patients to receive the BCG survived. Analysis of the results showed that those patients whose melanoma was confined to the skin recovered but those whose melanoma had struck deep into the body—particularly the brain—did not.

However, while orthodox cancer clinics have been prevented by lack of FDA approval from offering vaccine therapies, this is not the case with scientific pioneers who are forced to practice outside the USA. Vaccination plays a key part in the therapies offered by the ITL Cancer Clinic in the Bahamas, which is carrying on the work of Lawrence Burton. For more information go to www.immunemedicine.com. I have discussed this story at greater length in Section 3: *Cancer: Research and Politics*.

Bone marrow transplantation

There are two reasons why a patient may be advised to undergo bone marrow transplantation. One is allogenic transplantation, in which new bone marrow—usually from a close relative without cancer—is transplanted into the patient to help the body to fight the cancer. Identical twins are fortunate in having a walking supply of perfectly-matched bone marrow to draw on.

The more common autologous transplantation is used when the doctors want to use massive doses of chemotherapy—dose levels that would normally kill the bone marrow cells. In this case the bone marrow is taken out before the chemotherapy course and replaced afterwards.

Anti-angiogenesis agents

This is a new but promising area of attack. It is known that solid tumours need to develop their own blood supply—a process known as angiogenesis—in order to fuel their growth. By attacking this development of blood vessels, using an anti-angiogenesis agent, the tumour can, in theory, be prevented from growing. However, it still remains to be seen whether or not attacking the blood supply will be effective in eliminating tumours.

However, this approach opens up another interesting avenue. It is known that inflammation induces angiogenesis, which in turn increases the risk that a cancer will spread—and this may explain why physical trauma is associated with cancer. This has led some researchers to hypothesize that anti-inflammatory agents may help prevent increasing angiogenesis of pre-existing tumours. It should be mentioned that there are many natural anti-inflammatory agents (e.g., lavender essential oil, ginger, curcumin, fish oils, the Ayurvedic herb Boswellia serrata, and bindweed, among others).

Interestingly, among drugs being tested for anti-angiogenesis effects is the notorious Thalidomide.

Smart drugs

The latest scientific research buzz-word is 'smart drug'. The idea is that so much is now known about cancer that to talk of lung cancer, for example, no longer makes sense to a cancer researcher. He will want to know whether you are talking about lung cancer type A2 or Type B3. These different types are distinguished by molecular peculiarities. It is these peculiarities that are now becoming the focus of intense research activity. Drugs will target the specific molecular vulnerabilities of each different type of cancer. Great things, according to research spokesmen, are expected.

One new smart drug is a breast cancer treatment called Herceptin. It targets cancer cells that make too much of a protein called HER-2 which is found on the surface of cancer cells. This effect occurs in about 25 per cent of breast cancer cases. Herceptin is designed to slow or stop the growth of these cells. And has it been successful? Sadly, it is not a cure. It has demonstrated some short-term benefits in relation to tumour shrinkage but these benefits are not earth shaking. On its own, only 14 per cent of women taking it demonstrated a significant response. For patients taking it in addition to chemotherapy there was a slight improvement in life expectancy after one year (76 per cent as against 68 per cent of women taking chemotherapy alone).

Unfortunately, there is a big fly in the ointment. It is no longer possible to talk even of a lung cancer type A2, for example. Every tumour contains cells that are genetically heterogeneous. Put simply, there are many different types of cancer cell within each tumour. And your tumour is different from mine. In addition, the cells that leave the primary tumour—the ones that will eventually create the metastases that will, possibly, kill the patient—are different again. And not all cells that go on the journey away from the primary tumour will create metastases. Given this complex genetic cellular reality no one smart drug can possibly work. This is a case of researchers knowing more and more about less and less until they are close to knowing almost everything about virtually nothing. The level of focus is too precise. Scientists need to lift their eyes from these tantalizing details to look at cancer once again within the framework of its context.

What orthodox treatments are recommended for your particular cancer?

As cancers at various sites differ from each other in many ways, so too do the treatment protocols for these cancers differ. Chemotherapy may be very effective in treating some (e.g., testicular cancer), but totally ineffective in treating others, even though they may initially provoke a response. Remember, response rates are a meaningless measure of therapeutic effectiveness and have little if any correlation with long-term survival of the patient, or even with extending life. A tumour may respond initially but then return with renewed force.

The problem is that doctors are part of a system—and that system is wedded to the use of surgery, radiation, and chemotherapy. The availability of other therapies may only be open to patients who persist in looking for options, or for those who are considered 'terminal' and for whom the other therapies have been tried and have failed.

The medical establishment requires obedience by individual doctors to generally agreed treatment protocols. Doctors cannot, therefore, be trusted to be open and truthful about the impact of these therapies and the damage they can cause. Their careers—their ability to pay mortgages school fees, etc.—depend on going with the institutional flow.

The patient undergoing treatment should take note of the words of one of the founders of modern medicine, Sir William Osler: 'In today's system of medicine a patient has to recover twice: Once from the disease and once from the treatment.'

However, many readers will nevertheless want to know more about the latest treatments for their own cancers. Rather than attempt to provide inadequate summaries of these standard treatment protocols for the various cancers, I will here direct you to sources of information of the latest approaches.

The US National Cancer Institute at www.cancer.gov. provides detailed descriptions of the standard treatments and prognoses for each cancer. It is updated monthly, so you can be sure this is the very latest information.

Two books that are aggressively in favour of the orthodox protocols and which give an impressive amount of information are:

- *Everyone's Guide to Cancer Therapy*, by M. Dollinger MD et al., and
- *What You Really Need to Know about Cancer*, by Dr Robert Buckman

When reading these books, you should be alert to the fact that where there are no figures of success for a treatment, there is very likely little chance that this treatment will be effective. Where there is no standard treatment that means none has proven itself to be effective. That when it says clinical studies are ongoing, that means patients are being directed to treatments so that they can be studied. Also, it has been brought to my notice by a doctor that these books tend to recommend the most aggressive approaches and there are private clinics where less aggressive approaches are preferred.

A book you really should read before undergoing chemotherapy is *Questioning Chemotherapy*, by Ralph Moss.

Another book, one that is stridently in favour of orthodox treatments but which, blow by blow, describes how painful undergoing such cancer treatment can be, is *C*, by John Diamond.

Reducing the Side Effects

Although I have been very critical of standard cancer treatments—and have argued that surgery, radiation and chemotherapy are forms of treatment to be regarded with great caution, many patients have undergone these therapies, their tumours have disappeared (for the time being) and they appear, for now, to be living comfortable lives. In America alone it has been estimated that there are more than 11 million people who are living with cancer, many of whom have been treated and have apparently recovered having gone through some form of orthodox treatment. The therapeutic conveyor belt will continue to channel patients to these therapies in large numbers, and many patients will feel happy that their cancer is in the hands of experts who know what they are doing. For these and other reasons, radiation and chemotherapy will continue to be performed in large numbers for the foreseeable future. However, since these forms of treatment are extremely hazardous, anyone deciding to undergo radiation therapy or chemotherapy should consider the advice of a number of complementary therapists and take the following precautions before, during and after treatment. Let's deal with the issue of pain first.

Pain

One of the most effective pain relievers is the enzyme serrapeptase. Not only is it pain-relieving but it may help fight the cancer tumour by helping to digest the fibrin coating that cancer tumours produce to protect themselves against the body's immune system. There are a number of products available—high dose enteric coated capsules or tablets are best. Inholtra, a natural pain relief product designed for arthritis sufferers, has also been advised by David Walker, a biophysicist who cured himself of cancer.

According to Dr Earl Mindell, author of *The Vitamin Bible,* DL-Phenylalanine is as, or more, effective in relieving pain as morphine or other opiates, and does not have any of the dangerous side effects that a more potent analgesic has. It also has the ability to potentiate opiates so that if you are taking morphine you can boost its effectiveness by also taking DL-Phenylalanine. Cough suppressants containing dextromethorphan (aka DMX) also have this boosting effect. Of course, you must check all medication combinations with your doctor.

Some herbs that have pain killing qualities are: *white willow bark* and *cayenne*. Some herbal cures are also associated with pain-relief: Essiac and pau d'arco among others. Cabbage leaves also appear to have powerful pain-relieving qualities. I was told of one cancer patient in extreme pain who could only find relief by lying naked on a bed of cabbage leaves. Hydrazine sulphate also rapidly brings about relief from pain. The reason it does so is that it attacks cachexia. MGN3 and Pycnogenol have also had the same effects according to anecdotal reports. One other suggestion is to combine magnesium, the herb feverfew and the vitamin B6.

Some people are also making claims for a static-electricity approach to pain relief. The theory is that static electricity helps to normalise the body's own inter-cellular electrical currents. Get a pair of gloves such as a painter would wear and a one-foot section of PVC pipe. Rub the pipe vigorously with the gloved hand and then—when it is charged—sweep the pipe over the painful area. Pass the pipe down from the head to the toe about half an inch from the skin and keep repeating for three or four minutes—keep recharging the pipe every three passes. It is claimed that pain relief can be speedy and dramatic.

There are a number of energy machines that claim to be very effective in relieving pain. One is the Quantronic Resonance System which is a pulsed magnetic field therapy developed in Germany. Another is the SKENAR, developed by Russian scientists for use by cosmonauts in space. It has been described as a Star Trek-like device as it receives and sends back energy waves. Both these devices are available on the Internet and health claims are made for both machines beyond simply providing pain relief. Another machine used for pain relief (see www.naturalworldhealing.com) is the Tennant Biomodulator. For more information about these and other devices, see Section: *Cancer: Energy, Mind and Emotions.*

Linus Pauling discovered that megadoses of vitamin C given to terminal cancer patients not only increased longevity but also enhanced personal well-being. The lengthy pain-filled weeks of the normal terminal cancer patient were almost totally eliminated. Instead, patients on high vitamin C regimes tended to have a very sudden, speedy and virtually painless end after an extended period of well-being (see book 6: *Cancer: Vitamins and Other Supplements*).

Hydrazine sulphate, cesium chloride, laetrile, Willard water, colloidal gold and organic germanium are also considered to be effective relievers of the pain of terminal cancer.

For a pain-relieving bath, one recipe is to run a hot bath (as hot as is bearable) and add three cups of Epsom salts, 0.5l of hydrogen peroxide (six per cent solution) and the contents of a small container of baking soda. Enjoy.

One person has reported adding MSM to the Budwig Protocol (see Section 4: *Cancer: Detox and Diet*) and finding that this substantially reduced pain levels.

The case for taking vitamin C as an adjuvant therapy

The question of whether vitamin C interferes with chemotherapy and radiation is contentious with many oncologists insisting it interferes by helping cancer cells repair themselves. Abram Hoffer argues very strongly against this view. 'Well, what are the facts? The first fact is that there are no clinical trials which show that patients given vitamin C and chemotherapy fare worse than those not given this vitamin. On the contrary, all the published trials show just the opposite. I have treated over 1,100 cases with large doses of vitamin C and most of them had chemotherapy. I have examined the follow-up data and find that the mean difference on prolongation of life was heavily in favour of the use of the vitamins. In the first trials I published with Linus Pauling those patients on my program lived 10 to 20 times as long as the patients not receiving the vitamin.' The full article can be found at the Doctor Yourself website (www.doctoryourself.com/chemo.html).

Victor Marcial, MD, an oncologist in Puerto Rico, is in agreement:

We studied patients with advanced cancer (stage 4). 40 patients received 40,000–75,000 mg intravenously several times a week. These are patients that have not responded to other treatments. The initial tumour response rate was achieved in 75 per cent of patients, defined as a 50 per cent reduction or more in tumour size …. As a radiation oncologist, I also give radiation therapy. Vitamin C has two effects. It increases the beneficial effects of radiation and chemotherapy and decreases the adverse effects. But this is not a subtle effect, is not 15–20 per cent. It's a dramatic effect. Once you start using IV [intravenous] vitamin C, the effect is so dramatic that it is difficult to go back to not using it.'

Even if you don't take vitamin C during your treatment, you should certainly start taking it as soon as you can afterwards. Ralph Campbell, MD, a Montana paediatrician gives the following advice: 'More and more oncologists are admitting that a course of chemo disrupts the immune system to the point of allowing more cancer down the pike. It would seem reasonable for post-chemo patients to enter a regimen of high antioxidants intake as soon as they can.'

For serious damage

In the event that serious damage is caused by radiation, you should know that oxygen is considered to have enormous healing properties. One way to make use of this knowledge is to get a referral to a hyperbaric oxygen unit. These units use the oxygen chambers familiar to divers who rise to the surface too quickly and are in danger of 'the bends'. These chambers increase oxygen levels throughout the body and could be very beneficial for anyone suffering serious damage from radiation treatment. Similarly, drinking water containing a few drops of 35 per cent pharmaceutical grade hydrogen peroxide may be a simple way of achieving the same end. Some private clinics offer ozone treatments that are also said to be beneficial.

Damage prevention

Grapes. Doctors at The Institute of Cancer Research in London believe the antioxidants in grapes may protect against radiation fibrosis, a condition that causes tissue around the breast to become hard and stiff. It can be very painful. The problem can appear many years after the treatment. Eating grapes or taking grape seed extract appears to be highly effective as a preventative—but doctors are not entirely sure why.

Glutamine. This is a common amino acid. Supplementing 25–30 grams a day (or 0.3 grams per kilo of body weight) is highly recommended for anyone undergoing radiation or chemotherapy. Very important for healing. It is recommended to combine this with isoleucine, another amino acid.

Co-enzyme Q10 (CoQ10). CoQ10 provides important protection for the heart. For anyone taking Adriamycin/ doxorubicin or any other cardiotoxic drug, this is a must: 200–400mg a day.

Lactobacillus acidophilus. These are the friendly bacteria. L acidophilus and L bulgaricus have a noted effect in cleaning out the toxic wastes that result from these therapies. As a result, the toxic impact of the treatments is reduced. Start taking before any treatment is started.

Potassium. Radiation causes problems for the sodium-potassium balance of the body. Potassium is a very important mineral, which is essential for nerves, muscles, regulation of osmotic pressure, maintenance of the acid-base balance of the body and also for the proper levels of blood sugar. Ocean fish, seaweed (kelp, dulce, etc.), beans, whole grains and dried figs and bananas are good sources. For a protective effect, 3–6g a day is required. Overdosing can be a problem above this level, so it is best to monitor your intake carefully. A normal dietary intake (from fruits, vegetables, nuts and whole grains) should provide around 2–3g.

Magnesium. Magnesium deficiency can be caused by drinking too much milk, coffee, alcohol, and fluoridated water. Many chemotherapy drugs cause loss of this mineral. Deficiency can cause a loss of calcium and potassium, kidney disease, muscle cramps, irritability, depression and even heart disease. It is an important mineral and needs to be taken as a supplement unless your diet also includes a lot of sea vegetables, soybean products or nuts. The truth is most people are deficient in this vital mineral. For more information on the importance of magnesium go to www.mgwater.com.

Selenium. This has a protective effect against mercury—as in dental amalgam ('silver') fillings. It also helps protect against radioactivity. Although usually only required in small amounts, during treatment you should take up to 1–2mg a day (one ounce of Brazil nuts, the best food source, contains 0.5mg). Indeed it is one of the most significant anti-cancer minerals (and depletion of selenium has been associated with higher incidence of AIDS and many other diseases). It is advisable to avoid taking at the same time as vitamin C, as there have been some suggestion (not definitely proven) that vitamin C interferes with the absorption of selenium.

Iodine. Iodine deficiency can also occur as a result of radiotherapy, and some form of supplementation should be considered. Iodine in particular affects a large number of the body's metabolic processes. For this reason, it is recommended that seaweed products such as kelp or dulce, available at any adequate health store, should become a regular part of the diet—also green vegetables, and egg yolks. A tincture of iodine called Lugol's solution is recommended by some. If the local chemist shop won't supply it, try the Internet. Iodoral tablets are another useful way of taking iodine and potassium. These are easily available from Internet suppliers. Finally, many people advocate the benefits of Atomic Iodine, or Nascent Iodine as it is sometimes referred to. This comes in one per cent and seven per cent solutions. Cancer patients will want the seven per cent solution. As it is a liquid it can be administered to the skin as well as taken internally. Dr Albert Szent Györgi, the Nobel Prize-winning biochemist who isolated vitamin C, wrote, 'When I was a medical student, iodine in the form of KI (potassium iodide) was the universal medicine. Nobody knew what it did, but it did something and did something good.' In those days the standard dose was one gram—which contained 770mg of iodine. For more information on the health benefits of iodine go to: www.health.groups.yahoo.com/group/iodine.

Sodium alginate. Sodium alginate is another highly recommended substance, as it helps reduce the impact of radiotherapy on the bones and, in small doses, is known to act as a cancer preventative. Brown sea vegetables such as kelp are a good source of sodium alginate. There are a number of concentrated brown seaweed extracts—which incidentally also have strong anti-cancer activities: Modifilan and U-Fn Fucoidan are two such products.

Aloe vera. Some people recommend drinking aloe vera juice regularly for its healing properties. We have already noted the terrible impact of radiation on the intestines. It is also recommended that aloe vera gel should be rubbed into skin areas affected by radiation half an hour before exposure. In addition to its anti-cancer activity it also protects people with weakened immune systems against infection. It is a powerful protector against free radicals and is an excellent source of glyconutrients.

Slippery elm. Since damage to the mucous membranes lining all the hollow tubes in the body is inevitable, some complementary therapists recommend that radiation patients should constantly drink slippery elm, a herbal compound that should also be available at your local health shop, and olive oil. These are obviously intended to replace the natural mucous material lining the insides of hollow organs and so avoid the worst consequences of radiation treatment. Blackcurrant juice is also recommended for this purpose.

Transfer factors. There are stories of people sailing through chemotherapy and radiation with very few side effects because they were taking transfer factor supplements. (see Section 6: *Cancer: Vitamins and Other Supplements*)

Vitamin A. The main problem of both radio- and chemotherapy is that it attacks the epithelial cells that line the inside of the intestines and which produce the mucous membrane. Vitamin A is necessary for the growth and maintenance of epithelial tissue, and it is therefore necessary to take this vitamin, either as vitamin A or as beta carotene, in large quantities while undergoing either treatment; several glasses of fresh carrot juice a day throughout the treatment would be sufficient. For cancer patients, real Vitamin A is better than beta carotene, because conversion of beta carotene into vitamin A may be, and often is, problematic.

Vitamin C. Chemotherapy patients are often urged not to take any anti-oxidant vitamins, particularly vitamin C, during their chemotherapy, as it is believed these will reduce the effect of the drug. Critics, meanwhile, suggested that it was the chemotherapy that was interfering with the benefits of vitamin C!

However, a recent study shows that vitamin C not only supports the body but aids any chemotherapy regime by making cancer cells more sensitive to the toxic impact of the drug. If you need to, direct your doctor to the following reference: Abdellatif et al. 'Vitamin C enhances chemosensitization of esophageal cancer cells in vitro.' *Journal of Chemotherapy*, 2005; 17 (5):539–549.

Vitamin D. Important for healing and the immune system—10,000IU per day.

Vitamin E. This vitamin helps the body to recover from post-irradiation anaemia and helps to protect red and white blood cells. It has been found to protect the heart against damage and lower skin toxicity from the doxorubicin agents, and protects against lung fibrosis from use of bleomycin. Taking 1,600IU or more, starting one week before chemotherapy treatment, has a significant impact on hair retention. However, a number of alternative cancer therapists believe vitamin E protects cancer tumours and even promotes their growth. On the other hand, there is evidence that vitamin E in the form of vitamin E succinate does inhibit tumour growth. This demonstrates very clearly that all forms of any vitamin are very far from being equal.

Herbs. A number of herbs are useful as protective agents: Siberian ginseng, panax ginseng and chaparral. In the case of panax ginseng, a Korean study found that a normally fatal dose of radiation would leave five per cent of mice alive in the control group compared with 82.5 per cent in the group given the herb. Chinese herbs—especially blood strengtheners and kidney tonics—have shown great ability to support the body. Milk thistle and rosemary will help the liver.

Maharishi Amrit Kalash (MAK). This is an Ayurvedic food supplement made up of a variety of herbs and minerals. According to its manufacturers it has 1,000 times the antioxidant power of vitamins C and E. The All India Institute of Medical Sciences in New Delhi did a study comparing breast cancer patients, some of whom received only chemo while others had chemo plus MAK. The MAK was found to cut the number of people who suffered vomiting by almost half. It also helped reduce appetite loss and increase overall quality of life. It had no effect on hair loss, diarrhoea, mouth ulcers, and low blood counts. It is available at www.mapi.com.

Triphala. This is another Ayurvedic preparation that helps to maintain good health and which has demonstrated strong anti-cancer effects of its own.

Nutritional yeast. Nutritional yeasts bond with pollutants and heavy metals. Mixed with brown rice, this has protective value for the liver. Bio-Strath is a Swiss herbal product that contains a good yeast (saccharomyces cerivisiae) and 15 herbs. The production of Bio-Strath requires two months of fermentation. In one study, a group of radiation patients who took Bio-Strath suffered no weight loss, or depression of the haemoglobin. It also helped to enhance the assimilation of nutrients. It also has been shown to retard tumour growth in mice—and mice on a diet of Bio-Strath—did not develop as many cancers as a control group.

Bromelain. Pineapple enzymes that help reduce inflammation.

Reishi mushrooms. In Japan, drinking tea made with Reishi mushrooms (aka Ling Zhi) is also often recommended for radiation patients as it protects the white blood cells.

Green drinks. Green drinks based on chlorella, spirulina and barley sprouts and which also contain vegetables rich in chlorophyll such as green cabbage, broccoli and alfalfa have been shown to reduce radiation damage by 50 per cent in studies on guinea pigs. Chlorophyll is very similar in its molecular composition to haemoglobin. This should be near the top of the list. There are a number of different brands. I am familiar with Barlean's Greens and Green Defense, both of which are good.

Olive oil. When this comprises 15 per cent of total calories of a daily diet it provides optimal protection against radiation. In one study with mice which received from 0 to 30 per cent of their diet in the form of olive oil, those mice that had no olive oil all suffered radiation damage to liver, kidneys, lungs, skin and hair. Olive oil demonstrated strong protective properties.

On a side note, the incidence of skin cancer among Mediterranean populations is low, and it is speculated that this is because of the high olive oil consumption. Olive oil contains significantly higher amounts of squalene than seed oils. Extra virgin olive oil (cold pressed) applied to the skin after sunbathing may protect against skin cancer.

Olive oil may also protect against bowel cancer by regulating the enzyme diamine oxidase, which in turn may be linked to cell division in the bowel.

When buying olive oil make sure it states on the container that the oil was extracted by mechanical means and not by heat. Cold pressed extra virgin olive oil is best. Extra virgin olive oil is the only vegetable oil that does not go through chemical processing—peanut, safflower, and canola oil all go through chemical processing to remove toxic substances. Many cheap commercial olive oils may also have green dyes added to them to make them look more authentic.

Garlic. Garlic promotes healing and protects against radiation damage. It is a very powerful food medicine, and you should eat as much as you can tolerate. It contains two powerful substances: allicin oil and organic germanium. It also contains a substance that Russian scientists have called vitamin X, because its functions are not yet fully understood. Kyolic brand deodorized garlic capsules are highly rated and aged garlic extracts are reputed to be highly effective as protection against DNA damage that the radiation causes. However, there is nothing wrong (and a lot that is right) with eating fresh, preferably organic, raw garlic. Another product that claims to be very much more effective in crossing the stomach barrier is alkaline buffered garlic powder. This is available under the name, Real Garlic, from Purity Products: www.purityproducts.com.

DMSO. DMSO, dimethyl sulfoxide, an organic sulfur compound of great therapeutic value, has shown itself to be valuable both in alleviating the side effects of radiation and being an anti-cancer therapy in its own right. There is evidence that, when combined with low doses of chemotherapeutic agents, it is also highly effective against cancer.

Immune-system boosting drugs; isoprinosine. This is marketed under the trade names Methisoprinol and Inosiplex. It is used for anyone with a compromised immune system—AIDS and cancer patients—as it has demonstrated a strong anti-viral activity and is valuable for restoring and strengthening the immune system. It is even used to treat some cancers—particularly melanomas. It is often used postoperatively and with radiation and chemotherapy. Discuss the availability of these drugs with your doctor. It has few side effects—or as doctors like to put it, it is 'well tolerated'. The few side effects reported included: itchiness, dizziness, and problems with digestion (slight stomach pain, feeling full after eating only a small amount of food).

Seaweed. Lots of sea vegetables (seaweed) are recommended. Anecdotal evidence strongly suggests that side effects are much reduced if the patient takes large quantities of seaweed during treatment. Modifilan and U-fn Fucoidan brown seaweed extracts are highly recommended.

Ice-pack. Some people have suggested that keeping an ice-pack on the head during the chemotherapy sessions and for an hour or so after may prevent hair loss (as does vitamin E).

Lifewave patch and IceWave patch. One of the problems patients face with these gruelling treatments is that they feel completely depleted of energy. Lifewave patches, developed to enhance athletic performance, will give much needed energy. These are not transdermal patches in that nothing in the patch is physically absorbed through the skin. Instead, they use a proprietary technology involving minute quantities of certain organic compounds that are programmed to send frequencies into the body. These in turn stimulate the body to produce ATP, which is the fuel needed for cellular energy. The result is increased energy, stamina and strength. These patches are used mainly by athletes to promote performance—and they have testimonials from quite a few well known athletes such as veteran tennis player, Fred Stolle—but they will be particularly beneficial to those who are energy-depleted as a result of medical treatment. Go to www.lifewave.com for more information. The IceWave patch is based on the same technology and has been developed for pain relief.

Kinotakara foot patches. Two Japanese researchers Dr Takao Matsushita and Dr Kawase Itsuko have developed a patch that they claim gives a major boost to the wearer's energy levels while at the same time helping detoxification. The patches are placed overnight on the foot (usually) or anywhere else where there are swellings. In the morning, the white patch is generally found to be stained with toxins it has drawn from the body. The patches, which combine 'wood vinegar essence'—from oak, beech and sakura trees—with a number of other ingredients including pearl powder, tourmaline stones and negative ions. It may seem bizarre and exotic but they have become big business in Japan. For more information go to www.kinotakarafootpatch.com.

Traditional Chinese medicine/Ayurvedic medicine. Both these forms of traditional medicine—which use diet, herbs, breathing, exercise and other modalities such as acupuncture—are extremely helpful in countering the negative effects of chemotherapy and radiation. Look in the Yellow Pages for a local practitioner.

Visualisation. Finally, anyone opting for radiation and chemotherapy should develop a positive attitude to these treatments and visualize how they are working against the cancer.

Fasting. Apparently, fasting for two days before each chemo session allows you to cope much better, according to a study led by Valter Longo of the University of Southern California. Mice given a high dose of chemotherapy after fasting continued to thrive. The same dose killed half the normally fed mice and caused lasting weight and energy loss in the survivors. So, it is clear that fasting can have a major impact on your well-being.

Lymphoedema relief

The following suggestions come from a cancer forum on how to deal with lymphoedema.

Suggestion 1

'I use a machine called Light Beam Generator from ELF labs in America which is excellent to clear lymph nodes naturally. You can contact the company if they have any practitioners near you. To read more on these machines go to my website at www.bioenergy-rochdale.co.uk'

Suggestion 2

'I've seen and experienced tremendous results for ridding clogged lymph in my breast tissues, under my arms where there has been much pain and inflammation, if I take high doses of SOD (superoxide dismutase). I get the one from Biotec International. I actually use the BioVet line for animals and use the same for myself. Lots of carrot juice. Ginger and garlic juiced with everything aids in clearing toxic waste and lymph. Lemon juice juiced with garlic and ginger. I have had great results using raw cold processed hemp seed protein powder by Manitoba Harvest in Canada. You can probably find a good source in the UK.

'Lastly, I'm experiencing very good results taking powdered Humic Acid daily for detoxing and clearing infection. I bought 25 pounds bulk for $4 per pound. I bought it for my animals and soil as an organic agricultural supplement. The farmer I bought it from uses it as a tea daily. 1/4 teaspoon. He told me it's critical to make sure it's from a good source and no other ingredients are added. Humic Acid is ancient compost. Its age can range from hundreds of years old to millions of years old. A friend who introduced me to the source puts some in water and after his shower each morning sprays his whole body with this and some sea minerals added to the mixture. He says he feels incredible after he sprays his body. It's black so you only need a little in the spray. He advised me to use the 1/4 teaspoon daily.'

Suggestion 3

'I would highly suggest continuing the Budwig Protocol, Oleander, pancreatic enzymes, coffee enemas, etc. Obviously what you are doing is having an effect. I would also suggest performing a parasite cleanse and

adding something for yeast overgrowth since most with cancer have a concern with yeast. Oregano oil is a good choice along with a good colloidal silver. Also N-Acetyl-Cysteine. Adding more greens to your juicing is always a great idea. Be sure to keep your elimination routes open and working—we eliminate by breathing, sweating, urination, defecation (2–3 bowel movements daily is recommended) and for women menses. For exercise consider rebounding as this will help to keep the lymph system moving. Dry skin brushing is another suggestion.'

Marie emailed me with another suggestion that she says worked for her: a product called Herbal Release. 'I was on it for a month and my arm went down from 19 inches to 13 inches. There is only a one-inch difference between my arms now. I'm hoping that if I keep this up and I lose some extra pounds, I may be able to enjoy some of my favourite tops again!' She was so impressed she became an agent for the company—contact: marie@chrisbyrnesllc.com.

Dealing with 'chemo brain'

The American Cancer Society makes these suggestions for coping with 'chemo brain':

- Use a detailed daily planner. Keeping everything in one place makes it easier to find the reminders you may need. Serious planner users keep track of their appointments and schedules, 'to do' lists, important dates, websites, phone numbers and addresses, meeting notes, and even movies they'd like to see or books they'd like to read.
- Exercise your brain. Take a class, do word puzzles, or learn a new language.
- Get enough rest and sleep.
- Exercise your body. Regular physical activity is not only good for your body, but also improves your mood, makes you feel more alert, and decreases tiredness (fatigue).
- Eat your veggies. Studies have shown that eating more vegetables is linked to keeping brain power as people age.
- Set up and follow routines. Pick a certain place for commonly lost objects and put them there each time. Try to keep the same daily schedule.
- Don't try to multi-task. Focus on one thing at a time.
- Ask for help when you need it. Friends and loved ones can help with daily tasks to cut down on distractions and help you save mental energy.
- Track your memory problems. Keep a diary of when you notice problems and the events that are going on at the time. Medicines taken, time of day, and the situation you are in might help you figure out what affects your memory. Keeping track of when the problems are most noticeable can also help you prepare. You'll know to avoid planning important conversations or appointments during those times. This will also be useful when you talk with your doctor about these problems.
- Try not to focus so much on how much these symptoms bother you. Accepting the problem will help you deal with it. As many patients have noted, being able to laugh about

things you can't control can help you cope. And remember, you probably notice your problems much more than others do. Sometimes we all have to laugh about forgetting to take the grocery list with us to the store.

Three other suggestions have been suggested:

Tai Chi. A University of Missouri study seems to show that Tai Chi—done twice a week for an hour—had a significant impact in helping women improve their mental functioning after only ten weeks.

Wii. The interactive game system. Here is one story that appeared on a cancer forum telling of its beneficial effects: Mary Jane Zamora is a 50-year old woman who was diagnosed with breast cancer in February 2005. Weakened by chemo she was too tired to get off the couch. So her daughters had the bright idea of buying her a Wii for her to play. This is the story of the healing power of games. They force us to compete. The desire to win. And the fun of trying to win are powerful motivating forces. Although she found it 'exhausting' to begin with, she played every day and as a result she recovered faster than she otherwise would have.

'What this game did for me,' she said. 'Was encourage me that I could still do these kind of things. It came around when I needed it.' Zamora said that the Wii and its games helped her to visualize her new life, after cancer. 'My life is coming back. It's not about loss. It's about setting aside what I was and evolving into an even better person … this has been a cornerstone.'

Rosemary herb or essential oil: This is known to be beneficial to good mental functioning.

Summing up

Siddharta Mukherjee's best-selling book, *The Emperor of All Maladies: A Biography of Cancer*, makes for very sobering reading. Mukherjee is an oncologist and his book is the history of the conventional approaches to cancer. It was very interesting for me personally to see that all the concerns that I had identified were strongly reflected in his book. High-dose, multiple chemotherapy regimes have had, he argues, very good success against a limited number of cancers and there is some incremental improvement for many other cancers, but, nevertheless, overall, it is clear that this is not the route that is going to win any war on cancer. He does see a great deal of hope in the smart drugs, but here again, the ability of cancer to mutate quickly also places a limit on their likelihood of success. He concludes: 'But with cancer … no simple, universal or definitive cure is in sight—and is never likely to be.'

Let us now review what we have learnt in this section. In its early stages, before it has metastasized, cancer may be viewed as a 'local' disease. As such it is reasonable to consider the use of limited surgery (e.g. a lumpectomy) and/or radiation of this local area. Hodgkin's disease is amenable to being treated in this way and has a pretty good survival rate (about 85 per cent). However, once cancer has spread, then it becomes a 'systemic' disease—a disease of the whole system. Cancers spread in unpredictable ways. They do not only spread in a simple way by radiating out from the initial source of the disease—they also rapidly move to distant organs. Once this has happened, no amount of surgery or radiation is going to be effective, and so there is no justification at all for going down these routes even though you, the patient, might desperately want to be rid of this malignancy in your body. One surgeon has said: 'This blessed achievement [a cure for cancer] will, I believe, never be wrought by the knife of a surgeon.' (quoted by Siddhartha Mukherjee in his book, above). However, surgeons often can be prevailed on to do surgery that they know to be useless, because patients have begged them to do so.

The problem is that the patient can never know if his/her cancer has spread. It may therefore be best to assume it has. In this case, a 'systemic' approach to cancer treatment needs to be adopted. That is why most of the current effort to find cancer cures is focusing on chemotherapy, because that is a systemic approach. But we have seen how limited its successes are and how damaging it is. Following this logic, we should cast around for other systemic approaches—and when we do that, we see that this is exactly what the alternative approaches offer through diet, herbs and supplements. That these approaches offer real hope is clear from the 25 stories at the end of this book. These stories show that there is real hope, and that the road to health need not inevitably involve pain and damage.

Whatever decisions you decide to take, I wish you every luck and success: long life and good health.

Cancer: Research and Politics

This section helps you understand the wider context of cancer—why cancer research has not come up with a cure and most likely never will; why the medical profession is unable to recognise the value of herbs and supplements—if a herb or supplement can cure cancer you will never hear about it from the medical profession; and why we should all be worried by the erosion of our health freedoms.

You will also learn about the scientists who have bucked the system, and what has happened to them.

Until you understand the wider context of cancer you will not understand why there are so many disagreements as to how it should be treated and why, despite very obvious case histories of individuals who have become cancer-free using various non-conventional approaches—including diet, vitamins, herbs and a great deal more—doctors continue to be aggressively hostile to these other approaches.

This section aims to provide this wider context so that you can make sense of the real world in which medical decisions are made.

Part One
Cancer Research

Introduction

'People have this really weird conception of science. They think that it's the one reliable source for information that we have. They think that even if their public leaders are not to be trusted, and their newspapers are inaccurate, and cultural and religious morals are treacherously shifting, that science, at the very least, will provide a stable compass. But the problem is that science can't do that. Science is alive, it evolves. It occasionally establishes a fact, but, if given enough time, it'll probably refute that fact. Remember when the earth was flat? Remember when the Sun and all the other planets spun around the Earth? Remember when humans became sick because the gods were angry with us? Science just uses a kind of rhetoric that sounds authoritative. Just like any other form of communication, however, science is susceptible to abuse, inaccuracy and just bad interpretation.'

(Geologist, Vic Baker, University of Arizona and member of the US Department of Energy's Expert Judgement Panel—quoted by John D'Agata in his book About a Mountain [Norton, 2010].)

Underlying all orthodox cancer treatment is the belief that it is scientific in some way. Both patients and doctors base their faith in modern medicine on this credo. It is presumed that behind everything that doctors do there is a vast machinery of scientific expertise that is creating, testing and evaluating products and processes. And which, in the case of cancer, is going all out to find a cure, with no other consideration being allowed to hinder this effort. Certainly this is the picture that is created by news reports and advertisements for cancer research charities.

> 'Less than half of what doctors do now is based on solid scientific evidence ...'

But inevitably the truth is a little baser than this idealistic image. Even a casual look at modern medicine will find very little that is based on such scientific procedures. Dr Luisa Dillner, an assistant editor of the *British Medical Journal*, explains: 'Less than half of what doctors do now is based on solid scientific evidence .... This is not to say that doctors are lazy or incompetent. It is partly that medicine moves so fast it is hard to keep up with the latest evidence of what works and what does not.' (*Guardian*, October 1995) I can only interpret this statement as saying that many new developments in medicine are not based on any evidence. Other commentators have suggested that as much as 80 per cent of what doctors do has little or inadequate scientific support.

The simple fact (as seen in Section 2: *Cancer: Diagnosis and The Conventional Treatments*), is that there is no proof that surgery and radiation are effective methods of treatment of cancer. This doesn't mean that surgery and radiation are useless (though they may be useless or even dangerous—how would we know?). It just means that they haven't been tested in a way that allows us to say that there is proof that they do work. And by 'work', I mean that ten years down the line people who have undergone these procedures are better off than people who haven't undergone them.

Chemotherapy, on the other hand, has been very heavily tested by scientific methods of extreme rigor—and the results effectively amount to a disproof of the value of chemotherapy as a curative treatment for the vast majority of the cancers for which it is used.

The American analyst of medical statistics, Hardin Jones, presented a paper nearly 40 years ago arguing that his statistical analysis overall suggested that no treatment was better than any treatment—indeed it was four times better! People who received no treatment were likely to live four times longer than people who did receive treatment. There has been no marked change since then. That is the closest thing to a scientific analysis of the benefits of modern medicine as we are likely to get.

Yet doctors continue to insist on the necessity of treating cancer with the weapons of surgery, radiation and chemotherapy. Now, it may be that doctors and statisticians are looking at different things. Since doctors are focused on the tumour, not the patient, they may be able to claim successful treatment (talking of remission and regression— that the tumour is growing smaller, or even disappearing for a period of time) even though a patient's total life span may not be affected at all. The treatment was a success, even though the patient died.

Is medicine an art or a science?

The question of the interplay of medicine and science is a complex one. Should medicine be seen as an art or as a science? When doctors treat patients are they serving the cause of the patient's health alone or a higher god of scientific truth? Should a doctor, when all else fails, give a sugar pill under the guise that it is an effective medication, or refuse to give it on the basis that there is no proof that a sugar pill is beneficial?

Deepak Chopra tells the story that having cut open a patient he found that she was so riddled with cancer that there was no point in continuing with the surgery. He agonized over what to tell her and in the end he lied to her saying that he had removed the cause of her problems. He fully expected her to die within a matter of months. A long time later he found her once again a patient. He did some tests and found her cancer had completely disappeared. She confessed that she had previously feared that she had had cancer but that his reassurance had so cheered her up she had felt a new person altogether. So his lie had cured her. Is this science? Clearly then there is more to being a doctor than simply being a technician of health procedures. This is an extreme example of the placebo effect.

A placebo is an inert substance—like a sugar pill—that cannot have any direct biochemical effect. But it is well known that placebos do have an effect—and a sizeable one at that.

Many doctors actually feel that it is somehow wrong to make use of the placebo effect. It is unscientific therefore it is fraudulent. The patient of course doesn't care if the cancer has gone away as a result of a placebo effect. He is just damned pleased to be free of the cancer.

But science is of course central to what doctors do. We want them to be armed with the facts, with an understanding of the truth. Without that how could we trust them?

Science and medicine

How can we discover the truth of any matter?

I suppose we can say that what is true is what has been demonstrated to be true — demonstrated absolutely so that we can say it has been 'proved'. Let us now look at this question of proof in a medical context.

The concept of 'proof' and the clinical trial

Proof, in the context of medicine, has a very specific meaning. It means that something has been demonstrated to be true in a double-blind clinical trial. This is a specialized experimental procedure that is the end result of a series of other clinical trials. It will help if we have an idea of the whole process.

The double-blind clinical trial can, in theory, be applied to any practice or treatment. However, since most of these trials relate to the development of drugs, we will see how it is applied in this area.

Usually the initial idea is developed in the laboratory. A scientist has found a chemical agent that appears to be toxic to cancer cells in Petri dishes. This is tried out on rats or mice to see if the effect persists and also to see what dose levels might be appropriate for humans. This is the preliminary stage. Once a drug has passed this process, it is given a phase I clinical trial. About 20 humans are given the drug. They are terminal patients who have volunteered. The sole purpose of this trial is to determine dose levels. It is not expected that any of the phase I patients will actually survive.

The next step is to see which cancer tumours are likely to be the most responsive to this new drug. Different groups of about 20 patients each, all having the same type of cancer, are tested to determine what the response rate is. Does the drug work better for breast cancer or colon cancer or what? This is the objective of the phase II trials, which again are conducted on patients who have no further orthodox treatment options. They have been treated, the treatments have been ineffective and they are now considered terminal. If the results are acceptable, then the process moves to the last phase.

The phase III clinical trial focuses on one particular drug regime and applies it to thousands of patients—all with the same cancer—over a period of time. These patients are in two groups: the experimental group—which receives the new drug—and the control group, which doesn't. Instead this second group receives a placebo, which appears identical to the drug but which contains nothing of any known medical benefit. It is best if the patients don't know who is receiving the drug and who the placebo. This is known as a blind trial. The trial becomes double-blind when even the doctors dispensing the drug don't know who is getting the new drug and who isn't.

In very simplified terms this is the process that all new drugs go through in order to get approval for their general use. It is also the procedure used to assess the value of the drug. However, once a drug has been approved in this way, doctors will start using it in different unapproved ways. This is admitted by the authors of *Everyone's Guide to Cancer Therapy*, who write: '… many drug programs in standard use are not listed as 'approved'. They are used because experience with patients has shown they are effective.'

This applies to about half of all current uses of anti-cancer drugs in North America. Where is the science in this? The critic may ask. The treatment is based solely on 'experience'—and this experience must first have been obtained by applying the drug randomly in an empirical—let's see what happens if we do this—manner. Clearly at this stage, what they are doing may be rigorous, it may be analytical, rational and scientific but it is not based on proof or even evidence. (Furthermore, while this may very well be a valid way of proceeding, doctors are a little dishonest because they attack other people's use of 'experience' on the grounds that it is merely anecdotal evidence.)

For patients recommended to join a clinical trial, the key implications of all this has to be taken on board. First, they should understand that apart from the clinical trial, their doctors have run out of ideas about what to do with them. Their cancer is 'terminal' (I have put the word in inverted commas because some patients undoubtedly owe their lives to being classified as terminal. They have therefore been saved from gruelling radiation and pointless chemotherapy and they have been free to look at the unorthodox treatments). Secondly, patients should remember that no standard chemotherapy regimes have established themselves for the vast majority of cancers over the last twenty to thirty years. They have not established themselves because they have not been adequately successful.

Surely, new drugs are better than the older ones? Scientists are progressively making better and better drugs and these new treatments are better, aren't they? You'd like to think so, wouldn't you? But again, the truth is that new treatments that come on to the market are not necessarily better than the previous treatments. In fact, according to Iain Chalmers of the *British Medical Journal*, there is evidence that 'new treatments are as likely to be worse as they are to be better' than the current treatments. Amazing, isn't it?

'new treatments are as likely to be worse as they are to be better'

Since the clinical trials of the past two to three decades have not been successful, the chances of a new drug being successful are also remote. But why not? If the general theory makes sense, why haven't they been able to convert that into a practical cure? In short, how is it that rigorous scientific procedures are not producing the goods?

It is hard to imagine that there should be any problem with modern scientific research and the means it uses to advance knowledge and thereby, hopefully, help the development of cancer treatments. Unfortunately, a closer examination reveals fundamental flaws.

Flaw 1

Dr Gerald Dermer, who published his views in his book, *The Immortal Cell*, pointed out one major flaw, a flaw so great it invalidates all laboratory-based cancer research.

When most people talk about cancer they are thinking about the tumours in people's bodies. These tumours consist of rapidly reproducing cells, which have specific characteristics depending on what kind of cancer they are. If a breast tumour spreads to the lung, the resulting tumour is still composed of cells that have the characteristics of the original breast cancer cell. However, when cancer researchers think of cancer cells, they are thinking of the cells they observe in Petri dishes in their laboratories, cells that derive from cell lines.

What are cell lines?

In 1951, a woman by the name of Henrietta Lacks became a patient at Johns Hopkins Hospital in Baltimore, Maryland. She had cervical cancer and she eventually died of this disease. But her cells live on. Cells from her tumour were removed and placed in a Petri dish with a culture to feed them. All previous attempts at trying to establish living colonies of live cancer cells in a test tube environment had failed. Mrs Lacks' cells successfully made the leap from existence in vivo (i.e., in the living body) to existence in vitro (i.e., in a Petri dish). 45 years on, these cells—known as the HeLa cell line—continue to reproduce and continue to be used in research.

It is not easy to create a cell line. Tumour cells will generally live a short time in a Petri dish before dying off. But very occasionally, something else happens. One or more cells display different behaviour. They keep on dividing and do not die off. The result is a cellular culture that has evolved to living in a Petri dish. It is effectively immortal. It just keeps on dividing. This is the birth of an ancestral line of cells all of which derive from this individual parent. This is known as a cell line.

It is the fact that these cells grow quickly and are standardized that makes them attractive. Scientists can then conduct daily experiments on them and publish monthly papers. (The rule of the research game is 'publish or perish'.) Cell lines then provide an efficient source of cancer cells to work on. The alternative of using fresh tumour cells is less appealing. Malignant cells living in a tumour, just removed from a patient, are more difficult to work with. Real tumours do not just consist of malignant cancer cells. Various types of normal cells are also present. Another problem is that the tumour itself remains alive for only a short period of time, so it is difficult, if not impossible, to measure the effects of experimental procedures on these living cancer cells while they are alive. These difficulties slow the work and limit the kinds of experiments that can be performed. As a result, fewer papers are published by the even fewer scientists who study tumours than are published by the vast majority of researchers who study cell lines.

So using cell lines seems to make a lot of sense. However, in order for a cell to adapt to life in a Petri dish it has to change. It has to change at a very fundamental level. That change makes the cell very different from a normal tumour cell. It displays very different characteristics. Those changes completely invalidate the results gained from research on cell lines. The information gained applies to cell lines—but does not apply to real living cancer cells in real living tumours in real living people. This is a fundamental flaw.

> 'The cancer research community is almost devoid of people who understand human cancer.'

How different are cells in vitro from cells in vivo?

Dermer points out a number of differences. First, cancer cells in the body are genetically stable. Their characteristics remain fixed. A breast cancer cell that metastasizes in the lung five years later will be identical to the original breast tumour cells. In contrast, cells in cell lines are notably unstable at the chromosomal level. The number and structure of the chromosomes in the cells change in a random way over time. Scientists working with such cells assume the genetic instability derives from the original breast cancer cell. Pathologists know that's not true.

Another important difference is that cancer tumour cells taken from the body have clear sex chromosomes; cells in cell lines commonly lose these sex chromosomes altogether.

A third difference is that when fresh from a living human, a breast cancer cell is very different from a lung cancer cell and is different from a rectal cancer cell. In cell lines they are indistinguishable. This fact led to an amusing, but costly, result. For a decade or more many scientists who believed they were studying prostate cancer cells or liver cancer cells or bladder tumour cells were actually studying the HeLa line of cells. What had happened was that contamination had occurred and the HeLa line is a particularly dominating cell line. If a cell from HeLa gets into a Petri dish containing cells from another line, it quickly colonises the dish and annihilates the other cells. This is what had happened at a number of institutes—and they never noticed. They didn't notice because there was nothing to distinguish one cell line from another. It was only when the weight of anomalous results became apparent over a period of a decade or more that the problem was discovered.

But it may be that this contamination continues. Who knows? Who cares? As long as papers are accepted for publication, nothing matters. Except that the possibility of a cure remains forever a mirage and people will continue to die of cancer in large numbers. Dermer's comment: 'The cancer research community is almost devoid of people who understand human cancer.'

Flaw 2

If we then turn to animal studies, there would appear to be a great deal we can learn from these. They are based on a simple premise that all mammals share a great many physical similarities, and that what is true for one species has an increased chance of being true for another. The problem is that there are substances that are seriously toxic for rats that have no effect on mice. There are viruses that will devastate man, which are quite innocuous for other primates—AIDS being one; malaria is another. Almost every ape and monkey has its own susceptibilities to a different type of parasite—but very few species share susceptibilities with each other. In short, what is true for rats and mice has no necessary predictive value for man.

This is a serious issue. Unfortunately, most of the attacks on animal experimentation have focused on the emotive issue of cruelty. While this is an important issue it has rather left the public thinking that animal experiments are deeply unpleasant but nevertheless necessary if we are to properly test drugs to make sure they are safe for humans. The truth of the matter is that animal testing serves only two functions. It allows experimenters to produce research studies that can be published at a great rate—though everyone knows that these studies are useless as far as the development of drugs for humans is concerned. Secondly, animal experiments allow pharmaceutical companies to claim that they have done due diligence. Useful insurance for when things don't turn out as expected.

Testing drugs on rats, rabbits, guinea pigs and even chimpanzees provides absolutely no valid data in relation to the effect and effectiveness of any drug on a human being. Thalidomide, for example, was widely tested on animals before being approved. It simply does not have the effect on any other of the normal experimental species that it has in humans. Because of this, Thalidomide remained on the market even when everyone knew it was to blame for the damage it caused. The animal data, unfortunately, refused to validate this conclusion.

The reverse situation is also a danger. If penicillin, for example, had been tested on animals before being made available to humans, its devastating effect on guinea pigs would very likely have stopped research on this drug in its tracks. In fact the development of penicillin was delayed because it was tested on rabbits and found to have no effect whatsoever. It is odd to think that if Fleming had not taken a chance and tested it on a human being, the development of antibiotics might never have occurred.

Cancer research focuses an enormous amount of attention on cancer tumours in rats and mice. But, to take one example, a breast cancer in a rat or mouse is a very different thing to a human breast cancer. The biochemical context of the mouse provides lessons that are only applicable to mice. We are spending vast sums of money looking into cancers of mice and rats; very little into understanding the real cancers of human beings.

Animal testing is an enormous scientific cul de sac. But the name of the game for most scientists is to knock out papers. That is the currency of their careers. As long as this fact remains unchallenged the pressure to persevere with animal experiments will continue.

Scientists and medical researchers need to get their houses in order. If they don't, we will all suffer.

Flaw 3

And then we come to the human phase of the double-blind clinical trial. Medical science has built a cult around this specific test. Nothing else can replace this experimental procedure and hope to achieve acceptance. The reason for its status is that it is assumed to provide results that are irrefutable. But is this true? Can we rely on the results gained from double-blind clinical trials?

To answer this question I am going to compare two trials that were conducted to see if vitamin C was an effective agent in the fight against cancer. One of these trials was not double-blind, though it was a controlled study—that is, an experimental group was compared with another group. This trial was conducted by the famous vitamin C protagonist, Linus Pauling. The other trial was a double-blind clinical trial conducted by Dr Charles Moertel, a noted opponent of vitamin C—and of anything else that smacked of the unorthodox. These two trials came up with very different results. The former showed that vitamin C had the power in some cases to cure terminal cancer patients and for many others to extend their lives, and also to reduce the pain they were suffering. The latter appeared to show that it didn't have this effect at all.

The Pauling trial was conducted in cooperation with Dr Cameron at a Scottish hospital. Cameron, like Pauling believed in the efficacy of vitamin C. He could not therefore ethically refuse to give it to any of his patients for the purposes of a double or even a single blind clinical trial. However, he reasoned that the other doctors at the hospital did not share his views and since cancer patients were distributed to doctors on a random basis, he could simply compare his vitamin C-taking patients with the patients being seen by other doctors. In addition, he also asked another doctor to compare his patients against 1,000 past patients who had already received treatment and who were matched by age and disease with his patients.

Because the trial was not double-blind, the normal demeanour of the presiding doctor ceased to be a factor. Both Cameron and Pauling made a point of encouraging and exhorting their patients to feel hopeful about the potential for a cure. The result was very positive. A small number of these patients were still alive ten years later compared with none from any of the other groups.

The Mayo Clinic trial was, however, a true double-blind trial conducted by doctors sceptical of the value of the substance they were testing—and dealing with patients who had no idea what they were taking. So, in the Cameron-Pauling trial the patients became involved. They bought into it. Doctors and patients were partners fighting for the same cause. In the Mayo Clinic trial, on the other hand, the doctors remained aloof, patients remained passive. We can therefore assume that the patients in Cameron-Pauling's test felt better about their situation. This 'feeling good' response may have had a critical importance as we can see from the following.

It has been argued by Hans Selye in a book called *The Stress of Life* that the body goes through three stages in responding to stress:

- alarm reaction
- stage of resistance
- stage of exhaustion.

Most terminal cancer patients are in the final stage. Stages one and three are typified by overproduction of corticoid hormones. Corticoids are stress hormones and they depress the immune system. This explains the link between stress and illness. They make the body feel bad to tell the mind that it is time to take a rest. In the Stage of Resistance, however, corticoid hormone levels are normal. Now, vitamin C has among its many functions the regulation of the production of corticoid hormones.

So, in Stages 1 and 3, the vitamin C intake may be used to produce corticoid hormones rather than going to the aid of the immune system. It may therefore have no protective value to the patient. Indeed it may hasten death. The only way to make it valuable is to force the patient back from the stage of exhaustion into the stage of resistance. This can be done only by psychological means: the emotions reflect the physiological status of the body and, similarly, the physiology reflects the emotional status of the body. Happy, involved people are resisting. Tired, frustrated, depersonalized people are exhausted. Hopeful patients live, hopeless patients die.

And so double-blind studies, that deliberately keep patients in a state of uncertainty and helplessness, that see patients as mechanical objects not as active biological beings, cannot detect the value of chemicals that to be effective depend on the patient's own psychological attitude. People are not things but clinical trials assume they are. That is the flaw.

Having said this, it should be noted that Moertel's study has been heavily criticized by Linus Pauling (see Section 6: *Cancer: Vitamins and Other Supplements* for a fuller discussion).

Flaw 4

There are flaws of omission as well as of commission. The key flaw of omission is that the whole focus of attention is on the cancer cell—not on the person who has cancer. The biochemical terrain in which the cancer cell develops and lives is hardly considered. If we believe that the cancer cell arrives in the body as an act of God—and has no biochemical origin—this might make sense. This of course is one of the dividing lines between orthodox and unorthodox medicine. Orthodox researchers focus on the problem in its most reduced state—the chemicals in the cancer cell. Unorthodox researchers look at the whole body of the person who has cancer and seek to determine what is different about that body. As a result they have found that trace minerals and omega 3 oils, for example, are deficient in people with cancer. By restoring the balance of these chemicals they claim to obtain good results. But this is not mainstream research and so gets little funding.

To put this in another way, let us make an analogy. The modern scientific cancer researcher is in the position of a Martian who, seeking to understand the game of tennis, approaches the task by minutely analyzing a tennis ball. He may come up with fascinating information on the performance potential of the ball and the industrial processes required to produce it—but none of this will lead to any real understanding of tennis as a game.

Flaw 5

Clinical trials are a cumbersome method of progressing from one truth to another. Ultimately, they require vast resources of time, effort, people and money. If we were to depend entirely on clinical trials, scientific progress would slow to a snail's pace. Problems are subjected to a reductive analysis in order to ensure that all possible variations are controlled and that any result that emerges can have only one cause—and the means of action of that cause are clear. Requirements such as these enable science to take leave of common sense.

This point is well made by Harry Clayton, Director of Patient Experience and Public Involvement at the UK's National Health Service. He says: 'The randomized control trial can only ever answer one question at a time. To get a good answer to that question it eliminates all the variables. The problem is that in real life our health care is surrounded by variables. Although (it) remains the gold standard for pure scientific research, it is not necessarily better at answering the questions of what works in the real world.' (*Sunday Telegraph*, October 19, 2003)

There are also other requirements that have to be satisfied before and during the human phase clinical trials. One of these requirements is that the exact means by which the drug achieves its effect has to be described.

Some years ago, a report appeared in newspapers to the effect that some scientists at the University of Texas had successful results using certain un-named Chinese herbs against cancer. The project director was quoted as saying, 'We have something that works, or at least seems to. Our problem, however, is that we do not know why or how it works, and until we do, we cannot develop this as a modern medicine.' So, these Chinese herbs are kept away from patients even though there is scientific evidence—based on scientifically controlled tests—that they work. Is this a sane way to go about the management of our health profession? As consumers of the work of doctors we are entitled to ask this question. Clearly the risk-benefit question is not being applied to the problem: what is the risk involved? What is the potential benefit? The search for truth has deposed the original goal (i.e., the search for cures).

If 'proof' is the only acceptable standard then there is no reason for assuming that smoking causes cancer. The association of tobacco with cancer is statistical. No proof of a classical nature exists—yet 99.99 per cent of scientists believe that tobacco causes cancer. Thalidomide was withdrawn from the market—but there was never any proof that it caused birth defects—yet there is no doubt that thalidomide caused those defects. So when doctors and scientists insist on the necessity of proof, they are being seriously dishonest. Perhaps we need proof that the concept of 'proof ' is a useful concept.

Flaw 6

Even the results of clinical trials cannot be accepted uncritically. As Dr Steven Rosenberg, Chief of Surgery at the US National Cancer Institute says in his book *The Transformed Cell*: 'I think as many as 30 per cent of scientific articles contain results or conclusions that are wrong and are not reproducible. A good many more stretch their conclusions far beyond what their evidence will support.'

The misreporting of experimental results was a subject that Linus Pauling exposed in his marvellous book *How to Live Longer and Feel Better*. This book is a wonderful diatribe in which he analyses experiment after experiment and shows how the authors tailored their conclusions not based on the data they had discovered but to reflect prevailing professional biases.

Flaw 7

This is perhaps the biggest flaw of all. A method is successful only to the extent that it leads to a good result. The final flaw of the whole edifice of medical research as it applies to cancer is that it has not developed anything that remotely looks like a cure for cancer. I see it as a highway that is perfect in its proportions, made from the very best materials, precisely engineered in every way but which, in the end, leads nowhere—certainly nowhere very useful to you or me if we have cancer. Is a highway to nowhere a good highway?

But how is it possible that billions have been poured into research with no results? This frustration with the current state of research methods and objectives is shared by many others who have read widely around the subject. For decades now, the general public has been told that cancer research is getting closer and closer to finding a cure. But the sad fact is, despite the billions poured into cancer research, it is unlikely that there will be any sudden breakthrough in the near future. That is the simple truth but how is this possible?

A question of ethics

In addition to these flaws, there is growing concern about the ethical questions relating to clinical trials. Because of their size, large numbers of people need to be drawn into these trials. Many of these people are desperate. The existing protocols for most cancers are not curative so there is a constant search for new treatments. The result, as one leading British hospital, Addenbrooke's, explains on their website: 'Many patients who have cancer will be asked by their doctors whether they wish to enter a clinical trial or clinical study.' That is to say, the carrot of possibly benefiting from a new successful treatment is dangled in front of patients who are offered no other choice apart from the existing protocol of which the same hospital says: '… for many cancers, the commonly used treatments offer a smaller chance of cure than we would like.'

As we shall see, there are many very promising approaches to the treatment of cancer—but patients are not properly informed of these options (in fact, to the extent that doctors do discuss them it is simply to deride them). Instead patients are encouraged to take part in large scale trials in which they don't know which group they would prefer to be in: the experimental group which gets the new treatment (but which may be more dangerous, or less effective) or the control group which gets the 'standard treatment' which is admitted to be inadequate.

Given the size of trials and the expense of running them, many are now being subcontracted to specialist agencies who conduct their trials off-shore in third-world countries—especially India. Issues of whether patients are really given 'informed consent' have recently come to the fore. Many patients do not even know that they are taking part in a clinical trial. As one Indian patient explained: 'We just sign [the forms] because I believe the doctor takes the signature to help us. That's why I sign it … I don't know a lot about all these things. I am poor and I live in a small hut and I don't understand many things. The doctors are intelligent. They write the drugs for me so I have to take them accordingly.' (quoted in a BBC report, 22nd April 2006)

The problem of reductionism

Science is the rational analysis of reality using certain tools. Different sciences use different tools. Astronomy and physics use observations and calculations to arrive at hypotheses. Biochemists make use of experimentation.

Reductionism—the method by which much of science operates, reducing questions and concepts to simpler questions and concepts—is one of the most powerful of all scientific tools but it contains within it a fatal problem. Let me explain with an example.

Assume that it has been found that a certain plant product—for example the bark of the willow tree—has (or appears to have) the observable effect of reducing pain, then the scientist will argue thus: The willow bark contains a chemical that has pain-relieving qualities. I will proceed by finding all the chemicals in the bark and test them one at a time to determine which of them is the 'active ingredient'. When I have found the active ingredient I will then determine its chemical structure. Once I know the chemical structure I will be able to create a purified form using other process—and perhaps I will call it aspirin.

It all sounds so reasonable. And, as with the case of aspirin, sometimes this approach is useful. However, in other cases, this approach has lethal results. If we extract nicotine from the tobacco leaf and drop some of this purified extract on to our exposed skin then we will not have very long to live. Yet we can smoke this same nicotine, or chew it with enthusiasm, as some early baseball players seemed to have done, and we will not be so poisoned—not immediately, not so quickly.

Nicotine in herbal form acts differently from nicotine in purified extract. Presumably, its effect is moderated by its natural context. This is what scientists cannot explain by a reductionist method. Reductionism fails when it is confronted by complex interacting systems. This is why herbal combinations cannot be evaluated scientifically—not by scientists using reductionist methods. So if a herb or combination of herbs is curative we will not learn about it from scientists—we can only learn about it by hearing of other people's experiences and by experimenting on ourselves.

The problem of illogic

Another common failing of scientists is that you often find them arguing as follows: X can't work because the explanation you have made is stupid, therefore it doesn't work.

I hope you see the flaw in this argument. We see this in operation in the following:

1. Homeopathy cannot work because there is no possibility that a dilute homeopathic solution can contain even one molecule of the active ingredient—therefore it doesn't work.
2. Simoncini is wrong to argue that cancer is a fungus and therefore his sodium bicarbonate injections cannot work.

There is only one way to find out if something works or not and that is to test it. If it works it works whether or not our explanation for how it works is right or wrong.

Control of research by drug companies

How is it possible that after decades of research and billions of dollars spent, a cure for cancer still remains a mirage shimmering on the horizon? One answer that has been put forward is that pharmaceutical companies have no desire to find a cancer cure—unless it is a cure that they can profit from. It doesn't take too much cynicism to see the validity of this argument. If it became possible to turn the clock back 200 years when cancer incidence was in the region of 1–2 per cent of the population—compared with 40–50 per cent today— the pharmaceutical industry would suffer grievously. No industry will support the means by which its own profits will be threatened. On the contrary, it is very much in the pharmaceutical industry's interests to impede any such work. The most benign way in which this work can be impeded is simply to starve it of funds. In this way, interesting but unprofitable possibilities are sidelined in favour of research into patentable drugs.

Most cancer research is conducted under the umbrella of one or other of the pharmaceutical companies. They provide much of the financing and the means by which a drug can be developed. If their search for a pharmaceutical cure is fundamentally flawed then all the money put into this kind of research will be wasted. The pharmaceutical companies are very happy with the current situation as the profit margins on the anticancer drugs they are currently marketing are very fat. Cancer is good for profits.

Many people will consider such a conclusion to be overly cynical, even paranoid. And it may be that the truth is slightly more prosaic. One writer who knows the drug companies very well, who writes for *Fortune* and *The New York Times*, who according to the blurb on the back of the book in front of me 'has connections deep within the business and financial communities' and who has written in-depth studies on both drug companies and the US Food and Drug Administration (FDA), is Fran Hawthorne. In her 2005 book, *Inside the FDA*, she discusses a cancer drug, Erbitox. In passing, she makes this comment: 'Erbitox does not "cure" colon or rectal cancer. It did not even extend patients' lives significantly in clinical trials. Oncology drugs rarely do. But measured by the yardstick generally used for cancer treatments—how they shrink tumors—Erbotix seemed promising.'

> 'Erbitox does not 'cure' colon or rectal cancer. It did not even extend patients' lives significantly in clinical trials. Oncology drugs rarely do.'

Read that statement again, very slowly. 'Oncology drugs rarely do [extend patients' lives significantly.]'

It seems that the pharmaceutical companies have slightly but significantly changed the rules of the game. Success is measured in tumour shrinkage not cures. That's the word from as close to the horse's mouth as any of us will get.

If anyone should doubt the controlling influence of the drug companies on cancer research they should look at who is on the controlling boards of the largest cancer research institutions. Certainly, it is common for senior officers retiring from American regulatory bodies such as the FDA to be given directorships on the boards of the drug companies. So commercial interests and their influence in the halls of power must be accepted as one of the problems a new idea seeking acceptance must overcome.

The question of status

But money and commercial interests are not the only obstacles. Another obstacle relates to the status of the person demonstrating the proof or the institution where the work is undertaken.

We can see this clearly if we consider the following argument. It seems sensible to say that results emerge from effort and that therefore the greater the effort, the greater the results must be. If we follow this logic, then we can also argue that the greater the amount of money we spend on a project, the greater the amount of effort that will result. So it follows that the places attracting the largest amounts of research money must be the places where the greatest scientific advances will take place. And since those institutes will also be where the scientists with the highest reputations will be employed, because their presence will attract research funding, we have a very tidy and comfortable picture of scientific eminence and scientific breakthrough walking hand-in-hand.

Conversely, of course, a poorly-funded individual of little eminence cannot be expected to achieve much. Certainly, such a person cannot be expected to solve problems that elude the great minds supported by access to large resources.

As a result of this and related, possibly unconscious, prejudices, established bodies will not accept any 'proof' simply because it has been demonstrated. They will, instead, be highly suspicious of any evidence that does not come from certain accepted sources. This is quite explicitly stated by Dr Robert Harris of the then Imperial Cancer Research Fund (now part of Cancer Research UK) who rejected the value of the work of Dr Joseph Issels. 'But you must remember that millions of pounds are spent on cancer research every year, and you can't expect anybody in this field to seriously believe that somewhere in Bavaria there is a man who's got hold of something which has escaped the rest of us.'

Curiously, however, there does appear to be a consistent pattern where the poorly-funded individual of little eminence, either through rigorously logical reasoning, great genius, bold experimentation, rare opportunity, simple accident or plain dumb luck (or perhaps simply freed from the stultifying pressures of peer-group evaluation) does indeed find the answer— often only to be ridiculed or ignored by the great.

The most famous case in medical history concerns a Dr Ignaz Semmelweiss. It was in a Viennese hospital that Semmelweiss's attention was drawn to a curious fact. There were two maternity wards in the hospital. One was attended to by the doctors, and the other was attended by midwives. No doubt the wealthier ladies were favoured by the doctors while the poor had to make do with the midwives. Semmelweiss discovered that women patients who should have been clamouring for the attentions of the doctors were actually seeking to get admitted to the other ward. There were two possible reasons for this. Either it was a matter of modesty or ill-informed nonsense—as the Professors insisted—or the women's excuse that fewer women died in the midwives' ward had some merit.

To determine the matter Semmelweiss studied the records and observed the matter in person. The results were clear. The women patients were right. A great many of the women in the doctor's ward died of puerperal fever, relatively few from the midwives' ward did so. What could account for this strange fact? Semmelweiss saw that the main difference was that the midwives washed their hands while the doctors did not. Worse, the doctors when not attending to their patients were in the next room doing post-mortems on patients who had died of puerperal fever to discover the cause of death.

Semmelweiss started to wash his hands and the result was that few of his patients subsequently got puerperal fever. He therefore theorised that some form of invisible contagion was the cause of the disease—at that time, 1848—Pasteur had not yet convinced the world of the germ theory of disease. Puerperal fever was common. 40 per cent of women giving birth in hospital got it and more than a third of those died.

Semmelweiss, sought to persuade the other doctors of his findings—but he was a young provincial Hungarian in the best hospital in Vienna. His views were derided. When he published the results of ten years of observation in 1861, he suffered vicious attacks on his integrity and was forced to flee Vienna. He eventually suffered a complete psychological breakdown and committed suicide.

Semmelweiss couldn't prove he was right. He didn't understand why he was right. But he was right. The sad truth is that experts resist change.

And as a postscript to this story it should be noted that it was the women patients who saw the truth first. They saw the simple truth that medical experts refused to see for several decades longer.

Dr Eugene Robin calls events of this type 'iatro-epidemics'—large-scale attacks on public health caused by doctors or the medical system itself. He lists radical mastectomy and tonsilectomy as two other common, unnecessary procedures which resulted and continue to result, in unnecessary deaths. His calculation for 1984 was that one child in 10–15,000 died as a result of a tonsillectomy, and, as 400,000 such operations were conducted annually, the result would have been around 30 children dying needlessly each year in the USA.

Other doctors think radiotherapy will one day in the future also be seen as an iatrogenic episode. Biostatistician Dr Irwin Bross, who tried to investigate this question of whether radiation therapy was iatrogenic, had his research funding cut off by the National Cancer Institute. Bross wrote: 'It is almost impossible to get 'peer review' that will accept a study of iatrogenic disease …. For 30 years radiotherapists in this country have been engaged in massive malpractice—which is something a doctor will not say about another doctor.' (quoted in Moss, 1982)

The problem of conformity

So, why is it that simple evident truths—or interesting possibilities—are so hard for the medical profession to accept?

One answer is conformity. Medical researchers conform to the same goal—to seek chemotherapeutic agents that will kill cancer (they test out 50,000 substances each year). They conform to the same method—the use of cancer cells that reproduce themselves in Petri dishes; they conform in their funding sources—in America these must be approved by the National Cancer Institute, and in Britain by the Medical Research Council. These deciding bodies are run by groups of respected scientists who have a shared vision of how the goal of cancer cure will be achieved. Anyone who does not share that goal will not get funding. Indeed, as Gerald Dermer discovered, they will be cold-shouldered. In this way, an entire industry quickly develops a single perception.

Most cancer researchers wish to advance in their chosen careers. They wish to go from working as part of a team, to leading a team, to heading an institute. To do this they need to publish results. In order to publish results they must persuade their mentors to add their names to their research—only the previously published get subsequently published. Their articles must also receive the go ahead from colleagues under the 'peer-review' system. So, they need to know the right people, they need to say the right things. If there are any fundamental flaws in fundamental assumptions, perceptions or methods of research then these flaws will invalidate the work of the entire industry. The laws of conformity will ensure that everyone is wrong.

If this is true, then the individual working far from these centres and uncluttered by a ruling theoretical orthodoxy is the one most likely to come up with something interesting, something that works, something true. However, this scientist would not find it easy to inform the world about his discovery because the same people who fund science are those that also validate and publish its results. New discoveries that are foreign to normal practice tend to be ignored or sidelined. Peer-review journals will not publish papers that go against the prevailing ethos. Conferences will not accept such papers. Research-funding bodies will not provide the necessary funds to continue the work. So the new discovery has to wait in the wings for unconscionable periods of time before it gets accepted—if it ever does. If the researcher attempts to go public by announcing the discovery to the world at large, he or she is vilified. We saw this process in action when Dr Andrew Wakefield announced that he had evidence linking the MMR vaccine to autism, he was eventually forced to abandon his career. Whether or not he did in fact have such proof is still open to question, but the resulting actions were not scientific but political, and were deliberately punitive.

Finally, another force working against the development of new interesting ideas is that institutions are highly competitive. If the idea has emerged from a rival institution there will be a natural attempt to discredit it. If that doesn't work then it must somehow be taken over. Current research work is a highly prized secret that must not be revealed to the outside world. Failures are buried. Successes applauded unduly.

The authoritarian personality

The structure of the scientific and medical professions is very hierarchical, giving great power and authority to those at the top and requiring submissiveness from those below. At the bottom is the patient. Since doctors and scientists live and thrive in professions that are highly hierarchical and authoritarian, we must assume that they feel comfortable in such a structure. Science writer Richard Milton thinks this is the case. He believes that scientists with authoritarian personalities will tend to do better in the scientific world than scientists with democratic personalities.

He quotes the case of a postgraduate student in the 1980s seeking to get support from his professor for permission to study hypnosis. The professor refused to allow it on the grounds that it was not a respectable field for research. It was not respectable because there was no serious literature, and there was no serious literature because no one had done any research, and no one had done any research because it was not a respectable field of research. Joseph Heller coined the term Catch-22 to define this form of circular argument. In this case, a potentially serious study of a subject about which little is known is starved of funds and professional support because it contravenes conventional attitudes.

Compare this with the following words from Professor John Huizenga: 'It is seldom, if ever, true that it is advantageous in science to move into a new discipline without a thorough foundation in the basics of that field.'

Huizenga appears to be saying that we should study only what we already understand, and we should ignore what we don't understand. This is troubling because, at the time he made this statement, Professor Huizenga was co-chairman of a committee set up to investigate whether funds should be directed into new areas of research. Clearly, no new area of research can ever satisfy the requirements required to obtain funding.

The concept of an authoritarian personality was put forward by psychologists at Berkeley University in California in the late 1940s. The contrasted it with the alternative—a democratic personality. Among the characteristics associated with the authoritarian personality are the following:

- a rigid adherence to conventional values
- a submissive, uncritical attitude towards leaders of the group with which he or she identifies—they are imbued with idealized moral qualities
- a tendency to be over-sensitive to violations of the conventional moral order—and to react to these violations by condemning, rejecting and punishing people who violate them
- a tendency to be opposed to subjective feelings, the world of the imagination and to emotional generosity
- a tendency to think in rigid categories
- a preoccupation with power and dominance—leading to the idealization of, and submission to, power figures.

Doctors, and even entire medical establishments, have a history of allying themselves with the most authoritarian political structures within any given society. Hitler's death camps were designed and run by the German medical profession. Robert Jay Lifton studied this and reported his findings in *The Nazi Doctors: Medical Killing and the Psychology of Genocide*. In the introduction to this book, Lifton says: 'When we turn to the Nazi doctor's role in Auschwitz, it was not the experiments that were most significant. Rather it was his participation in the killing process—indeed his supervision of Auschwitz mass murder from beginning to end. This aspect of Nazi medical behaviour has escaped full recognition.'

The point here is not to point the finger of blame at the present medical profession for the mass murder in Nazi Germany; rather, it is to demonstrate that we are discussing a valid concept that has a profound influence on the medical and scientific professions. Russian doctors sent dissidents to mental hospitals. American doctors lobotomized the mentally ill and then there was the 'Tuskegee Incident' during with the US government sponsored a syphilis experiment conducted upon 399 African-American men from 1932 to 1972. Over the course of these five decades, the US Public Health Service sought to determine if the long-term effects of syphilis were different for black people than for white. During the trials, the doctors who conducted the experimentations intentionally denied these men treatment; never informed them of syphilis' destructiveness to their health; and ignored the fact that these men were infecting their respective wives and sexual partners with the disease. By the end of the experimentation, at least 28 of the men had died of syphilis; over 100 died of related complications; at least 40 of their wives had been infected, and over 20 of their children had been born with congenital syphilis.

These are extremely painful facts. Perhaps they can be dismissed by saying they happened in other places at other times. Yet they do establish a general tendency.

This tendency is also clear in the practice of their profession. The doctor and the surgeon like to be in charge. They don't like patients who do not cooperate immediately. As Dr Steven Rosenberg says: 'Too many doctors are comfortable dealing with patients only when they can assume an air of unquestioned authority. Surgeons tend to be particularly authoritative.' Knowing this, we can now see how a profession can persevere for 25–30 years with a treatment like chemotherapy that they know doesn't work for the majority of cancers, and that they also know will kill a significant number of their patients.

Some research has been done on medical students and their attitude to authority. This research has found that first and second year medical students have a strong sense of ethical sensitivity but that this deteriorates as they progress through the next three years of their medical studies. Obviously, the doctors that most patients first see, their GPs, have to a certain extent opted out of this hierarchical world but only at the cost of being permanently last in the medical pecking order. The views of a GP carry no weight whatsoever in the medical field.

Have doctors been brainwashed?

While it is fair to say that there is a great deal of controversy over whether there is such a thing as 'brain washing', religious cults do make use of mind control techniques that do appear to result in conversions and rigid adherence to the cult by cult members. Some of those techniques appear to be present in medical training. One is to subject people to long periods of sleeplessness while at the same time imposing humiliating punishments to coerce people into automatic obedience. How do you train doctors? You force them to undergo long periods of sleeplessness and make them operate within a highly authoritarian structure in which their careers are constantly under threat if there is variance from the desired norm. Does this explain why mainstream oncologists are so resistant to any rational debate on the merits or otherwise of natural therapies?

Ann Knox, who runs a UK health conference organisation called The Truth Matters, tells the story of how she refused conventional therapies and instead chose a detox and diet-based approach (she now says there is no sign of cancer). But her doctors opposed this decision rather aggressively. Here she tells what happened:

'After my initial consultation, I agreed to go for an MRI scan, which confirmed what had been detected via the mammogram. I explained to the consultant at the time that I was not wishing to have any further treatment, which they didn't take too kindly to and have actually made my life a living hell.

My own doctor continuously called me and told me that was I was in huge trouble should I not accept treatment and even arrived at the door of my home, armed with my health file under her arm and told me that I was reaching the time where conventional treatment would not be an option. All I had asked for was regular scans so I could monitor if the lump was becoming smaller/bigger and I was refused this each time. I would only be offered this on the grounds that I accepted the biopsy.

It got to the point where I was called and asked to visit with the head of my doctor's office. After a short period of talking to him about where I was with my health, he promptly told me that I was in big trouble as I had let too much time elapse. I asked for my blood to be tested, which I was refused and told that they could tell nothing through my blood and that if they detected anything untoward in my liver then it would be palliative care for me!

I was then told that my body was rotting inside and one day I would wake up, place my feet on the floor and I would go straight through the floor boards! I was devastated to be treated with such disdain due to my making a personal choice for my own body that differed with conventional treatment. I then asked to view my medical records and to my shock and horror discovered that my consultant had commented that I should be sent for immediate psychological counselling.'

This sounds like the actions of the Moonies or Scientologists rather than the sane, rational, thoughtful, compassionate doctors we would all hope to consult with.

The question (are doctor's brain washed?) is a serious one.

See Ann's story here: www.anh-europe.org/news/anh-feature-graced-by-breast-cancer.

Research as a game

Then there is the theory that medical research is like a game, a theory argued by Dr Ashley Conway. Conway distinguished between two types of expert. The Type 1 expert is like an engineer. He knows how to do something useful. If there is a problem he seeks to solve it. When he has solved it he moves on. The Type 2 expert doesn't know how to solve problems—he just knows a lot. Dr David Horrobin, who first proposed this distinction, suggests that the area of cancer research is dominated by Type 2 experts. As a result it has gone nowhere.

Ashley Conway explains the incentives of turning research into a game. It allows for status recognition within a hierarchical system which has developed rules about how status is acquired. It also provides security: 'You know where you are with the Game—it reduces uncertainty, maintains equilibrium, blocks intimacy and keeps an emotional distance, which achieves the important effect of making people predictable. The Game enables the Type 2 expert to avoid taking risks and therefore avoid being wrong.'

And what happens if a Type 1 expert comes along and solves a problem? One defence is simply to find a flaw in a minor detail and then to dismiss the rest of it on that basis.

And what would happen if someone came along and solved the problem of cancer?

'A solution to cancer would mean the termination of research programs, the obsolescence of skills, the end of dreams of personal glory. Triumph over cancer would dry up contributions to self-perpetuating charities …. It would mortally threaten the present clinical establishments by rendering obsolete the expensive surgical, radiological and chemotherapeutic treatments in which so much money, training and equipment is invested …. The new therapy must be disbelieved, denied, discouraged and disallowed at all costs, regardless of actual testing results, and preferably without any testing at all.' —Robert Houston and Gary Null

And lastly, those who still believe that 'scientific research' is an honest enterprise should look at the blog of Dr Aubrey Blumsohn at www.scientific-misconduct.blogspot.com.

> Why do cancer research charities constantly seek funds for cancer research while pharmaceutical companies make enormous profits from their research?

Let me explain this question. Pharmaceutical companies do research and out of this research come ideas that lead to drugs that eventually make it to the market and earn very good profits for these companies. How is it that the research undertaken by cancer research charities does not lead to drugs that make the cancer charities lots of money? Why do they keep coming to the public, asking us to donate funds to support their work?

Part of the reason must be that the cancer research charities hand over the money but do not retain possession of the results of the research. In this case it would seem that public donations to cancer charities end up subsidising, in one way or another, the highly profitable pharmaceutical companies.

Alternatively, the research paid for by cancer charities is not the kind of research that results in drugs or other treatments. When you or I donate money to a charity we expect that money to be used in such a way that it will lead to a 'cure'. So, if that is the case, we are being misled.

It is clear that cancer research charities do not properly project manage the cancer research they pay for. Instead they simply hand the money on to whoever applies for those funds. Nor do they do the ethical thing of paying specifically for research into herbs and supplements that the pharmaceutical companies do not do, because there would be no financial reward for doing so. This is, in my opinion, the only useful function that a cancer research charity can perform.

Conclusion

It is hard to escape the conclusion that modern, laboratory-based cancer research is unlikely to arrive at results likely to be of benefit to cancer patients. Not next month. Not next year. Probably not in a hundred years. This is a frightening conclusion to arrive at—but it seems inescapable.

Part Two
The Politics of Cancer

Introduction

The medical profession is socially and politically powerful. The scientific community is entrenched, competitive and defensive. The drug companies wield a great deal of financial clout. Together they are a formidable social force.

A war has waged in America for several decades between this orthodox establishment, on the one side, and proponents of alternative or complementary medicines on the other. The details of the war are far too long and complex to go into in this book. Anyone seeking a good account of its impact in the US should read *The Cancer Industry* by Ralph Moss, very much an insider's account, and for the way the war is being waged (with the full backing of the national 'quality' press).

One of the most extreme—even rabid—organizations hostile to alternative medicine is the Campaign Against Health Fraud, who consider themselves to be 'quackbusters'. They seek every opportunity to attack alternative treatments seeking always to pin the label 'unproven' on them.

For the non-aligned spectator, this is unedifying—and indeed worrying. If the general public, through charitable donations and taxes, are supporting the major cancer research charities, then surely they have a right to expect these charities to engage in testing all the unpatentable ideas that might show anti-cancer activity. Yet these charities appear to be locked into a dance with the pharmaceutical companies. If big pharmaceutical companies can make profits from anti-cancer drugs, surely cancer research charities, at the very least, can benefit from royalties on any patentable drug they find effective and at the same time plough these surplus sums into looking at vitamin C, colloidal silver, herbs and indeed anything else that comes along. It seems to me that the onus for doing basic research belongs to that very medical/scientific establishment that is rejecting alternative therapies until they are proven.

Whether or not the Campaign for Health Fraud is itself responsible, the war against alternative thought has intensified in recent years. The means used are the smear campaign and outright harassment. Harassment of alternative practitioners or of anyone associated with unorthodox ideas has also occurred. In the US, doctors who mention vitamins in a positive way are in danger of losing their license to practice.

In the USA, the FDA (the US Food and Drug Administration) frequently raids alternative clinics. This is why most alternative therapy clinics have had to move to the relative freedom of Mexico. There they cluster in Tijuana, just across the border.

Then there is the manipulation by the medical authorities of our legal freedoms. Over the last decade or more, there have been several attempts in the USA and Europe to limit access to high-dose vitamin supplements by changing the law. Constant vigilance is required to ensure some sneaky piece of legislation is not passed through on the nod (most senators and congressmen are far too busy to read and analyze all the legislation they are required to vote on). The politics of medicine are as vicious as politics in any other arena of endeavour.

'Unproven therapies' and 'evidence-based medicine'

As we have already seen, one of the key concepts in the dispute between orthodox medicine and alternative medicine is the concept of 'proof'. The idea is generally put forward that orthodox methods of treating cancer are 'proven' methods and that all other methods are 'unproven'. We have already seen that most orthodox methods are unproven by any standard. There is a widespread medical myth—that, in contrast to complementary therapies, conventional therapies are all evidence-based, founded on a bed rock of sound science. But even the *British Medical Journal*'s website Clinical Evidence (www.clinicalevidence.com) has reported that, of the 2,404 treatments they have surveyed, only 15 per cent are rated as beneficial, while 47 per cent are of unknown effectiveness.

However, the term 'unproven therapies' is used by the American Cancer Society (ACS) to label methods of treatment which it has decided to oppose. This term is used in much the same way that the word 'Communist' was used by Senator McCarthy in the 1950s. It is used as a slur.

'Unproven' of course means simply that no proof has been obtained. It does not mean that a therapy's effectiveness has been disproved. Yet many writers who put forward the establishment view appear to think it does. They also confuse the words 'evidence' and 'proof'. We may accept that there are very hard standards that have to be satisfied before proof is established—but on the way to proof we collect evidence. We collect this evidence through tests and observations. Where there are tests, these must follow accepted scientific procedures. It is common therefore to have scientific evidence without necessarily having scientific proof.

The term 'evidence-based medicine' is also now becoming more common. Originally, this was used as a way of confronting habit-based medicine or authority-based medicine, but the term has now been taken over and used against non-conventional therapies. The implication is that conventional medicine does have a basis in evidence (not proof!) while other approaches are not. But as we have seen a few paragraphs earlier, all is not well in the halls of medicine—nearly half of all treatments are of 'unknown effectiveness'.

There is something curious and indeed unacceptable about the speed with which therapies are rejected. Why are they being rejected? What is the agenda of the people rejecting them? These are valid questions which need to be answered. Yet there appears to be very little desire among the hundreds of thousands of scientists working in the field of cancer research, and medical doctors working in the leading hospitals of North America and Europe, to demand an answer or to challenge these rejections. One former official of the American Cancer Society, Pat McGrady, Sr has written:

> '[The American cancer establishment] has turned the terror of [cancer] to its own ends in seeking more and more contributions from a frightened public and appropriations from a concerned Congress. Still, undismayed by the futility of funds dumped into the bottomless pit of its 'proven' methods, it remains adamant in refusing to investigate 'unproven' methods.'

Every book written from a staunchly orthodox stance contains warnings to patients that they should not entertain any thoughts of going down the route of 'unproven' therapies.

'Keep in mind that accepted medical treatment for your cancer is the best scientifically tested treatment …. The best way to determine whether a treatment is proven or unproven is to ask your family doctor. Doctors rely on scientific proof before they use a treatment. Unproven methods lack such proof.' So says an American Cancer Society pamphlet.

Other warnings suggest that 'unproven' methods can cause harm either directly or indirectly, by seducing patients away from proper treatments. Dr Friedberg is so concerned to dissuade the potentially errant patient that he produces the ultimate argument.

> '[E]ven if the "treatments" are not in themselves harmful, a serious consequence of their use, and one that is insufficiently recognized by cancer patients and their families, is that those who use them are wasting valuable time.' (Friedberg, Cancer Answers, 1992—a truly despicable book)

They are, he goes on to say, wasting time that should be better used in continuing 'accepted' forms of cancer treatment but also, more importantly, time that should be spent getting used to the idea of dying. Clearly Dr Friedberg assumes that unproven remedies are necessarily ineffective. This is, as we have seen, an unscientific position to take.

The problem is that by having a list of unproven therapies, and by using this list as a blacklist to stop further funding, we have a self-fulfilling prophecy. They are unproven because there is no institutional will to seek proof. There is, instead, an institutional will to prevent such proof being established. Disproof is assumed. That is one of the rules of the game. Another rule is that anyone who proposes or uses an unorthodox approach has to be slandered as a 'quack' and/or a 'charlatan'.

Underlying this game of name-calling is a profoundly false assumption. It is one thing to say that a doctor needs scientific proof that a drug is effective—a point that is itself debatable—It is quite another thing to demand this of patients. Patients don't need proof—not when the price of proof is so high. Anecdotal evidence is quite sufficient for most aspects of life. If Mr Brown took substance X and was cured and Mrs Smith took substance X and was cured of the same thing, you can bet your bottom dollar I also will try substance X the next time the need arises. I wouldn't think of waiting thirty or a hundred years for science to get its act together to prove that it worked. To repeat a point I made earlier, patients perhaps need proof that 'proof' itself is a valid validating concept.

And then there is the question: Why can they not say that these alternative approaches have been disproven? It is in the interests of the medical establishment and the pharmaceutical companies to demonstrate that alternative methods don't work. You can be sure that if they have evidence—as indeed they claim to have from time to time—they would trumpet it loud and clear. Yet, while a great deal of research has been undertaken, that proof has not been forthcoming. And if you can't disprove the effectiveness of vitamin C, say, doesn't this suggest that it *is* effective?

Are we missing opportunities?

One of the first examples of a well-conducted controlled test was conducted in 1747, on twelve patients suffering from scurvy. Dr James Lind placed all of them on the same diet except for one item—the supposed remedies that he was testing: citrus fruits, cider, vinegar, sea water, a mixture of drugs. He gave each of these remedies to two patients. At the end of six days the two who had been given citrus fruits were well, while the others were still ill. Lind published these results in 1753. This was not of course a double-blind trial. Both Lind and the sailors knew exactly what they were receiving but as a trial it was rational, rigorously carried out and easily repeatable. It therefore has all the hallmarks of classical scientific testing. It is now hailed as the moment the cause of, and cure for, scurvy was established beyond doubt.

Yet, as we have just seen, such a test today would carry little weight with the elders of the accrediting committees that govern the practice of medical science. First, the elders would note that it was a lowly and insignificant naval doctor who had done the experiment and simply ignore it on that ground alone. If, however, they were feeling generous, they might admit the result was interesting but certainly not conclusive. It does not establish proof, once and for all, that lemons cure scurvy. Under current protocols, many more years of testing would be required to establish such proof. Scientists would need to know why lemons cured scurvy. The active ingredient would have to be isolated and then tested on cells in laboratories, in animal studies and then experimentally in human trials using double-blind procedures. This is where science and common sense start to follow different roads. All this time, the doctors would be warning patients not to take any form of unproven treatment—like lemons—for their scurvy.

As it happened, Dr Lind's demonstration that the answer to scurvy lay in the lemon was not accepted despite its elegance. On the contrary, since fresh fruits—and fresh fruit juices—were expensive there were pressures on ship owners and the established authorities not to accept the results. However, eventually, in 1795, over 40 years after Lind published his results, the British Admiralty ordered that a daily ration of fresh lime juice be given to all hands. As a result, scurvy disappeared from the Royal Navy. The merchant navy, however, was under the control of the Board of Trade. It wasn't until 1865, a full 120 years after the original experiment, that the Board of Trade also passed its own lime-juice regulations.

> 'The National Cancer Institute is not operated in a way as to favor the discovery of new methods of controlling cancer … In my opinion the NCI does not know how to carry on research nor how to recognize a new idea.'—Linus Pauling

Putting it all together

We can now appreciate what Linus Pauling meant when he suggested that there is a fundamental, organizational blindness that prevents science and medicine developing except along narrow, well-trodden, safe pathways through the confusing forests of reality. 'The National Cancer Institute is not operated in a way as to favor the discovery of new methods of controlling cancer … In my opinion the NCI does not know how to carry on research nor how to recognize a new idea.'

This, then, is the scientific research that is eating most of the money donated to cancer research. This is the research that despite an expenditure of thousands of millions of pounds has not resulted in any fundamental advance in cancer treatment for the last 20 years.

'It is gradually dawning on the donors that for the past 20 years practical benefits have not followed (from medical research). During that time there have been no substantial improvements in morbidity or mortality from major disease that can be attributed to public funding of medical research.' (Dr David Horrobin, 1982, quoted by Milton, 1994)

But one can also see the problem from the orthodox side. If surgery, radiation and chemotherapy are to be set aside, what can the doctor do to help the cancer patient? The answer appears to be nothing—especially if that doctor rejects all unorthodox approaches. How could the medical establishment possibly address the world and say: we have nothing in our techno-pharmaceutical armoury that is truly effective against cancer? The uproar would be deafening. The courts would overflow with lawsuits. We can see that such a situation is impossible. No establishment in its right mind would voluntarily bring such a response down on its own head. In brief, no matter how damaging and ineffective conventional treatments may be, the orthodox medical practitioner must persevere in directing patients down this path. He must do this, or change his specialty or leave the profession.

All of this is simple logic. From this it follows that the fact that a treatment is offered by a consultant in a leading cancer institute does not in any way indicate that it is necessarily effective. The patient must always ask for proof or evidence of effectiveness. Usually, as with chemotherapy trials, the result may or may not indicate increased survival—by a week or a month, by two per cent or four per cent. This is not worth fighting for if the previous six months are full of suffering.

If doctors are not going to change standard medical practice, then patients must. Every single one of us has the right to choose the therapy we wish for ourselves based on our own understanding of the facts and awareness of our needs, fears, desires and even prejudices.

But if patients are to reject one form of treatment they must have some idea of the options. And there are options: in fact there is a dizzying array of options. Many promise exciting results. For the patient with courage, the picture is not bleak.

Summing up

It is clear from the preceding discussion of orthodox approaches to cancer that on the whole, with about a dozen notable exceptions, chemotherapy is useless and extremely damaging. Surgery and radiation can claim to be more successful, perhaps, but they too can be very damaging, and they too may have results that are seriously negative.

And despite what you read in the newspapers, there is probably more hard science supporting so-called 'alternative' treatments than there is for the orthodox approaches. Think about it. Where do you think these alternative therapies are coming from? Many of them are coming out of research laboratories.

Last year, more than one million Americans were diagnosed with cancer and probably the same number of Europeans. With or without treatment, these people will not die immediately. Many will undergo orthodox treatments and feel saved when the cancer appears to have gone. For some of these people the cancer will never return but for most it will come back. They will undergo further treatment and again, for some, this treatment may be successful in the long term. There are therefore going to be many millions of people who will swear that their cancer has been cured by orthodox means—and that therefore this is the only sensible way to proceed. That is, of course, for each person to decide but, as we can see in Section 8: *Cancer Survivors' Stories*, many people have rejected conventional treatments, instead using diet and supplements, and they too have become cancer free.

> '... more than 80 per cent of all women with breast cancer report using CAM ... CAM use can no longer be regarded as an 'alternative' or unusual approach to managing breast cancer.'

These approaches have almost all been attacked as 'unproven'— but almost never as having been disproved—but survey after survey has shown that patients are moving very strongly in that direction. Almost everyone is already doing something that their doctors don't know about. It's a secret move away from orthodox medicine—and this movement is getting bigger and bigger all the time. Ask yourself this: If doctors had a good cure for cancer there wouldn't be a need for alternative therapies—so if more and more people are using CAM (complementary and alternative medicine)—what does that indicate?

Here's what University of Toronto cancer researcher Heather Boon discovered in 2005: '... more than 80 per cent of all women with breast cancer report using CAM (41 per cent in a specific attempt to manage their breast cancer), CAM use can no longer be regarded as an 'alternative' or unusual approach to managing breast cancer.' According to her, younger, more educated women, in particular, are more likely to have a high commitment to CAM therapies.

Cristiane Spadacio, another cancer researcher, says: '... there has been an exponential growth in interest in—and use of—complementary and alternative medicine (CAM), especially in developed western countries .... Studies show that the number of patients who use some form of alternative therapy after the diagnosis of cancer is high ... [and they experience] high levels of satisfaction with alternative therapies.'

Part Three
Cancer Pioneers and Outcasts

Introduction

It comes as a surprise to anyone researching the range of approaches to cancer just how many approaches have been developed—and we should note that many of these have been developed by scientists working within the fold of orthodox cancer research. Unfortunately, as soon as their ideas conflict with the interests of the major pharmaceutical companies, when they refuse to be bought out or relinquish control of their therapy, they find obstacles being put in their way. If they persist, then they are vilified and their work repudiated. They are called quacks or charlatans. Their research is misrepresented. If they work in America, then the FDA comes knocking on the door.

There are clear signs that the interests of the big pharmaceutical companies are being expressed in legislation and repressive legal action both in Europe and the US—and it is very difficult to get any critical analysis of cancer research by the media. Nor do the so-called 'quality press' discuss the general failure of orthodox cancer treatments or give impartial consideration of alternative approaches. Our 'free press' would appear to be firmly on the side of big money.

But not everyone has toed the line. From time to time scientists have developed new treatments based on new concepts—and they have wanted to be free to develop these ideas and to make them available to cancer patients without selling out to the big pharmaceutical companies. The stories in this section are of scientists who have bucked the system, some successfully, others not. Taken together, the work of the men and women described below make us understand something of the dynamic of the world of cancer.

And, lastly, it must be clear to any impartial witness that the men and women whose work is discussed below are extraordinarily stubborn and well-intentioned and that the label 'charlatan', with all its associations of deliberate fraud, is totally misplaced in this context.

Two early pioneers

Dr John Beard

In 1902, a Scottish embryologist by the name of John Beard published an article that caused a stir in medical circles. He had noticed that pregnancy, involving the embedding of a placenta in the mother's womb, and cancer were very similar, but that something happened in pregnancy to limit the uncontrolled growth of the placental cells (trophoblasts). He discovered that the growth of the placental cells stopped as soon as the pancreas had developed and started producing pancreatic enzymes. He therefore proposed that injections of pancreatic enzymes would be a cure for cancer. He proposed injections as he believed that pancreatic enzymes taken orally would be destroyed by the hydrochloric acid in the stomach. It has since been discovered that in fact this is not the case and these enzymes can be taken orally and still be effective.

This was the birth of the 'trophoblastic theory' of cancer. It suffered the usual fate of intense disapproval by the medical authorities and though, for a while, there was a frenzy of interest in it, it was soon shunted away into one of the curious cul-de-sacs that medical history seems so prone to. X-ray therapies became all the rage and John Beard's theory was quietly forgotten. Well, not quite. Over the years a number of others—notably the Drs Ernst Krebs and William Kelley (and Dr Nicholas Gonzalez who is carrying on Kelley's work)—continued to subscribe to the trophoblast theory and claimed good rates of success by combining a regime of large doses of pancreatic enzyme along with Bromelain, the pineapple enzyme which also digests proteins.

Drs Ernst Krebs

Drs Ernst Krebs—father and son—based in Carson City, Nevada—made their name by promoting a number of diet-based 'cancer cures' that were inevitably derided as quackery. They followed Beard in their support of pancreatic enzymes, promoting one in particular, chymotrypsin, as being effective. Later they isolated laetrile ('vitamin B17') and pangamic acid ('vitamin B15') from the apricot pit, and touted these too as cancer cures.

Laetrile has a long and interesting history (see my fuller discussion in Section 6: *Cancer: Vitamins and Other Supplements*) and Felicity Corbin-Wheeler, for one, claims that it did indeed cure her of her terminal stage pancreatic cancer (see Section 8: *Cancer Survivors' Stories*). Pangamic acid supplements have been banned in the USA, despite there being no suggestion of toxicity. However dimethylglycine (DMG), possibly the active ingredient of pangamic acid, is available and highly regarded as an immune booster—again refer to my book on supplements for further details.

Despite the disapproval of the US cancer authorities towards laetrile and pangamic acid, there has been a lot of interest in Russia and elsewhere in Eastern Europe, where they are considered to have powerful health benefits.

As a side note, I wonder if the Krebs took an interest in cancer because of their name (In German 'Krebs' means cancer (if they had Anglicised their name to Crabb the connection would have been less obvious—but remember the animal associated with the star sign Cancer is the crab).

Dr Ernst Krebs Jnr made a presentation to the second Cancer Control Society conference, in which he made some telling points:

'Cancer is a chronic, metabolic disease … that is obvious. It isn't an infectious disease, which is caused by bacteria or viruses. It is a disease that is metabolic in origin. A metabolic disease is a disease that is linked with our utilization of food. Most metabolic diseases have as their basis specific vitamins and minerals. Let me give you a categorical or axiomatic truth to take with you. One that is totally uncontradictable, scientifically, historically and in every other way. This is that no chronic or metabolic disease in the history of medicines has ever been prevented or cured, except by factors normal to the diet or

normal to the animal economy. There have been many erstwhile fatal devastating diseases that now have become virtually unknown. They have been prevented and cured by ingesting the dietary factors, and thereby preventing the deficiencies, which accounted for these diseases.'

After discussing a number of related diseases: scurvy (vitamin C—cured by eating lemons); pernicious anaemia (B12 and folic acid cured by eating chopped liver); pellagra (caused by a lack of B vitamins, particularly niacin (B3)—cured by eating brewer's yeast), pointed out that doctors almost always got it wrong when it came to isolating the causes of these diseases—all of which were invariably fatal if not corrected.

He quoted Sir William Osler who, in his *Principles and Practices of Medicine,* written at the turn of this century, said of pellagra, 'I was at Lenoir, North Carolina during one winter and this winter I visited the Lenoir home for the colored insane and there 75 per cent of the inmates died from the disease. It ran rampant through this institution and convinced me beyond any doubt that pellagra is a virus that is infectious.' Osler was wrong. The inmates simply had a grossly inadequate diet.

Krebs went on to say:

'So another fatal chronic metabolic disease found total resolution and cure through factors normal to the normal diet or the animal economy. We know that cancer is no exception to this great generalization and to date has known no exception. That is that every chronic metabolic disease that will ever be controlled by man, must be controlled by means that are a part of the biological experience of the organism. Chronic and metabolic diseases can never be controlled, prevented or cured by factors foreign to the biological experience of the organism.

'Let's make it clear by what we mean by biological experience to the organism. We refer to the experience that the organism has had over the million years of its evolution. The organism was exposed to water, air, carbohydrates, fats, amino acids and various salts and these factors became integrated with the evolving organism. And the evolving organism became integrated with these factors. And these factors with the evolving organism were incorporated into the beautiful machinery of 'life.' And the vital mechanism of life runs just like the parts of a fine Swiss watch only infinitely more complex.'

Lewis Thomas, a former president of the Sloan-Kettering Memorial Institute once wrote:

'I'm thankful that my liver works without my knowledge. I do not have the brains to commence to do one millionth of what my liver does. These things are automatic. So I swallow the food and this infinitely complex machinery takes care of itself. We could spend years telling you about this magnificent machinery and we still wouldn't touch the surface of this infinite ocean. We do know that there is nothing that we can do to improve upon it. We do know that in the history of medicine there never had been found anything foreign to the indwelling requirements of this machinery that will do the living organism any good. And we can go further to say there has never in the history of medicine been found anything foreign to the indwelling machinery of this infinitely complex system that will not harm the organism. There isn't such a thing as a factor foreign to the biological experience that is not harmful to the organism.

'There is nothing we can add to our air water and food to improve it. The most we can do is to look at some of our devitalized food and hopefully attempt to replace that which was capriciously removed from it in the process of food refining, manipulation or cooking. There is absolutely nothing that we can add to that food to improve it. These things are basic.

'There isn't any chemical or drug that medical science could suggest that would make us healthier or better adjusted or wiser or give us hope for a longer life. There isn't a single drug or molecule in nature that can unless that molecule exists in normal food. And this probably explains one of the reasons why there is so much resistance to laetrile, B17.

'The application of this science brings us face to face with a lot of things we do not like to face. We have become over-civilized. We are inclined in our delusory thinking to feel that, here and there, there must be a magic out. That there must be a simple way, a short cut, that somehow or other medical science or some other man-made forces beyond our comprehension will do for us those things we must do for ourselves. And it is slowly dawning on us, perhaps too slowly, that this thinking is fraudulent; that it is unsound.'

On the subject of laetrile, also called amygdalin and vitamin B17, which Krebs believed was the dietary item in which deficiency caused cancer, he had this to say:

'We hear a great deal about its use in terminal cancer, but the time to start with vitamin B17 is now before the disease becomes clinical. The time to start is the same with any matter of adequate nutrition and that is right now. You may start now by commencing to eat the seeds of all common fruits that you eat. The apricot and peach seed contain almost 2 per cent of vitamin B17 by weight. The apple seed, although very small, is equally rich in vitamin B17. So are the seeds of prunes, plums, cherries, and nectarines. The only common fruit on the hemisphere that lacks nitrilosidic seeds, are the citrus fruits. This lack has come about by artificial cultivation by breeding and hybridization, since the seeds of citrus fruits on the African continent still contain vitamin B17.

'Two more rich sources of vitamin B17 are the simple cereal millet and buckwheat. Macadamia nuts, although expensive and exotic, are very rich in vitamin B17 and so are bamboo shoots, mung beans, lima beans, butter beans and certain strains of garden peas. But for convenience, the simple source for your vitamin B17 are the seeds of the common fruit.

'We know something about the prophylactic dose of vitamin B17. For example, we know the Hunzas (a tribal group living in the north of Pakistan) represent a population that has been cancer free for over 900 years of its existence. This population has a natural diet, which supplies on the average between 50 to 75 milligrams of vitamin B17 a day. Hunzaland is a land that has sometimes been described as the 'place where apricot is king'. The Hunzakuts eat the fresh apricots for the three months they are in season and the remainder of the year they eat dried apricots. They never eat a dried apricot without enclosing the seed between them. This supplies them with better than average of 50 to 75 milligrams of vitamin B17 a day. There are many of us in the Western World who don't ingest this amount of vitamin B17 in the course of an entire year.'

More current innovators

Beljanski

Professor Mirko Beljanski was born in Yugoslavia in 1923. He emigrated to France and became a research biologist at the renowned Pasteur Institute where he worked for almost 30 years on DNA and RNA biology. However, he was eventually forced to leave when his innovative ideas drastically conflicted with those of the Institute's director.

After leaving the Pasteur Institute, though under-funded, he continued his research and continued to publish scientific papers, most of which were in French. But his problems didn't end there. The Ministry of Health took him to court for practising medicine illegally. His lab was raided, equipment destroyed and documents seized. The court put a legal gag on him, forbidding him to speak about his products in public. This became public knowledge and caused a big scandal and there were street protests. But in the end nothing came of these protests and Beljanski was effectively side-lined. Beljanski himself died in 1998 after years of persecution for his innovative ideas.

One of Dr Beljanski's key discoveries was that a part of the structure of DNA in cancer cells differs from normal DNA in that it contains some permanently open loops which have been caused by carcinogenic substances interfering with the hydrogen bonding between the two strands of the double helix.

Once these permanently separated sections have formed they allow more carcinogenic substances to come between the two strands of the double helix and the result is to lead the DNA in the direction of uncontrollable replication, resulting in the rapid and uncontrollable growth of cancer cells.

Continuing his work, he created his patented Oncotest that allowed him to ascertain whether or not a given chemical was cancerous or not. It also allowed him to work backwards and find substances that helped to strengthen the hydrogen bonds. He formulated a number of products based on certain herbs. Working with some sympathetic doctors he was able to show that his approach did result in cures. The website dedicated to his work www.beljanski.com contains a number of very persuasive testimonials for many different cancers, including brain cancers, which are notoriously difficult to cure.

His formulated products are sold exclusively by a New York-based company, Natural Source www.natural-source.com

Two of the products have an anti-cancer effect and two are designed to support patients undergoing chemotherapy and radiation. The two anti-cancer products are called PAO V and ROVOL V. The first contains an extract from the herb Pao pereira and the second from the herb Rauwolfia vomitoria. These are entirely non-toxic in normal doses to ordinary cells.

PAO V seems to be useful for all forms of cancer including brain cancers while ROVOL V seems best in hormone related cancers but not for brain cancers as the extracted molecule is too large to cross the blood-brain barrier.

Interestingly, Beljanski believed that low doses of chemotherapy and radiation are necessary to break open the cancer cells to allow both PAO V and ROVOL V to gain access to the DNA, while high doses of vitamin C, iron, ferritin and vitamin B12, and possibly other natural substances, interfere with PAO V. Iron of course is a no-no where cancer is concerned, as cancer cells need it in large amounts for cell division.

Burton's immuno-augmentative therapy

Lawrence Burton was not a medical doctor, his doctorate work was in experimental zoology. His specialisation was the relationship between the immune mechanism responses and cancer first in invertebrates, then in laboratory animals and finally, he took the perilous step, in humans. He graduated in 1955, and for the next eighteen years his life was that of any ordinary highly successful scientist. He published in the right places and had a solid job, eventually becoming the senior investigator and senior oncologist in the cancer research unit of the pathology department of St Vincent's Hospital in New York—a post he held until 1973. It is significant that his cancer research was based in a pathology unit. He was working with real tumours not cell lines, with real patients not laboratory rats.

Burton's work led to the development of a serum that would, he argued, inhibit the growth of cancer tumours. This serum was derived from certain proteins found in blood: a tumour antibody, a tumour complement that activated the antibody, an antibody-blocking protein and 'de-blocker' that neutralises the blocker. Burton, with an associate Frank Friedman, isolated these blood fractions. His theory was that when these four elements were in a balanced ratio in the blood, cancer cells would be routinely destroyed. His serum therefore was a way of bringing about this balance and so putting cancers into remission. He called this method of dealing with cancer 'immuno-augmentative therapy'.

The way it works is that the patient's blood is analysed every day for the ratio of these four proteins. A personalised serum is then made up to correct any deficiencies in the balance.

> 'They injected the mice and the lumps went down before your eyes—something I never believed possible.'

Burton's work came to the attention of Pat McGrady, who was an editor working for the American Cancer Society. McGrady later reported seeing Burton inject some mice with his tumour inhibiting factor. 'They injected the mice and the lumps went down before your eyes—something I never believed possible.' This demonstration was repeated in 1966 before a group of science writers. The result was a story in the *Los Angeles Times* under the headline: '15 minute cancer cure for mice. Humans next'. Oncologists present at the seminar claimed that Burton and Friedman were tricksters.

That's when the problems began. Eventually Friedman gave up in disgust and Burton was forced abroad. Despite political interference, the Bahamian government allowed him to set up a clinic in Freeport.

There, patients who could afford it made their way to be treated. There were frequent demands from establishment medical bodies for him to conduct clinical trials on his own—a request he spurned for the obvious ethical reason that, when dealing with the terminally ill, this is tantamount to murder.

In 1985 his clinic was summarily closed down. The NCI and other bodies had persuaded the Bahamian government that Burton's serum products were a source of hepatitis B and of AIDS. The evidence supporting this was of very dubious quality. None of Burton's 2,700 plus patients treated with hundreds of thousands of serum injections ever got AIDS. Many people are known to have caught AIDS and hepatitis B from blood transfusions but no blood transfusion service has ever been closed down. Impartial experts pointed out, also, that the serum had been put through the wrong test, a test that produces a large number of false positives.

As for hepatitis, only one of Burton's patients came down with this disease. Contrast this with the fact that, in 1976, in the USA, blood transfusions caused 30,000 cases of hepatitis of which 3,000 were fatal. Even before the advent of AIDS, blood transfusions were not a good thing, but the general public has not been kept fully informed of the dangers. According to Dr John Wallace, 'Blood should be regarded as a dangerous drug. There are now more than twenty viruses known to be transmissible by transfusion.'

A sign reportedly seen in Dr Burton's waiting room more or less sums it up: 'Just because you're paranoid doesn't mean they aren't out to get you.'

Outraged patients lobbied Congress and the result was that Congress ordered a study of alternative cancer therapies—a point that, in future years, may be seen as the year the tide turned in America in favour of non-orthodox medicine.

Dr Burton was allowed to reopen his clinic, which continues the work, even though Burton himself died of heart disease in 1993 aged 67.

And does it work? One patient, Curry Hutchinson, diagnosed as having metastasized malignant melanoma of the lung, told the authors of a *Penthouse* article: 'When I came here I was in a wheelchair. My mother had to care for me constantly. Two months later she was able to go home. I'm walking, jogging, swimming—alive …. My improvements are unbelievable. Burton's critics claim there's no proof his therapy works. I disagree. I'm proof.'

The Centre offers a number of other experimental therapies using a number of vaccines. Its website www.immunemedicine.com is admirably clear and straightforward about the costs involved.

Burzynski's antineoplastons

Dr Stanislaw Burzynski is both a doctor and a biochemist who works in Houston, Texas. His discovery is that a group of peptides and amino acid derivatives occurring naturally in our bodies have the effect of inhibiting the growth of cancer cells. Burzynski calls these peptides antineoplastons.

In Burzynski's view there is a biochemical defence system that allows defective cells to be corrected through biochemical means. Antineoplastons are at the heart of this defence system. Blood samples from cancer patients show that they have only 2–3 per cent of the amount typically found in a healthy person.

Burzynski's method simply requires the injection of antineoplastons into the blood stream. The result is tumour shrinkage and even remission. Often this occurs in a matter of a few weeks.

Burzynski has been treating patients since 1977. He does not claim to be able to cure all cancers in all patients—but there is strong evidence that many are cured. In one study of 20 patients with astrocytoma, a highly malignant brain cancer, mostly in an advanced stage, four went into early remission, two showed partial remission, and ten showed stabilisation (i.e., tumour regression of less than 50 per cent). Some of these subsequently went on to complete remission.

For a long time, Burzynski was considered to be a quack and a charlatan by the FDA and the American Cancer Society, but despite decades of extremely unfriendly attention, including the invasion of his clinic and seizure of patient records, he remains very much in business. He has played the system well and is now running over 20 FDA-controlled clinical trials at his clinic.

Burzynski is phlegmatic and considers all this harassment to be normal: 'Most medical breakthroughs have happened because there was some lack of suppression by the supervisors of people doing some innovative work.'

Burzynski's website is coy about the cost of his treatment. For further information go to: www.cancermed.com. However, a website has been set up by ex-patients, and this contains many persuasive testimonials. See www.burzynskipatientgroup.org

Dr Govallo and VG-1000

Valentin I Govallo, MD, PhD, Director of the Laboratory of Immunology in Moscow and author of 290 scientific articles and 20 books, including *The Immunology of Pregnancy and Cancer* (1993), is clearly no charlatan. His credentials are scientifically impeccable. But the results of his labour, a substance that is almost wholly non-toxic (it causes some slight fever and chills when first injected) and which cures over 75 per cent of late-stage cancer—has been totally ignored by the leading medical journals in America. And the whole world is influenced by what the leading American medical journals choose to publish.

Govallo's perception is that the biochemical way in which cancer develops in the body and protects itself from the body's immune system, seems to bear a striking resemblance to how an embryo protects itself from being attacked as a foreign object during pregnancy. Govallo had the brilliant idea of using a placental extract to immunize the patient against the foetus-like cancer. This is the basis of his anti-cancer vaccine which he has called VG-1000.

According to Govallo, in human trials, he has achieved a whopping 77.1 per cent five-year survival rate—remember, these were all so-called terminal cases, no longer responsive to surgery, radiation or chemotherapy. Unfortunately, as Govallo admits, 'it is not exactly clear how the placental extract effect works.'

And equally unfortunately, no-one in the American cancer establishment is interested in following up on this. Joseph M Miller, MD, who has written the only review of the treatment to date, wrote: 'If the results are accurate, this innovative approach could be one of the greater discoveries of the twentieth century.'

VG-1000 is a non-toxic, organic product that doesn't so much attack the cancer cell as simply turn it off. VG-1000 appears to be most beneficial in treating carcinomas and melanomas, and it is also indicated for some sarcomas and in leukaemia. Patients who have been subjected to chemotherapy or radiation tend to respond more slowly to VG-1000 as they have a depressed immune system. However, patients who have had neither radiation nor chemotherapy respond well. VG-1000 treatment is available at The Immuno-Augmentative Clinic in Freeport, Grand Bahamas and also CHIPSA (Centro Hospitalario Internacional del Pacifico, S.A.) in Tijuana, Mexico (www.chipsa.com).

In Europe, VG-1000 can be obtained from Autobiologics BV and from the affiliated organization, The Placenta Research Foundation. Director William H. van Ewijk, MD (MA) PhD, Autobiologics BV will make VG-1000 available to qualified doctors only. For more information contact Autobiologics BV, JOL 24–19, 8243 GN Lelystad, The Netherlands. Tel. +31 (0) 320 247 326 Fax. + 31 (0) 320 247 327. autobiologicsplacenta@wxs.nl

Dr Joseph Issels

Dr Joseph Issels, working in Bavaria, and basing his approach on Gerson's work, established what he called a whole-body therapy to deal with the whole-body problem of cancer. The therapy is in fact a combination therapy including ozone/ oxygen treatments, diet, fever therapy and even low-dose chemotherapy and radiation.

For Issels, the body has four interrelated defence systems. First, there are the lymphocytes and antibodies that are normally considered to be the entire immune system. Secondly, there are the eliminating and detoxifying organs: liver, kidneys, skin and intestine. Thirdly, there are the friendly bacteria in the epithelial tissues of the body, and lastly there is the connective tissue where organic salts are stored and toxins are digested or bound chemically to make them inert. He also made a big point of insisting that infected teeth and tonsils should be removed—including all teeth filled with mercury amalgam and teeth whose pulp has been removed through root canal treatment. He believes that these impair the immune system.

External observers have calculated that 17 per cent of his patients go on to long-term remission. Since most of them were diagnosed as terminal when they arrived at his clinic, this is an excellent result. The Issels Clinic currently claims an amazing overall 87 per cent success rate with early-stage cancers of all kinds.

But Issels was not left free to pursue his own therapies. He was blacklisted by the American Cancer Society in 1958. In 1960 he was arrested on charges of fraud and imprisoned without bail in a cell block containing only convicted murderers. This attempt to intimidate him eventually failed. After five years of court case after court case, he was finally acquitted of all charges. But in the meantime his clinic was forced to close.

In 1970, a documentary about his work was made by the BBC but the scheduled release of the programme was first cancelled under pressure from the British medical establishment then, in a response to criticism over censorship, eventually rescheduled. A re-edited version was aired. Nevertheless, great interest was aroused by the programme, so much so that the medical establishment moved more firmly to discredit Issels. They sent a five man team to Issels' Clinic. They arrived in January 1971 to do their study. Two of the team were outspoken opponents of Issels, and only two of them could speak German. They spent three and a half days at the clinic. On their return they rushed out a report that concluded his treatment was ineffective. One critic of the report had this to say: 'The sum of the team's arguments that Dr Issels cures are not really cures boils down to this—"we cannot accept the cures because cancer is incurable." … I hope readers will not have missed the logical imperfection in the team's reasoning.'

The loss of business and the constant weight of pressure—nuisance calls, refusals by medical journals to accept advertisements, internal criticism from his own staff, tampering with postal deliveries of medicines—eventually forced Issels to close his clinic in 1973.

Issels work is being continued at the Hufeland Klinik, Bismarckstrasse, Bad Mergentheim, Germany, Tel.: +49 (0) 7931 8185 and at the Issels Clinic in Tijuana, Tel.: +00 1 888 447 7357 from the USA and Canada, 001-480-585-6804 from Europe/Asia. Email: informationcenter@issels.com (see www.issels.com).

William Kelley

Kelley is the odd one out in this company in that he wasn't a doctor, cancer researcher or a naturopath. In fact he was a dentist from a small town in Texas who in the early 1960s discovered that he had terminal-stage pancreatic cancer. People generally don't survive long after receiving such a diagnosis. Kelley lived another 40 years.

He cured himself by a combination of diet, detoxification and, most important of all, the taking of pancreatic enzymes. According to Kelley, all cancers are really only a single disease caused by a deficiency of proteolytic, protein-digesting enzymes (i.e., pancreatic enzymes—particularly trypsin and chymotrypsin).

In his theory, cancer arises when three events coincide. First there is the presence on an ectopic germ cell, secondly there are female sex hormones, and thirdly there is a deficiency of active pancreatic enzymes. In this theory, the cancer develops in the same way that an embryo develops. This is known as the trophoblast theory and it has a long and distinguished history. But back to Kelley. In his view, cancer progresses because there is a lack of cancer-digesting enzymes in the body. The solution, therefore, is to get pancreatic enzymes to the place where the tumour is growing, in a concentration that is sufficient to stop the cancer's growth, but not too high as that would cause the tumour to break down too rapidly as that in turn would release toxins into the body faster than the body can cope with. What is required is a slow regular decrease in the tumour's growth. In addition, he recommended physical manipulation of the body (chiropractic, osteopathy and so on) and prayer.

An interesting side note on the possibility that cancer might be curable by chiropractic: Hanna Kroeger, now more famous as the founder of a respected herbal brand, claimed to be able to stop leukaemia in less than one week by making an adjustment to the tail bone. She apparently did this on hundreds of people. This may sound mad but we should remember that bone setting has a long history and was associated with curing disease, not simply mending bones. Chiropractic has managed to develop as a profession in the last 120 years despite enormous pressure from established medicine—it must have something going for it. For more information go to www.kroegerherb.com and buy her short book: *Free Your Body of Tumors and Cysts*.

Returning to Kelley's dietary regime, this was at first simple but then became extremely complex, based on a theory of metabolic types.

It would be nice to say that he grew old to be a wise healer. Sadly this was not the case. He did not have the personal resources finally to withstand the witch hunt that was launched against him, and he ended his days as a clinically paranoid racist. He became convinced that the world's supply of pancreatin—the main element of his cancer programme had been deliberately contaminated with a deadly bacteria by the US government.

Dr Nicholas Gonzalez, who first came across Kelley's work when he was a medical student, studied the records of those who had followed the Kelley programme and found that of his first 139 patients, representing people with all types of cancer, and all of whom had come to Kelley as a last resort for whom no further conventional treatment could be offered, 93 per cent were effectively cured.

Dr Gonzalez has taken this work forward and adapted it. He is now the leading proponent of the Kelley approach. He recommends up to 45 grams of pancreatic enzyme a day taken in a number of equal doses. He offers at his clinic a rather expensive therapy, but, as Kelley himself said, there is only one person who can treat a person's cancer, and that is the person who has the cancer.

For further information contact www.dr-gonzalez.com and/or www.drkelley.com. Pancreatic enzymes are discussed in Section 6: *Cancer: Vitamins and Other Supplements.*

Just as this book was going to press in November 2011, I read a report in a supplement to *The Times* discussing the very latest cutting edge research ideas for dealing with pancreatic cancer (a hot topic with the recent death of Steve Jobs). One of these ideas was to give pancreatic cancer patients pancreatic enzymes! Well, I guess they got there in the end.

Dr Catherine Kousmine's combination therapy

Catherine Kousmine (1904 -1992) was a Swiss-trained doctor of Russian origins who, from a very early age, felt strongly that dividing the body into specific areas of expertise was the wrong way to focus on the question of health. She therefore became a GP in order to work with whole body solutions.

Early on in her career, two distressing failures to treat children who had cancer led her to conduct her own small-scale animal research at home. She found that through dietary means she could protect animals that she subsequently injected with tumour extracts. She would inject them and they would reject the cancerous growths that were created. Despite enormous professional pressures and public criticism, she persisted in using her methods with those patients who took responsibility for their own treatment. She publicized her work in a number of books that have been translated from the French into Italian and German, but, interestingly, never into English. Her success rate? While no statistics are provided, and the picture is obscured by the fact that many if not most of her patients had already undergone surgery and radiation before coming to her, nevertheless, according to one doctor, 'Survival rates are much higher than what could be expected.'

Her view was that cancer is caused by a number of factors, one of which was stress, which she believed had a measurable impact on the micro-organisms in the body. Another cause is a diet deficient in vitamins, minerals and trace elements. In her view, surgery and radiation might be acceptable as a means of getting rid of the existing tumour, but they would not result in a cure for the cancer if the terrain in which the cancer had developed remained unchanged. And changing the terrain is not something that surgery or radiation can address.

Kousmine eventually established a system of curing cancer that rested on what she called the five pillars.

1. **Diet:** raw fruits and vegetables, whole cereals, the Budwig Protocol (flaxseed oil and cottage cheese [to which Kousmine added: the juice of a whole lemon, a mashed ripe banana or honey, and whatever fruits are in season])—no meat. (For details of the highly acclaimed Budwig Protocol see Section 4: *Cancer: Detox and Diet*).
2. **Intestinal Health**: she recommended regular fasts and enemas. A clean colon was, for her, of vital importance. She suggested daily enemas.
3. **Promoting a positive alkali/acid balance:** to achieve tissue pH to 7.5, she recommended the use of potassium and magnesium citrate.
4. **Use of supplements:** the supplements she advised were: vitamins B (no B12), E, C (high doses), selenium, zinc, polyunsaturated fatty acids (capsules of evening primrose oil and fish liver oil), and magnesium salts.
5. **Use of some low-level chemotherapy**: she recommended the chemotherapeutic drug, Endoxan (2x100mg pills a week).

Central to her therapy is the health of the liver. This can be promoted by means of relaxation, moderate sport, exercise, fresh air, sunbathing, sleep, a good diet of raw fruits and vegetables and good intake of vitamins. Liver health is compromised by stress (worries), lack of sleep, fatigue; poor diet, constipation, chronic and recurrent infections, too much alcohol, smoking and too many drugs, even simple pain killers such as ibuprofen, heavy foods (fats, eggs, chocolate, milk and any food treated with chemicals).

Kousimine was an important figure in continental Europe and it is surprising that her ideas have not received a wider audience in the English-speaking world, where she remains virtually unknown. For further information (in French) see www.kousmine.com.

Gaston Naessens and 714-X

Gaston Naessens was born in Roubaix, France in 1924 but has done most of his work as a pioneering scientist in Canada. Among his inventions was an extremely powerful light microscope —he called it a somatoscope—which used ultraviolet and laser technology and which was capable of very powerful magnification—up to 30,000×—and which, unlike any other microscope before (with the exception of that developed by Rife) enabled the viewer to examine living tissue. Unfortunately for Naessens the electron microscope, which is capable of even higher levels of magnification, was developed soon after. Nevertheless his invention remains the most powerful microscope capable of looking at fresh, living and moving, unstained blood and tissues. Naessens too believed that disease was caused by a microbe that was capable of changing size and at a certain time in its life cycle was a bacterium and at another was a fungus.

His contribution to cancer was the development of 714-X which is now available at a number of centres, is inexpensive and by all accounts very effective. However, it took years of pressure and persecution for practicing medicine illegally before it became available.

714-X? It sounds like a new jet fighter but is in fact a derivative of camphor, with an extra nitrogen molecule attached, combined with organic salts (according to one source, 714-X contains 'a mixture of camphor, ammonium chloride and nitrate, sodium chloride, ethanol, and water'). This substance was developed by Naessens on the theory that cancer cells require high levels of nitrogen. In order to protect themselves from the immune system the cancer cells release a substance which he calls co-cancerogenic K factor, or CKF for short. 714-X neutralises this factor. This prevents the cancer cells from being able to hide from the immune system. The result is that the cancer tumour is gradually eliminated from the body by the body's own natural defence system.

714-X is administered by injection into the lymphatic system, usually in the groin area. A course of daily injections for 21 days is followed by a three-day rest and then another 21-day cycle is begun. This continues for as long as necessary, but for cancer patients this usually means 7–12 cycles. AIDS patients are also benefiting from this treatment.

One patient, a Mr Ganong, receiving this treatment found that his tumour shrank so much after two months that his surgeon decided to operate. When he went in, he found the tumour: 'had been changed into an apparently non-threatening jelly-like mass he'd never seen the likes of before' according to his son (quoted in Walters, 1993). Another patient diagnosed with metastatic prostate cancer in 1977 was still cancer free in 1989 after using 714-X

Other doctors using this substance report very impressive results. Although it is administered through injections, the entire course is relatively inexpensive.

Information on doctors using this treatment and/or treatment with 714-X is available from the following organisations:

- Centre d'Orthobiologie Somatidienne de l'Estrie (COSE), 5270 Fontaine, Rock Forest, Quebec J1N 3B6, Canada, Phone: (819) 564 7883
- Canadian Institute of Alternative Medicine, 715 Bloor Street West, Toronto, Ontario M6G 1L5, Canada, Phone: (416) 530-0473

Dr Hans Nieper

Hans Nieper, 1928–1998, was a German doctor who achieved a great reputation as a natural healer. Being German meant that he was able to carry on his cancer work untroubled by the American medical establishment. At one time, he found himself in the interesting situation of treating Ronald Reagan's cancer while at the same time being persecuted by the FDA.

Nieper has sometimes been dismissed as a dreamer and not a serious scientist. Nevertheless there has been little investigation of his contention that mineral orotates, a kind of salt, are effective in transporting minerals such as potassium and magnesium into cells—particularly cancer cells—and that this helps to maintain cellular health. In his view, the taking of magnesium orotate would have the effect of reducing the recurrence of cancer by four-fifths. 'The rate of new cancerous diseases with long-term magnesium orotate therapy is perhaps less than 20 per cent of the frequency otherwise expected, at least for the first ten years of the observation period.'

He was an early promoter of bromelain, the pineapple enzyme, as a way of dissolving the protective shield around cancer tumours that protects them. He also promoted the use of iridodials—for details see Section 6: *Cancer: Vitamins and Other Supplements.*

Dr Matthias Rath

Dr Rath is the new star of the alternative medical universe. He worked for some years with Linus Pauling and since Pauling's death has taken on his mantle as the world's leading exponent for vitamin C. He is a research scientist.

Rath's answer to cancer seems very simple. According to him, all metabolic disease involves a collagen-dissolving process. Collagen is the substance from which all cell walls are formed. The key building blocks for healthy collagen production are a plentiful supply of vitamin C, L-lysine and L-proline. These also block the enzymes that do the work of dissolving the collagen and maintaining proper cellular health. Take these three supplements, increasing steadily until you are taking as high a dose as can be tolerated—and the cancer's growth will be checked, even reversed.

A final component of his protocol for cancer is a substance that is found in green tea, a polyphenol catechin known as epigallocatechin gallate (EGCG)— this is available in pure form only for the purposes of laboratory-based cancer research but it is a significant component of green tea extract.

A full explanation of his cellular medicine and cancer is available at his website as a free e-booklet. See www.health-foundation.org.

If Rath's answer to cancer is considered to be too simple a programme, we might respond by asking: why shouldn't the answer to cancer be simple? The answer to scurvy was simple (take vitamin C); the answer to beriberi was simple (take vitamin B1). Both of these were metabolic diseases that had complex symptoms that led eventually to death. Both were easily and quickly cured once the answer was discovered. Why should cancer not be the same?

Dr Wassil Nowicky and Ukrain

Dr Nowicky is another very stubborn research scientist, based in Vienna, who has persisted in the face of great opposition to develop, test and promote his answer to cancer: Ukrain, named after his native country. For the last twenty or more years he has been in the absurd position of being firmly backed by the Austrian Ministry of Science and blocked at every turn by the Austrian Ministry of Health.

Ukrain is a patented formula which combines a potent herb—greater celandine—with a chemotherapeutic drug called thiotepa (thiophosphoric triaziridine). It has been well studied—mainly in Germany, Belarus and Ukraine—and in Ralph Moss's words: 'What makes Ukrain so unusual is that this forced marriage of herb and drug yields a compound that is lacking in toxicity in normal cells. Yet it seems to have a strong affinity for killing cancer cells.' It is delivered by intramuscular injection.

The US National Cancer Institute tested it on 60 different cancer cell lines, and it was 100 per cent effective against all. Unfortunately, it has not been quite so successful in real cancer cases though results are still extremely impressive. Dr Wassil Nowicky, its developer, himself claims that in cases of terminal stage cancer it can be 30 per cent successful, and 90 per cent successful in early stage cancers.

So why isn't it being widely used in the cancer hospitals of the world? That is a question that the medical authorities should be asked—and indeed should be asking themselves. Details of his research and a record of the obstacles that have been put in the way of Dr Nowicky can be found at his website at www.ukrin.com.

Ukrain is a medium- to long-term treatment which has been shown to be very effective against all kinds of cancer. It has even cured cases of terminal-stage melanoma. It is administered by a doctor ideally in a clinical setting supervised by a doctor—however, patients can buy it directly.

Curiously, or perhaps not so curiously, the American Cancer Society has shown no interest in this therapy.

Ukrain is available only from the clinic of its inventor, Dr J Wassil Nowicky, and is produced by his company JW Nowicky Pharmaceuticals. Imitation products are apparently available on the internet but should be avoided. According to Nowicky, the alkaloids in the milk of greater celandine vary in quality depending on what time of the year they are harvested. Only he knows when to collect the herb. For further information contact Dr Wassil Nowicky at nowicky@ukrin.com.

Others

A number of other pioneers—Rife, Lakhovsky, Priore and others—developed anti-cancer approaches using electronic, magnetic or other energy-based equipment. I have discussed their work in Section 7: *Cancer: Energy, Mind and Emotions.*

Medicine and money

Our image of the doctor is an amalgam of *ER*'s frenetic interns desperately dealing with casualty victims and the calm competence of their family doctor or a senior consultant. Whatever the personal flaws of the individual, it's generally a picture of solid professionalism. But this image has in recent years come under strong attack—and the fiercest critics are themselves distinguished doctors, like Jerome Kassirer MD whose credits are hard to fault. He is Distinguished Professor at Tufts University School of Medicine, Adjunct Professor at Yale University School of Medicine and was for eight years Editor-in-Chief of the *New England Journal of Medicine*. His 2005 book, *On The Take*, has the following subtitle: 'How Medicine's Complicity with Big Business Can Endanger Your Health.' Another critic is Marcia Angell, MD, who is on the faculty of Harvard University School of Medicine and who is another former editor of the *New England Journal of Medicine*. Her 2004 book, *The Truth About the Drug Companies*, has the subtitle: 'How They Deceive Us and What To Do About It'.

These books are blunt and trenchant in their attack on the tight embrace of medicine and the pharmaceutical companies. These and other critics make the following points:

1. Doctors make a lot of money from complex incentive schemes designed to reward them for prescribing particular drugs. This is so endemic it constitutes a serious conflict of interest that negatively affects their relationship with their patients. This conflict need not be at the level of the individual doctor but at the level of the medical institution as a whole. Patients are directed to protocols that benefit pharmaceutical companies. (For cancer patients going to specialist cancer clinics, this spectre is particularly frightening.)
2. Pharmaceutical companies provide agreeable doctors with all-expenses-paid 'conferences' in exotic locations and pay large consulting fees. Often the drug companies write up the research findings on their own drugs and then go looking for doctors to put their names to the research. There is no shortage of doctors willing to engage in this practice. (The Lancet recently expressed concerns at this practice, suggesting that as many as half the articles they published were not in fact written by the person whose name appeared on them.) This means that the higher up the medical ladder a doctor goes, the more likely he or she is to be compromised.
3. Most continuing medical education is funded by the drug companies and is effectively a covert marketing strategy to promote their drugs. Studies show that doctors' prescription behaviour is influenced.

4. Most medical charities and patient activist groups receive a great deal if not most of their funding from pharmaceutical companies or companies with a potential interest, and this undoubtedly influences their behaviour. To take one obvious example: The American Council of Science and Health, which bills itself as 'a consumer education organization concerned with issues related to food, nutrition, chemicals, pharmaceuticals, lifestyle, the environment and health' is financed mainly by, as one critic puts it, 'corporations with specific and direct interest in ACSH's chosen battles'. Since its creation in 1978, it has stated:
    a. that there is no proven link between heart disease and a diet high in fat and cholesterol
    b. that there is no truth that saccharin is potentially carcinogenic. This research was financed by Coca-Cola, Pepsi, NutraSweet and the National Soft Drink Association
    c. that bovine growth hormone is perfectly safe, despite clear evidence that it substantially increases the IGF-1 (insulin growth factor) content. IGF-1 is known to be a risk factor in breast and prostate cancer.
5. Almost all research on any drug is done by doctors and scientists who are paid by the pharmaceutical companies who tie those researchers to contracts that prevent them from making public any negative findings—even where patients' lives are placed at risk. Negative findings are routinely hidden. Pharmaceutical companies also routinely request changes to results or changes of wording.
6. Universities have been known to fire faculty who raise issues about drugs or research that conflict with the views of pharmaceutical companies. University research funding is highly dependent on maintaining good relations with the pharmaceutical companies. When truth is the victim, who can we trust?
7. Many supposedly objective research studies published in major peer-reviewed medical journals are reviewed by peers who themselves have financial interests in the drug companies whose drug is being reviewed

What would happen if cancer researchers found a cure for cancer but couldn't patent it?

That of course is the big question. If they were ethical, of course they would do everything in their power to promote it for the general well-being of humanity. But of course, even if they did, their efforts would be useless unless someone came along to make the stuff. But in the real world, what they do is sit on the discovery until they can create a patentable version—by tweaking the molecule. If they can achieve this then they stand to make lots of money and a big reputation for themselves.

But, you might say, this is a hypothetical question. But is it? There are claims that a cure for cancer has been found and that it has been ignored. According to health writer, Bill Sardi, a molecule has been isolated that, when injected in minute quantities works 100 per cent of the time—and the cancer does not return even years later.

Sardi writes: 'The weekly injection of just 100 billionths of a gram of a harmless glyco-protein (a naturally-produced molecule with a sugar component and a protein component) activates the human immune system and cures cancer for good, according to human studies among breast cancer and colon cancer patients, producing complete remissions lasting four and seven years respectively [the length of the studies—ed.]. This glyco-protein cure is totally without side effect.'

This glycol-protein is called Gc macrophage activating factor (Gc-MAF). This is normally produced in the body when the body feels itself to be under attack. Cancer cells, however, secrete an enzyme known as alpha-N-acetylgalactosaminidase (also called NaGalase) that completely blocks this production. In this way, cancer cells escape detection and destruction by the immune system. By injecting Gc-MAF, the immune system is primed to attack the cancer cells—and it does so, apparently with 100 per cent success. A course of treatment would involve a weekly injection for up to a year.

Nobuto Yamamoto, director of the Division of Cancer Immunology and Molecular Biology, Socrates Institute for Therapeutic Immunology, Philadelphia, Pennsylvania, says this is 'probably the most potent macrophage activating factor ever discovered.'

Dr Yamamoto first described this immunotherapy in 1993. [*The Journal of Immunology*, 1993 151 (5); 2794–2802]. Since then there have been animal and small scale human studies all showing that it works—and that's it.

Twenty years have passed and millions of people have died while scientists try to develop the cash stream. Meanwhile the cure is there, it is known—and people are being denied access to it.

That's the answer to the question. If researchers found a cure for cancer that they couldn't patent, they would just sit on it.

Health freedoms

Are you free to treat your cancer in any way you want?

The answer to that question is not as clear as it ought to be. On the one hand you are, of course, free not to do what your oncologist recommends. The days are gone when doctors can say, as I have heard a doctor say: 'I make the decisions about what treatments my patients will do.' And yes, most people are now aware that they have the right to get second and third opinions (and indeed they are encouraged to do so). Where there is resistance is when a cancer patient chooses not to do what the doctors advise, but instead sets out to explore the world of natural and holistic therapies.

This resistance manifests itself in a number of ways. Suppose you were to say to the doctor 'Doc, I have decided to follow a dietary regime supported by herbs and supplements but I would like to continue to remain on your books so that I can have regular blood and urine tests to see if these approaches are effective.' You may very well find that the oncologists will respond in this way. 'If you don't follow the treatments we advise then we cannot help you any further.' There. No co-operation. You're on your own. For many patients that is a scary place and naturally they are often loathe to go there. But, nevertheless, you are free to go elsewhere. It's your decision.

What you are not free to do, however, is to make that decision on behalf of any child of yours who is still a minor. There have been a number of cases where the police have forcibly abducted children at the bequest of the social and medical services and forced them to undergo treatments that they do not want. They do so on the grounds that they are protecting the child. (I have discussed a number of cases where parents have successfully treated their children secretly, in Section 8: *Cancer Survivors' Stories*).

You are also not free to give—or particularly sell—someone a herb, say, that you might know absolutely can cure cancer—a herb such as bloodroot, for example—as Greg Caton has discovered very much to his cost—and ours. I tell his story below.

And you have no absolute right to choose the food you wish to consume—like raw milk for example.

Codex Alimentarius, EU and the USA

This is how Codex Alimentarius describes itself: 'The Codex Alimentarius Commission was created in 1963 by FAO and WHO to develop food standards, guidelines and related texts such as codes of practice under the Joint FAO/WHO Food Standards Programme. The main purposes of this Programme are protecting health of the consumers and ensuring fair trade practices in the food trade, and promoting coordination of all food standards work undertaken by international governmental and non-governmental organizations.'

This sounds very reasonable, but in fact the Codex is a highly contentious organisation. This book is too short to offer a complete picture of what is happening but a summary might go like this. There is a seemingly unstoppable move, both in the EU and in the USA, to restrict access to supplements and herbs by the simple act of making the rules that define drugs cover these other areas. But the cost of going through all the required hoops is prohibitive—and only makes sense if the product being tested can eventually be sold with a high profit margin. Herbs and supplements cannot do this so the end result will be an effective ban on the development of new products—and any product that cannot show that it was in general existence prior to 1994 will be affected.

Obviously there is a great deal of opposition to this development, and if you are interested in finding out more about what is happening on the ground then you should contact The Alliance for Natural Health at its websites: anh-USA.org or anh-europe.org.

State control of our children's health

Laurie Jessop's story started in February 2007 when Chad, her son, was diagnosed as having stage 4 melanoma. Her doctor—a general practitioner not an oncologist—insisted that immediate surgery was required, saying Chad was in imminent danger of dying. Laurie and Chad decided not to go down this route (after all surgery was very unlikely to be beneficial for a widely disseminated melanoma) and instead chose to treat the melanoma using bloodroot, which has a strong history of being beneficial (see Section 5 i: *Cancer: Herbs, Botanicals and Biological Therapies*). The doctor immediately reported her to Child Protective Services on the grounds of 'gross negligent child endangerment'.

In fear of the authorities, Laurie and Chad fled from their home and went to San Diego where Chad underwent a number of various alternative treatments including: ozone, hyperbaric oxygen chamber, hydrogen peroxide, energy work, Rife, nutritional supplements, and deep emotional work (see Section 7: *Cancer: Energy, Mind and Emotions* for a discussion of these approaches). Laurie also used 'black salve'—bloodroot—that she purchased from Canada to remove the visible malignancy. These treatments appear to have been successful. It took about two and a half weeks for the wound to heal from the bloodroot. When it was healed, Laurie took Chad to a Del Mar dermatologist for a biopsy. The test results were negative of any signs of melanoma. A second biopsy was done and again, no sign of cancer could be found.

Laurie returned home and was arrested, while Chad was sent to a children's home. What follows is a description of these events (widely cited on the Internet).

'The arresting deputy harassed her. When Laurie protested, the officer told her she didn't have to like her or be nice to her. After arriving at the county jail, her first telephone call had been to the social worker, David Harper, although he did nothing to get her out of jail, nor was he willing to help correct the record. Laurie was physically abused, they spread her legs twisting her knee, when she complained they called out 'Resisting! … Resisting!', then they pushed her violently to a cell wall (behind the cameras) causing her to twist her neck, shoulder and arm. After being worked over, they took away her jacket, shoes, socks, and toilet paper, and locked her up. Her holding cell was extremely cold and she was deliberately denied toilet paper. She asked for toilet paper, only to be answered it must have been taken for good reason and she was not getting any. She was denied toilet paper from approximately 3:30pm until 11:00pm. One has to wonder, what was she going to do with the toilet paper, hang herself? By 11:00 pm Laurie got taken to be assessed. She asked 'is this a madhouse run by animals, who is running this place?' Laurie told this officer her story for half an hour. He let her talk, then said he sees all kinds of characters, his job is to ascertain threats. He told her she has the fire, the spirit and the power to overturn the system and create a riot. He informed her she'd be put in solitary confinement, but she might get a roommate, probably a drug offender. She was forced to take a chest X-ray against her will, without any explanation. Laurie was eventually released after five days.'

After a lengthy legal dispute Chad was eventually allowed to make his own decisions. Laurie and Chad Jessop have since then set up a foundation—the C.H.A.D. (Choosing Health Alternatives Deliberately) Foundation—to press for changes to the law to enable greater freedom of choice in the state of California.

This story echoes an earlier story involving a boy called Abraham Cherrix. Born in June 1990, Cherrix was 16 when he became the object of a court case in Louisville, Kentucky, the objective of which was to force him, against his wishes, to undergo conventional medical treatment in the form of chemotherapy for his Hodgkin's Disease—one of the few cancers that is indeed responsive to chemotherapy. In 2005, Cherrix had already undergone a round of chemo treatments, but a year later he was told the cancer had returned and that he needed to undergo a second round. Initially he agreed and had one chemo session but then, because of the side effects, he decided to stop. His parents supported this decision and as a result they were taken to court for medical neglect of their child. They eventually won their case on appeal. This case eventually resulted in a new law—dubbed Abraham's Law—that increases the rights of patients aged 14–17 to refuse medical treatments in the state of Kentucky.

FDA attempts to suppress the alternative health industry

In August 2011, Natural News (www.naturalnews.com) reported on the US Food and Drug Administration's (FDA) 'long history of conducting armed, SWAT-style raids on farmers, cancer treatment pioneers and dietary supplement manufacturers.' They published a long list of raids, which they argued demonstrated 'a pattern of government-sponsored terrorism against innocent Americans and small business people; all done in the name of "protecting" the public from milk, walnuts, vitamins, plants or fruit extracts. The real reason behind all this, of course, is that the FDA has long waged a campaign of fear and intimidation against natural product providers for the sole purpose of destroying the natural products industry and thereby handing Big Pharma a monopoly over health treatment medicines.' *Further details of these farm raids can be found at the Farm-to-Consumer Legal Defense Fund* website at www.ftcldf.org/farm-raids.html.

Here are details of some of these raids:

1985, July 7. FDA agents raided the Burzynski Research Clinic (Texas), took 200,000 medical and research documents, and forced Dr Stanislaw Burzynski to pay for copies of these to be made of them. No official charges are ever filed by the FDA.

1987, February 26. 25 armed FDA agents and US Marshals stormed the offices of the Life Extension Foundation (Florida), terrorized employees and seized thousands of nutritional products, materials, computers, files, and newsletters. 80 per cent of these seized items were later determined not to even have been on the warrant. The FDA later filed 56 criminal charges against Foundation officers Saul Kent and William Faloon. After 11 years in and out of court all the charges were eventually dismissed.

1988, November. FDA agents raided Traco Labs (Illinois) and seized several drums of black currant oil as well as many containers of capsules. The FDA claimed the capsules that the oil was being put into were an 'unapproved food additive'. The judge ruled that the FDA's definition of 'food additive' was too broad, so that even water added to food would be considered a food additive.

1989, Summer. FDA agents seized the entire inventory and business records of Pets Smell Free (Utah), a company that produces a natural product for eliminating pet odour. The company later won a lawsuit against the FDA.

1990, October 6. Federal agents raided HA Lyons (Arizona), a home-based mailing service that published materials for vitamin companies. Armed agents seized all business records and literature, and even tried to steal the owner's cheque book and cash. The FDA eventually drove the company out of business.

1990, Autumn. FDA agents raided Highland Laboratories (Oregon), a company that produced vitamins and nutritional supplements. The agents did not present a warrant, but proceeded to seize everything except for the office furniture, and threatened the employees with violence if they failed to comply.

1990, March. FDA agents—without a warrant—raided Solid Gold Pet Foods (California), seized all pet food products, and shut down the store. Owner Sissy Harrington-McGill was later tried and convicted of violating the Health Claims Law, a law that did not exist at the time of the raid and was never passed by the US Congress. She was sentenced to 179 days in prison and fined $10,000 for, as Natural News put it, 'daring to say that vitamins are good for puppy dogs!'

1990. Agents from both the FDA and US Postal Service twice raided Century Clinic (Nevada), and seized chelation products, computers, and various other equipment. No official charges were ever filed against the clinic.

1991, Autumn. FDA agents raided Scientific Botanicals (Washington), a nutritional supplement company, and seized herbal extracts and literature. The company agreed to comply with FDA demands in return for the release of the seized products.

1991, December 12. FDA agents raided Thorne Research (Idaho)—a respected vitamin manufacturer—and seized $20,000 worth of vitamin products, and 11,000 pieces of literature. Unable to afford to defend a law suit, the company agreed to stop publishing literature.

1991. FDA agents raided NutriCology (California), a nutritional supplement company. All FDA injunctions against it were later tossed out of court.

1991. Bounty hunters, in collaboration with the FBI, kidnapped Jimmy Keller from Mexico, took him back to the USA where he was arrested for 'wire fraud' and sent to prison for two years. Keller having cured his own cancer through alternative methods had opened a perfectly legal clinic in Tijuana Mexico. The wire fraud charges resulted from telephone calls to patients living in the US.

1991. Agents from the FDA and the Texas Department of Health again raided the Burzynski Research Clinic (Texas), and seized products and materials. Dr Burzynski eventually won the resulting court case. Burzynski's war with the FDA was to continue for many years and a documentary of his battles has recently been made—see www.burzynskimovie.com for further details.

1992, May 6. Agents from the FDA and officers from the King County Police Department raided the Tahoma Clinic (Washington), a natural health clinic. Dr Jonathan Wright had been giving patients injectable B vitamins in high doses. Agents entered the clinic with guns drawn, and seized products, computers and records. The FDA showed no valid warrant to justify its actions and no court case resulted. Natural News commented: 'The purpose of the FDA raid was clearly not to arrest Dr Wright, who was never charged. Rather, the purpose appears to be conducting a campaign of terror: sending a message to the alternative medicine community that anyone engaged in nutritional treatments could be raided and shut down, with no legal justification.'

1992, June 30. FDA agents raided Nature's Way (Utah), a vitamin and nutritional supplement company, and seized bulk containers of primrose oil because the addition of vitamin E to the formula was allegedly 'unapproved'.

1992, June. The FDA prompted the Texas Department of Health to conduct raids on numerous health food stores throughout Texas. They seized natural oils, aloe vera, zinc, vitamin C, and other natural products. No valid warrants were presented, and no charges were ever filed against the stores. None of the confiscated products were ever returned. Later that year the FDA announced that they were going to ban a wide range of supplements, but 24 million people sent letters and made phone calls to their Congressmen to protest and the FDA withdrew the proposed legislation. Although there were further raids on vitamin producers during the rest of 1992 and into 1993 this setback eventually forced the FDA to redefine its goals. The new targets were largely organic farms and co-operatives selling raw milk.

2006, March 6. Ohio police, Ohio Department of Agriculture officials, FDA agents, and agents from unmarked vehicles intercepted a raw milk pickup in the Cincinnati area. They confiscated milk and harassed customers, leaving farm owner Gary Oakes so shaken up that he had to be hospitalized three times for panic attacks caused by post-traumatic stress disorder.

2006, October 6. Armed agents from the FBI and FDA arrived at Growers Express (California), a produce company, and began searching the premises for evidence that the company's bagged spinach might be linked to an E. coli outbreak. Agents never even tried contacting the company prior the raid, and found nothing in violation of any statute, regulation or law.

2006, October 13. Michigan Department of Agriculture agents and police officers stopped Richard Hebron on the way to deliver raw milk to cow share owners. Agents seized his cell phone and wallet, and proceeded to unload 453 gallons of fresh milk from his truck. A six-month investigation found Hebron innocent, but was charged a $1,000 'administrative' fee.

And on and on. The raids have continued.

Comment

We see that these raids are essentially a form of harassment—and the question has to be asked whether or not taxpayers should be paying the salaries of people who see their jobs as giving them the right to use extra-legal means to enforce corporate agendas—because the FDA is very much in bed with the big pharmaceutical companies. On retirement it is standard practice for senior officers of the FDA to get well-paid jobs as non-executive directors of major drug companies.

What also emerges from these stories is that the underswell of public opinion can be harnessed effectively, and that it has moved the game on. Vitamin suppliers are not being hassled as they once were. But the game will never be won absolutely as long as big corporations with government agencies in their pockets keep thinking of new ways to undermine health freedom.

The raw milk issue

'If we are not even free anymore to decide something as basic as what we wish to eat or drink, how much freedom do we really have left?'—Rep. Ron Paul

This is becoming something of an issue in the USA. Raw milk means unpasteurised organic milk. Some people believe that raw milk is healthier for you than pasteurised milk and they want to have access to it. Many people are participating in food co-operatives in order to have the raw milk they wish to have. There appear to be some minor health issues in relation to raw milk but the arguments are balanced by the fact that there is also evidence that children who drink raw milk are less susceptible to allergies. However, the FDA is so concerned about the issue that it has banned the interstate sale of raw milk for human consumption. The ban began in 1987, but the FDA didn't really begin enforcing it seriously until 2006. Since then there have been a number of incidents such as those that follow—none of which involve 'interstate sales' which is the limit of FDA's authority.

On 14 Oct 2010, an LAPD police squad raided Rawesome, an organic food co-operative, with guns drawn, because it was selling raw milk. The raid was conducted as if the police were raiding an illegal drug den and expected resistance. You can see a video of the raid at the Treehugger.com website. It would be funny if it weren't sad.

This was not the first raid on a food co-operative by armed police. On the morning of December 1, 2008, police raided The Manna Storehouse, an organic food co-op in LaGrange, Ohio owned and operated by John and Jackie Stowers. Law enforcement officers used force to enter the Stowers' residence without first announcing they were police or stating the purpose of the visit. With guns drawn, they swiftly and immediately moved to the upstairs of the home, where ten children were in the middle of a home-schooling lesson. Officers then moved Jacqueline Stowers and her children to their living room, where they were held for more than six hours.

A year later, the Stowers are charging the state and county with 119 complaints including unlawful search and seizure, illegal use of state police power, taking of private property without compensation, failure to provide due process and equal protection, and denial of their inalienable rights guaranteed under the Constitution, including their right to grow and eat their own food and offer it to others.

The reason I have mentioned these stories is not that I support the use of raw milk. I do however support the rights of others to drink raw milk if that's what they want to drink, just as I support the rights of parents not to vaccinate their children—another area of enormous contention. I believe we should all have certain rights to eat and drink what we wish to eat and drink. The desire of various police departments and federal US agencies to over-react in the way that they have is quite simply scary and needs to be resisted strenuously.

At the same time that the FDA is pressurising police departments to take these actions, it is resisting calls for tighter regulation of artificial colourings despite clear evidence that they can have a negative effect on children. The FDA argues that there is no proof that foods with artificial colourings cause hyperactivity in most children. Although it acknowledges that children with behavioural problems can worsen their symptoms by eating foods with synthetic colouring.

Consistency? Yes. The FDA has consistently sided with big business and has shown willingness in the top management echelons to bend regulations when pressured to do so by large corporations. This 'corruption' is so evident that even the FDA's own employees have protested publicly. In January 2009, anonymous FDA employees released a letter containing strong accusations of corruption. In the letter, the authors concluded:

> 'America urgently needs change at FDA because FDA is fundamentally broken, failing to fulfil its mission, and because re-establishing a proper and effectively functioning FDA is vital to the health of the nation.'

Further details of this letter can be found on the internet. The FDA itself has confirmed that the letter is authentic.

Greg Caton's story

I want you to imagine that you have found a herb that cures cancer. What would you do about it? If you were an ethical person you would certainly tell the world about your discovery. You might even make it available for people.

That is what Greg Caton did. He made a 'black salve' preparation, with bloodroot herb as its main ingredient, which he called Cansema. In 1999, the FDA took note of his actions and as a result of their investigations Caton was arrested, tried and found guilty. He was sentenced to 33 months in prison. When he was released he was put on probation for a further three years. While serving his probation, Caton discovered that an FDA agent was pressuring people to testify against him in order to have him convicted of further charges. Caton then fled to Ecuador where he established legal residence. Still he was not safe from the FDA. In 2009, he was effectively kidnapped and flown back to the USA, where once again he has been tried and imprisoned.

One fact that Caton has continually, but unsuccessfully, attempted to use in his defence is the fact that Cansema works. It cures cancer. As Dr Brian O'Leary, who was cured using Cansema has stated:

> *'On the larger issue of the suppression of alternative possibilities in the health, environmental and technology fields, we see a pattern emerging that the true geniuses of innovation are all too often violently suppressed by authorities who illegally, unethically and immorally punish these true pioneers of our time—solely because of powerful vested interests that are far less effective in solving the problems presented.'—Dr Brian O'Leary*

I couldn't have put it better myself.

Alternative cancer clinics

While some cancer clinics offering non-orthodox therapies appear to be able to operate in the USA, Germany, France, England and elsewhere, very often they find themselves blocked or harassed. This is particularly true of the USA. The result has been that a number of clinics have gone off-shore—mostly to the town of Tijuana, Mexico —a town conveniently located just across the US-Mexican border close to San Diego. Often there will be a presence of sorts in the USA. For example, Dr Vincent Gammill has offices in Solana Beach, near San Diego, California, registered as the Center for the Study of Natural Oncology (www.natural-oncology.org), where, as he says: 'Primarily we just research and problem solve.' However, he is associated with the San Diego Clinic in Tijuana (www.sdiegoclinic.com). I mention this, as Dr Gammill is very approachable and has a lot of fans. However, there are many other clinics, many of which also have their supporters. There are far too many to list here, but anyone looking for one will find lists of clinics at the following internet links:

www.cancure.org/directory_mexican_clinics.htm
www.cancure.org/directory_clinics_outside%20US.htm
www.cancertutor.com/Other/Clinics.html
www.cancercure.ws/clinics.htm
www.annieappleseedproject.org/gerclinstor.html
www.CancerControlSociety.com
www.ThirdOpinionGuide.com.

China is a beacon of freedom

I hope that heading got your attention. It's a sad day indeed when China can claim to be freer than the USA or Europe—but in the area of medical freedoms that is certainly the case. China's long tradition of traditional herbal medicine and other healing practices from acupuncture to qi gong ensures that these freedoms will persist—as they will also in Indonesia, Malaysia, Thailand and the other countries of South East Asia. That is why Chris Teo has been free to run his clinic in Penang without any official harassment. 'I could not do what I do if I were living in the States,' he told me. 'Here, in Malaysia, I'm free to say what I want. I can give herbs. I can say I can help people who have cancer with herbs. I can sell them the herbs. I'm very lucky that the situation in Malaysia is sane. What is happening in America is not sane. It is completely insane.'

How dangerous is the medical system?

'More people die in US hospitals every year from medical errors than they do from industrial accidents, car accidents or AIDS' says Lee Clarke, a sociologist at Rutgers University. Is this true?
The figures for 2007 are as follows:

Total Deaths:	2.4 million
Heart disease:	600,000 (25%)
Cancer:	560,000 (24%)
All accidents (car, work, home etc):	124,000 (5%)
Suicide:	34,000 (1.4%)
Murder:	18,000 (0.8%)
AIDS (figure not easily obtained)	estimated 18,000 (max)

And medical error? According to *Scientific American* magazine (Aug 10, 2009): 'Preventable medical mistakes and infections are responsible for about 200,000 deaths in the US each year' (around 8.5 per cent). This would make it the third major cause of death in the USA. On top of that, over 100,000 die from 'adverse drug reactions'—that is, they die from properly taking the drug properly given to them. But this is just the tip of the iceberg. According to the US Institute of Medicine (2006) at least 1.5 million Americans are 'sickened, injured or killed' by errors in prescribing, dispensing and taking medication.

We can see that Lee Clarke, quoted above, was not quite accurate in his statement. He should have said: 'More people die in US hospitals every year from medical errors than they do from industrial accidents, car accidents, murder, suicide and AIDS combined.'

In Britain, the NHS reported only 11,000 deaths or injuries due to medical error. In light of the statistics emanating from other countries, either Britain is a paragon of medical care or there is serious under-reporting going on. However, Charles Vincent, head of the clinical risk unit at University College London, estimates that the true figure is around 40,000 (or about eight per cent of the total).

An Australian Government report into the situation in that country found that not only was preventable medical error responsible for 11 per cent of all deaths (i.e. one death in nine) but that when you added in all the deaths from 'properly researched, properly registered, properly prescribed and properly used drugs' then the total of deaths due to medical practice came to about 19 per cent (one in five). (*British Medical Journal* Nov 11, 2000)

Summing up

There is a war out there—and in some ways it appears to be a very one-sided war. The entire apparatus of government and law appear to be aimed against anyone who wishes to make basic health decisions that are at variance with the officially-approved options. But, as always, the reality is a great deal murkier.

Firstly, there is an enormous groundswell—and a growing one—in which people are becoming more and more dissatisfied with the failings of medicine. They see it is not working. There will come a time when the orthodox medical views will be held in such overwhelming disrepute that change will come—and it will be revolutionary change.

Let's face it, Codex will never change the medical systems of India, China or even the more malleable nations of South-East Asia, for the simple reason is that their native herbal systems are so embedded in the fabric of their cultures that it will be impossible. The US government may be able to exert pressures on foreign legislatures but who will enforce them? We are, as ever, sitting on a rolling wave.

Already Sedgwick and a number of other towns in Maine have passed local laws guaranteeing their residents the right to 'food sovereignty'. The town declared its right, and that of its residents, to produce and sell local foods of their choosing, without the oversight of State or federal regulation. It is actions such as these that will bring us to a saner place a hundred years from now.

In the meantime, you have to protect yourself. And the only way you can do that is by educating yourself. I leave you with these words that have been attributed to the Buddha:

'Believe nothing just because a so-called wise person said it. Believe nothing just because a belief is generally held. Believe nothing just because it is said in ancient books. Believe nothing just because it is said to be of divine origin. Believe nothing just because someone else believes it. Believe only what you yourself test and judge to be true.'

Cancer: Detox and Diet

Detoxification and diet are the twin platforms for any long-term strategy for recovering from cancer. But what detox? What diets? And why? What's the rationale? What foods should we avoid? What foods are healing? What about the other food-based anti-cancer regimes? In this section I will be looking at the many forms of detoxification and the diets that you might wish to consider. Unless you believe cancer came from nowhere, and that removal or obliteration of a tumour has solved the problem, then you will want to put in place a regime that will lead to a state that can be described as free from cancer and a state where you will again feel alive and healthy. The first stop on the way to that place is by undergoing a regime of detox and diet. This section provides you with the options you should be thinking about.

Detoxification

The food and drink we consume and the air we breathe are all contaminated with chemicals that we would normally not choose to take into our bodies. The more toxic our bodies, the less able they are to be brought back to a state of health. If we want a cancer-free body, we need to help the body to become cleansed internally. That means detox. Here are some of the procedures people with cancer should be thinking about.

Colon cleansing

'There is a definite correlation between breast cancer and chronic constipation. My own observation leaves no doubt about this. There is hardly a case of breast cancer with good bowel function.'

Prof. Serge Jurasunas

Purification of the liver is the key step to a cancer-free existence. But before we look at liver detoxification, it is reasonable to ask what causes toxicity in the liver and so dysfunctional in the first place. The answer is poor elimination of waste in the colon. Poisonous materials are trapped in the large intestine and reabsorbed back into the bloodstream where they again go through an increasingly weakened liver. As it becomes less and less able to keep up the work of cleaning the blood, the whole body becomes more toxified. According to Professor Serge Jurasunas, writing in the Townsend Letter for Doctors and Patients, 'There is a definite correlation between breast cancer and chronic constipation. My own observation leaves no doubt about this. There is hardly a case of breast cancer with good bowel function.'

If you attempt to clean your liver, blood, or lymph system without first addressing a waste filled bowel, the excreted toxins will only get recycled back into your body. So, before attempting to detoxify the liver, you need first to cleanse the colon.

There are a number of different approaches to resolving this problem. Enemas help clean out the end of the colon, colonic irrigation helps clean the whole of the large intestine using warm water pumped in under pressure, and there is colonic cleansing which uses herbs or clay to achieve the same object.

The most famous exponent of colon health was Norman W Walker. On the first page of his book *Colon Health: the Key to a Vibrant Life* (1991), he says: 'Few of us realize that failure to effectively eliminate waste products from the body causes so much fermentation and putrefaction in the large intestine, or colon, that the neglected accumulation of such waste can, and frequently does, result in a lingering demise.'

Norman Walker's prescription for a healthy life included half-yearly colonics, vitamin C, and raw vegetable juices—particularly carrot juice. Since he lived actively to the age of 109, it is hard to argue with him. Clearly he was doing something right.

An efficient colon will eliminate food 16–24 hours after it has been ingested. Very few American or British intestines work at this rate. According to the Dunn Nutritional Institute at Cambridge, they average 60 hours, and five days is not unusual. In France, studies indicate that over 35 per cent of the population suffers from constipation regularly. According to the 1991 National Health Interview Survey, about 4.5 million people in the United States say they are constipated most or all of the time.

Colonic therapist Pauline Noakes, likens the situation to having the dustmen permanently on strike so that the rubbish piles up in the street.

'Many people don't realize they are carrying around impacted faecal matter in their colons and that their lack of energy, their irritability, their aches and pains … and various ailments are due to the toxic waste in the bowel.' (P Noakes, *Positive Health* magazine, April/May 1995)

There is evidence to support this view. Two doctors from University of California, Nicholas Petrakis and Eileen King, writing in *The Lancet* in 1982, reported that they had studied the breast fluids of 5,000 women. They had found that women who had two or fewer bowel movements per week had four times the risk of breast disease (benign or malignant) as those who had one or more bowel movements per day. They also found that the bowels of people who ate meat contained greater amounts of mutagenic (potentially harmful) substances than did those of people who abstained from eating meat.

Enemas can be undertaken at home with an enema kit bought at a pharmacy. Easier and more effective is to go to a colonic cleansing clinic, but make sure the person giving the therapy is a registered colonic therapist.

And how do you feel after a colonic? Carol Signorella, writing in *Cosmopolitan* magazine, October 1979 wrote: 'After a year of colonics, my appearance and energy levels were both radically improved. No more draggy mornings or late afternoon slumps. I seem to think more clearly now and I need less sleep. In a word my body and mind feel marvellously clean.'

Wouldn't laxatives work just as well? The answer is a definite no. Colonics clean out the large intestine but laxatives also interfere with the small intestine which is where digestion and absorption of nutrients occur. Also laxatives are, in a sense, addictive—for them to continue to be effective, you need to take larger and larger doses.

A word of caution: colon hydrotherapy is not suitable for people with the following conditions: severe cardiac disease, aneurysm, severe anaemia, severe haemorrhoids, cirrhosis, carcinoma of the colon, fistulas, advanced pregnancy, kidney problems and hernia.

There are perfectly good alternatives to a full colonic. One is to drink a colon cleansing treatment. A suspension of bentonite mud and dried psyllium husks does a good job of taking waste material out of the digestive system. Those who like a ready-mixed product will find any number on the Internet. One that boasts a lot of testimonials can be found at www.drnatura.com.

However, when doing colonic cleansing it is important to replace electrolytes, perhaps by drinking raw fruit and vegetable juices. This needs to be stressed: you must replace electrolytes after any form of detoxification procedure.

Magnesium oxide

Magnesium oxide is one of the best and easiest ways to flush out the intestines. When mixed with water it produces large amounts of oxygen. In the intestine, the effect of this is to promote healthy aerobic bacteria and at the same time inhibit the growth of unhealthy anaerobic bacteria and fungi (especially Candida albicans).

The freed oxygen in magnesium oxide reacts with hydrogen to form water in the intestinal tract. This helps to soften and cleanse the intestine's contents and walls. Unlike other laxatives, magnesium oxide is both safe and gentle.

Magnesium oxide is a white powder. Dissolve half a teaspoon in a glass of water. Add lemon juice or cider vinegar as desired and drink on an empty stomach. This can be repeated several times a day. The aim is to achieve two or three bowel movements a day.

It is safe to use on a regular basis but anyone doing so should ensure their potassium and electrolyte levels don't fall too low. Drinking fresh fruit juices will help achieve this.

Charcoal

Charcoal is a traditional remedy for many gastric and other ailments. It is used for resolving dysentery and eliminating stomach upsets. Less well known is the fact that has a wide ranging action that is both healing and detoxifying. For all types of skin ailments including cancer, it can be used externally in a poultice (mix olive oil and charcoal powder and soak a cloth in the mix. Add a heating pad to help absorption through the skin). Charcoal, taken both internally and externally, has been successfully used against a variety of cancers and can help reduce swellings of the lymphatic system. A good source of charcoal powder is www.buyactivatedcharcoal.com.

Castor oil

For a stronger purging of the contents of the intestines, castor oil is highly recommended. A few tablespoons mixed with juice or water should be sufficient. It has memorably been described as WD40 (a brand of household cleansing and lubricating oil) for the gastro-intestinal system.

Naturally, for obvious reasons, no laxative or purgative should be taken during pregnancy.

Once the colon has been flushed out, it is important to maintain a regular and frequent pattern of elimination. Twice a day is considered healthy. Unfortunately, constipation is a problem that seems to go hand in hand with the Western diet. Green drinks filled with enzymes (see below) are one answer to regular bowel movements. A couple of apples a day should also do the trick.

Castor oil as a healing oil

On the subject of castor oil, you should note that it is a healing oil in its own right—and can be applied continuously—particularly to any tumour on the surface but also for cancers lying below the surface. Famously, castor oil was promoted by the mystic Edgar Cayce, whose instructions on how to make a castor oil pack was as follows: 'Heat the oil; dipping two, three to four layers of flannel in same, wring out and apply directly to the body.'

Castor oil is also a solvent, so it is possible to add other ingredients to the oil and these will also soak into the tissues through the skin. Some use raw crushed ginger and I personally have used tea tree oil, propolis and the grapefruit seed extract, Citricidal, to very good effect against a fungal infection. Herbalist Dr Richard Schulze promotes the use of cayenne pepper tincture. There are stories on the Internet claiming that castor oil has cured even deep seated cancers such as carcinoma of the kidneys.

Cellular drainage therapy

The argument for cellular drainage therapy is this: once we have flushed the colon out we can now start to address the problems of the liver. Can you mop up a pool of water with a soggy sponge? Obviously not. You first have to eliminate all the water from the sponge before it can useful help mop up further water. The cells of the liver are the same. If each cell is full of toxic matter, then these cells need to be regenerated first before any other detoxification activity is initiated. Cellular drainage works on detoxification at the level of each individual cell.

However, even good hydration will not necessarily eliminate all toxins. If blood circulation is sluggish, and organs such as the kidney and liver are compromised for any reason, then toxin loads may build up within cells. To help drain these toxins from the cells, certain herbs are used that help to stimulate blood flow and release toxins. These will be given as homoeopathic remedies.

Naturopaths and homoeopaths can advise you which drainage remedies might be suitable. Although there are a number of websites that sell products for those wishing to self-treat, it is more common to find a naturopath who is able to do a meridian stress assessment using EAV (electro-acupuncture) equipment. They will then be able to assess the specific toxins that need to be eliminated and, in addition, also provide the remedies.

If all of this seems altogether too esoteric, you might want to consider using as a cellular flush a form of water, marketed under the name of Crystal Energy. I describe this more fully in the discussion on water below.

Panchakarma

Panchakarma is essentially a detoxification process—and is central to Ayurvedic medicine. The first step in Panchakarma is the use of herbal oils (either internally or using massage) to initiate the purification process. The second step is to heat the body using specific steam and warm oil therapies.

This therapeutic heat is intended to drive toxins out of the tissues into the intestinal tract. The third step is to eliminate the toxins that have accumulated. This is accomplished by the use of gentle herbal enemas, known as bastis, and gentle cleansing of the upper respiratory tract and sinuses, known as nasya. The Panchakarma treatments are administered over a period of several consecutive days (up to 14 days), and are said to have a profound detoxifying and deeply purifying effect.

A growing number of Ayurvedic resources can be found on the Internet. A good website for Ayurvedic information is www.ayurvedacancercare.com.

Liver flush

'Cancer can be reversed and controlled only if we regenerate the liver.'

Dr Harold Manner

The liver is the largest internal organ of the body. It processes all pharmaceuticals and supplements. However, the liver can be weakened by the overload of toxins. When the liver no longer is able to do its job, you will feel this in a number of ways: low energy levels, digestive problems, depression, headaches, dizziness, joint pain, sleeping disorders, dry skin or eczema, irritability, PMS—and cancer.

The purpose of a liver flush is to flush poisons out of the body and so help its own regeneration.

Orthodox surgeons pour scorn on the idea that a poorly functioning liver has anything to do with the development of cancer, but most complementary health practitioners disagree. So, in fact, do some orthodox doctors. Dr Harold Manner has absolutely no doubt that liver dysfunction is the root of the problem: 'The livers of cancer patients have become clogged with many of the poisons they were meant to eliminate …. Cancer can be reversed and controlled only if we regenerate the liver. Fortunately for us, the liver is the one organ in the body capable of regenerating itself.'

Herbalist, Christopher Hobbs, in his book *Foundations of Health*, recommends the following flush.

1. Squeeze oranges or grapefruit or other citrus fruit to make a cup of liquid.
2. Add 2 cloves of garlic freshly squeezed and a small amount of ginger juice—made by grating fresh ginger and squeezing it in a garlic press.
3. Add a table spoon of good quality olive oil.
4. Shake it vigorously and drink.
5. Follow with one or two glasses of herbal tea made with the following: equal parts of fennel, flax, fenugreek and peppermint with one quarter parts of burdock and liquorice. Simmer in water for 20 minutes.

He recommends drinking this mixture first thing in the morning after some stretching exercises and then not eating for at least an hour. He suggests doing this for two cycles of ten days at a time separated by three days at least twice a year but more frequently as required.

Epsom salts

Epsom salts are a more drastic way to flush the liver, specifically to eliminate gallstones. It is recommended that you have a bath in dissolved Epsom salts every day for a week or more before taking them internally so as to allow the body to absorb magnesium—magnesium deficiency being very common.

Another liver flush suggestion

Drink two glasses of organic apple juice every two hours for two days, eating only fruits and vegetables. At the end of the two days, have one to two tablespoons of Epsom salts dissolved in water, followed by half a cup of olive oil with lemon juice at bedtime.

Apple juice is high in malic acid, which acts as a solvent. Epsom salts relax smooth muscle and will relax and dilate the bile duct to enable larger solid particles to pass through. Unrefined olive oil stimulates the gall bladder and bile duct to contract and expel its contents.

Herbs and liver support

A number of herbs are also specifically recommended to support liver function, particularly burdock, dandelion, milk thistle, rosemary and sage. A number of herbal combinations are sold as specific liver cleansers.

Having said all this, there are many who think a liver flush is too extreme—and should not be done if there is any risk that the cancer has spread to the liver. Instead of a flush, a diet of fruit and vegetables—no meat, dairy or grain—will be naturally detoxifying in itself. Freshly juiced carrots and beetroot are also very beneficial to the liver.

Liver detox using coffee enemas

The doctors who treated my wife found the concept of coffee enemas to be particularly worthy of ridicule. However, it is an established method favoured by many, if not most, alternative practitioners for helping to cleanse and stimulate the liver and so help it in its work in removing toxins. It is particularly associated with the Gerson approach discussed later in this section.

It is important to remember that if cancer tumours begin to break down, they release toxins into the body and an already weakened liver may easily become overloaded. People have died in this way from the overly powerful healing effects of vitamins and herbs. There is a direct connection between the lower colon just before the rectum and the liver. Coffee that is taken in as an enema is held for as long as possible—15–20 minutes. The coffee helps to cleanse the liver. Several enemas a day may be required. There are a number of re-usable enema kits on the market which come with clear instructions on how to use them. There are also special coffees designed to be used for this purpose. A Google search for 'coffee enema' will provide many sources of equipment.

Having said this, however, you should not do more than one or two enemas a day at most (unless directed by a practitioner). The rectum is very efficient at absorbing whatever is put in it—hence the value of suppositories. Coffee enemas can result in a sudden lowering of blood levels of sodium, potassium and chloride electrolytes. This can have very harmful consequences. Dr Robert Buckman, in his book *Magic or Medicine*, blames over-zealous use of coffee enemas for two deaths. It was not the coffee but the water that had the negative impact. As with colonic cleansing, it is important to replace electrolytes, perhaps by drinking raw fruit and vegetable juices immediately afterwards.

Warning: coffee should be mildly tepid (not hot!)—some people have suffered painful rectal burning by doing enemas with hot coffee.

Castor oil packs

Castor Oil packs have been around for a long time—and perhaps because castor oil seems, well, so common, that we under-estimate its healing potential. There is a strong view held by many doctors following natural therapy, that what kills cancer patients is a toxic overload of the liver. One way to relieve this overload is to place a cotton tea towel or piece of t-shirt soaked in castor oil (preferable slightly warmed—but take care not to burn yourself!) and then to place it at the lower back area—held in place by kitchen wrap and a heating pad on top (hot water bottle?). This will draw toxins out and at the same time you will get the other benefits of castor oil.

MSM

MSM (or methylsulfonylmethane) is a natural sulfur that is found in fruits and vegetables. This organic sulfur is lost when food is processed, heated or dried. High sulfur foods include asparagus, broccoli, red pepper, garlic, and onion, but cooking tends to destroy it, so many people take MSM as a convenient replacement.

MSM has a detoxing effect—and quite a strong one. Many people taking it complain of headaches—but as MSM also naturally occurs in the body there is little danger of overdosing—the headaches are a Herxheimer reaction to toxins being released into the bloodstream from the liver. So feeling bad (temporarily) is a sign that things are improving (hopefully long term). Other negative side effects are stomach discomfort and slight diarrhoea. Drink plenty of water as this will help your body flush out the toxins easier.

MSM also makes cell membranes more permeable. This helps in the delivery of nutrients as well as the removal of toxins from cells. People who take it report an immediate increase in energy, which is why it is best to take it in the morning rather than late at night. MSM is best taken with vitamin C and CoQ10.

In terms of dosage, start with one tablespoon of powder a day and slowly increase this until you experience a negative effect then cut back.

Cleansing the lymph system: lymphatic massage

Lymph is a clear fluid that travels through the body's arteries and tissues to cleanse them. It circulates through the lymphatic system.

Lymph nodes are the filters along the lymphatic system. Their job is to filter out and trap bacteria, viruses, cancer cells, and other unwanted substances, and to make sure they are safely eliminated from the body.

Lymphatic massage is a light touch technique used since the 1930s to promote health and aid recovery from illness. It is also called lymphatic drainage. Lymphatic massage is used to promote general wellness. It is a gentle technique which prevents or reduces fluid retention, and enhances the removal of toxins from body tissues.

The lymph vessels are just under the skin, so moving the lymph requires a very light touch. Lymphatic massage is widely available and is practiced by most massage therapists.

However, for the cancer patient, lymphatic massage is best done with extreme lightness of touch—preferably under the guidance of a trained professional—as there is a danger—theoretical but not proven—of promoting the spread of cancer cells. However, this danger should not be exaggerated. Lymphatic massage promotes the movement of lymph towards the chest where it becomes exposed to highly oxygenated blood capillaries that surround the lungs—which in turn are likely to kill off any circulating microscopic metastases. The dangers of a static lymphatic system are far more serious.

Also, for those who have had some form of radiation or removal of lymph glands there is a danger of promoting or worsening any existing oedema—which is caused by lymph being unable to drain away, so causing painful swelling. Further suggestions for dealing with lymphoedema can be found in Section 2.

Strong massage is contraindicated only in association with high-dose enzyme therapy, with melanoma, or if someone is immune-compromised from chemotherapy or radiation, or suffers from a clotting disorder. But even those patients can have a light massage.

The importance of human touch is well-known. Babies die if they are not properly cosseted. Massage is an important therapy that should not be neglected.

The benefits of rebounding

Bouncing on a rebounder—a mini-trampoline—is another good way of getting the lymphatic system moving and boosting the immune system. You don't have to bounce energetically, just raising and lowering the heels to set up a rhythmic bounce is sufficient. Some people do this for 30–60 minutes a day while watching television. Some have taken to calling this exercise 'lymphasizing'—exercising the lymph!

Oil pulling

This is a simple Ayurvedic technique for which powerful long-term health benefits are claimed. Using only sesame or sunflower oil, take a tablespoon of oil into the mouth and suck, swirl and swish it round the whole mouth for around 15 minutes. Then spit the oil out (it has become toxic). This is particularly recommended for anyone with gum disease but is beneficial to everyone who is ill in any way. It is well accepted that oral infections and gum disease have a powerfully negative impact on the heart and may be implicated in cancer. This is a cheap and simple health-promoting practice.

Skin brushing

The skin is the largest organ of the body, and is responsible for a quarter of the body's daily detoxification. Brushing the dry skin is a simple way of helping the lymph system to eliminate toxins. It also strengthens the immune system, stimulates the glands and even improves digestion. Skin brushing should be done with a long handled bristle brush made of natural materials. The skin should be dry, not wet, when brushed. Some practitioners recommend that the abdomen should be brushed in an anti-clockwise direction and other areas should be brushed towards the heart. Brush each part of the body several times vigorously—though breasts should be brushed lightly, avoiding the nipples which should not be brushed at all. Start with the soles of the feet because the nerve endings there affect the whole body, then the ankles, calves, and thighs, up across your buttocks stomach and chest. After the brushing session you can have a shower.

Hydrotherapy

Water is a powerful cleaning agent and the skin is an important organ for elimination of toxins. Putting these two together we get hydrotherapy. There are many forms. Saunas and steam baths are one form of hydrotherapy. Spend at least half an hour in the heat—but not continuously. Five- to fifteen-minute sessions are the norm. The purpose is not only to sweat out the poisons in the body. The heat itself acts as an immune system stimulator. Some health clinics will offer a hydrotherapy treatment involving wrapping the body in hot towels, but a hot bath at home—as hot as can be borne—can work just as well. Add one pound of baking soda and one pound of sea salt or deep mine salt (not standard table salt which is totally ineffective). Rock salt is not so good. Stay in the bath for 20–50 minutes and then have a quick shower to rub off the soda and salt. This is known as a detox (detoxification) bath. It is important with all these forms of hydrotherapy to drink lots of water—distilled, reverse osmosis or natural spring/mineral water—before, during and after the hydrotherapy sessions.

Water should also be drunk in large quantities every day. Many health experts warn that many of our problems arise from the fact that we are semi-permanently dehydrated. We drink coffee and tea and beers and so on, all of which are diuretic, causing water to be expelled from the body. Our blood and body's cells are absolutely dependent on an adequate supply of fresh, clean water. We need at least four pints (2.2l) a day. Some people think that many illnesses arise directly as a result of inadequate intake of water: asthma, allergies, diabetes, arthritis, angina, all intestinal problems and many degenerative diseases.

However, too much water can also be bad for us too, as that can dilute the sodium salts our cells need, so don't overdo it.

Water massage

Most spas offer water massage treatments in which you are massaged by jets of water, There are also 'dry hydrotherapy' machines that claim to boost oxygenation of the blood, eliminate toxins, reduce pain and muscular tension.

Alternating hot and cold showers

This is not a detox regime but a way of stimulating the metabolism of the body. Isolate the area where the tumour is located, and alternate showers of very cold and very hot (not scalding) water. Do this at frequent intervals.

The water question: what kind of water?

Up until now I have discussed a number of water-based procedures without confronting the elephant in the room—what kind of water? This is a subject that has created an enormous debate—so, let's look at the whole question of water.

First, it is strongly believed by many that tap water, chlorinated and/or fluoridated or simply heavy in calcium, is extremely unhealthy and interferes with the absorption of nutrients. The option generally argued for is pure distilled water. However, there is an opinion that distilled water leaches minerals from the system and would therefore lead to inevitable mineral deficiencies. Others say that if it does, it only leaches inorganic minerals that are potentially toxic to the body and so distilled water is doing the body a favour by removing them. Most health systems in fact promote the use of distilled or ionized water as the only water that should be drunk. However, there are others who are vehement that distilled water should be taken regularly only for a short period of time, because it does deplete the body of organic minerals—and also because distilled water is likely to be slightly acidic in its pH. There are also concerns that it is 'de-energized', unnatural and distorted in its molecular structure.

You see, there is no consensus. The danger of depletion of trace minerals is a serious matter—one proposed cure for cancer is to take in large amounts of trace minerals (see Percy Weston's story in Section 6: *Cancer: Vitamins and Other Supplements*). It has been pointed out that people who drink lots of bottled soft drinks (made with distilled water) are almost always mineral deficient.

Others have recommended various mineral or bottled waters—however, the plastic containers they come in contaminate the water with infinitely small amounts of chemical that act like the female hormone oestrogen (oestrogen mimics) and the heavy metal antinomy—and that is very bad news.

Also most mineral waters contain inorganic minerals that are of no use to the body. Bottled 'Spring Water' may be just tap water, or may come from a polluted source.

However, there are those who say that the answer is tap water fed through a simple home-based reverse osmosis filter, which filters out all the impurities. If this is the solution you opt for make sure you change the filter regularly. However, one applied kinesiologist I know has reported that reverse-osmosis water has been tested as dead and should be avoided. Perhaps better than a filter is to have an ozonating machine and run ozone through the water—this kills all microbes and at the same time substantially increases the oxygen content of the water—a big plus when we remember that cancer thrives in low environments characterized by low oxygen levels. Water heated in a microwave machine should be avoided at all costs.

To test the quality of water you are taking in you can plant seeds in two or more containers and water each container with a different type of water. Compare the health of the plants that grow from these seeds.

However, to leave the discussion there would be doing a great deal of disservice to water's potential as a healing agent in its own right. First of all we need to meditate on a simple truth: We are water. Or at least 70–80 per cent of us is water. Yet we tend to think of water, if at all, as something simple. Water is very far from being simple. In fact it is unique in many of its characteristics: It is one of the few natural substances whose solid form is lighter than its liquid form. It is also an extremely powerful solvent. Without these two characteristics life on Earth would be impossible.

As our bodies are composed very largely of water, dehydration is a matter of some concern. And there is strong evidence that the majority of people are almost permanently dehydrated. This is the conclusion of Dr Fereydoon Batmanghelidj, who argues in his book, *Your Body's Many Cries for Water*, that almost every ailment known to man can be cured by drinking half your body weight (as measured in pounds) in ounces of water. For example, a 200lb (90kg) man should drink 100 ounces (2.8l) of water a day, which is 12–13 standard 8-ounce (0.25l) glasses.

In addition for every cup of coffee or alcohol, you should drink two more of water. Further, for every four glasses of water you should take in a quarter teaspoon (1.25g) of unprocessed, mineral-rich sea salt. In fact, you can use this salt liberally on food as well. That's it. It's free and according to those who espouse it, it works. Dr Batmanghelidj claims that this can cure heart disease, asthma, rheumatism and many other conditions. He makes no claims with regard to cancer—but that is no surprise: cancer is a dangerous subject. In any case cancer cannot be cured in isolation from the health needs of the rest of the body.

Incidentally, Dr Batmanghelidj thinks ordinary tap water is generally fine.

Not all agree, however, that simple tap water will do. The problem, they say, is that no amount of drinking tap water will prevent this dehydration. Tap water is not taken into the cells efficiently. However, there is an opinion that the water melt from glaciers is an almost perfect form of living water containing suspensions, it is asserted, of trace minerals but no mineral salts. In this state, it is said, the water is able to saturate cells very quickly. So this source of water can be used as a form of cellular drainage therapy.

Two types of water have been developed that also help saturate cells fast. The first, developed by an American scientist, Dr Patrick Flanagan, is made by adding a microcluster of colloidal minerals to distilled water. This product has been patented under the name Crystal Energy. The result is a form of water that contains no dissolved mineral salts but contains a colloidal mix of many trace elements—just like the glacial melt waters on which it was modelled. For more information go to www.phisciences.com.

Another form of water that is claimed to be capable of saturating cells is known as Willard Water. This was initially developed as an industrial cleaner but it was discovered incidentally to have powerful pain-relieving qualities and an ability to speed up the healing process. This product is also known as catalyst-altered water. For more information about this product go to www.dr-willardswater.com.

Both of these waters are added to normal filtered water. For one thing, they ensure that nutrients are taken in by the cells very efficiently. In both cases, users are warned that drugs will act faster when taken in conjunction with either of these two forms of water.

There is a third treatment of water that is also of interest to the cancer patient: electrolysed (or ionized) water. This is a product that has been widely used in Japan for more than 25 years. Essentially, water is passed through an electrolytic process, which produces acidified and alkalized solutions. The acidic solution is a general all-purpose anti-microbial treatment that can be sprayed on food to keep it free of mould, and can be gargled or rubbed on the skin to treat herpes, acne, athletes foot and so on.

Of more interest to us is the alkalized water. As we shall see when we come to the discussion of diets, an acidic body state is unhealthy. Conversely, an alkaline state is good. For those with cancer, one mode of thought is that a quick fix is to speedily raise the pH value of the body's tissues. Cancers, according to this theory (for which there is a great deal of evidence), cannot survive in a highly alkaline bodily terrain. Drinking electrolyzed water is one way to raise the pH very quickly. At the time of writing a 32oz bottle costs around $20, which will provide about five days worth of water.

It is possible to purchase an ionizing water purifier that will allow you to create your own ionized alkaline water. There are many models on the market costing from $500–$2,000. There is also a water-vitalizing system which, according to the marketing blurb, creates hexagonal water which is more easily absorbed; see www.thewolfeclinic.com for details.

However, all these machines are very expensive and, arguably, are not needed at all. There is a very cheap and simple way to create an alkaline solution using tap water. All you have to do is dissolve a teaspoon of sodium bicarbonate in it. Best done last thing at night so it doesn't disturb digestive acids. And it will help you sleep well.

These different waters are options, each of which appears to solve the same problem, that of getting water into the cells to flush out toxins and to replenish the healthy cellular medium.

The issue of what water to drink has recently been enlivened by a Japanese researcher, Masaru Emoto, who has written several books extolling an almost mystical message. In his view, water is the mirror of the soul. Emoto believes that, in addition to all its other unique qualities, water has another characteristic that has not yet been widely recognised. It carries in it vibrational information.

Emoto claims to have found that water will recognise the word 'love', for example, and will respond by producing a beautiful crystal shape. However, if we give the word 'hate' it will produce a very deformed crystal. Interestingly, he found that chlorinated tap water was incapable of forming crystals—he used distilled water for those experiments where he compared the effect of external influences (such as microwave ovens) on water's ability to make crystals—not good in the case of microwave ovens.

Emoto believes that we should respect water and show it respect. He believes that the words we use to address water will change it in a subtle way and make it more healthy for the body. He therefore recommends thanking the water, to express gratitude to it, before we drink it.

His interest was sparked when he decided to freeze water in order to study the crystalline shapes that appeared when it melted. He took photographs of these crystals. The results can be seen in the photographs in Emoto's books—*The Secret Life of Water*, *The True Power of Water* and *The Hidden Messages in Water*—which have become international best sellers.

According to an article in *New Scientist* magazine (8th April 2006), scientists are taking a closer look at water and finding that it has interesting energetic properties which may explain why a homoeopathic solution (which may be so dilute that not one molecule of the original substance remains) retains its effectiveness. According to Cambridge University researcher, Felix Franks, genes and proteins cannot function without the presence of water. 'Without water, it's all chemistry,' he says. 'But add water and you get biology.'

If DNA needs water to function properly, we can see the necessity to ensure the proper hydration of every cell.

As a postscript to this discussion of water, an American company, Oculus Innovative Sciences, has developed a form of ion-hungry, super-oxygenated salt water that is extremely hostile to bacteria, viruses and fungal infections. Called Microcyn, it is hoped that it will prove to be an effective agent against hospital acquired infections. As fungal infections appear to be connected in some way with cancer—either as cause or effect—and as this water is super-oxygenated, it may also be beneficial for cancer patients. It is sold for external use but is non-toxic to animals or humans if ingested. For more information see www.oculusis.com.

Infra-red sauna therapy

Infra-red light is light that is invisible to us, at the opposite end of the visible light spectrum from ultraviolet light. (Factoid: approximately 80 per cent of the sun's rays fall into the infrared range.) Compared with a traditional sauna, the far infra-red sauna is much lower in ambient temperature, does not use water and is better at promoting whole body detoxification. The toxins are eliminated through sweat.

It is claimed that in addition to its detoxification benefits, far infra-red saunas also directly help stimulate the immune system, improve oxygenation of tissues, and make cancer cells more vulnerable and so easier to kill. This is a long-term therapy. Ideally, one or two sessions a day for up to two years is suggested. After each session a shower is essential to clean off toxins that have been expelled and to prevent them from being reabsorbed.

Some claim that even better than far infra-red saunas are infra-red electric light saunas. These use a different way of emitting the infra-red light. Whereas far infra-red saunas use ceramic or metallic elements for heating that mainly emit radiation in the far infrared range, infrared electric light saunas use incandescent infra-red heat lamps for heating. These emit red and orange light and near, middle and some far infra-red light. Dr Lawrence Wilson is a leading proponent of this therapy. For further information go to his website at www.drlwilson.com.

EDTA chelation

Chelation is a method by which unwanted metals are purged from a system by putting another substance through the system which binds to the metals and so flushes them out. The need for such a chelating substance was strongly felt before the war by industry: paint, rubber, petroleum and electro-plating industries: all needed substances that would bind to and eliminate corrupting substances. Research in pre-war Germany came up with an extremely good substance: ethylene-diamine-tetra-acetate, known since then as EDTA for short.

Its first use for medical purposes was in 1947, to clear the bloodstream of a cancer patient suffering toxic side effects of chemotherapy. It did the trick. In the early 1950s, EDTA was used in a number of circumstances where workers were suffering in large numbers from heavy metal poisoning. In every case it worked marvellously, according to Harold and Arline Brecher who have written a number of books on chelation therapy.

> *The treated [men] spontaneously reported unanticipated health benefits. Among the varied improvements were increased endurance, improved stamina, better memory, enhanced vision, hearing and smell, clearer thinking, fewer headaches, less anxiety. Those with early signs of arthritis or atherosclerosis enjoyed even more extraordinary recovery—increased mobility, reduced leg cramps, easier breathing.' (Brecher, Forty Something Forever, 1992)*

Since then, hundreds of studies have consistently shown the benefits of chelation therapy particularly for atherosclerosis—a problem for which the heart bypass operation was designed.

Additionally, it appears that chelation therapy has a possible cancer preventative action. The evidence? A Swiss study investigating the link between lead-based gas fumes and cancer incidence by Drs W Blumer and T Reich, based on the health records of 231 Swiss citizens living next to a heavily used highway. Blumer and Reich were in a position to compare long-term death rates in a matched population of chelated and non-chelated patients. They found a significant mortality difference between the two groups. Of the 231 people in the study, 59 adults had chelation, 172 matched controls did not. Only one (1.7 per cent of the chelated persons) died of cancer, as compared with thirty (17 per cent) of those untreated. After exploring all possible explanations for this statistical disparity in cancer mortality, the authors concluded that chelation was the sole reason for the 90 per cent decrease in cancer deaths.

This supports the experience of doctors who use EDTA chelation in their practices. One, Dr E W McDonagh, founder member of the International Academy of Preventive Medicine, found that of 25,000 patients that he had treated with this chelation only one of those who had not previously had cancer was later diagnosed as having cancer. Taking this as an interesting indication of EDTA chelation's merits, he looked for cases of Vietnam veterans who had been severely poisoned by Agent Orange. This group is known to suffer very high incidences of cancer. He found 63 cases who had also, later, had EDTA. Not one of them subsequently developed cancer. But a word of caution, chelation may not be so effective if cancer has already started to develop before the chelation treatment started.

How does EDTA chelation work, if it does, against cancer? First, by removing toxic metals, it is removing a source of free radicals. It is therefore a preventive measure. For patients who already have cancer, it improves blood circulation by clearing arterial obstructions and so allows greater supplies of oxygen to reach the cancer site. Cancer tumours do not like high-oxygen environments. One interpretation is that EDTA strips away the protein coat that surrounds tumour cells—this protein shield is what protects the cancer cells from T-lymphocytes, the white blood cells whose job is to kill invaders. Because of the protein layer T-lymphocytes do not identify the tumour as an enemy to be overcome. Once the protein layer has been stripped away the T-lymphocytes can start to do the job.

During EDTA chelation, the patient is hooked up (for 2–3 hours per session) to an intravenous drip which contains not only EDTA but also megadoses of vitamins. Increasing numbers of people are undergoing chelation treatments as a general preventive health measure.

One caution is that chelation needs to be carefully administered as there can be kidney complications from the extraction of too much toxic metal in a short time. A careful graduation of chelation treatments is therefore required. A standard treatment will include 20 sessions. Also high supplementation of zinc and selenium is needed as good metals are taken out with the bad. Some infrequent effects of EDTA chelation may include: low blood calcium, cardiac arrhythmia, fever, headaches and inflammation of the vein. However, these side effects are not common. EDTA chelation is contra-indicated in the cases of damaged kidneys, liver disease, TB, brain tumours and pregnancy.

It is also possible to self-administer a chelation program by taking an oral chelation course of capsules. Karl Loren is a long-time advocate of this and he sells his oral chelation Vibrant Life capsules from www.oralchelation.com. Calcium disodium EDTA is available from www.naturodoc.com. Another product that has been recommended can be found at www.thedoctorwithin.com. Chelation can also be done using a suppository—see www.detoxamin.com.

Ionising footbaths

These are hydrotherapy devices in which you place your feet in a footbath containing a saline solution. The water is charged with negative ions which draw out the positively charged toxins from the body. The process gently detoxifies the body of excess heavy metals, toxins, and infectious agents. It also helps to reduce inflammation and improve liver, kidney and colon function. A 20–30 minute session will result in the initially clear water round your feet becoming murky as toxins are removed. By removing the toxins through the bottom of the feet, the detox sickness caused by most detoxification protocols is avoided. That, at least, is the claim.

There are a number of ionic footbath systems on the market: Aqua Chi, BioCleanse, Ion Cleanse and others. Many testimonials attest to their energising and health promoting effects. Most systems cost over $1,000 and there are parts that need to be replenished regularly, so this is not a cheap option.

Bentonite clay

Bentonite clay is so named because it was first mined near Fort Benton in Wyoming USA. It contains high concentrations of a medicinal mineral called montmorillonite, which comes from weathered volcanic ash. This name derives from Montmorillon, France, where the medicinal mineral was first identified. Sometimes mineralogists use the term smectite instead to describe the same substance.

Bentonite, then, is a powdered medicinal clay which happens to be one of the most effective colon cleansers available—it scrapes the interior lining clean so that it is capable once more of absorbing efficiently the nutrients that pass down it . At the same time it is a nutritional supplement in its own right as it contains many important minerals and trace elements. The clay itself passes through the intestines without being digested. It absorbs all types of toxin from heavy metals, pathogenic viruses, moulds such as aflatoxin, and pesticide residues. One of the reasons it is so effective is that bentonite's minerals are negatively charged electrically and they bind with toxins which tend to be positively charged.

Bentonite has many general healing abilities: providing relief from both constipation and acute diarrhoea (no matter what the cause), ulcers and much else. A tablespoon of dissolved bentonite clay taken two to three times a day for two to four weeks will have a strong regenerating effect on the entire body—as can be seen from the improved colour of the whites of the eye, improved vitality and emotional well-being.

The best way to drink clay is on an empty stomach, at least an hour before or after a meal.

The clay is also available as a thick, more-or-less tasteless, greyish gel, but this form is best avoided. It tends to come in plastic containers and there are fears that bentonite, being such a potent attracter of toxins, may leach out toxins from the plastic. However, it also comes as a powder, which is better.

Start with one tablespoon daily for a week, perhaps mixed with a small amount of juice, if this seems comfortable, then increase to two spoons a day. The maximum dose would be four tablespoons a day. You can also sprinkle bentonite in a bath and let it soak in through the skin.

Zeolite (clinoptilolite)

Zeolites are naturally existing, negatively-charged minerals, formed by the fusion of glass-rich volcanic rock with either fresh water or seawater. They have a number of rare properties. Clinoptilolite, the zeolite that we are concerned with, has the demonstrated ability to capture and eliminate free radicals, heavy metals, carcinogenic chemicals such as nitrosamines, and even viral particles.

So far so good, and if this was all that claimed for Natural Cell Defence (NCD), it would be worth taking for these properties alone. And anyone taking it should know that it is generally recognised as having no ill effects whatsoever, as long as it does not amount to more than two per cent of total food intake. The only caution is that anyone taking it should make sure they are fully hydrated at all times.

However, the big buzz surrounding zeolite is not its detoxification ability but rather its anti-cancer effects. In animal studies conducted by Ljiljana Bedric PhD, at the Faculty of Veterinary Medicine in Zagreb, Croatia, 51 dogs with various cancers were treated with zeolite. All the dogs improved some having a dramatic reduction or elimination of their tumours. In only one week, six dogs with prostate cancer were found to be completely tumour free. In human studies, 114 patients were given 10–20 grams or more of Megamin capsules containing a specially processed form of zeolite, with the following results:

The terminal brain cancer patients showed some improvement in their condition within three to four weeks. Almost all of the forty lung cancer patients experienced decreased pain and improved respiration within the same time frame. Another fifty-three patients with terminal gastrointestinal cancers improved but at a much slower rate.

Another group of 16 cancer patients were treated by doctors at the Svecnjak Polyclinic with only Megamin therapy for a period of three years. At the end of the three years, 13 (81 per cent) of the patients were in complete remission. This patient group included three with liver cancers, four with metastatic melanoma, two with bronchial carcinoma, one with bladder cancer, and one with hepatocellular carcinoma. The other three patients had obtained partial remission and stabilization of their cancers (two lung cancer and one breast cancer).

Megamin can be obtained from www.megamin.net.

Zeolite is also available in liquid form from multi-level marketing company, Waiora, with their product, Natural Cell Defence. Destroxin is a powdered form, which has the further advantage of being much cheaper. This is available from www.cutcat.com. Another zeolite product called Denali Green is currently getting a lot of word-of-mouth support. Do an Internet search for the latest info and for suppliers. There are testimonials relating to its ability to kill tumours over time. One indication of its power is the fact that many testimonials refer to a Herxheimer response (the onset of negative symptoms as the first sign of healing). As always, when this happens, cut back the dose or stop taking the product for a few days until the symptoms go.

Removal of parasites

Are we harbouring many parasites that have negative impacts on our health? It depends who you talk to. But increasingly, among the alternative health community, it has become commonly accepted that 80–90 per cent of us are carrying a load of parasites in the form of various worms and flukes.

To get rid of them Hulda Clark, the person most associated with this treatment recommends the following regime involving three herbs: black walnut hulls, wormwood and common cloves.

'These three herbs must be used together. Black walnut hull and wormwood kill adults and developmental stages of at least 100 parasites. Cloves kill the eggs. Only if you use them together will you rid yourself of parasites. If you kill only the adults, the tiny stages and eggs will soon grow into new adults. If you kill only the eggs, the million stages already loose in your body will grow into adults and make more eggs. They must be used together as a single treatment.' (Hulda Clark, *The Cure for all Cancers*)

These will, she says, eliminate over 100 types of parasites with no side effects.

Eliminating fungi and yeasts

Another kind of parasite are the fungi and yeasts that live in our bodies and which, when the immune response is weakened, can take over. These, like cancer, live and thrive in tissues that are poorly oxygenated. They can therefore be seen as an early warning system. To eliminate them, we can attack them directly or we can eliminate them indirectly by making the tissue environment healthier. This is done by increasing oxygen levels.

It is important to eliminate fungi and yeasts not only because they are a sign of systemic ill-health but also because their by-products overload and weaken the immune system.

One way to eliminate them is through diet (see the anti-candida diet below).

Like cancer, fungi and yeasts also thrive on sugars, so the first step to elimination is to halt intake of all sweet foods. Secondly, yeast-containing foods should be avoided: bread, fermented beverages (beer, wine, brandy, scotch, etc.) mouldy cheeses, processed and smoked meats, and so on. There are a number of herbs that have an anti-fungal effect: wormwood, garlic, grapefruit seed oil among others. These should be taken on a rotating basis. Acidophilus and the use of good digestive enzymes are also recommended. For infections on the skin, tea tree essential oil can be applied liberally directly on the infestation with good results—mixed with castor oil and propolis. Also colloidal silver can be useful. And then of course there are the anti-fungal drugs that your doctor could prescribe.

Dietary Approaches to Healing Cancer

Introduction

If diet can cure cancer, we will not hear about it from doctors.

The idea that food might have something to do with cancer prevention or cancer cure is one that has not always been encouraged by the US National Cancer Institute: 'There is no diet that prevents cancer in man. Treatment of cancer by diet alone is in the realm of quackery.' Dr Michael Shimkin wrote in 1975. For decades, spokesmen for the leading American cancer institutions poured scorn on 'food faddists' who promoted 'wonder foods'. Yet, now, these voices are not so loud. It is now accepted, for example, that a high fibre diet is important for intestinal health. However, nutrition still plays a very minor role in the education of a doctor. Most doctors go through their medical training without touching on the subject. One doctor told me that the word 'vitamin' had never been uttered during his years as a medical student.

But this neglect of nutrition is a modern attitude. Two and a half thousand years ago, Hippocrates said: 'Let food be your medicine and medicine be your food.' Six hundred years ago, Paracelsus talked of curing cancer by natural means. 'In the hand of the physician, nutrition can be the highest and best remedy,' he said. Unfortunately, he didn't keep statistics. By the 20th century, this idea that nature does not need to be over-ridden by drugs had become derided—and still is derided by large numbers of doctors. But people are voting with their feet and scientists from the US National Cancer Institute are belatedly finding evidence to support their concerns.

One American study published in 1994 reported a sharp drop in the incidence of colon cancer between 1985 and 1988—eight per cent for men and 11 per cent for women. 'The most salient risk factor for colorectal cancer is diet,' the authors reported; dietary fat, particularly animal fat, was associated with a high risk, and dietary fibre, particularly insoluble or grain fibre, was associated with low risk. Fruits, vegetables and vitamin D were also seen to have a protective effect while a sedentary life-style and obesity were correlated with a higher incidence of colorectal cancer. An eight to 11 per cent drop in incidence over three to four years. This is a very significant development.

Evidence that diet and environmental factors could be the key to all cancers is, of course, implicit in comparisons of cancer rates in different countries. We know it is not genetic because immigrant families, after a generation or two, develop the cancer profiles of their host countries. We can see this clearly by comparing the statistics of death rates from various cancers round the world.

What do we find? Higher cancer incidences in northern Europe. Very low rates in poor countries where the diet is largely cereals and vegetables. Here is clear indication that the diets of prosperous countries, high in animal fats, are to blame for significant numbers of cancer cases. Wealthy Hong Kong, for example, compares badly with neighbouring China. It can't be genetic. If it's not food-related, what else could it be? It might of course be climatic. Poor countries tend to be warmer countries. It may be the amount of food eaten rather than the type. Whatever the case the evidence is clear that cancer is caused by environmental factors.

Colon cancer (%)	Men	Women
USA	16.7	11.4
England and Wales	20.2	13.7
Ireland	23.2	15.1
Scotland	20.6	15.2
Germany	21.1	15.2
Denmark	22.8	17.5
France	17.3	10.3
Spain	13.2	9.2
Italy	15.6	10.3
Greece	6.8	5.5
Japan	15.1	9.7
China	7.9	6.5
Hong Kong	14.8	10.7
Mexico	3.3	3.1
Argentina	13.7	9.3
Chile	7.0	6.0

[Age-adjusted death rates per 100,000 population for colon cancer (1988–91)

Colon cancer, of course, has obvious links to food. But what about other cancers? Do the death rates for these other cancers also support the view that diet is a major factor? The next table, below, shows breast and lung cancers.

The lung cancer figures may not at first appear to support the argument (certainly the figure for Chinese women is anomalous—the result almost certainly of the double whammy of a husband who smokes and low quality charcoal used for cooking)—but the Chinese, Japanese and Greeks are ferocious smokers and certainly a far larger proportion of the male population in these countries smokes than in the USA. Yet their death rates are much lower. How can this be? Diet is the obvious answer.

	Breast cancer (%)	Lung cancer (%)	
	women	men	women
USA	22.4	57.1	24.7
England and Wales	28.7	57.0	20.5
Germany	21.9	48.7	7.8
Spain	17.1	45.2	3.4
Greece	15.2	49.8	6.9
China	4.6	34.0	14.5
Japan	6.3	30.1	8.0
Mexico	8.1	16.5	5.9
Argentina	20.9	39.2	5.8

[Age-adjusted death rates per 100,000 population (1988–91)

If we compare the top five with the bottom five for *all forms of cancer* we get the following:

ranking	Men	Women
1	Hungary	Denmark
2	Czechoslovakia	Scotland
3	Uruguay	Hungary
4	Poland	Ireland
5	France	New Zealand
...		
42	Israel	Mexico
43	Venezuela	Greece
44	Mauritius	Japan
45	Ecuador	Puerto Rico
46	Mexico	Mauritius

Relative poverty, a diet heavy with vegetables, olive oil or tofu—add in sunshine, music and laughter. These are, it has been argued, the ingredients for a cancer-free life. The Mediterranean diet of olive oil, pasta, vegetables with a little wine and lots of grapes has been put forward by some as a healthy diet that we should adopt. Certainly it is a tempting one.

These epidemiological comparisons of countries are one basis for the argument that diet can help protect against cancer. And given the impact of diet on cancer incidence it seems reasonable to suggest that the huge and continuing increases in cancer incidence are due to changes in the diet we eat or the quality of the food we ingest.

There is general agreement from all sides that 70–90 per cent of all cancers are caused by lifestyle and environment, and of this at least half are in some way related to diet and nutrition, while a further 30 per cent are the result of cigarette smoking. Some studies supporting a nutritional approach to prevention are summarized here:

A large-scale study in New Zealand published in 1994 showed that vegetarians had less than half the cancer risk of their meat-eating friends.

A 50-year study in England and Wales found that breast cancer mortality fell from the beginning of World War II because intake of animal fats and sugar fell due to rationing. In 1954, consumption of these items returned to pre-war levels. However, breast cancer rates did not return until about 1969, suggesting that there is a 15-year time lag between ingestion and development of the disease. This is close to the 20-year time lag reported between increase in smoking habits and increased incidence of lung cancer.

Seventh Day Adventists, of whom roughly half are vegetarian, have significantly lower cancer levels than average, 84 per cent less cervical cancer and 30–44 per cent fewer cases of leukaemia.

The Hunza people of northern Pakistan are renowned for their freedom from degenerative diseases. Dr Robert McCarrison who visited the area from 1904–11 said, 'I never saw a case of cancer.' He attributed their health and longevity to their diet of whole-wheat chapattis, barley, maize, green leafy vegetables, beans and apricots. Later experimenting on rats, he found that rats fed on the Hunza diet remained healthy and free of disease, while rats fed on the normal Indian diet contracted heart disease, cancer and other ailments.

The China study

'The genes that cause cancer were profoundly impacted by the consumption of protein.'

T Colin Campbell

The China Study is the title of a remarkable book by T Colin Campbell who was involved in the study of diet in relation to cancer and other diseases across China. There is an enormous range of diet from one region of China to another, and also enormous differences in cancer rates. His interest in this subject was sparked by an obscure piece of research conducted in India that had a rather remarkable result. In the study, two groups of rats were given diets high in aflotoxin, which is known to cause liver cancer. One of the groups was fed a diet containing 20 per cent milk-based protein and the other group a diet with only five per cent protein. The result was that 100 per cent of the rats in the high protein group died of liver cancer while zero per cent of the rats in the low protein group died of liver cancer. He repeated the test and found the results had been accurately reported. On analysis he found that the protein activated enzymes responsible for metabolizing the aflotoxin—and it was the resulting chemicals that caused the cancer. In the absence of protein the aflotoxin was not metabolized and so did not cause problems. However, plant-based protein did not have this effect. Campbell's conclusion is that all meat-sourced protein should be avoided.

One other point that Campbell makes is in relation to the supposed genetic basis of cancer. This is an area that receives enormous funding. And of course it is true: at one level all cancers are genetic in origin—that is to say that a genetic change occurs before a normal cell can become cancerous. But genes are not fully expressed until they become activated. If they are dormant they have no effect at all. And what is it that activates the genes? Their cellular environment, which in turn is affected by diet.

It's not possible to adequately summarize this book here but I do urge you to read it.

But can diet cure cancer?

This suggestion is strongly condemned by the orthodox profession. The authors of *Everyone's Guide to Cancer Therapy* say flatly: 'Following a certain diet or eating certain foods will not make cancer go away …. None is known to be helpful. Many result in nutritional deficiencies …. Moderation is still the best approach to diet for all medical problems.'

This sounds authoritative but it is not. This is simply the unsupported opinion of surgeons and oncologists who have no training or experience in the nutritional sciences and who have done no research on the subject. The need for evidence and proof cuts both ways. We are free to make up our own minds on the matter.

Interestingly, one study of 200 cancer patients who had experienced 'spontaneous regression'—that is, the inexplicable disappearance of cancer tumours without any obvious cause—found that 87 per cent had made serious dietary changes, which were mostly vegetarian in nature, and many others had undergone some detoxification program or used nutritional supplements.

It is clear that proactive cancer patients are making dietary changes and that these are having an effect.

Indeed, if you read Section 8: *Cancer: Survivors' Stories* you will find compelling anecdotal evidence that dietary changes are at the heart of many cancer cures.

But before looking at the various diets that have been proposed let us look at the effect the absence of food can have on cancer.

Fasting

Fasting is generally seen simply as a system of detoxification, but, for the cancer patient, it is also potentially a very powerful anti-cancer therapy.

Doctors, by and large, take it as an article of faith that it is important to eat well in order to maintain the health and vigour of the body. Even Max Gerson, whose dietary regime is discussed below, opposed the idea of fasting because it would result in vitamin and mineral deficiencies and so weaken the body further. However, there is a great deal of evidence that fasting, either voluntarily or involuntarily, can have a positive effect on the body's health.

Fasting as a way of achieving physical and spiritual purification is a common aspect of religious life. Fasting is frequently mentioned in the Bible. Moslems fast at Ramadan. The ancient Greek philosophers were also frequent fasters. Before anyone could be accepted as a student by Pythagoras, he had to undergo a forty day fast. Jesus also underwent a forty-day fast in the wilderness. In addition to its therapeutic value it was, presumably, a means of determining who had the necessary discipline for study. Asclepius is the Greek God of Healing. Healing through fasting was a regular feature of life at his temples. All the great doctors from Hippocrates to Avicenna have recommended healing fasts. Even the non-medical Mark Twain approved of fasting: 'A little starvation can really do more for the average sick man than can the best medicines and the best doctors. I do not mean a restricted diet. I mean total abstention from food for one or two days. I speak from experience. Starvation has been my cold and fever doctor for fifteen years.'

The masterwork on fasting is Herbert Shelton's *The Science and Fine Art of Fasting*, which was first published in 1934. In a foreword to this edition, Shelton describes the case of Henry Tanner MD, who, in 1877, felt he could no longer cope with the pains and illnesses that were plaguing him. It was an accepted fact at that time that to go without food for ten days was a certain way to enter the beyond. So Tanner, preferring to ease his way to the next world, rather than to commit an act of violence against his person, took to his bed and refused all food. So far from dying, he found that, by the 42nd day he had recovered. When he announced this to his colleagues, he was denounced as a fraud. To prove he was not a fraud, he undertook another forty-two day fast under the supervision of the United States Medical College of New York. He was placed in a fenced off area and a watch was kept on him by 60 volunteer physicians. 'During the first fourteen days of the fast I drank no water and breathed air in the hall that would vomit an Arizona mule.'

Amazingly, he didn't die of dehydration! He was eventually allowed access to water and fresh air. On the eighteenth day, he got into an argument with a medical student over which was the best source of food: oxygen or beef. He challenged the student to walk around the hall until one of them dropped out. The medical student dropped out puffing and panting on the eighteenth lap, leaving Dr Tanner a clear winner.

Shelton describes the case of an overweight 53-year-old English businessman who was blind in both eyes due to cataracts, had no sense of smell and who had heart trouble. He went on a fast from October 31st 1932 to February 8th 1933—101 days. He lost 89lbs, regained his sight and his sense of smell. His heart trouble was much improved. He had started the fast as an experiment, intending only to go on it for ten days. After that he had just continued from day to day, gradually feeling better. But those who go on fasts to lose weight should know that the weight lost is very easily regained especially if ravenous eating follows the diet.

Shelton argues that fasting, far from being an abnormal reaction to ill-health is actually a very natural one. He points to the fact that wounded or ill animals very often refuse food until they are well on the mend. When we are ill we very often feel no appetite at all for food. The obvious implication is that the body does not wish to have food—and since the body is credited with healing powers, what it wants is probably good for it. Animals will also go for months in hibernation without any food or drink of any kind.

Fasting works against cancer because of a process known as autolysis, self-digestion. This autolysis is a controlled process by which the least essential parts of the body are self-digested. This is also true in starvation. The body seeks to preserve the most essential organs and tissues by allowing the least essential to be digested first. This is very important when it comes to cancer. Cancer tumours are recognised as being the least essential tissues in the body and so are easy victims of the autolytic process.

Shelton gives a number of examples of people who were cured of cancer by means of a fast, but he cautions that there is a wide variation in response from person to person. In some people the tumour will be devoured quickly, in others slowly. In one case a cancer cure required a fast of 21 days followed shortly after by another of 17 days. This was considered by Shelton to be abnormally long. Another woman had a speedier response: '(after) exactly three days without food, the "cancer" and all its attendant pain were gone. There had been no recurrence after thirteen years and I think that we are justified in considering the condition remedied.'

Shelton does accept that, when a cancer tumour has grown very large it may take years of on and off fasting to absorb it—and even then it may not be possible. But on the whole he is extremely optimistic about the cancer curing potential of a fast.

Is fasting hard to do? Apparently not. After a few days, it seems that the hunger goes. Many fasters experience clear improvements in their mental abilities. Shelton says: 'All of man's intellectual and emotional qualities are given new life.'

Having said this, anyone undergoing a fast must expect to experience in the first week a number of unpleasant sensations: headaches, nausea, etc. which is the body's response to accumulated poisons that are being eliminated.

Is there any more modern evidence that fasting works? Certainly there is evidence that low calorie diets are health-promoting.

In 1942, Albert Tannenbaum, cancer researcher at Michael Reese Hospital in Chicago, found that mice on a low calorie diet had substantially lowered incidences of induced breast tumours, lung tumours and sarcoma than mice on an unrestricted diet. He also found that mice on a high-fat diet had a significantly higher incidence of spontaneous breast cancer. Tumours also appeared much earlier in mice fed with a high-fat diet.

In 1944, cancer researcher J Saxton reported that a special strain of laboratory mice having a high leukaemia rate fed only 40 per cent of a normal diet reduced their leukaemia incidence from 65 per cent to ten per cent. A 1947 study found that the opposite effect also occurred. A high-protein diet increased leukaemia incidence.

A 1982 study at UCLA found that mice fed 28–43 per cent fewer calories lived 10–20 per cent longer than their controls and had fewer tumours of the lymphatic system.

> *'Calorie restriction—coupled with the correct macronutrient composition—is far more effective than any drug in the prevention or treatment of cancer.'*
>
> *Barry Sears*

Dr Virginia Vertrano, who took over Shelton's clinic reports: 'I kept a lady alive for ten years longer than the doctors said she'd live by fasting her once a year and keeping her on an all raw-food diet between the fasts. She had a very malignant breast tumor.' (quoted by Richard Walters, 1993). However, she cautions that some tumours return once the fast has finished.

At the end of the fast, you should not go for a sudden blow out. A juice diet should be the first step on the road to a normal diet with some thin oatmeal porridge or vegetable soup working slowly up to a vegetable stew.

As a postscript I would like to offer the following story. Shortly after the first edition of this book came out I was visiting a friend whose father, Dr Solomon Bard, is well known in Hong Kong as a medical doctor, archaeologist and musician. He told me a story from his own experience in support of fasting. At that time he had been a medical student at Hong Kong University. In 1941 Hong Kong fell to the Japanese and he was interned. With him in the camp was a man that he knew only had weeks or months to live. This man had an aggressive testicular cancer which had been treated with radiation but which had returned and there was nothing more the doctors could do about it. Obviously, any kind of medical intervention was made impossible by his imprisonment. But the man didn't die. He was alive at the end of the war—and still alive ten years after that in perfect health. Dr Bard told me he had drawn the conclusion that if he had ever been diagnosed with cancer he too would have gone on a Japanese camp diet of rice and vegetables (mainly cabbage) in quantities just sufficient to maintain life.

Even more interestingly, when I publicized this story in Hong Kong another correspondent told me he knew of two men who had been cured of syphilis by the Japanese prison camp diet!

Animal studies have also shown that a hunter-gather type diet, which involves long periods of famine between moments of glut, is also highly protective against cancer—and this may be because of the autolytic process described above.

Finally, Barry Sears, biochemist and author of *The Zone*, has this to say: 'calorie restriction—coupled with the correct macronutrient composition—is far more effective than any drug in the prevention or treatment of cancer.' Read that sentence again. It is very important. The correct macronutrient composition, according to Sears, involves low levels of insulin-producing foods (cakes, biscuits, etc.), low in total fat, high in activated omega 3 oil, EPA. One should take three grams of protein for every four grams of carbohydrate, with most carbohydrates coming from fruits or fibre-rich vegetables.

The Australian herbalist, Walter Last, promotes what he calls urine fast in which nothing is eaten or drunk except one's own urine. For further details of urine therapy go to Section 6: *Cancer: Vitamins and Other Supplements.*

Fasting for many people will seem to be problematic in that it will take great will power to refrain from eating. There is a South African plant called hoodia, which the Bushmen of the Kalahari Desert eat to keep away hunger pangs. This is available on the Internet as it is being marketed as a useful weight-loss tool.

The Breuss juice fast

According to Rudolf Breuss, an Austrian healer, cancer can live only on the protein of solid food. He therefore advised cancer patients to drink nothing but vegetable juice and teas for 42 days—the length of time, according to Breuss, that it takes for a cancer tumour to die.

His 'Breuss Juice' consists of 50 per cent red beetroot, 20 per cent carrots, 20 per cent celery root, five per cent raw potato, five per cent radishes.

For a daily juice requirement, he recommends the following amounts: 300 grams of red beets, 100 grams carrot, 100 grams celery root, 30–50 grams of raw potato, 30–50 grams radish.

These should be juiced and strained to get rid of sediment. The juice should be eaten by the spoonful, and while sipping slowly and before swallowing you should salivate strongly. Half a litre of Breuss juice is considered appropriate for a day's intake.

This is the core of the Breuss cancer cure. In addition to the juice, you are recommended to drink special herbal teas. For the first three weeks of the six week program, a cold kidney-enhancing tea is recommended for first thing in the morning followed an hour later by two cups of warm tea containing the following herbs: St John's Wort, peppermint, and lemon balm. This is followed an hour later by the drinking of a little juice—after a lot of salivating. You should then take the juice ten to 15 times throughout the morning but only when you feel like it. Sage tea can be drunk throughout the day. Also one cup of cold cranesbill tea (Geranium robertianum) should be drunk every day throughout the 42-day juice fast. During the complete treatment you should not take any food other than the vegetable juice mixture.

According to Breuss, sage tea drunk every day will keep you free of almost all illness. It is made by putting two teaspoons of fresh sage in half a litre of boiling water. This should be boiled for three minutes, left to steep for ten minutes and then drunk.

One person who followed this diet successfully commented that for several weeks during this diet he felt extreme weakness but that his strength recovered towards the end.

The five-week juice fast cure

In her book *Cancer Battle Plan*, Anne Frahm describes how, for eighteen months battling her breast cancer, she went through every form of conventional therapy—surgery, chemotherapy, radiation, hormone therapy and finally, a bone marrow transplant. They all failed. She was told that she had at most a few weeks to live. Her cancer had metastasized to the spine—and even to the bone marrow. A more hopeless case it is impossible to imagine. However, she refused to 'lie down and play dead' and instead went to see a nutritional counsellor. Alongside her dietary changes, she had a daily enema and was forbidden by her nutritionist from taking in any animal product. By following a strict juice diet, she claims, all signs of cancer quickly left her. 'Within five weeks after starting a strict program of detoxification and diet under the guidance of a nutritional counsellor, my cancer had packed its bags.'

Her recovery was begun by going on a juice fast that looked like this:

8:30 am	grapefruit juice with olive oil. She brewed a pot of Jason Winters' Tea to sip throughout the day.
9:00 am	apple juice with fibre cleanse, plus enemas
10:00 am	green-drink with vitamin C powder
11 am	apple juice with fibre cleanse
Noon	carrot juice, acidophilus
1:00 pm	green drink with vitamin C powder
2:00 pm	apple juice with fibre cleanse
3:00 pm	carrot juice
4:00 pm	green drink
5:00 pm	apple juice with fibre cleanse
6:00 pm	carrot juice
7:00 pm	green drink with vitamin C powder
8:00 pm	carrot juice
9:00 pm	green drink with vitamin C powder
10:00 pm	apple juice with fibre cleanse

(Note: Jason Winter's Tea is a proprietary blend of a number of unknown herbs.)

The ingredients for the juices were organically-grown apples and carrots and they were mixed 50:50 with distilled water. No tap water was allowed. The juices have to be drunk soon after they are made as the nutrients quickly oxidize. (Eating two apples a day has been suggested as a good cancer preventative.)

As for the 'green drink', in an interview she reveals that she used Kyo Green but there are a number of different green drinks on the market containing a mix of barley and wheatgrass sprouts, chlorella, spirulina and other green vegetable products. These are discussed below.

For Anne Frahm, this was the start of a program that would lead on to a largely raw vegetarian diet supported by enzymes, amino acids and vitamin and mineral supplements; strengthened through morale boosting activities and exercise. And, if we believe what she says, by following this diet rigorously all signs of her cancer were gone in five weeks. Anne lived for another ten years.

Anne Frahm's story is enlightening. It is clear evidence that it is never too late. That even someone on the brink of death can return to full health. Anne Frahm's experience is clear evidence demonstrating that food alone can cure cancer in a person who is still prepared to fight despite gloomy medical predictions.

Schulze's 30-day incurable's program

Richard Schulze is a prominent American herbalist who believes that even terminal cancer patients can cure themselves if they are prepared to stick to a 30-day raw-food diet or preferably juice program supplemented with herbs, colonics every other day, hot and cold showers, warm castor oil packs, exercise and sunlight. To order his book and a month's supply of supporting herbs, superfoods and so on, go to his website at herbdoc.com.

Diets

A large number of diets have been proposed for cancer patients. Here I will look at the best known. However, before looking at the diets, we should look at the act of eating itself.

Chewing food slowly

As we saw with the Breuss Juice fast (above), the manner of eating may itself be an important fact to which we should focus attention. It is also a key tenet of the macrobiotic approach to health. The thinking behind it is very simple. First, the body has two basic modes: tense and relaxed. For most people the body is in a state of more or less constant tension from morning to evening. When the body is tense, adrenalin is released which triggers the fight or flight response. In this mode, the body is not prepared to absorb all the nutrients in the food. Rather it is ready for the speedy elimination and only partial digestion of the food. Even the food that is digested is not made use of because the body's cells have other priorities. A relaxed body, however, is able to benefit from the nutrients taken in.

It is advised that a little prayer of thanks to those around you and to the world and the forces that have produced the good food you eat will relax the body and harmonise the mind. Slow chewing maintains that state. Additionally, chewing food until it is completely dissolved—each mouthful should be masticated up to 200 times—allows the powerful digestive enzymes in the mouth to predigest the food before it hits the stomach. This allows much better absorption of nutrients. One last benefit of slow chewing is that the body becomes aware of its state of fullness in time to have an impact on the amount of food eaten.

With that point made let us now look at a number of diets that have been proposed as powerful healing strategies.

The grape diet

Basil Shackleton was a very ill man when he came, almost at the end of his tether, to the grape diet. His one remaining kidney was diseased and would not respond to drugs. He had been chronically ill for over 40 years, having caught bilharzia as a young boy growing up in Africa. In despair he turned to a cure that he had only vaguely heard about—a diet of grapes. In his book, *The Grape Cure*, he explained what happened: 'There is magic in the world—and there are miracles! ... after twenty-three days on the treatment … I came through … looking and feeling twenty years younger—and I was completely and permanently cured! My body became charged with a new vitality. I felt radiant and whole.'

This grape cure is probably an ancient Mediterranean folk cure. It is nothing more or less than the eating of grapes—all of the grape (skin, pips and all)—and nothing but the grapes—for a period of four weeks or longer. No drugs, no other foods, no liquids other than hot or cold water—hot for those times when you will feel nauseated. The water may be drunk at all times but not within an hour after eating the grapes as this will only dilute the strength of the natural chemicals in the grapes. The grapes must of course be washed thoroughly—and soaked two or three times—to wash off any pesticides that might be on the skin. Organic grapes would of course be better but these are not so easy to get hold of. During the grape cure there must be at least one bowel movement every two days—if not, then an enema or colonic is necessary—because the faeces is the main channel for the elimination of toxic matter. Shackleton also recommends a glycerine suppository for the purpose of encouraging a bowel movement. However, he added that in his experience it wasn't necessary!

The importance of crunching the grape seeds needs to be emphasised. Seeds are designed to pass undisturbed through the digestive tract. The chemicals contained in the seed have been found to be powerful anti-cancer agents and these need to be released. Nowadays it is difficult to find grapes with pips so you may need to supplement with grapeseed extract (Note: grapeseed oil contains very little of these chemicals as they are not fat soluble. An article published in the October 18, 2006 issue of the journal *Clinical Cancer Research*, based on research at the University of Colorado Health Sciences Center in Denver reported that grape seed extract inhibits the growth of human colorectal tumours in cell cultures as well as in live mice. So remember, crunch those pips.

Anyone following a toxin-removing regime is likely to suffer badly in the first week from headaches, but these symptoms will gradually disappear. The headaches are a barometer of your condition. The worse they are, the more toxins you have in your body that need to be eliminated. Shackleton ate between four and five pounds of grapes a day and after four weeks—having started the diet near death's door was able to say, 'All forms of irritability and frustration—from which I had suffered for so many years—had completely disappeared. It was quite impossible for me; it seemed, to get angry! All negative symptoms recorded before the treatment had completely vanished. I was [even] able to read a newspaper without glasses.'

The idea of a grape cure has been around for many centuries but it is associated in most people's minds with the name of Johanna Brandt who, shortly after the World War 1, left South Africa for America to popularize her 'grape cure' which involves fasting, eating grapes, and drinking grape juice.

Brandt claims that she was diagnosed with stomach cancer in 1916. She treated herself by fasting but that the cancer came back each time she started to eat normally. Eventually she stumbled on the grape cure and this time the cancer was indeed cured. She also claimed that the grape cure had demonstrated effectiveness against arthritis, diabetes, gallstones, cataracts, ulcerated stomach, tuberculosis, and syphilis. Her story was published in book form in 1928 as *The Grape Cure*. In this book, Brandt wrote: 'The grape is highly antiseptic and a powerful solvent of inorganic matter deposits, fatty degeneration, morbid and malignant growths. It acts as a drastic eliminator of evil while building new tissue.'

Brandt noted that unsweetened grape juice may be substituted for grapes and, in the very weak patients, may be the treatment of choice. Where fresh grapes are not obtainable, unsulfured raisins may be added to the grape juice to give bulk to the diet.

Grape juice contains several major cancer killing nutrients, such as: ellagic acid, catechin, quercetin, oligomeric proanthocyanidins (OPC) or procyanidolic oligomers (PCO), originally called: pycnogenol (in the seeds), resveratrol (in the purple skin), pterostilbene, selenium, lycopene, lutein, laetrile (in the seeds), beta carotene, caffeic acid and/or ferulic acid, and gallic acid!

Modern proponents of Brandt's version of the grape cure say it is advisable to fast from 8pm to 8am so that the cells are really hungry when they get their grape juice. The cells therefore gorge themselves on the lovely sugars they find in the grape and these sugars contain the arsenal of cancer poisons that kill the cancer.

During a grape fast no other food is allowed at all and only distilled or other form of natural, non-chlorinated water is allowed.

In general, the 'Grape Cure' diet cannot be mixed with other alternative cancer treatments. However, some grape diet advocates say it is allowed, indeed recommended, to add chlorella and spirulina, which contain many necessary nutrients that grapes do not have. These should be taken at the same times as the grapes.

Modern proponents of the diet also suggest that most grape juices now available are simply not acceptable—either because they have been pasteurized or because they have at some time come in contact with tap water.

One further warning: The first ten days on the grape diet produces some fairly toxic smells as the intestine and stomach are cleaned out. It is at this time that you may also feel some distressing symptoms as toxins are released into the system. These will not last long. Substantial weight loss is also to be expected in the first few weeks.

Contemporary practitioners of the grape cure talk of staying on the grape-only diet for six to ten weeks at a time, rather longer than Basil Shackleton recommended.

Not all grapes are the same. The Muscadine grape is an older variety, closer to the wild original. Although lower in resveratrol than normal grapes, it is higher in other healthy phyto-chemicals and research has shown that Muscadine grape skin extract has a powerful anti-cancer effect in the laboratory.

At the end of the diet you should ease off it by adding uncooked, whole vegetables and fruits to your diet.

Dr A Ferenczi and beetroot therapy

From 1950, Alexander Ferenczi, MD, a Hungarian cancer therapist, at the Department for Internal Diseases at the district hospital at Csoma, Hungary, began putting patients on a diet of red beetroot (raw or juiced) which they ate in addition to their normal diet. Patients ate up to 1kg daily. The patients he worked with had all previously received chemotherapy and radiation but were, at the time he started to treat them with beetroot juice, mostly at the final stage of their disease.

Brief details of this treatment were reprinted in the *Australian International Clinical Nutrition Review* in July 1986.

One case study he reported was a 50 year old man referred to as D S, who had a lung tumour 'After six weeks of treatment the tumour had disappeared …. After four months of treatment he gained 10kg (22lbs) in weight …. The improvement lasted for about six months.' All other tests confirmed that he had the symptoms of a clinical recovery. However, he discontinued taking the beetroot, the cancer returned and no further treatment could save him.

Ferenczi worked with a number of patients and in all cases there was clear clinical improvement from the use of beetroot. Beetroot was, in one case, so successful in attacking the tumour that the patient died from the toxic overload that resulted. This suggests that anyone following this regime should accompany it with a daily detox—perhaps the coffee enemas that Gerson recommended.

From this, two lessons must be taken on board. People with cancer should start the beetroot therapy as early as they can, perhaps building up slowly from 250 grams a day to a kilo, reducing the intake in the event of nausea, but maintaining the beetroot intake for years as a maintenance regime. In fact, for those of us who do not yet have cancer, regular beetroot consumption is clearly to be recommended.

The active ingredient is believed to be the purple colouring chemical anthocyanin. Anthocyanins are widely present in fruit and vegetables particularly those that are dark red and purple and research is showing that they have many health benefits. In addition to being an anti-cancer agent, it is useful as a way of protecting the body from the damage caused by radiation and chemotherapy.

However, a word of warning from the Cancer Nutrition Center (www.cancernutrition.com): 'Beets clean up cancer faster than the liver is capable of processing all the wastes dumped into it at any one time. Consequently, the internal administration of beetroot needs to be staggered out somewhat, and closer attention given to detoxifying the liver and colon at the same time the beetroot therapy is commenced. Never drink beet juice by itself. Pure beet juice can temporarily paralyze your vocal chords.'

The Gerson diet

The story of what happened to Dr Max Gerson is the kind of story that can break your heart. It demonstrates without a shadow of a doubt that when the medical authorities wish to crush someone they can—and that they will do so if they consider someone to be a threat to their interests.

Max Gerson was a Jewish doctor of rising eminence who fled Nazi Germany for America— only to find himself persecuted there for his methods of treating cancer. He had become well known in Germany for having cured a number of incurable diseases—lupus, tuberculosis—with the help of diet. Among his patients was Albert Schweitzer's wife whom he cured of tuberculosis by dietary means. On his death in 1959, Schweitzer said of him: 'I see in him one of the most eminent geniuses in the history of medicine.'

Apparently, Gerson started looking at diets to treat his own migraines. A few years later, a migraine patient informed him that not only had his headache disappeared but so too had his 'incurable' disfiguring skin disease, lupus. This success brought him some recognition—even in the American medical journals. At first, when he was dealing with obscure diseases the American medical journals were happy to record his achievements. But when he claimed to be able to cure cancer by diet alone his articles were rejected by these same journals. Then he was accused of keeping his methods secret. When, frustrated with these obstacles, he went to the press, he was vilified.

Max Gerson then wrote his book: *A Cancer Therapy*. This was a summary of 30 years of cancer work using dietary means. The Gerson diet, because it aims at the healing of the whole body, can, it is claimed, heal many of the major chronic health conditions including coronary heart disease, diabetes and even premature senility. Gerson stated his fundamental principle in this way: 'A normal body has the capacity to keep all cells functioning properly. It prevents any abnormal transformation and growth. Therefore, the natural task of a cancer therapy is to bring the body back to that normal physiology, or as near to it as is possible. The next step is to keep the physiology of the metabolism in that natural equilibrium.'

Gerson's diet consists of fresh juices of fruits, leaves and vegetables; large quantities of raw fruit and vegetables; vegetables stewed in their own juice, compotes, stewed fruit, potatoes, oatmeal and saltless rye bread. Everything must be prepared fresh and salt must be completely excluded. After six to twelve weeks, animal proteins can be added in the form of pot cheese (saltless and creamless), yoghurt made from skimmed milk, and buttermilk. The original Gerson diet also included raw veal liver juice. This, however, has been discontinued at the Gerson Institute because modern farming techniques have destroyed the value of the liver and calves are being born with diseased immune systems.

One underlying principle is to exclude sodium as far as possible and to enrich the body's tissues with potassium—'to the highest possible degree'. Gerson was in favour of Lugol solution (half strength) to provide potassium and iodine. Developed by the French physician, Jean Lugol, in 1829, it is a transparent brown liquid consisting of ten parts potassium iodide (KI), five parts iodine and 85 parts of (distilled) water. It is an effective bactericide and fungicide and general antiseptic.

'High potassium/low sodium environments can partially return damaged cell proteins to their normal undamaged configuration,' he wrote. Potassium deficiency has been shown by others to be present in the following diseases: cancer, leukaemia, diabetes, glaucoma, chronic arthritis, acute and chronic asthma and sinusitis.

This aspect of the Gerson diet needs to be stressed. The high-potassium, low-sodium balance is well accepted as being one of the key cornerstones of good health. But before you reach for your potassium capsules, you should be warned that there are real dangers associated with sudden potassium overload—dangers to the heart, the muscles and the kidneys. You should only take potassium supplements under the guidance of a nutritionist. The best way of taking in potassium is through foods: almonds, apricots, avocados, bananas, lima, mung and pinto beans, dates, dried figs, hazelnuts, raw garlic, raw horseradish, kelp, blackstrap molasses and brewer's yeast. In fact brewer's yeast, on its own, is considered to be a powerful anti-cancer agent.

On the Gerson diet, the following are forbidden: tobacco, spices, pickles, salt, tea, coffee, cocoa, chocolate, alcohol, refined sugar, refined flour, candies, ice cream, cream, cake, nuts, mushrooms, soybeans and soy products, cucumbers, pineapples, all berries (except red currants), avocadoes, all canned foods, preserves, sulfured peas, lentils and beans, frozen foods, smoked or salted vegetables, dehydrated or powdered foods, bottled juices, and all fats (except flaxseed oil), and oils.

Some food items are forbidden at the beginning but may be introduced to the diet later. These include: milk, cheese, butter, fish, meat and eggs. When cooking, aluminium pots must not be used—only stainless steel, glass, enamelware, or earthenware pans and containers. In addition to diet, hair dyes are also forbidden.

Almost everyone following this diet will suffer some degree of nausea, headaches, gas, depression and even vomiting. Gerson recommends peppermint tea served with some brown sugar and a bit of lemon as a cleansing drink to take away any bad tastes or inability to stomach the diet.

Patients also have to expect 'flare-ups'—a sudden incidence of unpleasant symptoms—which do not last more than a few days. These are considered to be essential to health as they indicate that the body is expelling toxins. It was, and remains, a key aspect of the Gerson approach that without these flare-ups the patient will not be cured. The more poisoned the body was prior to treatment, the more serious the flare-ups. These flare-ups are the result of a toxic release and the body must be detoxified with the use of coffee enemas to ensure that the patient is not damaged by them. It has been argued that it would be very dangerous to combine the Gerson diet with any other effective regime as this might bring on an unexpectedly quick flare-up of dangerous intensity.

Beata Bishop is one person who has been cured by strictly following the Gerson regime. In her case, it took about eighteen months before she was certain she had beaten the disease. Her book: *Triumph over Cancer* starts with these words:

'I should have died of malignant melanoma, one of the fastest spreading cancers, around June 1981. Today I am healthy in the full sense of the word; not just not-ill but enjoying great well-being and energy.'

I met with Beata and you can see my televised interview with her at my Facebook Cancer Recovery site (scroll to the bottom of the page), and at www.cancerfighter.wordpress.com.

Gerson also recommended niacin 50mg, six times daily, for six months. As for vitamin B12, he was undecided, but he was against the administration of other vitamins because he noticed they sometimes had the effect of causing a tumour to grow back. This is because, he says, non-cancerous tissue in a cancer patient does not react in the same way as normal healthy tissue. That is to say, vitamins may normally be very healthy—but they can have negative effects in people with cancer.

And what evidence did Gerson put forward to support his claim that his diet was effective as a cancer treatment? In his book, *A Cancer Therapy*, he provides case histories of 50 patients that he cured.

One of these cases, Case No. 46, was a Mrs E B, aged 48, married with two children. She presented with a cervical carcinoma which was showing signs of invading neighbouring tissues. The biopsy showed clear malignancy. By the time she reached Gerson she had already had radiation treatment but the tumours had returned. He started her on the diet and she kept to it faithfully for 18 months. At the end, she had no sign of cancer. She slowly weaned herself off the diet and eleven years later was still cancer-free.

How successful is the diet? Various estimates have been given—ranging from as low as five per cent to as high as 80 per cent. One of the problems is that the Gerson diet is extremely rigorous and the extent to which ex-patients of the clinic have maintained the diet is unknown. But in one small retrospective study of melanoma, the results were extremely good: 100 per cent of the stage 1 and 2 melanoma cases surviving for five years—in fact none of them died of melanoma, and one was still alive 17 years later. For stage 3 cases the results were 82 per cent, compared with 39 per cent reported by the American Cancer Society. It appears that the Gerson diet is particularly helpful for people with melanoma. There are suggestions that it is less successful with other types of cancer. For further information contact: The Gerson Institute, P.O. Box 430, Bonita, California 91908. USA Tel 1-(619)-685-5353 www.gerson.org or Gerson Research Organization www.gerson-research.org.

The Moerman diet

In 1938, Dr Cornelis Moerman developed a diet that he used to treat those cancer patients that came to see him. He had to suffer professional ridicule for several decades but eventually, in 1987, the Dutch Ministry of Health publicly recognised the Moerman therapy as an effective cancer treatment. Moerman, like many others favouring nutritional health, lived rather longer than most of his colleagues. He was 95 when he died in 1988.

Moerman first became involved when a man by the name of Leendert Brinkman came to him seeking his help. He had a stomach tumour that had spread to his groin and legs. The doctors had given up on him. Moerman told him to eat as many oranges and lemons as he could. He ate them 'by the truckload until I was up to my eyes in vitamin C'. A year later he was free of tumours. He went on to live to a healthy old age, dying at the age of 90.

This success led Moerman to develop his nutritional ideas. Eventually he came to believe that there were eight substances of vital importance to ideal health. These should be taken in supplemental form as well as through dietary means. The required doses of the eight substances were as follows:

Substance	Dose
1. Vitamin A	50,000IU–100,000IU
2. B-complex vitamins	2 large dose tablets
3. Vitamin C	as much as can be tolerated
4. Vitamin E	400–2,200IU
5. Citric Acid	3 tablespoons (of solution: 10–15g Acidum citricum in 300g of water)
6. Iodine	1–3 drops of 3 per cent iodine solution in 300g of water
7. Iron*	
8. Sulphur	1g

* Iron is now generally contraindicated with cancer (see Section 6 Cancer: Vitamins and Other Supplements for a full discussion). However, blackstrap molasses (generally considered healthy) contains iron, so 1–2 tablespoons of this should meet the requirements of the Moerman diet.

Citric acid helps the blood flow, iodine is important for stimulating the thyroid gland. It also works with sulphur to help oxygenate cells. Iron is needed to prevent anaemia. It should be noted that Moerman's liking for iron is not universally accepted among the vitamin and mineral supplement crowd today. Iron has also been implicated, in other studies, as a cancer-promoting agent. Cancer tumours have a great need for iron and some approaches to cancer are based on depriving it of this mineral—so with the regard to the iron, caution is strongly advised.

Moerman's diet allows selection of any of the following:

Grains: whole-grain breads and pastas, brown rice, barley, oat bran, wheat germ, corn flakes

Dairy: butter, buttermilk, cream cheese, cottage cheese, egg yolks, plain live yoghurt

Vegetables: most vegetables lightly steamed. Highly recommended: beet juice and carrot juice, limited intake: Brussels sprouts, cauliflower, parsley

Fruit: most fruits. Most recommended: mixed fresh orange and lemon juice.

Others: bay leaf, garlic, herb tea, nutmeg, cold-pressed olive and sunflower oil.

Prohibited foods:

All meats, all fish and shellfish, alcohol, animal fats, artificial colourings, beans, peas, lentils, mushrooms, potatoes, red cabbage, sauerkraut, cheeses with high fat and salt content, margarine and other hydrogenated oils, coffee, cocoa- or caffeine-containing teas, egg whites, sugar, salt, white flour and tobacco.

Is there any proof that it is effective? A number of doctors sympathetic to Moerman's diet set up a research project which followed 150 patients who had used the Moerman diet either alone or in combination with other therapies. They found that 115 (76.66 per cent) of the patients were cured—60 (40 per cent) using the diet alone.

Results of small studies like this are open to many objections but the results certainly indicate that further research should be done.

The macrobiotic diet

Modern macrobiotics was developed in Japan at the turn of the century. Two educators, Sagen Ishitsuka, who was himself a doctor, and Yukikazu Sakurazawa, cured themselves of serious chronic illnesses by changing their diets to one consisting of brown rice, miso soup, sea vegetables and other traditional foods. Sakurazawa went to Paris in the twenties and—using the name George Ohsawa—began to spread the word.

Ohsawa's macrobiotic diet is based on Eastern philosophy and takes its starting point in the idea of Yin and Yang, the dark passive female and light active male forces which must be maintained in a state of harmony. The body, as with everything else in the universe, must also maintain a healthy balance between these two forces. As each person is unique, the point of balance will be different for each person. Individual cancer tumours also have yin and yang characteristics. For example, while cancer of the tongue is yang, all other tumours of the upper digestive tract are considered to be yin.

From a macrobiotic point of view, cancer is simply a sign, one among others, that the body is in a disharmonious state. The objective, then, is simply to restore the harmony. The only way we can achieve this is through dietary means, such as that recommended by Michio Kushi and Alex Jack, in their book: *The Cancer-Prevention Diet.*

One of the surprising features of the macrobiotic diet is its avoidance of fruits. This avoidance isn't absolute, but fruits are advised only occasionally and only in the proper climatic zone and in the proper season. A person in Europe in winter should not be eating bananas or even oranges. Also to be avoided, in addition to red meats, are dairy products and any form of processed food, are cooking spices and herbs, butter or margarine, iodized salt, ginseng, eggs and yoghurt. Another surprise is the ban on any kind of vitamin or mineral supplement.

Food item	Percentage of daily intake
Whole grains	50–60 per cent. These should be eaten in whole form—and not cracked. Brown rice should be pressure cooked rather than boiled. Breads should not contain yeast, so chapattis and tortillas and sourdough bread are recommended.
Soup	5–10 per cent. One or two bowls of miso or tamari soup. Miso is a kind of fermented soybean paste. Miso should have aged more than 1.5 years and be made of organically grown soybeans.*
Vegetables	25–30 per cent. These should be fresh. Up to one-third can be eaten raw.
Beans and sea vegetables	5–10 per cent
Oils	Unrefined sesame, corn or mustard seed oils are best. Unrefined safflower, sunflower, soy and olive oils can be used occasionally.
Others	Sea salt—though meals should be neither too salty nor too bland. Sea salt should be used in the cooking and not at the table.

* Note: It is known that miso contains a number of anti-angiogenesis substances that interfere with tumour growth.)

Is there any evidence that the macrobiotic diet is effective? Kushi and Jack offer a number of stories of people being cured. One was Jean Kohler, a 56-year-old pianist and professor of music. One summer, he suddenly became aware of an itch that spread up his leg. After several tests were conducted the doctors discovered a massive tumour on his pancreas. Pancreatic tumours are almost always fatal. He was told nothing could be done and that he had anywhere from one month to three years to live. He accepted chemotherapy but after a few days decided that he didn't want to continue with the treatment as it was too debilitating. He started to look for an alternative therapy and was referred to the Kushi Institute in Boston. He started a macrobiotic regime and within six months all signs of cancerous activity had ceased. This was confirmed by medical tests.

Kohler lived another seven years and died of something else entirely. He publicized his case whenever he could and even wrote a book about it.

In another case, Dr Vivien Newbold, an emergency care doctor in Philadelphia, became interested in macrobiotics when her husband had a metastatic cancer of the colon. He reduced the cancer by 70 per cent by going on a macrobiotic diet. She subsequently wrote an article detailing the effect of a macrobiotic diet on six cases in which the five cases who stuck with the diet went into total remission for over five years. This article was rejected by three professional magazines. She was also told by the American Cancer Society's director: 'It is of no interest to us.'

In 1993, however, the *Journal of the American College of Nutrition* published a study of the effects of the macrobiotic diet on people with pancreatic cancer. After one year, 52 per cent of those on the diet were still alive compared with only ten per cent of the controls—a 500 per cent increase in one-year survival rates.

For further information contact: Kushi Institute, PO Box 7, Becket, MA 01223, USA.

Barry Sears, a biochemist and pioneer in biotechnology who wrote a best-selling book, *The Zone*, analyzed the macrobiotic diet and praised it for the fact that it has low overall fat, especially bad omega 6 fats, but is rich in the activated omega 3 fatty acid EPA (fish and sea vegetables), but he faults it for being too high in grains. He characterizes the diet as being 'like taking two steps forward and one step back' .

The alkaline pH diet

The foods we eat, once they have been digested and the useful food elements extracted, leave a residue, or an ash, in our bodies and this ash will either be acid, alkali or neutral. The acidity or alkalinity of any substance can be determined by comparing it to a pH scale. If it tests at below 7.0 on the scale then the substance is acid. If it tests above 7.0 then it is alkali. A healthy state of being is slightly alkali (7.35–7.45). Unfortunately, for most people living on convenience foods, the body's tissues are increasingly tending towards an acidic, disease-vulnerable state.

In a famous analysis, which was to lead to a Nobel Prize, Dr Otto Warburg described the environment of the cancer cell. A normal cell uses oxygen to convert glucose into energy by the process of oxidation. When there is insufficient oxygen around the cell to be used for this purpose, the cell reverts to a more primitive process, converting glucose by fermentation. This fermentation process produces lactic acid as a by-product and the acid lowers the cell's pH (i.e., it makes the cell more acidic) and this in turn makes the cell unable to control its own cell division processes. The result is cancer. At the same time, the lactic acid causes intense local pain and destroys the cell's enzymes. From this we can see that an acidic state is essentially cancerous and an alkali state is healthy. We can also see that a cancer cannot continue to exist when the surrounding tissues are highly alkaline (that at least is the theory).

The following two lists show the foods that leave an alkali ash (good) and those that leave an acidic ash (bad).

Alkali-ash foods

Almonds, apples, apricots, avocados, bananas, dried beans, beetroot, blackberries, broccoli, Brussels sprouts, cabbage, carrots, cauliflower, celery, chard leaves, cherries (sour), cucumbers, dried dates, dried figs, grapefruit, grapes, green beans, green peas, lemons, lettuce, goat's milk, millet, molasses, mushrooms, onions, oranges, parsnips, peaches, pears, pineapples, sweet potatoes, white potatoes, radishes, raisins, raspberries, rutabagas, sauerkraut, green soybeans, raw spinach, strawberries, tangerines, tomatoes, umeboshi vinegar, watercress, watermelon.

Acid-ash foods

Bacon, barley grain, beef, blueberries, bran (wheat and oat), bread (white and whole meal), butter, cheese, chicken, cod, corn, corned beef, crackers, cranberries, currants, eggs, flour (all types), haddock, lamb, dried lentils, lobster, macaroni, oatmeal, oysters, peanut butter, peanuts, dried peas, pike, pork, rice (white and brown), salmon, sardines, sausage, scallops, shrimp, spaghetti, winter squash, sunflower seeds, turkey, veal, walnuts, wheat germ, yoghurt.

Refined sugar and olive oil are neutral ash foods that nevertheless have an acidifying effect on the body.

The pH of the body is also affected by emotions and activity—stress and aggressive sports create a more acid environment; relaxation and relaxed exercise create a more alkaline environment.

Drinking a teaspoon of sodium bicarbonate in a glass of water at night is also recommended as a way of raising alkalinity. In fact sodium bicarbonate has been used as a cheap and effective way of attacking cancer cells by introducing it as close to the tumour as possible by intravenous injection or vaginal flush. An Italian doctor, Dr Tullio Simoncini, has claimed a high degree of success using this method.

What I like about this diet is the fact that it is simple to understand, and does not rely on the inspiration or intuition of one man based on multiple understandings. The object is to become as alkaline as it is possible to be, the foods needed to achieve this are known. Just eat those foods. Simple really.

Baking soda

Another approach to curing cancer by raising pH levels, originally promoted by an Appalachian folk healer in the 1930s, is to heat one part of baking soda with three parts of pure maple syrup (or some prefer organic blackstrap molasses) for five minutes, stirring briskly. When this mixture is consumed, the theory is that the cancer cells suck up the glucose along with the baking soda that is bound to it. The sudden increased alkalinity in the cell kills it. Some critics point out, however, that maple syrup cannot chemically bind with sodium bicarbonate. However, Bill Henderson, who has experimented on himself, says he experienced clear and indeed powerful demonstrations that this mix had a healthy impact on his bowel movements. Whether it also has an anti-cancer effect is still very much in the realm of anecdote and folk lore—but there are animal studies showing that sodium bicarbonate inhibits metastases—so slowing down if not reversing the spread of cancer. This is not a stand-alone cancer therapy but it is one that can cheaply and usefully be followed.

The one issue with bicarbonate is that, because of its alkalinity, it should not be taken within a couple of hours of a meal as it will have a negative impact on the stomach acids needed to digest food.

'Sodium bicarbonate happens to be one of our most useful medicines treating as it does the basic acid-alkaline axis of human physiology. Sodium bicarbonate is a 'nothing-to-lose-everything-to-gain' treatment for cancer as well as the general acid conditions behind a host of modern diseases.'

Dr Mark Sircus

Oxalic acid diet

This is a diet whose aim is to increase the oxalic acid concentration of the blood, according to the man whose inspiration this is: Colonel Joe Hart, a retired American army officer. This will, he claims, help cure you of cancer and a number of other health conditions.

Before starting this discussion, however, it is important to note that oxalic acid is a powerful poison and should never be ingested in its purified chemical state. 600mg per kg body weight is lethal.

Col. Joe—Francis J Hart—has noted first that a healthy body has a high oxalic acid presence in the blood—an odd fact given that it is toxic. Also he notes that the foods that are most commonly focused on as being beneficial against cancer (carrots, cabbage, beetroot, etc.) are precisely those that contain oxalic acid—and he believes that oxalic acid is what keeps the blood clear of cancer cells.

His diet consists of eating vegetables selected from the following list: snap beans, Brussels sprouts, beets, carrots, cassava, chives, collards, garlic, lettuce, parsley, purslane, radish, spinach, sweet potato, turnips and watercress. Nuts—especially walnuts—are also a good source and contain fatty acids (oleic and linoleic), which will increase the intestinal absorption of the acid. He also advises that all cooking be done with olive oil (cold pressed extra virgin is best). Chocolate is also good—but not the milk and sugar that goes with it.

Unfortunately, the benefits of oxalic acid can be blocked by other dietary and non-dietary items such as citric acid, calcium, cow's milk (and milk based products), vitamin B6 (pyridoxine) and alcohol—though if you like a tipple then choose a cheap red wine which is high in oxalic acid. The danger of citric acid comes not from ingesting too many oranges but from its use as a preservative in most processed foods (all of which must be avoided). The non-dietary blocker that most concerns Col. Joe is radiation—from cell phones, irradiation of food and from every other source of radiation. For further information and for testimonials go to Col. Joe's website www.coljoe.com.

The anti-candida diet

Fungi and yeasts are associated with cancer and can themselves harm the body with their toxins. To get rid of them, Philip Day, author of *Cancer: Why We're Still Dying to Know the Truth*, suggests the following diet.

Eliminate: all cow's milk products and derivatives including yoghurt; all yeast-containing products: including alcohol, bread, vinegars; mushrooms; processed and smoked fish and meats; all sugar products including honey and artificial sweeteners; nearly all fruit; root vegetables with a high sugar content: carrots, parsnips, sweet potatoes, potatoes, beetroot.

Other foods to be eliminated are: all pastries, cakes, cereals, fast food snacks, white rice, corn, pasta, chick peas, dried beans, lentils and pinto beans, coffee, all soy products, all sauces, all hydrogenated oil products.

Instead you should eat plenty of the following foods:

Vegetables:	Bean sprouts, bell peppers, broccoli, Brussels sprouts, cabbage, cauliflower, celery, chinese greens, cucumber, endive, fennel, garlic, green beans, hot chilli peppers, kale, lettuce, onions, parsley, radishes, spring onions, spinach, Swiss chard, turnips, yellow beans.
Meat, etc.:	Free-range eggs, fresh fish (deep sea, wild), lamb, veal, chicken, turkey.
Herbs:	Culinary herbs and spices are permitted.
Oils:	Avocado oil, cod liver oil, fish oil, flaxseed oil, grape seed oil, hemp oil, olive oil, evening primrose oil.
Fruit:	Only one apple, pear or kiwi fruit a day.

Raw-food diet

The main problem with cooking food is that not only does it destroy some of the vitamin and nutrient qualities of the food, it also destroys the enzymes that help to digest that same food. Raw food is therefore generally much healthier than cooked food.

The raw food diet is vegetarian—raw steak has no place here. The vegetables and fruit can be eaten either raw or as a juice. The foods that have been identified by the other dietary regimes above are all suitable for this diet. A number of people claim to have cured their cancers simply by turning to an all raw-foods diet, among them a number of doctors. This diet was promoted by the Danish doctor Kristine Nolfi. She cured her own cancer with a 100 per cent organic and vegetarian raw-food diet, and then continued to cure cancer patients in the same way on her health farm.

When she discovered that she had cancer, she wrote: 'I started immediately, going to a small island in the Kattegat where I lived in a tent, ate raw vegetables exclusively and sunbathed from four to five hours a day when weather permitted. When I felt too warm, I plunged into the sea. My fatigue continued throughout the first two months, and the tumour in my breast did not diminish. But then my recovery began. The tumour grew smaller as I regained strength, and I felt better than I had for several years.'

She eventually lost her medical license for using 'dangerous' and unapproved methods but her fame nevertheless spread throughout Scandinavia. It should be noted that after a year she went back to a diet that was only 75 per cent raw vegetables, and soon afterwards she felt the tumour return.

A New Zealand doctor, Eva Hill, successfully treated her basal carcinoma following a raw-food diet—becoming a well-known advocate in the antipodes. She had to overcome a few legal barriers before it became accepted that she should be allowed to treat cancer patients in any way likely to be successful. And, in Britain, Dr Barbara Moore successfully cured herself of leukaemia in the same way. She subsequently went on to publicly demonstrate the health of her vegetarian diet by walking the length of Britain from John O'Groats to Land's End.

Lactic acid diet

Lactic acid is a natural preservative in that it inhibits pathogenic bacteria. It is a by-product created by the breakdown of sugars and starches by lactobacilli—a family of bacteria that includes the well-known acidophilus. These living lactobacilli produce many helpful enzymes, antibiotics and anti-carcinogens. Lactic acid, their by-product, promotes the growth of healthy flora throughout the intestine as well as preventing the growth of harmful bacteria. It is also an extremely fast fuel that is vital for ensuring that our bodies get a steady supply of carbohydrates. Athletes use drinks containing lactates.

In the 1950s, German cancer therapist, Dr J Kuhl, used a diet high in lactic acid fermented foods with good results. It was Dr Kuhl who discovered that there was an important difference between 'healthy' lactic acid and the lactic acid produced by cancers. He noted that lactic acid produced by a tumour rotates light to the left and enhances tumour growth. Lactic acid produced by lactic acid bacteria, on the other hand, rotates light to the right and inhibits tumour growth.

A lacto-fermented diet consists of foods like sauerkraut, olives, pickles, vegetable juices, dairy and naturally fermented soy products like miso. But note that not all soy sauces are good—some commercially-produced soy sauces contain dangerous chemicals.

To make your own fermented vegetable preparation: shred green or red cabbage, grated beetroot, diced Brussels sprouts, red peppers, chillies, cucumbers and add either sea salt or, if you prefer not to use salt, add some strong alcohol and water (but not tap water as chlorine interferes with the process). Mash the mixture for several minutes and then bottle it in sealed glass containers. Leave some space between the top of the mix and the top. Leave for at least three days at room temperature before refrigerating—but the longer the better. Do not open at any time as oxygen interferes with the fermentation. When it's ready, eat it.

The Dries cancer diet

Dr Jan Dries is a leading Belgian naturopath and active promoter of a vegetarian diet. His starting assumption is that wild animals do not get cancer, that we are a monkey and that wild monkeys live mainly on a diet of fruit and nuts—and this answers all their nutritional needs. Another basic principle behind his anti-cancer diet is that the consumption of natural foods is, in effect, the consumption of sunlight—the more sunlight a food has absorbed, the more powerful it is as an enhancer of the immune system.

The Dries cancer diet, unlike almost every other anti-cancer diet, promotes the consumption of large quantities of raw fruits, particularly tropical fruit such as pineapple and mango. In addition, the diet includes some raw vegetables, seeds, yoghurt, buttermilk and some oils. These foods are chosen on the basis of their bio-energetic value measured in bio-photons.

All chemicals whether they are preservatives, fertilizers or pesticides, undermine what he calls the 'bio-energetic value' of food. So too does cooking. The Dries cancer diet promotes the eating of raw, preferably wild or organic, fruits. The Dries diet divides foods into seven groups of decreasing bio-energetic value. The first group consists of the foodstuffs that, according to Dries, have the greatest bio-energetic value. But food from all seven groups should be eaten.

Group I:	pineapple, cactus fruit, avocado, raspberry, honeydew, melon, pollen, comb honey
Group II:	bilberry, kiwi, cherry, persimmon, apricot, melon, mango, papaya, almonds, chervil, mushrooms, honey
Group III:	feijoa, red currants, blackcurrant, strawberry, lychee, passion fruit, red and green grapes, medlar, peach, sunflower seeds, pumpkin seeds, wheat germ, germinated wheat, sprouts, liquid brewer's yeast, Panaktiv*
Group IV:	banana, gooseberries, green melon, Brazil nut, coconut, vegetables, dairy products
Group V:	oranges, mandarins, apples, pears, plums and grapefruit.
Group VI:	this group consists of common vegetables
Group VII:	avocados, nuts and seeds

*Panaktiv is a liquid brewer's yeast developed by a Dr Metz—see www.drmetz.de for further details.

Group 1 foods should be eaten at every meal. Foods from the other groups should be eaten with decreasing frequency depending on their place in the hierarchy. It is recommended that you follow the Dries diet exclusively for three months.

The result, according to those who have undergone this diet, will be a very obvious detoxification of the body—bad smells and so on for a few weeks. But once this is complete there are no further negative impacts. Personal testimonials refer not only to the healing potential of the diet but its ability to help patients undergo radiation and chemotherapy with very much reduced levels of side effects. You can expect substantial weight loss.

If there is an issue with this diet it is the apparently high intake of sugars—in the form of fructose. However, while refined white sugar will cause a sudden leap in blood sugar levels—it is known as a high-glycaemic food—fructose, despite being a sugar, is in fact one of the lowest-glycaemic foods there are. Fructose is, it must be admitted, a dietary issue, but not when it is packaged in the form of fruit. As endocrinologist Robert Lustig states: 'When God made the poison he packaged it in with the antidote.'—the antidote is fibre. Fruit therefore is good, for all sorts of reasons that have nothing to do with the fructose (and the amounts of fructose in fruit is not a matter of concern)—but high-fructose syrup is a poison. Unfortunately, it is a poison in virtually every form of processed food you can buy in the supermarket. Everything that needs to be made sweeter is done so with high-fructose syrup. This is what is making us all fatter. For an excellent discussion of this go to Lustig's 90 minute video and watch it right through. It will astound you. (www.youtube.com/watch?v=dBnniua6-oM).

Dries is not alone in advocating a raw fruit and/or vegetable diet. It has been pointed out that such diets are high in water and bulk fibre content and result in low nutritional intake. Since cancer growth appears to be directly related to food intake, this is good news. In experiments using mice fed on raw fruits and vegetables, the benefits of the raw diet were lost when soy protein or other dietary 'improvements' were added. So this diet, in the guise of being a diet, may be just another way of fasting.

Contact details: Jan Dries, Avicenna Health Centre, Schepersweg 112, 3600 Genk, Belgium, Tel: 32 89 396 169 Fax: 32 89 355 307

The longevity diet

The following diet is not proposed as an anti-cancer diet but as one that will boost longevity in a healthy way and one which will promote weight loss (and being over-weight adds to one's risk of getting cancer). It is a strategy that can be combined with any of the diets previously discussed.

The benefits of a low calorie diet have long been known. Animals given low calorie diets tend to live about one-third longer than similar animals on normal diets. They didn't just live longer, they had clearer arteries, lower levels of inflammation, better blood sugar control, their brain cells were less likely to get damaged and the rates of diseases linked to ageing all dropped. We also know that war-time Britons were in general much healthier on their calorie-restricted rations than they were before or after. The problem is that, in this time of abundance, it takes an iron will to reduce calorie intake by the required amount.

It has now been discovered that the same benefits can be achieved by alternating days of normal intake with days of very low calorie intake. One day on, one day off. That means you don't have to go on a permanent starvation diet.

Krista Varady, assistant professor of kinesiology and nutrition at the University of Illinois, Chicago published the results of a ten-week trial of 16 patients, all weighing more than 14st (90kg).

On one day, they ate 20 per cent of their normal intake and, on the next, a regular, healthy diet. Each lost between 10lb (4.5kg) and 30lb (13.5kg) over the ten weeks. 'It takes about two weeks to adjust to the diet and, after that, people don't feel hungry on the fast days,' she said. On the fasting days, dieters should only consume around 500 calories—equal to three bowls of unsweetened porridge or around 700 grams of potatoes.

Dr James Johnson, author of The Alternate-Day Diet, who has now been doing the diet for a number of years 'I've always been a bit overweight. When I first started, I lost 35lb in 11 weeks. Now I use the diet to keep my weight stable. If it starts going up, I'll just go back on it for a few weeks. The evidence says this is about the most healthy thing you can do for yourself.'

In another study with ten obese asthmatics showed that after eight weeks they had lost eight per cent of their body weight and their levels of inflammation was down by 70 per cent and the level of free radicals by 90 per cent.

British researchers led by Dr Michelle Harvie, of the Genesis Breast Cancer Prevention Centre in Manchester are looking at the benefits of the diet in preventing breast cancer in high risk patients. 'We've found a very low 800 calories-a-day diet dramatically lowers the enzymes that metabolise fat and glucose in breast tissue,' 'These enzymes are always raised in breast cancer patients.'

It seems that a specific gene (SIRT1) is the reason for the diet's success as it prevents other genes involved in storing fat.

The weight-loss benefit could also be due to the way the diet tricks the body's metabolism. In the case of most diets the body will respond after about 48 hours by slowing down the metabolism but that doesn't happen if you only 'diet' for a day at a time. The other advantage is that when you come off the diet the body doesn't rapidly put the weight back on.

One woman who had lost 15lb (7kg) on the diet found that nine months later she had only put 2lb back on. Going back on the diet for another month she lost a further 10lb.

The rules of the diet are as follows:

1. For the first two weeks, try to keep calories intake on fasting days to 500 calories—then you can go up to around 700–800.
2. On normal days eat normally—but try not to compensate by eating more.
3. Drink plenty of water and exercise regularly.

Conclusion

It will be seen that there is a great deal of difference between one diet and another—and since different diets are based on different principles and have different objectives it is not necessarily a good idea to mix and match. Nevertheless, there is also a strong degree of overlap and as you can see from the stories of cancer survivors in Section 8: *Cancer: Survivors' Stories*, diet plays a big part in any cancer recovery program.

Other Food-Based Therapies

The Budwig protocol

This is the most highly-regarded of all dietary approaches and supporters of the Budwig protocol claim a 90 per cent success rate against all forms of cancer. Dr Johanna Budwig, an eminent German biochemist, was the first person to promote the health benefits of flaxseed oil.

Budwig was among the first scientists to take a close look at an area that had previously been lumped together and ignored—the fats. She soon discovered that although some fats, the saturated fats, were harmful, others the 'natural electron-rich, vital, highly unsaturated fats' had enormously beneficial properties. The saturated fats tended to clog cells and organs and the result of this process, eventually, is diabetes, arthritis, heart disease and cancer. The most highly unsaturated fats are those Budwig grouped together under the heading 'linoleic acids'. By this she meant both linoleic acid (an omega 6 oil) and alpha-linolenic acid (an omega 3 oil). It is now known that omega 6 oils, in excess, promote inflammation and cancer, while omega 3 oils are healing.

These so-called 'essential' fatty acids are vital for the proper oxygenation of the body. For Budwig the key element that made these unsaturated fats life promoting was their electrical charge created by a surrounding field of electrons. Unfortunately, industrial handling of these fats strips away this field of electrons and destroys their vitality. She likens them to a battery that has run flat.

These de-activated unsaturated fats along with the saturated fats are no longer able to travel through the small capillary network of the blood system. The result is that they clog the capillaries and as a result the tissues these capillaries serve become de-oxygenated. As cells accommodate themselves to this new low-oxygen environment, cancer can be the end result.

The solution, according to Budwig is to take in flaxseed oil (also known as linseed oil) which contains an excellent mix of 4 parts alpha-linolenic-acid (ALA) to one part linoleic acid. However, in its pure form it is not so easily absorbed by the body. Looking around for a protein-based substance in which to dissolve the flaxseed oil and allow it to become water soluble (and so more easily absorbed by the body) she found in succession skim milk, quark and low-fat cottage cheese. Some nutritionists are now proposing that yoghurt or an undenatured whey concentrate might be equally good.

One tablespoon of flaxseed oil (liquid, never capsules) should be hand blended, very thoroughly, with one or two spoons of soft low-fat cottage cheese or, preferably, quark. This can be taken once a day for normal health maintenance and six to ten times a day to cure cancer. Cayenne pepper and garlic can be added for taste (and because they are also beneficial). People with advanced liver cancers may not be able to tolerate such quantities straight away so dose levels will have to be built up slowly.

This is the core of the Budwig protocol, which should be supported by a diet that contains fresh, preferably raw (and consequently enzyme-rich) fruits and vegetables, unprocessed cereals, and fresh cold water fish, six to eight glasses of bottled distilled water and herbal teas. Starting the day with freshly home-made sauerkraut is a key recommendation. Foods to avoid include all processed oils, fried foods, sugar, artificial sweeteners or any processed food containing preservatives, or chemical additives. In addition, as much time as possible should be spent being exposed to the sun's rays without sunblocks. In her booklet, *Flax Oil as a True Aid Against Arthritis, Heart Infarction, Cancer and Other Diseases*, she discusses in great detail the electromagnetic benefits of light on the body.

She also recommends a number of oils, called EL-DI (short for electron-differentiation) oils that can be rubbed on the skin. They are available from: Gesundheitsprodukte-Reformwaren, Tel: 07441-2877 (011 49 7441 2877 from USA and Canada); email: Wolfgang.Bloching@t-online.de.

However, as some people have discovered, it is not a good idea to take powerful anti-oxidants like vitamin C or ellagic acid at the same time as the Budwig protocol, as these tend to deactivate the benefits of flaxseed oil. Even too many citrus fruits should be avoided. In fact, Budwig was opposed to the taking of any man-made supplements.

In most cases, according to Dr Budwig, this protocol will be sufficient to cure cancer, arthritis and heart disease. What's more, there are large numbers of testimonials to support this claim. She and her supporters claim a 90 per cent success rate with all forms of cancer. However, in a small number of cases the body lacks certain enzymes and nutrients and so is unable to process the flaxseed oil. In this case, fish oils should be added to the diet along with Brewer's yeast. (In fact there is a record of a 78-year-old man who recovered slowly—it took him six years—from a widely spread lung cancer by taking 15 grams of fish oil a day. This was reported in an article by Dr Ron Pardini of the University of Nevada.)

It has been said that strictly speaking the Budwig protocol, as it is known, does not attack cancer, it merely corrects a previous deficiency in omega 3 oils. Armin Grunewald, MD, Dr Budwig's nephew has commented, 'Dr Budwig's approach is not a method of healing cancer but a technique which strengthens the body's own immune defense against cancerous cells.' In 1990, oncologist, Dr Roehm concluded: 'this diet is far and away the most successful anti-cancer diet in the world'. This Budwig protocol has claims to be a very powerful anti-cancer tool as the many testimonials on the Yahoo health groups flaxseed oil page demonstrate. For more information go to: www.health.groups.yahoo.com/group/FlaxSeedOil2/files/

Another very useful information site is www.healingcancernaturally.com/budwig_protocol.html.

It should be noted, as a postscript, that flaxseeds are one of nature's more potent anti-cancer plants, and not just because they are the richest plant source of omega-3 fatty acids. Flax has at least 100 times more lignan precursors than any other known edible plant. Lignans are natural plant compounds that possess strong anticancer properties. One of these lignans is secoisolariciresinol diglycoside (SDG) which on its own has been shown to inhibit metastases.

However, lignan-enriched flaxseed oil is not advised by Budwig purists. The process of adding lignans to the already lignan-rich flaxseed oil has negative consequences for the quality of the oil.

Also, there is a new flaxseed strain called Linola that has been developed to provide oils for the food industry. Sadly, this form of flaxseed oil is very low in ALA, and so it too should be avoided. In the USA, Barleans brand flaxseed oil is highly regarded and I am informed that if you contact them directly and tell them you have cancer, they will give you a substantial discount. To enquire, call them at 1-800-445-3529 or www.barleans.com. Flaxseed oil is sold at most health food shops. It must be kept in dark bottles and kept in cool places. It quickly loses its potency in light conditions.

As a postscript to the flaxseed story, Steve Martin, who runs a very interesting site at www.grouppekurosawa.com, quotes the case of an 83-year-old man who had terminal prostate cancer. Taking a flaxseed product, he saw his PSA score drop from 155 plus to 14.5 over a few weeks. According to Martin, the lignans in flaxseed oil cause cancer cells to die through apoptosis. The product he recommends is Jarrow Formulas Omega Nutrition Cold-Milled Flaxseed, which is organic, and provides 105mg of lignans per tablespoon.

Controlled amino acid therapy (CAAT)

This is a combination dietary regime, accompanied by supplements and a specially formulated amino acid mix. The regime is customized for each patient.

Formulated by Dr Angelo P John, this therapy is offered exclusively by the A P John Institute for Cancer Research. The object of the therapy is to create a diet that deprives the cancer tumour of certain amino acids and carbohydrates (which are converted into sugar during digestion—and cancers love sugar). This approach has a great deal of experimental support.

The whole therapy program lasts six to eight months and costs approximately US$1,200 a month. For further information go to www.apjohncancerinstitute.org.

The dairy-free diet

Prof. Jane Plant was diagnosed with breast cancer at the age of 42. At the time she was a successful geochemist (she subsequently became chief scientist of the British Geological Survey). She went on a vegetarian diet. She had a mastectomy. She had radiation. But the cancer kept coming back. At its fifth recurrence, she underwent a course of chemotherapy but was told that she had at most a few months to live. She had by this time an egg-sized tumour on the side of her neck.

All this time she was researching and looking for answers. Then, one night, brainstorming with her husband about why breast cancer rates in the west were so high and yet were extremely low in China, it suddenly occurred to them both that one of the key differences in diet was that the Chinese don't eat dairy products.

Plant immediately eliminated all dairy products (including goat and sheep) from her diet. Six weeks later, the tumour had disappeared. Since then she has stayed on her dairy-free diet and has remained clear of cancer.

Giving up dairy products was only part of a health regimen she has followed since then. She now advocates taking folic acid and zinc supplements, drinking filtered water and never consuming anything that had been packaged in plastic (phthalates, harmful carcinogenic chemicals, leak from soft plastic into food).

She is not alone. Hearing of her success, over 60 other women decided to follow her regime and also recovered. As a result of these experiences, Plant wrote her book: *Your Life in Your Hands*.

The reason for milk's deadly effects is that it contains insulin-like growth factor (IGF-1). This chemical occurs naturally in women to help their breasts develop. Plant found that pre-menopausal women with the highest IGF-1 concentration in their blood had a far higher risk of developing breast cancer (other studies have found a link between IGF-1 and prostate cancer).

This correlation of breast cancer, in particular, with increased use of dairy products has a lot of support from epidemiological studies. Plant has also found that pasteurization appears to result in the production of free oestrogens, and these may stimulate IGF-1 activity resulting in long-term tumour growth. Milk also contains dioxins and other environmental toxins that come down the food chain, as they are fat-soluble and end up particularly concentrated in milk.

Instead of dairy products, Plant recommends soya milk, herbal tea, hummus, tofu, nuts and seeds, non-farmed fish, organic eggs and lean meat (not minced beef, which tends to be dairy cow) and plenty of fresh organic fruit and vegetables (in salads, juiced, or lightly steamed). Below, we will see that not everyone agrees with her that soy products are good.

Traditional Chinese medicine (TCM) and diet

TCM encompasses a number of different practices: diet, herbs, acupuncture and qigong. Here we will look at the dietary aspect.

TCM views the body in a way that is hard to reconcile with Western perceptions. First it has a concept of five elements: fire, earth, metal, wood and water. Then there are the five bodily systems: heart, spleen, lungs, liver and kidney.

Each person varies in the extent to which these elements influence their bodily systems. The elements are in dynamic relationship with each other as are the bodily systems.

In addition there are opposed pairs of dynamic forces: yin (female) and yang (male). All of this is infused by 'qi' (pronounced 'chee') energy, blood and other bodily fluids; and then there are the pathogenic factors: the bodily systems can be hot or cold, damp or dry. TCM assesses these systems and forces to determine whether there is a state of deficiency, balance or excess.

The bodily systems (heart, lung, etc.) are not the same as the Western organs of the same name. When the TCM doctor talks of kidneys, for example, he is not referring to the physical organ that we know as the kidney but to a range of functions.

All of this can easily sound bizarre but we should remember that the Chinese are among the most pragmatic people in the world. If something doesn't work, they don't persevere. TCM has been around for well over three thousand years. We must therefore assume that it has been at least moderately successful at what it does.

However, in relation to cancer we must understand that TCM does not, generally speaking, recognise cancer, it only recognises the imbalance of the bodily systems. The one exception to this is breast cancer which was isolated several hundred years ago as a specific ailment with a specific cause:

liver qi stagnation. This is interesting in that many (if not all) alternative practitioners point to poor liver function as a major contributory factor of cancer.

The TCM doctor's approach is to seek to bring the body back into a harmonious state of health. If he can manage that, it is possible the cancer will depart. However, the general consensus is that, in relation to attacking cancer tumours specifically, TCM is not particularly effective. TCM doctors that I have talked to see the role of TCM as supportive of other therapies and as a way of protecting the body, or particular organs or eliminating specific symptoms: nausea, for example.

There is no such thing therefore as a TCM anti-cancer diet (though there are websites that put forward supposedly TCM anti-cancer diets). There are only patient-specific diets. These diets need to be specially formulated depending on the specific signs and symptoms that the particular patient exhibits. For some people, raw foods may be beneficial, but for others, they may be harmful—similarly grapes will be appropriate for some but not to those who have a 'hot' constitution).

Since the assessment of the situation is crucial to deciding what particular diet should be followed, it follows that you need to be careful in selecting an appropriate TCM doctor. The minimum requirement is that they have completed a five-year full-time university course.

In China today all proper TCM doctors have to study for five years followed by a year of practical work. This then is followed by advanced training of about three years. Each province in China has a specialist TCM university, but the best is the China Academy of Traditional Chinese Medicine in Beijing. Anyone wishing to go to Beijing can contact the Guang An Men Hospital, which is affiliated to the Academy (Email: gamhkycy@netchina.com.cn for details).

Dr Luke Tian, a TCM doctor practicing in Rockville, Maryland, specialises in treating cancer, and he has a number of testimonials from patients that he has helped with chronic lymphocytic leukaemia (CLL). For further details see www.lukeacupuncture.com.

See also the interesting website at www.tcmtreatment.com.

Ayurvedic medicine and diet

There are many similarities between TCM and Ayurvedic medicine. Ayurvedic medicine also has a five-element concept (air, fire, water, earth and ether) but it also has a concept of three basic body types or doshas: kapha, pitta or vata. If you are more drawn to an Indian dietary approach then you should seek out an Ayurvedic practitioner to develop a dietary strategy which may be your central anti-cancer therapy, or a support for other therapies.

Much of the discussion of TCM also applies to Ayurvedic medicine. Any diet that is formulated will be specific to each patient.

Again, the question of how you can assess the professional ability of an Ayurvedic doctor needs to be asked. First, of course, there is the normal personal assessment. However, for many people, it is a surprise to learn that Ayurvedic doctors, like doctors of TCM, are not folk healers but are university trained. In India today there are close to 200 undergraduate colleges of Ayurveda offering a five-year degree course in Ayurvedic Medicine, including one-year internship, part of which is spent in conventional medicine departments. In addition there are 55 postgraduate colleges of Ayurveda offering a three-year MD PhD in Ayurveda.

The pre-eminent institution is the All India Institute of Medical Sciences (AIIMS) (address: Ansari Nagar, New Delhi 110029, Tel.: +91-11-660110,6864851 Fax: +91-11-6862663. Email: pkdav@medinst.ernet.in).

Another centre in Kerala, the Athulya Ayurvedic Medical Research Centre, has a website with details of patients whose cancers have been successfully treated using Ayurvedic medicine. For further details go to www.ayurvediccancertherapy.com.

The Healing Attributes of Individual Foods

Vegetables

Asparagus

There are a number of anecdotal reports that asparagus could be a cure for cancer. Here is an example: 'Case No. 1, A man with an almost hopeless case of Hodgkin's disease (cancer of the lymph glands) who was completely incapacitated. Within one year of starting the asparagus therapy, his doctors were unable to detect any signs of cancer, and he was back on a schedule of strenuous exercise.'

The problem with unspecified anecdotal reports like this is they cannot be relied on. Indeed the above case history appears to be in an article by an author who doesn't exist. Nevertheless asparagus is a healthy plant to eat and does contain chemicals that have been shown to have an anti-cancer effect. So anyone deciding to take the risk of asparagus overdose should cook and blend as much asparagus as they can afford and drink a few soup spoons (or even bowls?) of the stuff every day. Canned asparagus appears to be OK.

Beetroot

From 1951, Alexander Ferenczi, MD, an Hungarian cancer therapist, at the Department for Internal Diseases at the district hospital at Csoma, Hungary, began putting patients on a diet consisting almost entirely of eating large amounts of red beetroot (raw or juiced). Brief details of this treatment were reprinted in the *Australian International Clinical Nutrition Review* for July 1986.

One case study he reported was a 50 year old man referred to as D S, who had a lung tumour 'After six weeks of treatment the tumour had disappeared …. After four months of treatment he gained 10kg (22lb) in weight.' All other tests confirmed that he had the symptoms of a clinical recovery. The active ingredient is the purple colouring chemical anthocyanin. Anthocyanins are widely present in fruit and vegetables particularly those that are dark red and purple and research is showing that they have many health benefits.

Bitter melon

This is a light-to-medium-green Chinese melon recognisable for being 6–8 inches long with knobbed ridges—a very bumpy vegetable! Its botanical name is Momordica charantia. In Cantonese it is known as Fu (bitter) Gwa, or Leung (cooling) Gwa. When lightly fried or steamed, it has a sharply tart but not unpleasant taste. It is very popular in summer months when it is eaten to cool the body down. This 'cooling' effect may be felt as a cleansing or purifying process. It is not recommended for pregnant women as it can have the effect of inducing spontaneous abortion (and as we know, anything that can cause spontaneous abortion can also help eliminate tumours, and vice versa). For cancer patients it is suggested that the bitter melon fruit and leaves are eaten together in large daily quantities. The bitter melon fruit (i.e., the part that is normally eaten) has a powerful ability to lower blood sugar—and as sugar is cancer's main fuel, this is very good news.

Bitter melon is being recommended by a number of AIDS activist groups as an immune support for people infected with HIV. For these purposes, the fruit of the bitter melon is not used. A 'tea' is made from boiling a pound of leaves and vines with two litres of water, brought to the boil and then simmered for 60–90 minutes (stirring every 20 minutes) and then cooled. Alternatively leaves and water can be put through a blender. In both cases the resulting 'tea' is strained to remove solid particles. It is then taken into the body through the colon in the form of a retention enema.

This way of taking bitter melon may also be beneficial for cancer patients. Bitter melon tea appears to be, like garlic, a powerful anti-viral agent and is also effective against the Herpes simplex virus. One source of bitter melon tea is www.charanteausa.com.

Cayenne pepper

Cayenne pepper is known to be very effective for heart problems and can even stop a heart attack. Herbalist Dr Richard Schulze also claims that it has powerful anti-cancer effects. He tells the story of a man who had an inoperable brain tumour. He went home, did a colon/liver detox and then started a regimen of ten cups per day of cayenne pepper tea. In three months he returned to his doctor and his X-rays showed a dried up, dead tumour in his head. In countries that have some very hot cuisine, Thailand for example, you find significantly lower cancer and heart disease rates.

In March 2006, the journal *Cancer Research* published the results of a study undertaken at the Los Angeles Cedar-Sinai Medical Center, demonstrating that capsaicin, the ingredient that makes peppers hot, has the effect of causing cancer cells to die by inducing apoptosis (natural cell death).

Schulze recommends one teaspoon of organic cayenne pepper, or an equivalent number of drops of a good cayenne pepper tincture, in a glass of hot water three times a day for almost everything. It may, however, be necessary to build slowly to that level if you are not used to hot foods. Capsules should be avoided as the interaction of the cayenne in the mouth is an important feature of its benefits.

Cayenne has an immediate impact in widening the blood vessels, which allows more blood and oxygen to reach distant sites—this means that besides being effective in itself it will also speed the delivery of other drugs and herbs you take at the same time. If cayenne is not immediately available then chillies will be good, but sweet paprika is an extremely weak substitute, having a heating potential of less than 1,000 Scoville units compared to Cayenne's 50,000 units plus.

I make my own tincture by adding a cup of cayenne pepper (strength 140,000 heat units) to a bottle of cheap vodka and shaking it repeatedly every time I go near it. A splash every morning goes into my health mix that I have every morning.

Cruciferous vegetables

This vegetable family which includes broccoli, cauliflower, cabbage, Brussels sprouts, collards, kale, mustard greens, turnips and turnip greens contains a number of compounds that have shown inhibitory action on cancers in animals. Communities that eat higher amounts of these vegetables show reduced incidence of cancer. Large amounts of cabbage and broccoli are particularly recommended.

The potential of cabbage as an anticancer treatment was known over 2,000 years ago. The Roman statesman, Cato the Elder (234–149 BC), in his treatise on medicine wrote: 'If a cancerous ulcer appears upon the breasts, apply a crushed cabbage leaf and it will make it well.'

A key compound that has been isolated from broccoli and cabbage is indole-3-carbinol and this is available as a supplement. Recommended minimum dose 300–400mg. This supplement must not be taken by any woman who is pregnant. It has been shown to have anti-cancer effects for a number of cancers—particularly cervical and breast cancers.

Garlic

Garlic is a very potent anti-pathogen. Recent tests at the University of Alabama Medical School suggest that it is as powerful as many modern anti-bacterial and anti-viral drugs—with minimal toxicity—'the only toxicity is social' said one commentator wryly. To beat the social side effects chew on parsley leaves or take garlic in de-odorized pill form. Kyolic brand garlic pills are highly regarded because of the quality of attention paid to the soil that the garlic is grown in and the quality of the cold-aging process that the whole cloves of garlic undergo. In China, garlic extract is used in intravenous infusions to treat systemic fungal infections.

One or two cloves a day can be sure to keep the doctor away. Garlic is also a potentially useful protective agent for the liver. It may be relevant that garlic is a very good source of selenium, germanium, amino acids and enzymes among other things. Garlic is the most potent member of the onion family but the other members are also associated with good health. Apart from garlic and onion, this family includes asparagus, chives, leeks, and sarsaparilla.

Garlic can also be applied externally with good effect. A poultice of finely chopped or juiced garlic, slippery elm, pokeroot—a wild plant common to the southern states of America whose leaves appear in salads—castor oil, vinegar, water and, on open wounds, cayenne pepper. Place this mixture with any additional herbs desired on a gauze pad and apply it to the skin closest to the tumour site. The poultice should be washed off in a shower every 12 hours and the area under the poultice allowed to breathe for 1–2 hours before a new poultice is applied. The result will burn the skin and may even raise a blister. These burns can be treated with lavender essential oil, aloe vera or comfrey. DMSO can be added to the poultice to aid absorption through the skin. This is claimed to be a very powerful anti-tumour treatment.

Ginger

Ginger has a broad range of health benefits. One anecdotal report of its anti-cancer effects is this:

'When I had prostate cancer and also colorectal cancer that blocked my colon, I tried ginger. I took up to six capsules (50mg five per cent gingerol extract plus 450mg of gingerroot powder per capsule)[this product is no longer available], four times a day. I was very lucky. It worked! How can I be so sure that it works? Because the cancer returned three years later, this time it was also in several new places—in my bones, sinus, and the bottom of my spine. I used the ginger treatment at full dosage for three days and then another three days a week later. It seemed that nothing happened, but the pains slowly went away and my body functions returned to normal within a month except for my kidneys that took about six months to get back to feeling normal. Also, after my cures, results from research began to make the news that confirmed that ginger does have anti-cancer properties.'

The writer then went on to comment:

'The reason I am making this document public besides the primary reason of saving lives is because when my oncologist found out that I was cured the response was "I don't believe it, I don't want to hear about it." Well I thought, with that kind of attitude how many people will die needlessly. I will not let that happen.'

Rather than take expensive ginger extract capsules you can just dice a few slices of ginger and steep them in hot water. You can make a big jug of it and sip it throughout the day. It makes for a very refreshing drink.

The Kelley Eidem 'cure'

Kelley Eidem claims to have cured his own cancer in five days using the following protocol.
   Grate one habaneros (or Scottish Bonnet—or whatever is hottest) pepper each day, putting it on a slice of bread. Grate two cloves of garlic each day, putting them on the same piece of bread. Add 1–2 tablespoons (14–28ml) of emulsified cod liver oil each day (he explains: I used the cod liver oil because I was not losing any weight or dealing with fluid retention. If I had either of those conditions, I would have used evening primrose oil or borage oil instead of the emulsified cod liver oil.) Finally, smother the grated garlic and habaneros peppers with real butter and eat it. No margarines of any type, including Smart Balance, etc. You can replace the pepper with freshly grated ginger—or simply add ginger to the mix.
   In support of this protocol, Eidem points to the fact that there is research supporting the benefits of hot chillies and ginger (and of course garlic) against cancer.

While a hot chilli pepper, garlic and ginger mix has a lot to recommend it—and the cod liver oil too—there doesn't seem to be much to recommend with the bread and butter. And to talk of a five day cure is nonsense. This is just hype with a core of good sense.

Sea vegetables (seaweed)

We call them seaweed but the Japanese, in particular, have a liking for these edible plants that grow in the sea. One seaweed extract marketed under the name Viva Natural has been found to be active against lung cancer and leukaemia. There is also some evidence that these vegetables may be active against breast cancer. Kelp and dulse are widely available seaweed extracts. Kombu, however, should be eaten in moderation as it contains very high iodine levels and can induce temporary hyper-thyroidism which stops when levels of iodine are reduced.

U-fucoidan, also marketed as Modifilan, is an extract of various brown seaweed (kombu, wakame, mozuku, and hijiki) that contains a polysaccharide known as fucoidan. Japanese researchers have found in laboratory studies that it causes cancer cells to self-destruct. For more information see www.modifilan.com and www.glycoscience.org.

Limu Moui is essentially the same product but coming from Tonga rather than Japan. For what it is worth, Tongans and Okinawans both eat a lot of brown seaweed extract and have low cancer incidence rates. There are a number of other fucoidan products available on the Internet.

Tomatoes

The humble tomato has been found to be a rich source of lycopene which has been shown to have strong anti-cancer effects. Interestingly, the lycopene levels of cooked tomatoes are over ten times higher than their levels in raw uncooked tomatoes. No one understands why this should be the case.

Watercress

Watercress has recently come to the fore as an anti-cancer superfood. It is the richest natural source of a compound called PEITC (phenylethylisothiocyanate) which has been shown to have powerful anti-cancer properties. PEITC is not just a potent inhibitor of cancer, it also has the ability to kill cancer cells. As if this wasn't enough, it has also been found to prevent cancer-causing agents being metabolised into carcinogens and also has the ability to stimulate the enzymes involved in the detoxification of carcinogens.

An American scientist, Stephen Hecht, demonstrated that smokers eating only 2oz (57g) of watercress with each meal were protected from a key carcinogen (known as NKK) which is associated with tobacco and implicated in lung cancer. It is now known that watercress also contains another compound—methylsulphinylalkyl glucosinolate—more usually found in broccoli and Brussels sprouts, and that together these compounds form an extremely powerful anti-cancer weapon.

Super greens

There are a number of words used to describe this group of food products: phytofoods, green foods, superfoods.

These terms have been applied to a number of plant sourced whole foods that are 'nutrient-dense' (i.e., they are packed with vitamins, minerals and a lot more). No matter what else you plan to do as part of your anti-cancer strategy, you should make sure these foods play a part.

Barley Green Essence and wheatgrass

Barley Green Essence is the concentrated extract of young barley, rye and oat shoots which have been allowed to grow until the leaves have become dark green. This was developed by a Japanese scientist Yoshide Hagiwara to support his own health. Wheatgrass is a variation which was developed independently in America by Ann Wigmore. Both consider their products to be effective components of a holistic anti-cancer dietary regime. There are now a number of similar products on the market containing additional herbs, enzymes and so on.

Hagiwara believes 'the leaves of the cereal grasses provide the nearest thing this planet offers to the perfect food.' Green Barley Essence is available as a powder and in capsule forms though he personally recommends the powder form as better. The potassium content of this product is very high, which makes it a good food for people working under high stress—when blood potassium levels will show a marked tendency to fall. Potassium is therefore being used up at a high rate and needs to be replaced. If it is not replaced then the result is fatigue. Green Barley Essence is also very high in vitamins. It has six times as much beta carotene and three times as much vitamin C as spinach. It is high in folic acid and nicotinic acid (important B vitamins) as well as biotin, chlorophyll and choline. Chlorophyll, which in plants is the substance that transforms sunlight into food, is very close in chemical structure to the haemoglobin in our blood—the only difference being one of its mineral components. Blood is bonded with iron while chlorophyll is bonded by magnesium. Hagiwara believes that the blood can be reinvigorated by eating chlorophyll.

Barley Green powder is also a very powerful alkalising agent, which as we have learnt is a good thing. Finally, it contains all the enzymes the body needs.

Cancer survivor Bob Davis believes that dried green barley leaves, in pill form (he takes 20 x 200mg a day), cured him of his cancer within ten days. His story can be found at www.cancer-success.com.

Chlorella and spirulina

It is believed that these two freshwater algae contain every single nutrient required by the human body. They have been called 'the perfect whole food'. It is also claimed that they can reverse a wide range of diseases including all types of cancer.

The range of health benefits claimed for chlorella is extensive: it supports and reinforces the immune system; it detoxifies the body by ridding it of heavy metals and pesticide residues; it improves digestion and helps elimination; it normalizes blood sugar and blood pressure and it balances the body's pH, and it fights cancer by stimulating the body's own anti-tumour resources.

Marine phytoplankton

The surface waters of the oceans of the world contain vast colonies of microscopic plant life, marine phytoplankton. These are at the bottom of the food chain for all ocean life. They convert sunlight, water and minerals of the sea into nutrients, using chlorophyll in the same way that other plants do. In short, they are a complete food source. As with their fresh water cousins, chlorella and spirulina they have a strong alkalizing, detoxifying effect. These too can very usefully be added to the diet. There are claims of very rapid healing benefits for a wide range of chronic conditions including cancer.

Green drinks

There are a large number of formulas containing a mix of chlorella, spirulina, wheatgrass, barley sprouts and many other ingredients: herbs, vitamins, enzymes, and fruit and vegetable extracts. You should compare the ingredients of the various products as they are all significantly different. Some of the more popular formulas are: Barlean's Greens, Green Defense, Kyo-Chlorella and Barley Power.

I would personally recommend that you take one of these as they have a very powerful alkalizing effect which is essential for anyone seeking to maintain or regain good health.

Medicinal mushrooms

Mushrooms are well known for their potent medicinal qualities. Even the standard mushrooms that can be bought in the supermarket are considered beneficial. However, most of the mushrooms promoted for their anti-cancer activity are part of the herbalist's armoury rather than the food nutritionist's, so a fuller discussion of these mushrooms appears in Section 5: *Cancer: Herbs, Botanicals and Biological Therapies*.

Fruit

Fruit, particularly berries, should be a significant component of any anti-cancer diet. The following fruits are considered to be particularly rich in healthy nutrients.

Apples

We all know that 'an apple a day keeps the doctor away', and there is good reason for that. Sadly, many of the commercial varieties of apple found in our supermarkets are not so good as the old 'heritage' varieties. Apples contain many phytochemicals that are medicinally beneficial and some reports suggest that eating two or more apples a day could help prevent cancer. Apples contain one chemical, phloridzin, indeed they are the only major source of it, which modulates sugar transport in the intestine and has the effect of slowing the absorption of sugar. Given the huge need for sugar that cancer tumours have, this could be very good news. The varieties that have the best phytochemical content are Hetlina and Monty's Surprise but if you take a rough and ready guide that four or five Red Delicious equal one of the above, you will not go far wrong. Note that half the benefit of the apples is in the skin.

Oranges and lemons

You may remember that Dr Moerman's first patient (under 'Diets', above) ate oranges until they were coming out of his ears. It's not just the vitamin C but also the citric acid that is effective. But the benefits of oranges and lemons are not restricted to the juice of this fruit. The peel also contains a potent chemical, D-limonene, for which there is strong evidence of anti-cancer activity. Researchers at the University of Wisconsin found that when D-limonene was added to the diets of rats that had developed tumours, 90 per cent of them had their tumours disappear completely. So make sure you juice the peel as well as the (organic) fruit.

Finally, an interesting point: citrus fruits, although acidic outside the body, have a very alkalising effect once they are consumed.

Cranberries

Powerful inhibitors of cancer cell division.

Exotic fruits

Besides grapes and apples, a number of fruits (usually exotic) have been promoted, often by multi-layer marketing companies, as being enormously beneficial to health. However, although it is reasonable to be somewhat cynical, most of these fruits and their juices do have health-supporting qualities. It is very unlikely that any on their own will cure cancer but they will help move the body to a place of nutritional health and may very well support someone who is undergoing chemotherapy or radiation.

Any dark-coloured red or blue nutritious fruit, grown in a place where there is strong sunlight, will have many beneficial qualities. However, the quality of the purchased product may be affected by many factors such as sweeteners, fillers, preservatives, colouring agents and other additional ingredients. Use your common sense when purchasing. Read the labels carefully.

Here are some fruits that have attracted recent attention.

Noni

Noni fruit has been used in general folk healing wherever it grows. There is strong anecdotal and experimental support for its anti-cancer effects.

In 1997, Dr Stephen Hall, author of a book on noni, reported: 'A 75 y/o male with metastatic prostate cancer, most recent PSA of 55, I added … Noni to his conventional treatment regimen and within two weeks, his PSA was 1.1. There is simply nothing else I am aware of that could possibly reduce prostatic specific antigen from 55 (indicating uncontrolled cancer) to a normal 1.1, and do it in just two weeks.'

Noni juice has been the subject of some controversy, because interest in this product has been driven by a powerful multi-level marketing scheme operated by the Morinda Corporation, which has dominated information relating to the noni fruit. The problem has been to what extent we can accept statements like Dr Hall's. It appears that everyone touting noni juice is also profiting from it.

Nevertheless, Japanese researchers have conducted independent animal experiments that clearly show a strong anti-cancer effect for noni juice.

Whether or not Tahitian noni is better than Hawaiian noni or noni from other sources is a matter for debate.

Acai, goji, mangosteen, papaya and pomegranate

Acai: (pronounced 'ah-sy-ee') is a small purple fruit that grows in the Amazon rainforest and tastes 'like a cross between blackberries and chocolate'. Its concentration of anti-oxidants is greater even than the blueberry (itself one of nature's healthiest fruits). Studies on the acai fruit have found that it enhances the immune system, helps protects the heart, controls cholesterol and can reduce prostate enlargement.

Goji: The berries of this Himalayan fruit, cousin of the American wolfberry, are rich in polysaccharides. It has a role in traditional medicine against inflammation, and one of the polysaccharides has demonstrated anti-cancer effects in the laboratory. It also has anti-coagulant properties, so anyone taking blood thinning drugs should treat this fruit with caution.

Mangosteen: This is a fruit common to Southeast Asia. However, it is the rind of the fruit that contains the highest concentration of xanthones, the chemicals that are considered most active medicinally. There is some evidence that it has anti-bacterial, anti-fungal, anti-tumour effects and that it promotes the healing of wounds. This fruit product is available as a drink (which has a high fruit content) and as capsules (which have a high rind content).

Papaya: If you were forced to choose only one fruit to eat, my choice would be the papaya. The enzymes and antioxidants make this a powerful immune booster. Note that the enzymes are largely in the peel of the fruit, so you should eat the whole fruit peel and all, or blend it into a juice. Note that unripe papaya has more of the enzymes than ripe papaya and so is more beneficial. The benefits of papaya leaf are discussed in Section 5: *Cancer: Herbs, Botanicals* and *Biological Therapies.*

Pomegranate: This fruit is native to the Middle East. Pomegranates are known to possess anti-inflammatory agents, which make them very interesting as potential anti-tumour agents. And in fact research has shown that it has a strong anti-cancer effect as well as supporting heart health. The BBC reported a senior researcher, Professor Hasan Mukhtar as saying: 'Our study … adds to growing evidence that pomegranates contain very powerful agents against cancer, particularly prostate cancer.' (BBC September 28, 2005) A glass a day could be very beneficial both as a preventative and as a treatment. Of all the heavily touted fruits, the pomegranate has the best supported claims and is also the cheapest as it is not part of a multi-level marketing scheme.

Strawberries

Strawberries have demonstrated a strong anti-cancer effect under experimental conditions. Researchers at Ohio State University were able to show that freeze-dried strawberries slowed the growth of dysplastic, or precancerous, lesions in about 30 people who consumed the fruit for six months. While this effect has been demonstrated only for those with oesophageal cancer, it is reasonable to assume the effect is of a general nature. Oesophageal cancer is the third most common gastrointestinal cancer and the sixth most frequent cause of cancer death in the world.

Other berries

All dark berries (raspberries, blueberries, blackberries, loganberries and so on) are beneficial and should be eaten in large portions.

Miscellaneous

Nuts: almonds and Brazil nuts

Almonds have a wide range of health benefits but, in relation to cancer, it is the fact that they are rich sources of the extract commonly referred to as laetrile, amygdalin or vitamin B17 that makes them so interesting—eat up to 50 a day. Brazil nuts are the richest natural food source of organic selenium—and selenium is known to be protective against cancer, and possibly even curative (see Section 6: *Cancer: Vitamins and Other Supplements*).

Vinegar

Acetic acid is a natural ingredient found in all vinegars. It is also the product of the normal metabolism of fats and carbohydrates when they are broken down in the body. Although it is an acid, it has important health benefits; its acidity is not an issue. It is calculated that the human body derives more than 80 per cent of all its energy from acetic acid. Interestingly, while acetic acid is necessary to fuel the activities of normal cells it interferes with the process of glycolysis, which is the process by which cancer cells get their fuel. Acetic acid effectively blocks the glycolic process. Glycolysis is the metabolic process by which sugars are broken down in the body—and remember, cancer feeds on these sugars. Any interference is a good thing.

The most favoured type of vinegar is apple cider vinegar as it contains some of the benefits of apples along with the benefits of the vinegar. Personally, I take a splash of vinegar diluted with water as a regular thirst-quenching drink. Bragg's organic unpasteurised vinegar is the most highly regarded—and they have a special deal for people with cancer. Enquire to www.bragg.com.

There are a number of very favourable comments about the impact of apple cider vinegar on the prostate at the website earthclinic.com—and even on improved erections!

Organic blackstrap molasses

Although blackstrap molasses are essentially a sugar product, high in iron, it is (despite this) highly recommended. It is loaded with 'good' sugars and trace minerals. Again many men suffering from various prostate problems appear to have seen these disappear quickly once they have incorporated a couple or more daily tablespoons of organic blackstrap molasses into their diet. According to one testimonial, Pam from UK writes: 'my daughter was diagnosed with an inoperable brain tumour 13 years ago. I was told she had not long to live. I gave her black molasses after reading a book. last week she was told the tumour was still there but had not grown in 13 years.'

Virgin coconut oil (VCO)

Virgin coconut oil (not coconut milk) has a lot of anecdotal support for a wide range of symptoms from heartburn and acid reflux to thyroid and adrenal exhaustion. It is an energizer and helps fight microbial, yeast and fungal infections. There are also animal research studies showing a strong anti-cancer effect, though as yet what that effect is, is not clear. However, in animal studies, rats fed coconut oils did not develop the cancers they were expected to develop when fed coconut oil. Naturopath Barry Fife, author of *The Coconut Oil Miracle* claims that he has seen melanomas dissolve when coconut oil was smeared over it.

VCO in-take should be built up slowly from one teaspoon (5ml) a day, to as high as feels comfortable. It appears to be a potent detoxifier, so eat too much and you will feel negative symptoms.

Whey

There has been some interesting research that suggests that whey protein can help protect against cancer—and is an important dietary support for anyone seeking to undergo radiation and chemotherapy. Whey protein appears to selectively deplete the cancer cells of their glutathione, while increasing or at least maintaining the levels of glutathione in healthy cells. No other proteins have this effect. Whey protein also contains branch chain amino acids which are known to aid healing and impede cancer growth. High glutathione levels are needed to maintain health. However, the denatured whey products sold to body builders is not what you need. You need 'undenatured' whey, that is to say, whey that has not been denatured and pasteurised.

Food controversies

Food, like religion and politics, is a subject about which there are opposing views and it is up to each individual to assess for him-or-herself where the truth lies. Here then, are some other key areas of disagreement.

Coffee: good or bad?

Almost all the anti-cancer diets ban coffee while at the same time espousing the benefits of coffee enemas—which cannot help but lead to the absorption of caffeine. This schizophrenic attitude now needs to take into account the results of a study published in May 2007, conducted at the University of Ferrara in Italy, which has found that caffeine inhibits three factors: VEGF, HIF-1 and IL-8, all of which are associated with the development of the blood supply that cancers need to develop if they are to grow. This process is known as angiogenesis. This means that caffeine is an anti-angiogenesis factor. This is very good news for coffee drinkers. It was already known from other studies that caffeine was associated with reduced levels of colorectal cancer. So maybe coffee isn't so bad?

Epidemiological studies have confirmed this: those who drink most coffee have the lowest incidence of prostate cancer. Apparently it didn't matter whether or not it was decaffeinated.

Meat: good or bad?

Meat generally has a bad press. Almost all anti-cancer diets are vegetarian, if not vegan. But there is a movement arguing in favour of meat as long as that meat is organic, free range meat—grass-fed beef, for example. Everyone agrees that standard, industrially-produced meat products—pumped full of hormones and antibiotics—are to be avoided at all costs. But organic meat provides a good source of cysteine, and that is essential for glutathione production.

Many people lay the blame for inflammatory diseases and diseases of aging on inadequate glutathione production in the body. What does glutathione do? It has a wide range of actions. It eliminates free radicals, detoxifies and removes heavy metals like lead, mercury and cadmium out of the body, recycles oxidized vitamin C back to useful vitamin C, and protects cells from damage against free radicals and oxidative stress. The key element of why glutathione is important is that it is stored inside individual cells. Healthy cells have good stores of glutathione. And it appears to require good levels of ATP, the fuel that cells use for their energy needs, to transfer from outside a cell to inside the cell. Cancer patients are known to manifest low glutathione levels. Many people suffering a variety of ailments get almost instant energy improvements from taking injections of glutathione and ATP combined.

But here's the thing, don't go out and buy glutathione supplements. The body needs to manufacture its own from three amino acids: L-cysteine, glutamic acid and glycine. Of these cysteine is the most essential—and that's where meat comes in.

Undenatured whey is also a good source of cysteine—but don't buy the whey powders that are sold to body builders. This is very much a denatured product. Colostrum is another good source of glutathione precursors.

Ian Clements, (whose story is told in Section 8: *Cancer Survivors' Stories*) eats meat every evening. He found that despite being on a vegan diet and juicing regularly, his cancer markers were going up. His current regime involves eating meat and his cancer markers are now down.

Oils: good or bad?

Generally speaking oils get a bad press but in fact they are essential to our good health. But not all of them.

Olive oil is most people's idea of a good oil—particularly if it is 'extra virgin' and extracted by cold pressing and not with heat. If it doesn't say on the bottle 'cold extraction' or 'cold pressing' then it is extracted by heat. But olive oil is essentially a source of omega 9 oils, which are not considered to be particularly beneficial or harmful (although the olive fruit and olive leaf are both packed with many health-promoting phytonutrients).

The omega 3 oils are generally seen as been absolutely necessary for health (see the Budwig protocol above), and these are found in flax oil and fish oils (and more recently krill oil). But the ocean-sourced oils are now getting attacked from some quarters as being over-processed and providing poisonous levels of DHA which have negative impacts on the immune system.

Then we come to the omega 6 oils. For a long time these were attacked as they appeared to be linked to inflammatory processes, but more recently they are being promoted—by Brian Peskin in particular (www.brianpeskin.com)—as being even more important than the omega 3 oils. In his view we should be taking in three times as much omega 6 oils. The reason these oils are beneficial is that they aid the transport of oxygen to the cells. Low oxygenation causes cancer.

Peskin is very hostile to processed oils that contain what he calls essential fatty acid derivatives (DHA, GLA, CLA, EPA). The only oils that should be taken for their omega 6 content are raw, unprocessed, organic oils: sunflower oil, safflower oil, evening primrose oil and possibly the best of all (in that it has a perfect 3:1 ratio of omega 6 to omega 3 oils) is pumpkin seed oil. Others rate hemp seed oil as also containing a good ratio (also 3:1).

Canola oil and soy oil are absolutely to be avoided. On this everyone is in agreement. All processed foods that claim to be omega 3 enriched are also to be avoided. These are 'dead oils', as Budwig described them.

Salt: good or bad?

Everyone knows—because of the anti-salt propaganda in the media—that salt is bad for you. So it must be true, right? Well, not entirely. Certainly everyone agrees that cheap table salt (purified sodium chloride) is not good. They also agree that all the salt in pre-prepared foods is bad for you. But sea salt, or Himalayan salt, or any other form of salt that still contains all the minerals found in the sea, is a very good source of trace minerals; and this may, for many people, be the only source of many of these trace minerals. The sea is the medium in which life on earth first arose, so it makes sense that this environment will be one that maintains our health. Read Percy Weston's cancer cure story in Section 8: *Cancer Survivors' Stories*, as an example of how important these trace minerals are.

The soybean: good or bad?

Throughout the 80s and 90s the soybean was lauded widely, as many things from the East were. It was noted that in China where tofu was a major part of the diet, that cancer rates were much lower. But in Japan, curiously, cancer rates are high (higher than in the US) particularly in the cancers most closely related to diet: stomach, colon, oesophagus, liver. However, more recently, there has been a strong backlash. The soybean has been attacked for containing a large number of dangerous substances called phytates, one of which is phytic acid. Soybeans contain very high levels of this organic acid. These acids block the body's ability to take up essential minerals like calcium, magnesium, iron and especially zinc and iodine. Soybeans are very resistant to phytate-reducing techniques, such as long, slow cooking.

Soybeans also contain a number of potent enzyme inhibitors that block the uptake of trypsin and other enzymes that the body needs for protein digestion. Cooking does not completely de-activate inhibitors.

Soybeans also contain haemaglutinin, a clot-promoting substance that causes red blood cells to clump together. This has the effect of preventing proper absorption of oxygen for distribution to the body's tissues.

However, these concerns relate to unfermented soy products. Fermented soy products do appear to be healthy, as the fermentation process neutralizes the phytic acid. The fermentation also creates good bacteria—'probiotics'—which help assimilation of important nutrients. In fact miso soup, a fermented soy product, has been shown to be highly protective against breast and prostate cancer—three bowls a day cut cancer risk in half.

Some doctors recommend fermented soy products for hormone-dependent cancers such as prostate, breast and some others for the reason that the soy products block the hormone receptors.

Haelan and soy essence are fermented soy drinks for which strong anti-cancer claims are made. These are discussed in Section 6: *Cancer: Vitamins and Other Supplements*.

For further information see www.mercola.com/article/soy.

It has been noted that some vegetarians have a very high soy intake and this may make them vulnerable to cancer. Children should absolutely not be given soy-based drinks. Children consuming such drinks have a much higher risk of thyroid and other auto-immune disorders. And if these drinks are not good for children why do we think they might be good for adults?

Sprouts: good or bad?

Here I refer to the freshly sprouted seeds of a number of plants such as adzuki, alfalfa, clover, fenugreek, lentil, mustard, radish, sunflower, watercress and others including wheat, rye, millet and oat seeds. Simple sprouting equipment can be set up at home to ensure a regular and extremely cheap supply of sprouts. These can be eaten as they are or juiced with garlic.

The value of sprouts is that they are extremely rich in vitamins, minerals, enzymes and amino acids. In addition, according to advocates, they are 'biogenic' (i.e., capable of transferring their life energy to the bodies of those who eat them).

> 'When you eat a sprout you are eating a tiny, easy-to-digest plant that is at its peak of nutritional value. The seed releases all of its stored nutrients in a burst of vitality as it attempts to become a full-sized plant.' (Wigmore, 1986)

Experiments with mice show that injections of sprout extracts have a strong inhibitory effect on cancer cells and are completely non-toxic at even large doses. Lentil, mung bean, and wheat sprouts were those tested with positive results.

However, there is an opposing view on the subject of sprouts. According to Charlotte Gerson, daughter of Dr Max Gerson and the force behind the Gerson Clinics: 'Sprouted alfalfa and other bean or seed sprouts are high in L-canavanine, an immature amino acid that is responsible for immune cell suppression. Also, patients with no prior history of chronic joint pain have developed the sudden onset of arthritic symptoms upon ingesting alfalfa sprouts. Healthy monkeys have developed lupus erythematosus from alfalfa sprouts in their diet.' The main culprit appears to be alfalfa.

Starch: good or bad?

The received wisdom is that starchy foods are basically sugar in disguise and that therefore they should be avoided at all costs. However, there is a strong argument against this point of view.

Take the case of Chris Voigt who went on a 60-day potato-only diet. His objective was simply to prove it was a nutritious food. The result? 'Besides sleeping well and remaining full of energy during the day, I benefitted from this all-potato diet in other ways, according to my blood tests and other measurements.'

	Before	**After**
Weight:	197	176
Blood glucose:	104	94
Cholesterol:	214	147
Triglycerides:	135	75

Chris claims he did not experience hunger and indeed was so worried about the weight he was losing that he ate as many potatoes as he could—but he still lost weight!

Someone else who has lived on a largely starchy diet for more than six years is Burgess Laughlin:

'[Because of various ailments] I avoid all animal products and all "seeds" (legumes, grains, nuts, etc.). I eat about 25 pounds of starchy "roots" per week: sweet potatoes, American yams, rutabagas, and (mostly) Russet potatoes, as well as other starches such as winter squash. I also eat plenty of vegetables and fruit. The one nutrient missing is B12, for which I take a supplement. I have been eating this way for six years. At 66, I am thriving on my root-starch centred diet. Medical tests (CAT scan, heart monitor, X-rays, blood tests, etc.) have revealed no problems: no heart disease, cancer, diabetes, osteoporosis, kidney problems, or others. My past inflammation problems are gone. My eyesight has returned to what it was around 1983. I sleep well. I walk two hours per day and climb stairs. I have a big appetite (three large meals, with no snacks).'

I took the question of potatoes—and other starches—in relation to cancer to Ruth Heidrich, (whose cancer story I tell in *Cancer: Survivors' Stories*). She had this to say:

'Potatoes, as you read in vegsource.com, are an excellent food for everyone, even people with cancer, but the problem is usually that people feel the need to add "bad" things to them such as butter, sour cream, bacon bits, etc. or worst of all, deep-fat fry them! They are best just baked and eaten plain. The US's National Institute of Fitness, which specialized in weight loss, encouraged people to fill up on them and they would lose weight!

Pasta, of course, is usually a very refined food and I suggest avoiding it as it's not any better than white bread. Even wholegrain pasta is still a refined, processed food which I recommend avoiding. Rice, of course, must be cooked and it takes a long time, especially if it's brown rice, which would be the only rice I'd recommend.'

The Irish, famously, thrived so well on a diet of potatoes and little else that the population doubled over a period of 60 years from 1780 to 1840, from four to eight million. As one writer commented, 'Accounts of Irish society recorded by contemporary visitors paint the picture of a people as remarkable for their health as for their lack of sophistication at the dinner table, where potatoes typically supplied appetizer, dinner and dessert.'—Jeff Chapman, *History Magazine*

Summing up

Most cancers are systemic by the time they are diagnosed. That means the cure must be systemic too in its nature. There is nothing more systemic to our bodies than the diet we eat. Our health is utterly dependent on our diet. Although it may be that some people have conditions that for one reason or another cannot be returned to full health through dietary means, this is not true for the majority of us. Diet is everything.

Not everyone believes that that diet has to be completely meat free. In fact some people believe that since we all have different 'metabolic types', we should have diets designed for us—and for some people that designer diet may have a high meat content. But, whether or not meat is entirely eliminated, there is general agreement on what a good healing diet consists of: at least 95 per cent vegetarian, supported by adequate intake of omega 3 and 6 oils. Foods to be avoided are dairy, sugar-heavy and soy products and it should also be unprocessed, raw (as much as possible) and organic. Anyone going completely meat free should make sure that they get vitamin B12 from time to time (only minute quantities are needed and the body usually holds enough for a couple of years).

The food that is taken in should be organic where at all possible. Not only is organic food free (one hopes) of pesticides and other chemical pollutants, but it is also (hopefully) richer in minerals and vitamins. Where there is doubt about the quality of the diet, then additional measures need to be taken, to take in the important minerals and vitamins If meat is eaten, that too should be organic, free-range meat—factory-processed meats are high in chemicals, antibiotics, drugs designed to increase animal weight and so on—and these are not good.

Instant processed meals should be avoided.

In cooking the food, the general rule should be the less cooking the better. Crispy vegetables are far superior to their soggy, over-cooked cousins.

It is really all a matter of common sense. For the person with cancer, making dietary changes is vital if true health is to be regained, whatever other decisions are made in relation to cancer treatment.

Cancer: Herbs, Botanicals and Biological Therapies

In this section I explore the important place herbs should have in any comprehensive anti-cancer strategy. Many herbs and herbal mixes have powerful anti-cancer effects. This section provides you with the options you should be thinking about. It also discusses the issues and dangers relating to herbs—and the arguments supporting their use in contrast to drugs. We also look at a number of biological therapies—with an extensive look at the different homeopathic strategies that have been developed.

Herbs and Botanicals

Introduction

That plants have medicinal properties is not a subject about which there is any disagreement. The medicinal qualities of many plants are well known. Hippocrates used to prescribe willow bark for a number of ailments—later, the active ingredient was isolated and marketed under the name of aspirin. However, with the rise of science, single-substance drugs became the order of the day, and herbalism to a large extent went underground. It became a woman's area of expertise. Old women's recipes were handed on from mother to daughter.

In eighteenth-century North America, a woman by the name of Mary Johnson came to the attention of the medical authorities. It appeared she was working as a healer and was claiming success in the treatment of cancer. The House of Burgesses of the General Assembly of Virginia appointed a committee to look into the case. Mary Johnson's medicine was a mixture of garden sorrel, celandine, persimmon bark and spring water. The committee took evidence over a period of six or seven years, 1748–54. They listened to the testimony of many witnesses who had taken the remedy and who had been cured. The result? Mrs Johnson was awarded 100 pounds to aid her work.

This is a rare tale of diligent and generous assessment. The outcome of the investigation would be very different today—for the simple fact is that herbs represent a fundamental challenge to the ruling medical paradigm.

This ruling paradigm argues in a reductionist way as follows: If there is anecdotal evidence that a herb has a specific medicinal property, then it is possible that the plant in question contains a specific chemical that can be called the active ingredient. The plant is then studied to determine what its chemical contents are, and these are tested one at a time until the active ingredient is identified. Then this isolated substance can be tested scientifically to assess its range of action and ideal dosage. It will also, incidentally, be possible then to manufacture the chemical directly in large quantities without having to go through the arduous and expensive process of extraction from plant sources. This illustrates the fact that the ultimate aim of chemical research is to create, on an industrial scale, single chemicals in pure form.

By contrast, Mary Johnson proceeded by mixing a number of herbs together—in what proportions is not known. She was operating according to very different principles. While the scientist is looking for pure unadulterated chemicals, the herbalist is seeking to blend combinations of many different chemicals.

There is no evidence, in relation to the work of healing and curing, that single-substance chemicals are superior to herbs. In fact, there is good reason to believe they may be inferior. Why? For three reasons. First, there is the problem of resistance. Invading organisms such as bacteria and viruses are able to resist pure chemical forms quite effectively. That is why bacteria are increasingly becoming resistant to antibiotics, and it's also why the body is able to resist chemotherapeutic drugs—and doctors are now mixing these chemotherapeutic agents. That is, they are starting to mimic the herbalist.

Secondly, the negative side effects of purified molecular forms—which are the basis of all drugs—are rarely present when herbs are used. This is not to say that herbs are always safe. They aren't. But such side effects as there are tend to be muffled by the presence of the surrounding chemicals in the composite herbal structures found in nature. The following two examples demonstrate this point clearly. Smokers take into their bodies a great deal of nicotine every time they light up a cigarette. 60mg of pure nicotine is enough to kill a 68kg (150lb) man—it is more poisonous than arsenic or strychnine. Nicotine in herbal form takes 20 or 30 years to achieve the same result.

Marijuana, to take another example, besides being an illegal drug has clearly demonstrated medicinal qualities. It is known among other things to reduce the effects of nausea. Scientists have extracted the active ingredient THC from the marijuana plant. Unfortunately, not only was this less effective than the original herbal marijuana but its side effects were such that half the patients testing it said they preferred to throw up than continue with it.

The third, and perhaps the most important, reason why herbs are to be preferred to drugs is the fact that the concept that a healing plant has a single active ingredient is almost certainly wrong. It is much more likely, in any herbal substance, that one dominant active chemical is boosted by the presence of others. When separated from these surrounding molecules, it may no longer have the expected effect. The process by which two chemicals contribute to a more pronounced effect is known as synergy. We can even imagine a situation where none of the ingredients of a particular plant have any effect on their own—but when present in an organic whole, they combine to have an effect.

This point about 'organic wholes' is central to the herbalist's credo. In the herb, compounds are interconnected in a coherent structure and have certain qualities both separately and together that are entirely absent from all artificially created chemicals.

Some people demonstrate the difference between organic and inorganic forms by using the metaphor of music. If you press the A key on a piano, you will create three kinds of vibrations. One is the vibration that creates the note A, but mixed with this will be overtones that make it clear to any listener that the note A comes from a piano and not a violin or clarinet. In addition, there will be other vibrations that stem from the interaction of the particular musician and the particular instrument. The writer Dean Black, in describing this fact, makes the point that if the music were a herb, then the active element would be the A note—it is the most noticeable property of the sound and it's the only one that can stand alone.

'[However,] None of the three vibrations define the note's entire function, and some of the note's most interesting properties—it's 'piano-ness' and its 'tone quality'—don't exist anywhere except as they somehow emerge like magic when the vibrations blend together.' (Dean Black, 1988)

Herbalists believe that the chemical properties of a whole plant operate in much the same way and that we lose these properties when we break the plant up.

However, there is one criticism of herbs that does carry some force. The problem is consistency. Whereas drugs from one batch will always be identical to drugs from another, this is not true of herbs, which contain too many ingredients in variable concentrations. One ounce of ma-huang grown in America may be very different in quality from an ounce of the same herb grown in China. Because of this variability, they argue, it is impossible to adequately test the precise effects any herb might have. Because these objections don't apply to drugs, they say, drugs must be better. Some herbal companies have taken note of this criticism and it is now fairly common to find mention of standardisation (i.e., that what they offer in one batch will not differ from what they offer in another batch produced months later). Nevertheless, this standardisation will apply only to some of the herb's chemical contents, not all.

The conflict of herb versus drug is, in miniature, the war between factory and nature, between West and East, between 'scientific' techno-medicine and holistic healing. How is it that there is no official recognition that herbs play a part in the treatment of cancer? Because it is impossible to prove this effect under the conditions of proof currently laid down—and it would cost US$200–300 million to attempt to do so. No herbal or pharmaceutical company would consider spending that kind of money on an unpatentable medicine. The rules of the scientific game have been designed with this objective in mind.

So, let's understand this clearly. Cancer research cannot ever arrive at a conclusion that a herb can cure cancer—even if people using that herb find that their cancers go away. The rules of the research game have been set in a way that will prevent such a thing happening. So cancer patients seeking the support of herbs in their fight against cancer must understand that there will never be any strong scientific support for the herbs they choose to use.

Herbs and the cancer patient

Let us now turn our attention to what it is the cancer patients may be seeking to achieve with herbs.

There are two main reasons for using herbs. The first is to aid wellness. The second is to attack the cancer in some way.

As an aid to wellness

It is known that organic wellness depends on a good digestive system and an efficient liver. The liver is central to good health. So it makes a lot of sense to take herbs that will help ease digestive issues—acid, constipation or what have you. It is also extremely important to nurture and strengthen the liver. Many naturopathic doctors believe that cancer starts with a distressed liver. Among the herbs that appear to be liver-supporting are milk thistle, rosemary and sage.

As a weapon against cancer

In order to understand the potential of various herbs to act against cancer, it is useful to understand the different ways in which a cancer cell can be killed.

Necrosis

This is what happens when a cancer cell is directly attacked by toxins, drugs, radiation beams and so on. It is death by assault from external factors. It also results in the leakage of the dead cell's contents, which are likely to be toxic to other cells nearby. So necrosis is not a very desirable result—it can result in the liver being overloaded with toxins.

Apoptosis

This is what happens when normal cells die, as they do continually as part of the general upkeep of the body. Healthy cells reach a point in their life cycle when they grow old. At that point they trigger their own death. This is what apoptosis means—normal cell death. This process is controlled by rod-like structures in the cell called mitochondria. Unfortunately, when healthy cells turn into cancer cells the mitochondria are switched off. This means the cancer cell cannot trigger its own normal cell death program. And this is why cancer is so dangerous—the cells multiply but cannot die. Gerald Dermer calls them immortal cells. If we can turn the mitochondria back on, then the cell will trigger its own death and be cleared away and replaced in the normal manner that does not cause toxicity to surrounding cells.

Blood starvation

Cancer tumours need a good supply of blood to enable them to grow. One way to attack them is by interfering with the development of this blood supply. The development of blood vessels is called angiogenesis. So the approach that seeks to limit this is referred to as anti-angiogenesis. Some herbs appear to be helpful in this way.

Important warnings

Safety

Once we accept that herbs are a soundly-based approach to medical treatment, we need to know which herbs are recommended for the prevention or cure of cancer. Before that a warning is in order. Herbs cannot be presumed to be safe just because they are herbs. Some herbs are poisonous. Pregnant women, in particular, should not take a herb without consulting a professional herbalist. Pregnancy and cancer have a number of features in common and anything that will act against cancer has a good chance of causing miscarriages in women. Anyone taking a herb should read up on it first. Not everything that is 'natural' is safe. Remember, Socrates committed suicide by drinking a herbal concoction of what was undoubtedly organic or wild-crafted hemlock.

However, it should be remembered that many herbs and other treatments will cause a negative reaction of a temporary sort. This is known as a healing crisis. As the herbs work on the liver, toxins are released that cause all kinds of negative reaction from headaches to skin eruptions. These healing crises—known as Herxheimer reactions—are usually short-lived and should not last longer than a week or so. Persistence of ill effects after this duration should be taken as a strong indication that whatever herbal preparation you are taking should be discontinued. It is also a good idea to drink lots of water to flush these toxins out of the system as quickly as possible. If a healing crisis seems to be particularly uncomfortable, then it makes sense to take a rest from the treatment for a number of days to avoid over-taxing the body.

Pregnancy

There are three conditions in which rapid cell division occurs in the body: cancer, the healing of wounds, and pregnancy. This means that any herb that is effective against cancer is very likely to be contra-indicated for pregnant women.

Drug/herb interactions

This is a minefield of an area. Drugs and herbs will interact in some ways. This is obvious. Doctors may be able to give advice as to whether the interactions are likely to be problematic—but the truth is, as one doctor explained to me, no-one knows enough about all the potential problems to be able to give an expert opinion. In some cases it may be reasonably clear—a herb may have a known effect that runs counter to the effects of a drug. But mostly you will have to accept you are on your own. This means each of us who follow this route have to monitor ourselves. How do we feel? How do we interpret these feelings? Then we can fiddle with our intake of the drugs and herbs as we see fit.

Intensity of impact

When building up an anti-cancer program, you should plan a gradual increase of weaponry rather than doing high doses of everything you can think of all at once. Build up gradually. Put a diet in place, then add a herb; later you can add another herb or supplement. Leave three or four days between each step and assess yourself—how do you feel? If things appear to be alright, then add something else. In this way you can assess the value of each element in your program of recovery. Avoid injecting anything unless you are absolutely sure it will be safe to do so.

The Herbs

Some herbalists claim that there are over 3,000 herbs displaying some form of anti-cancer effect. The following list therefore does not pretend to be exhaustive.

Aloe vera

Aloe vera helps the body fight infections and malignant cells. It is also a detoxifier.

Aloe vera may or may not, on its own, be a cure for cancer, but it has demonstrated a strong ability to enhance the immune system's response to cancer, and it eliminates toxic wastes. This has a revitalizing effect on the body. It is also important for immune system defence.

Most products make use of the inner gel, which is heat processed. This destroys many of the benefits. Look out for a whole-leaf, cold-pressed aloe vera product. Or get an aloe plant and grind up a leaf or two a day.

Historical side note: One aloe vera based serum, called Albarin, given intravenously, was used in the Medical Center for Preventive and Nutritional Medicine in Tampa. One patient reported that she had seen 'baseball-sized tumours' disappear from patients using Albarin. The head medico at the centre told authorities that in his experience, Albarin therapy was 93 per cent effective. Elsewhere, there are claims that Albarin cures 'over 80 per cent of all cancers'. These are astonishing statistics considering that the Food and Drug Administration and several other health organizations maintain that aloe-based serums are potentially dangerous and ineffective. In 1997 two terminally-ill cancer patients are reported to have died shortly after injecting an aloe-based serum. In any case, in response to prompting from pharmaceutical companies the FDA raided the centre and impounded the Albarin. Currently it is impossible to get this treatment anywhere.

Aloe arborescens

While everyone knows that aloe vera is a health supporting plant—Aloe arborescens, a close relative, is even more beneficially active. The current interest in this plant stems from the work of a priest in Brazil Fr Romano Zago. He has developed a product based on Aloe arborescens and raw honey. For details follow the link www.aloeproductscenter.com.

It seems his first version of the drink was using aloe vera leaves. This is what he recommends for cancer. '0.5kg of pure bee honey, three small (or two big) leaves of Aloe vera, 3–4 spoons of cognac, whiskey or any distilled alcoholic drink. After cleaning the leaves and cutting the thorns very carefully and gently blending everything in a liquidiser you get a creamy substance. And that is it … the remedy that cures cancer.' Presumably, the current product follows the same recipe but substitutes leaves of Aloe arborescens.

Astragalus

Astragalus is used widely in Chinese medicine. It has the effect of boosting the immune system and increasing energy. It improves digestion, and is often used to synergistically support other herbs, as it boosts their effectiveness. Astragalus does not directly attack cancer but it is often recommended for use by people undergoing chemotherapy and/or radiation. People taking astragalus have been found to recover faster and to live longer than patients who don't. It is also used as an anti-aging herb and it is good for the adrenal glands which are generally depleted in cases of cancer. So all in all, this herb offers a wide range of benefits to people with cancer, whatever else they decide to do, but it is not a standalone anti-cancer herb.

Bindweed

RECNAC ('cancer' spelled backwards) is a progressive cancer therapy centre in Wichita, Kansas, based at the Center for the Improvement of Human Functioning International, www.brightspot.org.

Bindweed came to the attention of their research team as an anecdotal report from a woman who claimed that an Indian shaman had given her a tincture of bindweed (*Convolulus arvensis*) with instructions to use the substance daily. She did so and a few months later was found to be cancer free.

Their research showed that bindweed is a powerful anti-angiogenesis factor—about 100 times stronger than shark cartilage. They also found that this effect is even stronger when bindweed is used in conjunction with an immune stimulant combination, muramyl polysaccharide-glycan complex (MPGC). An anti-angiogenesis factor interferes with the development of the blood supply that cancer tumours need to grow.

Proposed doses are six capsules of bindweed (250 mg) plus six capsules of MPGC (250mg) a day. These products can be purchased from Aidan, Inc. by telephone at 00-1-800-529-0269. Bindweed is sold as C-Statin and MPGC is sold as ImmKine. Other sources are available on the Internet.

Black pepper

Black pepper is one of the most common culinary spices worldwide. It is also frequently included in Ayurvedic prescriptions—for the reason that it contains a very important phytochemical—piperine.

Piperine has the effect of enhancing the bio-availability of other herbs—and is often recommended, in particular, to be taken alongside curcumin. Piperine increases the potency of all herbs dramatically. It is also an inhibitor of inflammation and at the same time it appears to interfere with the signalling systems between cancer cells, and so impedes tumour progression. In addition to its direct anti-cancer effects it also boosts the immune system and is rich in anti-oxidants. So it makes good sense to sprinkle black pepper generously over whatever it is you are eating, and add it also to whatever other herbs you decide to take.

Black seed (also called black cumin and Nigella sativa)

This herb is available as seeds, herbal extracts and as an oil.

Black seed appears to have very strong immune strengthening and anti-fungal qualities that make it very interesting for cancer patients. However, it is not recommended for pregnant women.

'Calling black cumin a magical cure would certainly be an exaggeration, but it is almost impossible not to exaggerate its effectiveness.'—Peter Schleicher MD

Researchers at Thomas Jefferson University in Philadelphia have discovered that an extract of Nigella sativa seed oil, known as thymoquinone, can remedy one of the most virulent and difficult to treat cancers: pancreatic cancer. The extract does this by blocking pancreatic cell growth, and actually enhancing the built-in cellular function that causes programmed cell death, or apoptosis. Nigella sativa has also been shown to help against colon cancer. This doesn't mean it is not useful for other cancers. It just means it hasn't been tested with other cancers.

Bloodroot

Bloodroot is a herb that has demonstrated very powerful anti-cancer properties. Bloodroot, (*Sanguinaria canadensis*), is native to the woods of north-central United States and Canada. Its tap root exudes a blood-coloured juice from which its name derives. It was one of the most popular herbal remedies among Plains Indians, who used it internally for sore throats and respiratory ailments and externally for growths on the surface of the body. It is this last property that makes it interesting for people with cancer—especially for those with melanoma or other surface tumours. Quite simply, bloodroot dissolves any form of malignant growth while leaving healthy tissue alone.

There is a long history of bloodroot being used as a herbal salve from the 1750s on promoted by a succession of doctors and healers.

Dr Andrew Weil, author of *Spontaneous Healing*, used some on his dog, who was suffering from a large surface tumour. For three days he smeared a small coat of paste on the tumour. He stopped on the fourth day because he was alarmed to see blood. It seemed that the tumour was separating itself from the flesh around it. He disinfected the wound and kept an eye on developments. Two days later the entire tumour fell off, and the raw flesh around it quickly healed up. 'The end result was a perfectly circular, slightly depressed area of skin, with no trace of tumour. The bloodroot had removed it more neatly than one could have done with a scalpel … the dog had shown no signs of discomfort.' (Weil, *Spontaneous Healing*, 1995)

An extraordinary set of photographs showing this effect can be seen at www.silvermedicine.org/clay-cansema-silver1.html and also at www.cancerx.org.

Here then is a herb that directly attacks cancers while leaving normal healthy tissue unharmed. It forms a scab over the cancer and expels it from the body. No secondary infections follow. One of America's leading experts on salves used against cancer, Ingrid Naiman, has written: 'Bloodroot has been researched and determined to be a potent anticancer agent. Besides the laboratory tests, tens of thousands of people have been treated by lay practitioners as well as medical doctors for at least the last 150 years. Of these, roughly 80 per cent experienced remission of malignancy and longer life expectancies than people with similar conditions who chose different treatments.'

Bloodroot is easily and quickly absorbed into the body so it is possible that the bloodroot will seek out tumours and eliminate them even though they are not on the surface.

TumorX Salve and Cansema are both products that contain bloodroot. Cansema brand products are available from Alpha Omega Labs. TumorX salve is available through cancerX.org (they also provide bloodroot for internal use). In fact there are a number of other websites offering black salves of various kinds. Perhaps the most interesting is blacksalveindonesia.org where they also sell an even stronger 'red salve' that contains a number of Indonesian herbs.

As these sources may or may not still be operating by the time you read this, I am including the following instructions for making one's own bloodroot paste.

1/2 cup powdered bloodroot (Sanguinaria canadensis)

1/2 cup zinc chloride, crystals or liquid

1/2 cup common white flour

1 1/2 cup warm water

100ml chaparral extract or 100g of powdered chaparral (Larrea mexicana)

Pre-mix all but the water, thoroughly, before adding to the water. Use a stainless steel double boiler. Put in water, and then stir in the other ingredients. Stir in well using a wooden spoon. Cook for thirty minutes over boiling water, stirring constantly.

Application is much the same as Cansema. Apply a thin layer (2–3mm) of the paste over the affected area and cover for 24 hours. Then remove the covering but do not disturb the lesion at all, do not attempt to pull the cancer out at any time, it should fall out in ten days or so. Some people with sensitive skin put Vaseline around the cancer so that the paste does not irritate the skin.

Some people have reported that using bloodroot has caused them excruciating pain while others have said that it is essentially painless. The pain, if there is pain, will not last for more than a few days—and is certainly far less severe than the pain associated with conventional therapies.

Boswellia

Boswellia has an anti-angiogenetic effect on cancer, interfering with the tumour's development of a blood supply system. However, it has another effect whose value appears to be particularly directed to men of advancing years who are more and more likely to get prostate cancer. One way to protect against prostate cancer is to inhibit an enzyme known as 5-LOX, which inflames the prostate and which is promoted by a diet that is rich in meat. An extract of Boswellia, known as AKBA, has been shown to be specifically useful in the suppression of 5-LOX. It can be obtained in a product called 5-LOXIN available from www.lef.org.

Frankincense (and myrrh)

Frankincense is an aromatic resin of a number of varieties of Boswellia, famous for being one of the gifts brought by the three magi at the birth of Jesus Christ. Researchers at the University of Oklahoma Health Sciences Center found that frankincense oil is able to discriminate between normal and cancerous bladder cells in culture, and more importantly it is able kill cancer cells 'by activating multiple cell death pathways'.

If frankincense is good, what about myrrh? Myrrh, one of the most important perfumes in ancient times, also has demonstrated anti-cancer effects in cases of breast and prostate cancer. It is also used in salves for the purpose of healing wounds.

Frankincense and myrrh are most generally available as pure essential oils.

Cannabis

Cannabis and the family of chemicals it contains—the cannabinoids—have generally been used as an anti-nausea treatment. However, cannabis has also been found to have direct anti-cancer effects—by inducing apoptosis and by preventing the development of a blood supply to tumours. Cannabinoids have also been shown to have the impact of reducing resistance to chemotherapy drugs, so helping make chemotherapy drugs more effective.

The benefits have been shown in the case of a wide range of cancers—including breast and lung.– but the main benefits might be most readily seen in the case of glioma and other brain cancers for which there are few other options. Cannabinoids are toxic to glioma cells while, at the same time, helping to protect normal brain cells, known as astrocytes, from oxidative stress.

The medicinal use of cannabis is legal in some countries and states, but not all.

How to take it? Smoking is the traditional way but there are two more effective ways of getting cannabinoids into the system. One is by vaporizing the herb, and inhaling the resulting vapour. There are many cannabis vaporizers available for sale online. The other method—promoted by Rick Simpson who has a number of highly recommended videos on You Tube about the health benefits of cannabis particularly in relation to cancer—is to eat cannabis oil. One of Simpson's videos describes the process for making 'hemp oil'. On his videos you can see testimonials from people who have been cured of a wide range of ailments by ingesting hemp oil. Or you can simply gently dissolve cannabis in olive oil and drink the resulting mixture.

Note that the hemp oil and other hemp products available in many health stores and supermarkets are not the right kind of hemp. You need the stuff that makes you high. Having said that, standard hemp oil does have a good mix of omega 3 and omega 6 oils so it shouldn't be utterly avoided.

Cat's claw (Uncaria tomentosa) and samento

Cat's claw is a woody vine found in the tropical jungles of South and Central America, which derives its name from its claw-shaped thorns. Studies have shown that cat's claw stimulates the immune system, prevents mutations, stops the spread of cancer cells, inhibits the development of leukaemia cells, kills viruses, reduces inflammation and helps cell healing. It was also used as a contraceptive by the local people whose original use led to its discovery. Cancer patients taking it have found that it is helpful in reducing the side effects of chemotherapy and enhancing vitality.

The effective part of the plant is the inner bark. Apparently some cat's claw products also contain outer bark, which is ineffective. The herb has a high tannin content that may cause gastric, liver or kidney problems. When taking, avoid milk or other dairy products.

The recommended dose is 3–6g per day (9 x 350mg capsules in three doses, 30–60 min. after a meal).

A very powerful form of cat's claw is called samento; samento extracts are also available on the Internet.

Chaparral

Chaparral is a desert plant covering large areas of southern California and Arizona. It has small brittle leaves and these have been used by the native American people to make a health tonic tea. It has an extremely unpleasant, pungent smell and bitter taste.

One dramatic case of a cancer cure using chaparral alone occurred in 1967–8. The patient was a man by the name of Ernest Farr, an 87-year-old man who had had four operations on a malignant melanoma and had been told there was no point to further interventions. He drank chaparral tea over a period of four months. The cancer shrank almost entirely away and was still very small nine months later. Clearly something in the chaparral had worked. Scientists investigated and found the chemical substance NDGA. This was already a well-known chemical as it was used to preserve butter in the tropics. It is a very powerful anti-oxidant. It is not known whether it works for all cancers—one test found little activity against breast cancer, while another found it to be effective against gastrointestinal cancer.

However, there is a caution: according to one anecdote, a woman taking chaparral in large quantities suffered severe liver damage. Ernest Farr took 7–8g of fresh chaparral leaves and steeped them in a quart of hot water. He drank 2–3 cups a day. Farr lived to the age of 96 when he died of the same melanoma. It appears that his doctor had refused to allow him to continue taking chaparral tea. As with other herbal cancer cures, chaparral needs to be continued after the tumour appears to have disappeared.

Curcumin (turmeric)

While turmeric is available as a food spice, for healing purposes it is best to take the purified extract, which is called curcumin. Studies show that curcumin can block cancer-causing enzymes and interfere with the development of new blood supplies; in other words, it is anti-angiogenetic. It is also an anti-inflammatory and helps maintain the health of the liver.

Evidence that it is highly beneficial comes from comparing cancer rates in Sri Lanka where the cancer mortality rate per 100,000 is 26.1 for females and 29.3 for males. This compares with US rates or 138.6 for women and 206.0 for men per 100,000. This difference is highly unlikely to be due to genetic or hereditary factors, for two reasons: 1) the population of Sri Lanka is ethnically very varied, and 2) the cancer rates of Sri Lankan immigrants to North America and Europe rise considerably within just a generation or two.

In Sri Lanka, a typical diet includes large amounts of turmeric. However, for the cancer patient, pure curcumin is required and a dose of 4–5 grams a day is recommended. However, curcumin capsules are useless, as the curcumin needs to be dissolved in fat before being ingested. The best way to take it is to buy curcumin powder, and dissolve it in warm coconut milk (or coconut oil), or cream and drink it. This has the effect of targeting the dissolved curcumin at the lymphatic system which is where it is needed.

Pregnant women should note this: because it acts as an anti-angiogenesis factor it must be avoided during pregnancy!

Recent research at the M D Anderson Cancer Center in Texas confirms that curcumin is a powerful anti-cancer agent which encourages normal cell death (apoptosis). Curcumin works synergistically with vitamin D (or natural sunlight).

Feverfew

Scientists have found that parthenolide, an extract of the feverfew plant (Tanacetum parthenium), is a highly effective agent against malignant stem cells. The first laboratory investigation found that it was potentially curative in cases of myeloid leukaemia — without harming normal, healthy blood cells. Because the focus of feverfew's activity is against stem cells, such a result indicates that feverfew—also known as bachelor's button—is likely to have an impact on all cancers. Until now, feverfew has been mainly associated with reducing fevers and treating migraines.

More recently, it has been suggested that pathenolide should be taken in combination with a prescription drug Sulindac to inhibit expression of nuclear factor kappaB (NF-$\varkappa$B), a transcription factor essential for cell division. It is activated in response to a number of factors that impose stress on the body: inflammation, viruses, etc. and, importantly for us, by cancers and carcinogens. Interestingly, radiation and chemotherapy also provoke activation of NF-$\varkappa$B, and so these conventional treatments are potentially carcinogenic.

One approach to attacking cancer is to prevent cancer cells from dividing—and inhibiting expression of NF-$\varkappa$B is one way to do this. A simple way of achieving this, according to Stephen Martin, PhD is to combine the feverfew extract parthenolide and the prescription drug, Sulindac—a non-steroidal anti-inflammatory drug also known as Clinoril. Martin recommends mixing the contents of ten capsules of Nature's Way feverfew herb (which is standardised at 0.7 per cent pathenolide) with some form of fat, say coconut milk. Do this twice a day. In addition take a 200mg tab of Sulindac three times a day. This combination will, he claims, have a strong inhibitory effect on cancer cell division. To further enhance the anti-cancer effect, Stephen Martin recommends taking vitamin E succinate.

Interestingly, the combination of curcumin (4–8g/day) and feverfew (4g/day) both dissolved in some form of cream or coconut milk is also considered to be effective. One user of this regime has dubbed the combination 'Curfew'—it's lights out for cancer.

Incidentally, high intracellular levels of vitamin C also appear to inactivate NF-κB—yet another way in which vitamin C in very high doses appears to work against cancer. (For a full discussion of vitamin C read Section 6: *Cancer: Vitamins and Other Supplements*.)

Graviola

Graviola is a South American plant with a wide range of medicinal uses. It has recently come to the fore as a very potent anti-cancer herb. In a 1976 plant screening program by the National Cancer Institute, the leaves and stem of graviola showed active cytotoxicity against cancer cells, and researchers have been following up on this research ever since. We can assume that their long interest in this plant is itself an implicit validation. But since they are not interested in validating herbs, but rather in the extraction of pure chemicals that can be patented, much of the research on graviola focuses on a set of phytochemicals called annonaceous acetogenins, which have been shown to have potent antitumor (and pesticidal) properties. Graviola produces these natural compounds in leaf, bark and twig tissues. Suggested dose: four capsules (600mg/cap) a day.

N-Tense is a branded formulation that has received a lot of attention in alternative cancer circles. It combines graviola with seven other herbs, including cat's claw. The ingredients are graviola (50 per cent), guacatonga, mullaca, vassourinha, espinheira santa, mutamba, bitter melon, and cat's claw. There are other liquid extracts of graviola on the market. Pawpaw, a cousin of graviola, is considered to be even stronger.

However, Marc Swanepoel, advocate of oleander therapies believes that all apoptosis therapies are ineffective in late-stage cancer. Here are his comments:

'From my reading of the research, pawpaw, graviola, and many other substances can help with cancer in the beginning stages by promoting the process of apoptosis. They work because they reduce the production of ATP which results, so the theory goes, in the death of fast growing cells that require a lot of ATP—preferably cancer cells. However, the alternative theory of cancer, that it (cancer) is a protection mechanism for cells that are under certain stresses, holds that this apoptosis period is relatively short and that the cancer cells have their own ways of overcoming it. Apoptosis requires that the mitochondrial membranes remain permeable to calcium ions. In cancer cells, these membranes get locked very quickly, especially after the cancer has metastasized. Oleander and NAC (N-acetyl cysteine), unlike pawpaw, graviola, etc., act to normalize the levels of glutathione in the body. This, in turn, unlocks the mitochondrial membranes and the mitochondria revert to normal. In summary, my personal take on pawpaw, graviola, etc. is that they are OK for cancer in the early stages, but that they should then not be taken with NAC, whey protein, or anything that promotes the levels of glutathione or ATP production in the body. Once cancer has spread, or in the case of very advanced cancer, my opinion is that pawpaw, graviola and other apoptosis-promoting substances based on reduced ATP production, will simply not work.'

This statement needs to be explained a little. The mitochondria are the rod-like structures in a cell that act as energy control centres. When the mitochondria revert to normal they trigger apoptosis (normal cell death). The argument here is between strategies that lower ATP (Graviola etc.) and those that raise it. But what is ATP? ATP (adenosine triphosphate) is the energy fuel that cells need to live and function.

My own feeling is that an ATP-promoting strategy as long as it is combined with good levels of glutathione is a healthier long-term anti-cancer strategy.

Green tea

A number of studies have shown that green tea helps protect against a variety of cancers, such as lung, prostate, and breast, but the mechanisms for these effects are not known. It is now suspected that EGCG (epigallocatechin gallate), a powerful antioxidant, may be the reason for its effectiveness. EGCG binds to a protein found on tumour cells and dramatically slows their growth. According to researchers, the concentration of the antioxidant having an anticancer effect was equivalent to that found in the body after drinking only two to three cups of green tea. This is a key component of Matthias Rath's anti-cancer protocol (see Section 3: *Cancer Research and Politics* for details).

Herb Robert—Geranium robertianum

In February 1953, *Natura*, a Portuguese magazine, published a story about a woman, aged 83, who was diagnosed with bowel cancer. She refused the surgery her doctors were insisting upon and instead went to a healer who prescribed a mixture of powdered leaves of St Robert's Wort and fresh raw egg yolk. The patient took this and, in time, was healed. A journalist became interested in this story and discovered that there were many other people—who had had a wide variety of cancers—who claimed to have been cured taking this same preparation. For more information go to: http://thehealingjournal.com/node/153.

Hypericum perforatum (St John's Wort)

Hypericum is a popular, safe and effective herb used mainly for its anti-depressant effects. It has also demonstrated strong anti-cancer effects in laboratory and animal studies—causing death by apoptosis and inhibiting angiogenesis in a wide range of cancers. It also appears to have the effect of reducing blood levels of drugs and so, if you are doing chemotherapy, you should discuss the impact of taking hypericum (as indeed you should discuss your use of any herb). Hypericin is one of the bio-active chemicals in the herb and this is highly reactive to light so you may find that one side effect is photo-sensitivity when in strong sunlight.

St John's Wort is taken orally. Suggested intake: dried herb: 2–4g as an infusion three times daily, or as a liquid extract: 2–4ml (1:1 in 25 per cent alcohol) three times daily.

Jergon sacha (Dracontium loretense)

This is a South American herb made from the roots of the plant (a member of the Araceae family, many plants of which have healing benefits—including the taro). It is used particularly as an anti-inflammatory and anti-snake bite remedy. In Peru, Dr Roberto Inchaustegui has used it against AIDS—and claims that many former AIDS patients are now free of HIV after six months. Inchaustegui also claims that it has strong anti-cancer effects. It is available in Peru in pill form and as a tincture. It has been widely used in Eastern Europe for several decades but is only now becoming more widely known in the West. For further information and to buy this herb go to www.rain-tree.com. Like keladi tikus, described below, this is a glutathione-boosting herb so should not be taken at the same time as graviola or pawpaw which are glutathione depleting herbs.

Keladi tikus (Typhonium flagelliforme)

Chris Teo, who now runs a cancer centre in Penang, started his healing work when, having recently retired as Professor of Botany (he is Malaysia's leading authority on orchids), he was approached by a man who asked him if it would be easy to propagate a particular plant. Chris said it would be easy and then asked him why he wanted to do so. The man told him it had powerful healing properties. Shortly afterwards he gave a root of the plant to a friend who had cancer—and the man recovered. The healing plant was keladi tikus—rodent tuber—which is also a member of the Araceae family of plants.

A keladi tikus product called Typhonium Plus is available from a number of Malaysian suppliers. Further details can be found at www.keladitikusubatkanser.com and www.cancerhelps.com. For cancer patients, a dose of two capsules three times per day is recommended. I have discussed Chris Teo's centre in more detail later in this section.

Lemongrass

Israeli researchers at Ben Gurion University of the Negev discovered in 2005 that the molecules that create the lemon aroma in herbs like lemongrass also kills cancer cells in vitro, while leaving healthy cells unharmed. Citral is the key component that gives the lemony aroma and taste in several herbal plants such as lemongrass (Cymbopogon citratus), melissa (Melissa officinalis) and verbena (Verbena officinalis). It also causes cancer cells to undergo apoptosis—programmed cell death. Patients are advised to sip lemongrass tea throughout the day. Each glass can be made with one gram of fresh lemongrass steeped in hot water. Lemongrass is also available as an essential oil, generally used to keep mosquitoes at bay.

Lobelia

Lobelia herb is a powerful brochodilator, which means it helps people breathe more easily, which helps oxygen intake, which could—and I stress 'could'—mean that there is more oxygen circulating in the system and that is good for cancer patients.

One contributor to a yahoo chat group provided this info: 'It will clear out years old mucus from the lungs. Dr Schulze recounts a story of being called to the bedside of a man dying of black lung, totally unable to do more than gasp for air through a liquid sound from his lungs. With nothing to lose, Schulze gave him a two ounce bottle of lobelia to drink. Now, lobelia is potent and usually taken in drops or only one dropper full. The bottle did nothing for the man. So Schulze gave him another one. Again, it did nothing. After drinking the third bottle of lobelia tincture, the man started throwing up all sorts of nasty, foul smelling black mucus. This went on for quite a while. When he was done, his skin tone was pink and healthy, and he was able to breathe normally and he lived for many more years without any coughing or gasping for air at all.

'As for seizures, a lady I knew on a herb group had a disabled adult son. The only thing that would bring him out of his seizures was a few drops of lobelia tincture rubbed into the back of his neck. Once rubbed in, he would immediately come out of his seizure.

I would never discount lobelia. It is a potent nervine. Schulze says that he carries a bottle of pure cayenne tincture in one pocket and a bottle of lobelia in the other, as these will cover most situations. Cayenne is given when a person is in shock or bleeding, and lobelia is given when they are hyper and too excited. And, when he doesn't know what the actual health problem is, he gives both cayenne and lobelia, one after the other—allowing 20 to 30 minutes between doses—because one is a stimulant (cayenne) and one a relaxant (lobelia) which will often pump blood in and out of any congested area anywhere in the body.'

Milk thistle

This is an important herb for strengthening the liver, and the livers of people with cancer need strengthening. The active ingredient—the one that protects the liver—is known as silymarin. Silymarin keeps new liver cells from being destroyed by toxins such as alcohol. It reduces inflammation (which is why it is often suggested for people with liver inflammation or hepatitis), and is a strong antioxidant.

But, in addition, it appears to have a number of direct anti-cancer effects. Silymarin and other active substances in milk thistle appear to stop cancer cells from dividing and reproducing, while at the same time reducing the blood supply to tumours. This is a strong candidate for any anti-cancer herbal mix.

An extract of milk thistle, silymarin-phosphatidylcholine complex, may be absorbed more easily than regular standardized milk thistle. Phosphatidylcholine is a key element in cell membranes. It helps silymarin attach easily to cell membranes, which may keep toxins from getting inside liver cells.

Dose levels. In divided doses: milk thistle, 500mg; silymarin extract, 200–400mg/day.

Mint

Mint has a wide range of effects that makes it beneficial for people with cancer—and Moroccan women who drink a great deal of it have low rates of breast cancer (though whether this is because of the tea is not known).

Mint has been shown, in laboratory animal studies, to protect against lung cancer—and even more suggestively, mint is used in certain folk cultures to induce abortions in the case of unwanted pregnancies. Anything that has that effect is likely to have an anti-cancer effect as well. Men should note that mint tends to lower testosterone levels and therefore libido. While it doesn't appear to increase estrogens levels itself it can promote the estrogens-increasing activity of drugs—and this may be a matter of concern for women with hormone related breast cancers.

The two most common ways of taking mint is in a mint tea or using peppermint essential oil.

Moringa olifeira

Moringa is a herb that is found in many parts of the world from Africa to the Philippines. Everywhere it grows it is used in traditional medicine as a general health support. Interestingly it is a powerful anti-inflammatory, and so beneficial to people suffering from arthritis—even rheumatoid arthritis which is notoriously problematic—as well as blood pressure and blood sugar levels (so beneficial to diabetics). For cancer patients, the news is that lab tests have shown it to induce apoptosis (normal cell death) in cancer calls and additionally it provides a chemical obstacle to cancer cell proliferation.

Oleander

An extract of oleander has been shown to cause autophagy—that is, it makes cells eat themselves and this self-digestion leads to cell death—in pancreatic cancer cells by research undertaken at M D Anderson Cancer Center. However, the oleander plant is poisonous if you don't know what you're doing. There are two oleander preparations described in this book: Anvirzel and Sutherlandia OPC. These come highly recommended. See below for details.

Papaya and pawpaw

The fruit that Americans know as the pawpaw (*Asiminia triloba*) is not the same fruit as the papaya (*Carica papaya*)—which confusingly is also known in Australia as pawpaw. However, both have an important part to play as anti-cancer therapies.

The papaya

The papaya is an excellent fruit. It contains more vitamin A than carrots and more vitamin C than oranges. It is particularly noted as the source of the enzyme papain (but only in the unripe fruit and the seeds of the ripe fruit) which has powerful anti-cancer properties in its own right. Barbara Simonson, author of *Papaya: Healing with the Wonderfruit*, recommends eating and juicing the skin as well. She claims it can cure cancer. 'I have a friend, Halima Neumann, who was healed from stomach cancer by drinking the juice of papayas for six months, half a litre each day, and after that eating half-ripe papayas every day.'

But this does not exhaust the potential of the papaya. Harald Tietze, an Australian who has actively promoted the health benefits of the papaya, reports that the leaves of the papaya plant have cured a number of cases of cancer.

He recommends that a handful of leaves can be put in a saucepan with boiling water and left to simmer for an hour. The resulting 'tea' can be diluted and drunk throughout the day. One man who read Tietze's advice, mentioned it to a friend: 'I told him to 'stuff a handful of pawpaw leaves into a saucepan and fill with water; boil, simmer for one hour and drink it till it comes out of your ears'. The friend followed this advice and, according to the anecdotal report, five weeks later he 'had no trace of cancer whatsoever'.

Papaya leaves and other products can be obtained from The Kombucha House, which also sells other papaya concentrate products. For further information go to www.kombucha-house.com.

The pawpaw

Let us now turn to the North American pawpaw, the fruit of which looks somewhat like a thick, short banana. This herb too is considered to have powerful biologically active effects against cancer—but in this case it is not the leaves but the bark and twigs. When buying 'pawpaw extract' from a North American herb supplier, it is this product that you will be getting.

Pawpaw extract contains a group of chemicals called acetogenins—which interfere with the production of ATP, a chemical that is necessary for cellular energy. The impact on ATP is more critical for cancer cells than normal cells and results in the reduced growth of blood vessels that nourish cancer cells. Very importantly, it is one of the few herbs that has shown itself to be effective in inhibiting the growth of MDR (multiple drug resistant) cells.

Pawpaw is a cousin of the graviola, guanabana, and soursop trees. However, the acetogenins extracted from pawpaw are reportedly even more active against cancer than those extracted from these other sources.

Pawpaw is also effective against viruses and reduces the side effects of chemo. A number of people have found it useful to combine pawpaw with CanCell. One reported the benefits in this way: 'It [pawpaw] stopped pain and bleeding and when later I added Protocel (a branded version of CanCell) I saw a tremendous lysing [disintegration]. The pawpaw had broken down a huge amount of waste and the Protocel went in and flushed it all out.' (For more details of Protocel/CanCell see Section 6: *Cancer: Vitamins and Other Supplements*.)

Jerry McLaughlin, professor of pharmacognosy at Purdue University, claims that pawpaw extract, which contains over 40 cancer-fighting compounds, is many times more potent than the leading chemotherapy drug Adriamycin, and yet, at the same time, totally without toxic side effects to normal healthy tissue.

Four capsules of standardized extract of Pawpaw are taken per day, until cancer goes into remission. While taking pawpaw, it is important to avoid at the same time taking megadoses of vitamins A, C and E; alpha lipoic acid; CoQ10; SOD; and 7-Keto, as these inhibit the effectiveness of the pawpaw. It is helpful, however, to supplement with concentrated doses of protease (a protein digesting enzyme) and other natural immune-enhancing supports such as noni juice, beta glucans, arabinogalactan, colostrum, reishi and maitake mushrooms, and cordyceps.

Warning: some people taking pawpaw have reported that it either caused or exacerbated severe depression.

As with graviola this is an ATP-reducing herb (see under graviola above for a full discussion of implications).

Pau d'arco (lapacho, taheebo)

In 1967, the Brazilian newspaper O'Cruzeiro reported the story of a cancer-stricken girl from Rio who continually prayed for a cure. In a dream or vision, she saw a monk who told her that she would recover if she made a tea brewed with the bark of the pau d'arco tree. The monk returned in a second vision and told her which specific pau d'arco trees she was to use. Whether these visions were true—perhaps a response to a subconscious recognition of the medicinal powers of this tree—or whether they were simply a necessary guise in which to cloak a desire persuasively, the girl was given the tea she required and she recovered.

She was not alone. Many others have claimed their cancers have gone into long-term remission after drinking pau d'arco tea. Anecdotal evidence and folk practice throughout South America appears to justify the claims made for this tree bark. Besides cancer, it is supposedly effective against diabetes, ulcers and rheumatism to name a few—and applied to the skin is good for burns. The inner bark of the tree contains many chemicals that are known to have anti-tumour effects: tannins, quinones and triterpines and others. There are many different varieties of the pau d'arco tree—and each variety seems to have its own range of medicinal characteristics. Its anticancer effects have been demonstrated in a number of animal studies. Pau d'arco—also known as lapacho and taheebo—is available as a bark, in powdered form, and as an alcoholic extract.

Unfortunately, there have been suggestions that a lot of the pau d'arco on the market is of poor quality. A number of studies on the alcoholic extracts commercially available in Europe and North America consider them to be medically useless as they do not appear to contain the active ingredient, lapachol. Others argue that looking for a single active ingredient is wrong: pau d'arco contains at least 12 quinones of which lapachol is only one.

To make a tea, add six tablespoons of the bark to four cups of boiling water. The water is kept boiling until it reduces to three cups. This takes about five minutes. The tea is then cooled and then filtered. Three to eight cups a day should be taken, each cup sipped slowly but steadily. The tea not being drunk should be kept refrigerated. Toxicity is low. The symptom to expect from over-consumption is a slight skin rash.

The following websites have been suggested as good resources and sources of good quality herb: www.pau-d-arco.com; www.princetea.com; www.herb-care.com and www.atlantishealthcenters.com.

Poke root (Phytolacca americana)

Poke root is a native American herb that helps as a blood cleanser and as a metabolic stimulant helping the absorption of nutrients from foods. This herb is particularly beneficial for glandular and lymphatic conditions and many herbalists believe that it can significantly speed up recovery times.

For the cancer patient, the key benefits are immune enhancement and the fact that it is a powerful anti-inflammatory. As with all herbs, and this reminder should be made frequently, recommended dose levels should not be exceeded with impunity. Herbs are powerful agents for healing but they are also potentially toxic if abused. This caution needs particularly to be made in relation to poke root. It is available as a tincture or as dry herb. One recommended dose level is a quarter teaspoon of dry herb in a cup of water, simmer for 15 minutes and drink when cool. Do this three times a day.

Pycnogenol

Pycnogenol is derived from the bark of the French maritime pine tree (*Pinus maritima*), and is a complex of more than 40 antioxidant compounds. It has been called the most powerful antioxidant discovered by science. However, it is not just an antioxidant but has shown direct and powerful anti-cancer activity. In one anecdotal report by Dr Lamar Rosquist, a Canadian doctor who is actively promoting pycnogenol, a woman with terminal breast and lung cancer started taking pycnogenol in large quantities (200mg three times a day) along with colloidal silver and aloe vera. One month later she was cancer free. Pycnogenol is being taken very seriously and a number of clinical trials are in progress to evaluate its effectiveness.

Rosemary

Rosemary is one of the best liver-strengthening herbs. It is also a notable source for betulinic acid which has demonstrated strong anti-tumour activity.

Sage

Sage is the name given to the leaves of the plant Salvia officinalis. It has been found to have antiseptic, antimicrobial, antioxidant, anti-inflammatory, antifungal, antiviral, and anti-mutagenic (i.e. it protects DNA against mutation) properties. Sage contains numerous biologically active compounds and has a wide range of benefits particularly for diabetics. It has also been shown to arrest human colon and prostate cancer cell development at different phases of the cell cycle. Animal studies have also shown beneficial impacts on melanoma in mice.

Some herbalists, however, recommend caution in the use of sage tea for women with breast cancer as this herb has complex and little understood impacts on the lactation process. This caution may be unnecessary as it is perfectly possible that sage has beneficial impacts on breast cancer as it does for other cancers.

Sage has many uses in Chinese medicine—notably, to treat irregular menstruation, cardiovascular problems, and inflammation. It is also used as a tranquilizer.

While the most common way of taking sage is as a herb tea, it is also possible to buy sage essential oil. This is a powerful oil and should never be used without dilution.

Sage should be avoided by anyone who suffers from epilepsy, and this herb also has the potential to increase liver damage from some prescription medications, and for that reason sage should never be taken during chemotherapy.

Salvestrols

These are phytonutrients found in fruits and vegetables—and more so in organic produce—which have only recently been isolated and studied. The results are exciting for people with cancer. The way it works is this: cancer cells contain an enzyme protein called CYP1B1. If this protein is triggered it causes the release of chemicals within the cell that will quickly kill it. And this is what salvestrols do. They activate this enzyme. Professor Burke, the co-discoverer of these phytonutrients, likens this protein to a Trojan horse. Unfortunately, the content of salvestrols in food is generally too low to provide enough to be medically beneficial. A concentrated salvestrol extract, called Salvestrol, has been developed. It is cheap and widely available on the Internet. It is so cheap that it has been proposed that people of all ages should take it simply as a cancer preventative.

Saw palmetto

This is the herb for anyone with prostate problems. It is usually considered useful for mild to moderate prostate enlargement. However, in-vitro studies have shown it to have a general anti-cancer effect with prostate cancer cells responding most readily. When purchasing, make sure the strength is 85–95 per cent fatty acids and sterols. Take 160 mgs twice daily.

A note on prostate health

In addition to saw palmetto, a number of other herbs are useful in maintaining a healthy prostate gland: pygeum, stinging nettle, isoflavones (genistein and daidzein), rye pollen, phytosterols (e.g., sitosterol), and lycopene. In one reported case, a 62-year-old man with advanced prostate cancer experienced regression of his tumour after taking 10mg of lycopene per day and 300mg of saw palmetto three times per day. Researchers attributed this effect more to the lycopene than the saw palmetto.

People with prostate cancer, in addition to the saw palmetto, should take zinc (50–60 mgs daily), because their prostate fluids are low in this mineral. Magnesium has also been shown to be beneficial for the prostate.

Wormwood (artemisinin)

Wormwood has long been used by herbalists as a bitter herb to improve digestion, to fight worm infestations (as its name suggests) and other parasites and as a useful remedy for liver problems. An extract from wormwood, artemisinin, which was known to the ancient Chinese as a malaria cure, has recently re-emerged as an anti-cancer treatment on its own.

Artemisinin works because it interacts biochemically with iron, a mineral which is needed by cancer cells as it is necessary for cell division, and for that reason usually advised against as a supplement. The surface of a cancer cell has many more iron-attracting receptors than the surface of a normal, healthy cell. When artemisinin comes in contact with the iron a reaction takes place, releasing a burst of free radicals that kills the cell. Although it is normally not advisable to take iron supplements in the case of cancer, when taking artemisinin, the reverse is true, as we wish to flood the cancer cells with iron.

In one study, researchers fed rats a substance known to induce multiple breast tumours. All the rats were then fed a normal diet, but half were given a 0.02 per cent dose of artemisinin. Over 40 weeks, investigators monitored tumour formation in the rats. Ninety-six per cent of the rats that did not get artemisinin developed tumours. In those that did receive the substance, only 57 per cent developed tumours. In addition, artemisinin-fed rats had smaller and fewer tumours.

Artemisinin has a good safety record because it has been used extensively against malaria. The problem is that wormwood herb has variable levels of artemisinin—and indeed a particular batch may not have any at all. It is therefore better to take a standardised extract. 1–2g per day per 100 pounds (45kg) of body weight, divided into four doses, is considered appropriate in the case of cancer, but it can be toxic at very high doses, so any negative side effects should indicate that a reduction in dose levels is desired.

In TCM (Traditional Chinese Medicine), wormwood is considered to be a 'cooling' herb. If you find yourself tingling (too cool), you might want to reduce the dose. Artemisinin should be taken with food. Using an essential fatty acid (flax oil, cod liver oil, lecithin, or wheat germ oil) will help absorption. Artemisinin is not considered a stand-alone cancer cure, but part of an overall, aggressive, anti-cancer program—possibly including high doses of pancreatic enzymes (on an empty stomach), CoQ10 and a detox program. A source can be found at: www.altcancer.com/artemis.htm.

Medicinal mushrooms

Mushrooms are well known for their potent medicinal qualities. Here are the ones most useful for the person with cancer.

Agaricus blazei murill (ABM)

This Brazilian mushroom, discovered only in the 1970s by Western scientists near Sao Paulo, has demonstrated remarkable anti-cancer properties. Normally, the polysaccharides found in fungus only affect solid cancers; however, the polysaccharide in agaricus (also known as ABM) is effective against almost all cancers. The polysaccharides appear to activate white blood cells known as macrophages, which filter the blood by destroying viruses, bacteria, and perhaps even cancer cells. Shiitake, maitake and reishi (see below) also contain these polysaccharides. In one Japanese study, ABM was found to eliminate all cancerous tumours in 90 per cent of the experimental mice. In another study the mice were fed agaricus as a preventative and then injected with a very powerful cancer-causing agent 99.4 per cent of them showed no tumour growth.

ABM contains much higher levels of beta glucans than the other medicinal mushrooms (maitake, shiitake, and reishi) and it stimulates NK (natural killer) cell activity at a rate higher than MGN-3. Japanese oncologists are in no doubt as to its benefits and Japan is now buying over 90 per cent of the available ABM from Brazil.

RAAX11. One extract from ABM is RAAX11. It is currently being studied in Brazil and has demonstrated some astonishing results for breast cancers.

Daily dosage for normal body maintenance and prevention is about 6g (about a quarter of a dry mushroom) or 40g (approximately. two mushrooms) for serious illness. Tea is also a popular way of taking the mushroom. Use about one mushroom per litre (two pints) and simmer it for an hour. Drink a cup a day, warm or cold. Taking vitamin C promotes absorption.

OPC. OPC is a combination of ABM with oleander, cat's claw and pau d'arco. It was developed in South Africa and anecdotal reports testify to its effectiveness. Note that although dramatic long-term effects have been seen with OPC, there may be some short-term negative side effects. Marc Swanepoel, who is the patent holder, gives the following list: slight nausea and vomiting, diarrhoea, pruritus, pain at a tumour site, tachycardia and arrhythmias. Because of its blood-thinning properties, people on medical blood-thinning preparations should consult their doctors before using the OPC. People on heart-active drugs, such as digoxin (Lanoxin), digitoxin or anti-arrhythmics should also speak to their doctors before using the mixture. No other drug interactions have been reported. Pregnant women should preferably not use the mixture due to its anti-angiogenesis effect. Other short-term detoxification symptoms like a slight rash, runny nose, pimples and slightly painful joints, may be experienced.

Recent research conducted at M D Anderson Cancer Center has shown that oleander attacks cancer in a number of different ways: it inhibits angiogenesis, promotes apoptosis, stimulates the immune system, reduces the power of cancer cells to defend themselves and promotes autophagy, a process where cells consume themselves. So, all in all, a very powerful weapon.

Sources: Agaricus and other mushrooms can be obtained from www.mitobi.com. ABM freeze-dried extract in capsules is available from www.hplus.com and to order mushrooms in bulk, wholesale from China go to www.abmcn.com. RAAX11, along with branded mixtures RF1000 and are available on wholesale terms from: www.takesun.com or www.agaricus.net. OPC is also available at less cost from Marc Swanepoel who can be contacted at www.sutherlandiaopc.com.

Maitake

This mushroom is arousing a great deal of interest as it appears to have powerful anti-cancer effects, as well as being helpful to people with AIDS, diabetes and high blood pressure.

Maitake has been found to contain grifolan and beta-D-glucan, two important beta-glucan polysaccharides—molecules composed of many sugar molecules linked together. These have been shown to have a strong effect in activating microphages, which have been described as the heavy artillery of the immune system.

Laboratory studies have shown that maitake extract can block the growth of cancer tumours and boost the immune function of mice with cancer. It has also been shown to reduce tumours in people with stomach cancer and leukaemia. Cancer research on this mushroom is still in a very early stage but the initial signs are encouraging.

Reishi (Ling Zhi)

The Japanese call it 'reishi', the Chinese call it 'Ling Zhi', the Russians call a closely-related mushroom 'chaga' (mentioned in Solzhenitsyn's great novel *Cancer Ward*). It was highly revered by Taoists in search of the elixir of immortality. Of course, any herb associated with long life is very likely to have shown clear evidence of general medicinal value. There are a number of varieties, the most potent of which is considered by the Chinese to be the red fungus—but this may simply be because the colour red has very positive symbolism in Chinese culture. Reishi mushrooms are very high in polysaccharides and these may be responsible for its immune system stimulation effect. The Chinese view it as a tonic that boosts the vital life energy they call 'qi' (pronounced: chee).

Studies have shown that reishi mushroom extracts can kill staphylococci and streptococci bacteria. This makes it a very useful treatment for pneumonia and hospital acquired infections. Interestingly, low doses of the mushroom appear to be more effective than large doses. The optimal dose appears to be 4g a day. One Japanese cancer surgeon, Dr Fukumi Morishige, stumbled on this by chance when a woman who was dying of cancer suddenly appeared to be cured. He discovered that her husband had been giving her fresh reishi mushroom tea every day. Morishige now prescribes a daily intake of 4g of reishi tea with 10g of a special form of vitamin C known as nucleic acid ascorbate. Morishige discovered that large doses of vitamin C prevented the diarrhoea caused by taking in too much reishi. He therefore reasoned that the vitamin C was having the effect of increasing its absorbability. In this way he was able to increase the dose of reishi to 9g a day. Reishi can also be taken effectively by intravenous injection. Morishige has treated and cured a number of cancer patients using nothing else but this combination of vitamin C and reishi mushrooms.

Studies undertaken by the National Cancer Research Centre shows that mice injected with reishi extract showed tumour regression between 50 and 100 per cent, depending on the dose.

People who take reishi mushrooms show a marked increase in blood oxygenation levels, and for this reason it is also used as an antidote to altitude sickness. The importance in cancer treatment of having high tissue oxygen levels has already been mentioned and this may be one of the ways in which reishi has an anti-cancer effect.

Some healers use it in combination with shiitake mushrooms and astragalus. It is used to treat asthma, allergies as well as insomnia. It can have a few unpleasant side effects: dizziness, light-headedness and itchiness. These can be dealt with by lowering the dose and then slowly increasing it. There have been no signs of toxicity in many studies—even up to levels equivalent to a human taking 350g a day.

Reishi is very bitter and not eaten as a food. It is cut into pieces and brewed in hot water: 5g/l. The water is simmered until it is reduced to one-third of a litre. It is then drunk. The vitamin C has to be taken separately as it is destroyed by heat. Reishi is also available in capsule form. At present it is quite expensive and as a result a great deal of fake Ling Zhi has made its way on to the market.

Apart from its claimed anti-cancer effects, it is recommended in Japan as a way of reducing side effects for patients undergoing radiation and chemotherapy.

Shiitake

The shiitake mushroom (Lentinus edodes) is the other well-known Japanese medicinal mushroom. Among its many excellent qualities is the fact that it contains ergosterol, which can be converted by sunlight into vitamin D–a potent cancer fighter in its own right.

In traditional Chinese and Japanese medicine, shiitake is considered to have a powerful and positive impact on qi energy. It is also considered to be a food that promotes longevity, protects the immune system, promotes good circulation and prevents liver disease.

Scientists are now studying an extract of shiitake known as lentinan for its potential anti-tumour effects. It works by stimulating certain types of white blood cells important in immune function rather than by directly attacking cancer cells. One wholesale source for lentinan and other mushroom extract powders is alibaba.com.

RM-10™ combination mushroom product

This is a combination of ten certified organic medicinal mushrooms (including agaricus, reishi, shiitake, maitake, Cordyseps sinensis, and Coriolus versicor, among others), extracted through an enzymatic enhancing process and combined with aloe vera and the herb Uncaria tomentosa (cat's claw).

It was developed by Jordan Rubin, who was motivated to help his grandmother who was diagnosed with advanced metastatic disease. She agreed to follow his regime and is now cancer free. Independent researchers and alternative therapists have confirmed that it is highly effective—and is very helpful in minimising the toxic effects of chemotherapy. It is sold by Garden of Life Vitamins as helpful for a number of immune-compromising illnesses. There are a number of Internet suppliers.

Sun soup

Sun soup is a product containing shiitake and other mushrooms, soy, and a number of Asian herbs. Developed by Alexander S Sun, PhD, a biochemist from the University of California, Berkeley, who did research at Mt Sinai Medical Center, New York, and Yale University, in order to help his mother survive cancer. Despite poor prognosis she did indeed recover with the help of this soup. Independent research indicates that it does have tumour-inhibiting qualities. For further details see www.sunfarmcorp.com.

Active hexose correlated compound (AHCC)

AHCC is made from a combination of hybridized Japanese medicinal mushrooms. There are reports that a number of cancer patients suffering from breast, prostate, and other forms of cancer have experienced dramatic improvement and even full remission after taking AHCC.

Most of the research has been done in Japan where AHCC was developed. In one study of five breast cancer cases given three grams of AHCC a day, two (40 per cent) had gone to complete remission by the end of the eight-month study. It should be noted that participants in these kinds of study have usually been considered terminal. This is an astonishing result. AHCC is widely available from Internet herbal suppliers.

There are a number of other mushroom extract formulations that have shown effectiveness either alone or, more commonly, as supporting therapies for people undergoing chemotherapy. Among these are PSK (This is the Japanese name. It is also known in China as PSP), Ganoderma, MycoSoft and others. There appears to be clear evidence that these formulations make chemotherapy more bearable and at the same time improve survivability rates. One source for these mushrooms is www.mushroompatc h.com/herbal_powder.htm.

A study by scientists at Memorial Sloan-Kettering Cancer Centre looked at the ability of a number of substances to induce immune reactions in laboratory mice. They found the following to have consistently significant activity:

Coriolus mushroom extracts (especially PSK)
Alcohol extract of astragalus
Yeast β-glucan
Maitake mushrooms.

Herbal Formulas and Combination Therapies

Alsihum (alzium)

Alsihum—also called alzium—was developed by a biblical scholar, Chaim Kass, based on 500-year-old Hebrew and Arabic texts that contained herbal recipes for cures for colds, flus and other ailments. These were tested and found to be effective. They were subsequently tested on cancer patients with some limited success. In the first study, two out of 30 terminal patients had long-term remission. Alsihum is a 100 per cent natural herbal compound developed by researchers at CED Tech Health in Jerusalem, Israel. The formula consists of nine herbs in a base of water and alcohol. The formula includes cone flower, myrrh, skullcap, burdock, saffron and cayenne. For further information and to order, contact info@cedtechhealth.com.

Anvirzel

The oleander is an extremely poisonous plant which nevertheless has been widely used in several folk medicines. Its use against cancer has been reported in the Caribbean, North Africa and India. A Turkish doctor, Dr Huseyin Ozel, developed a herbal cure involving oleander extracts, which he trademarked under the name Anvirzel. The roots, leaves and flowers are treated in such a way that the resulting liquid is entirely non-toxic. The product received a US patent in 1992 and a company called Ozelle Pharmaceuticals started work to try and get approval for the drug. It has since been trialled in Ireland with good results. No side effects were reported and it had clear anti-cancer effects along with pain-relief. According to a report on the trial quoted by Moss, 1998: all 46 patients 'have shown improvements that have surpassed or defied expectations of conventional treatments'.

Other reports indicate that this is a very highly effective anti-cancer treatment for all cancers, and, unlike the oleander plant, completely non-toxic. Anvirzel is administered either orally or by daily injection. It appears to be only available at present from Salud Integral Clinic in Honduras www.saludintegral.hn. (For another oleander-based herbal combination see OPC.)

Curaderm (BEC5)

This is a cream that has demonstrated strong healing activity against a number of skin cancers. It was developed by Dr Bill Cham, an Australian biochemist, and is based on a plant—*Solanum sodamaeum*—which is known in Australia as Devil's apple or Kangaroo apple. It is not a burning salve like bloodroot, but its effectiveness has been demonstrated in a number of studies at reputable London hospitals. The cream is also promoted as beneficial for psoriasis and eczema.

BEC5 can eradicate non-melanoma skin cancers, specifically basal cell carcinoma (BCC) and squamous cell carcinoma (SCC). It is also effective against benign tumours and other skin irregularities, including keratoses, sun spots and age spots.

One important point to note is that it is vital to use the cream before any surgery has taken place. This is because cancerous tissues on the skin are connected to cancerous tissues below the surface. The cream can then eliminate all these cancerous cells one after the other. Surgery may eliminate surface cells without impacting on the cells below the surface. The cream then cannot get access to the deeper lying cells.

It is available from www.curaderm.net and a number of other websites.

Skin cancer warning

If you have skin cancer, be very careful what the oncologist recommends: One skin cancer medication, Aldara, which contains the chemical imiquimod (IQ), has been known since 1986 to be itself a cause of cancer. 'It is so dangerous that the American Cancer Society, The National Cancer Institute, and others have determined it is a carcinogen, and have placed it on their lists of most hazardous chemicals. IQ has even been listed as a laboratory chemical hazard by the US Occupational Safety Health Agency. Yet, doctors worldwide are prescribing it, willy-nilly, to 'cure' skin cancers' (Elaine Hollingsworth, an Australian skin cancer patient who nearly died using it, writing in *The Townsend Newsletter*, May 2006) See also her own website: www.doctorsaredangerous.com.

Other creams recommended for skin cancer

PDQ Cream has been recommended by a person with skin cancer as being beneficial. Look at www.behealed.biz for further details. Another useful product is Raspex SPF-30 skin gel, which is made from meeker raspberries and has a strong ellagic acid content. See www.smdi.org/products.htm.

Danggui longhui wan

This is a mixture of Chinese herbs that is used in Chinese medicine, particularly against leukaemia. The active herb was found to be indigo, which contains indirubin, purified extracts of which have been shown to be potent inhibitors of cell proliferation (i.e., they help stop the growth of cancer tumours). Indirubin is a component of a number of herbs, and extracts of these herbs may be found through a normal Internet search. Interestingly, one easily available source of indirubin is available at no cost whatsoever—in one's own urine.

Eli Jones syrup

Dr Eli Jones (1850–1933) was one of the earliest doctors to consider that cancer could be treated by medical means (i.e., with medicines) rather than by surgery or radiation. His comment: 'Four-fifths of the cancers I have seen in the past forty years had been operated on and the cancer returned worse than before. Other cases have tried the x-ray, radium, escharotics and hypodermic treatments, etc., etc., before I saw them, with the same results.' (quoted in Moss, 1998)

Dr Jones formulated a herbal syrup which he called Compound Syrup Scrophularia. It contains poke root, figwort, may apple and a number of other herbs. This can be obtained from Dr Ingrid Naiman, www.cancersalves.com.

Essiac

The official story of Essiac starts in 1922, when a young nurse by the name of Rene Caisse was given the names of a number of herbs by an old woman who had cured herself of breast cancer by drinking a tea containing these herbs. This old woman had got the remedy from a native Ojibwa Indian. Sometime later, her aunt was diagnosed with terminal stomach cancer and given six months to live. Caisse remembered the herbs and, with the doctor's consent, gave them to her aunt, who went on to live another 21 years. She was given more cases and these also healed. The doctors were so impressed they petitioned the Canadian government in 1926 to give Rene Caisse facilities for research. The result? They tried to arrest her for treating cancer without a medical license. Fortunately for her she had the support of nine very eminent doctors so they desisted.

She gave the Essiac combination (named by reversing her own name) not only in the form of tea but also—in a modified form—by injection in the site of the cancer. She found this to be quicker and more effective.

In 1938 a Commission of Enquiry conducted an investigation. Unlike Mary Johnson, Rene Caisse did not receive a generous appraisal. It concluded that all of the patients who came to testify on her behalf, none had ever had cancer—despite their X-rays and medical documentation. Despite harassment, she continued to give patients her herbal treatment—without making any charge. In one case she records that her treatment for cancer had the interesting side effect of also curing the patient's diabetes.

There are currently a number of variations of the same basic Essiac formula on the market—Essiac, Tea of Life and Flor-Essence and possibly others—but they all share the same official ingredients, which are burdock root, turkish rhubarb, slippery elm and sheep sorrel. Additional ingredients found in commercial Essiac teas are: red clover blossom, kelp, blessed thistle and watercress. The tea can be drunk both as a treatment for cancer or as a preventative health tonic.

Rene Caisse died in 1978 at the age of 91. In 1983, Bruce Hendrick, Chief of the Division of Neurosurgery at the Hospital for Sick Children in Toronto, wrote to the Canadian Minister for Health and Welfare asking her to authorize clinical trials on the effectiveness of Essiac tea. In his letter he said: 'I am most impressed with the effectiveness of the treatment and its lack of side effects.' Further support for its effectiveness comes from Dr Charles Brusch, personal physician to President John F Kennedy, who also claims to have been cured of his cancer using Essiac.

The Canadian Cancer Society nevertheless maintains a cool distance. It considers Essiac to be a questionable or unproven method of cancer treatment. Canadian health laws prohibit it from being marketed as an anti-cancer treatment but they accept that it is not harmful and it is available on prescription—but the prescribing doctor must first get authorization from the Deputy Director of the Health Protection branch. They warn that Essiac may cause some nausea or diarrhoea. They also warn that it is not established that the commercial brands named above are in fact made with the true Essiac recipe. Nevertheless, the manufacturers of Flor-Essence and Tea of Life are able to produce testimonial letters from people who claim to have been cured by the herbal tea. One of the main constituents—Burdock root—has demonstrated anti-tumour activity on its own but, as with all herbal formulas, it is the synergistic effects that are important and which remain largely unexplored.

Essiac is widely available from Internet health supermarkets such as www.vitacost.com and www.iherb.com.

Green sap

This is a secret herbal formulation created by a Uruguayan oncologist that contains a high triterpine content and which claims to have strong anti-cancer activity. It is unsubstantiated by any large scale studies, but they offer a number of case histories of people who have been cured. For further information go to www.gotitas.com. It is claimed to be non-toxic supportive for people undergoing chemotherapy and radiation.

It is certainly true that triterpines, a family of essential oils found in many plants, seem to be one of the most potent ingredients in many herbs and plant extracts associated with long life. And, of course, long life can be seen simply as a life not shortened by cancer. The following are known to contain significant quantities of triterpines: Siberian ginseng; liquorice root; ginkgo leaves; gotu kola; and, interestingly, soybeans. These herbs have shown significant anti-tumour activity in studies in the US and Finland. Gingko has also been shown in animal studies to make aggressive cancers significantly less aggressive.

In addition, olives contain oleanolic acid, a triterpine, which is being examined with great interest by the Japanese as a chemopreventive of cancer.

HANSI

HANSI is an acronym for homeopathic natural activator of the immune system (it works better in Spanish!) The story is that Argentinean botanist, Juan Hirschmann, using his knowledge of plants created a number of homeopathic-concentration cures for a number of diseases. He called his product HANSI. It contains homeopathic concentrations of ten or so plants including cactus, aloe, arnica and licopodium, along with lachesis derived from the venom of the bushmaster snake. From his Buenos Aires clinic, he has treated tens of thousands of cancer patients—representing every type of cancer. He claims to have achieved a great deal of success, supported by reviews and testimonials. He markets his products from the Bahamas.

There are injectable and oral versions (the injectable versions are apparently more effective). In one study involving 87 terminal-stage pancreatic cancers, 60 were still alive after one year even though the standard prognosis was for death to occur with 3–6 months. It is also claimed that HANSI allows patients to tolerate radiation much better. Promotional material for HANSI quotes a medical researcher, Darryl M See MD as saying: 'Over the past two years I have been involved in screening various herbs and homeopathic preparations for in vitro immune-stimulating effects. Among the 200 or so that I have tested, HANSI proved to be among the most effective in increasing natural killer cell function.'

HANSI sells for US$1,300 for a 90-day supply. Critics of HANSI question this cost and ask what raw materials they are using—in undetectable homeopathic quantities—that could possibly justify that price. For more information contact www.angelfire.com/in3/hansi or email: hansiargentina@hotmail.com.

Hoxsey formula

In 1840, a man by the name of John Hoxsey had a horse with a cancerous growth. Thinking there was nothing he could do he turned the horse loose on a pasture. Amazingly, the cancerous growth soon began to shrink and eventually it fell off. Hoxsey observed the horse and saw that it liked to go to a certain part of the pasture and graze on the plants in that place. If we accept that animals have an instinct for healing plants—and there is a great deal of evidence that they do—then there is nothing strange about this story. Hoxsey collected the plants in that area and experimented with them in various combinations. Eventually, he made a formula that was handed down from father to son until it reached Harry Hoxsey in 1919.

Hoxsey began opening cancer clinics around the USA. He had seventeen when the cancer establishment started to crack down. Morris Fishbein of the American Medical Association offered to take over the treatment. His deal was that Hoxsey would receive nothing for the first nine years and after that, he would receive ten per cent of the profits. Not surprisingly, Hoxsey said no. Fishbein then arranged through his powerful political connections to have Hoxsey arrested 125 times in 16 months. The charges all dealt with practicing medicine without a licence. The cases were all thrown out of court. But eventually, Hoxsey was forced to close down.

In 1963, his chief nurse opened the Bio-medical Center in Tijuana, Mexico, and Hoxsey's herbal treatment is still available there. The current formula includes the following:

Red clover (Trifolium pratense)
Burdock root (Arctium lappa)
Barberry bark (Berberis vulgaris)
Liquorice root (Glycyrrhiza glabra)
Buckthorn bark (Rhammus purshiana)
Prickly Ash (Zanthoxylum americana)

Chaparral (Larrea tridentate- a late addition to the formula)
Stillingia (Stillingia sylvatica)
Cascara amarga (Picramnia antiderma)
Potassium iodide

Patricia Spain, who did a study of the herbs for the US Congress Office of Technology as part of its assessment of alternative cancer therapies, wrote in her report: 'More recent literature leaves no doubt that Hoxsey's formula … does indeed contain many plant substances of marked therapeutic activity.'

While there are a number of formulas on the market, one that combines the main Hoxsey herbs with other herbs of known efficacy is marketed as Blood Support and is available at www.baselinenutritionals.com.

The Hulda Clark 'cure'

The Clark cure, put forward by Hulda Regehr Clark, is very radical. Indeed, if she is right, the entire cancer research industry can switch off its lights and go home. It is her view that cancer is caused by a parasite—the human intestinal fluke. This causes no major problems in the gut where it normally resides But by some means as yet unknown—but associated with the presence of propyl alcohol—it can move to other organs where it starts creating problems. The problem it creates, if it gets to the liver, is cancer. Her test for cancer is to test for the presence of the marker ortho-phospho-tyrosine (OPT).

'All cancer patients (100 per cent) have both propyl alcohol and the intestinal fluke in their livers. The solvent propyl alcohol is responsible for letting the fluke establish itself in the liver. In order to get cancer, you must have both the parasite and propyl alcohol in your body.'

Just as the cause is simple, so is the cure that she proposes: black walnut tincture, wormwood, and cloves. The first two kill adult and developmental stages of over 100 parasites. The cloves kill the eggs. They are to be taken as follows:

Black walnut tincture. This should be taken in a glass of water four times a day. Start the first day with one drop each time and increase the dose by one drop a day until on day 20 you are taking 20 drops in water four times a day. Then reduce to 20 drops once a day for three months—and then reduced to 30 drops once a day, two days a week. It should be taken on an empty stomach (viz., half an hour before a meal).

Wormwood. This herb is made from the leaves of the Artemisia shrub. It is also available from herbalists as part of a combination of herbs. It should be taken once a day before the evening meal increasing daily from one capsule to fourteen. Then maintain this level twice a week forever. As we have seen, studies have shown that wormwood on its own has demonstrated anti-tumour effects.

Cloves. Obtain whole cloves and grind them up. Cloves that have already been ground do not work. Fill capsules (preferably, size 00 but any vitamin capsules will do) with the ground cloves and take three times a day before meals building up from one capsule a time to three capsules a time. Continue until day ten and then reduce to three capsules once a day for three months—and then just twice a week forever.

Dr Hulda Clark was a Canadian physiologist (not a medical doctor) who published details of her cure with 100 case studies in her book: *The Cure for All Cancers*. She believed that many, if not most, ailments, from asthma and AIDS to heart disease and schizophrenia, are the result of parasitical infection, and the formula she gave above is one that she believed would rid the body of many of these. She accepted that other formulas will also work. But, in her view, the parasite is only half the problem, the other half is the propyl alcohol. Most people can process this effectively, and so it causes no problem whatsoever. But people developing cancer have an impaired ability to do this. For this, she blamed the presence in the liver of aflatoxin B. This is a known carcinogenic substance found in mouldy food.

One way to deal with the problem, she argued, is to eliminate propyl alcohol from the system. Unfortunately it is a common ingredient used in the food and cosmetics industries. Check the items in your bathroom and you will find most contain one of the following ingredients: propanol, isopropyl alcohol, isopropanol and so on. Even if not listed, she claimed that propyl alcohol is so commonly used for cleaning industrial equipment that it will very likely be present in minute quantities in a wide range of modern retail goods—but for those people with an impaired ability to break it down, even these quantities are sufficient to cause cancer. She particularly fingered hair and cosmetics products, sugar, carbonated soft drinks and even bottled water, fruit drinks, and vitamin supplements. She made an exception for vitamin C as this helps the liver to break down propyl alcohol by directly attacking the aflatoxin.

Her four-point plan for regaining health is simple but extreme: remove every unnatural chemical substance from your mouth, from your diet, from your body and from your home.

Before her death, ironically of cancer, Clark became very famous and was probably number one on the FDA's ten most wanted list. And there are grave doubts about her facts. Scientists point out that there is no evidence at all that the human intestinal fluke is present in epidemic quantities in the USA; quite the reverse. They dispute the validity of her test for the presence of cancer and point out that very few if any of her claimed cures are in any way validated independently.

However, a degree of support for a parasitic cause of cancer comes from parasitologist Dr Raphael D'Angelo who I will quote at length:

> *'Doctors believe that most people do not really have parasites. This is fostered by the large number of stool parasite tests that are reported negative by conventional labs. As a medical lab technician in my earlier years I can tell you that the responsibility to examine specimens for parasites under the microscope is relegated to a low time and effort priority given all the other testing that labs must accomplish in the course of a day. This is really unfortunate because parasites are present in most people when the specimens are prepared properly and adequate time is spent examining multiple microscope slides thoroughly.*

'This brings us to the connection between parasites and cancer. A true statement is that chronic inflammation is a seedbed for chronic degenerative diseases including cancers. In my work with cancer patients, I found that at a certain point in recovery, the healing process will plateau and not advance until we uncover the specific parasite problems and correct them.

'Parasites come in many forms. Some are actual worms such as tapeworms and roundworms. Others are flukes. Many are single celled protozoans. The fungi such as yeast and molds along with pathogenic bacteria and viruses are parasites. All fulfil the criteria that part or all of their life cycle requires the human host for protection, nutrition or reproduction.

'All parasites produce toxic waste. Some of them destroy our cells. Some invade our tissues. Some steal our food. Some do all of these things. As tissues become inflamed from such things happening, cancers can arise. One way to think of cancer is an attempted healing response gone awry.

'Gastrointestinal symptoms commonly found with parasites are flatulence, diarrhea, abdominal bloating, abdominal cramping, constipation, malabsorption, maldigestion, bloody or odorous stool, mucus and leaky gut. Systemic symptoms can be one or more of the following: fatigue, nervous/sensory disorders, pain, skin disorders, allergies, nausea, muscle weakness/pain, immune deficiencies, headache, fever, insomnia, night sweats and weight changes.

'Who needs a good parasite exam? The truthful answer is—we all do.'

My own view is that Clark definitely did not satisfactorily prove her case, but it may be that she is on to something—and as we have noted, wormwood has demonstrated anti-cancer activity. I would invoke the risk-benefit analysis and argue that since the herbal part of her cure is cheap and not harmful we can happily do this—but only as an add-on to a more substantially-supported therapeutic regime.

Imupros

This is a concentrated formulation of a number of herbs, vitamins, minerals and other substances. It is used in Holland and Germany as part of a general anti-prostate cancer protocol.

Prof. Ben Pfeifer, Director of Aeskulap Cancer Center, Switzerland has had great success in treating patients with prostate cancer with a combination therapy that includes Prostasol, MGN-3 (Biobran), curcumin complex (3g a day) and Imupros. He quotes a success rate of two-thirds of his patients showing clear beneficial responses—whatever that means.

Imupros is a combination of vitamin E (tocopherol succinate), vitamin C, cholecalciferol. epigallocatechin gallate (EGCG), calcium carbonate, selenium, genistein, lycopene and zinc.

302   Cancer: Herbs, Botanicals and Biological Therapies

Iscador

This therapy is closely associated with institutions associated with Rudolf Steiner's Anthroposophyl movement. It is well-known in Germany.

Iscador is the trade name for a number of preparations made with different types of mistletoe that grow on different kinds of tree and therefore exhibit different properties. These are further combined with homeopathic doses of such metals as silver, copper and mercury. Although condemned by the American Cancer Society, it is approved for use in Germany and Switzerland. The Lukas Clinic in Arlesheim, Switzerland is the major centre where this therapy is carried out.

However, any doctor can procure the capsules. Contact www.lukasklinik.ch.

The Iscador is given by subcutaneous injection at a site close to the tumour, starting with low doses and gradually increasing them until the patient reacts by showing a clear objective or subjective improvement in general health, the tumour slows down, or there is a fever reaction. This is seen as a good sign.

Does Iscador work? A lot of evidence suggests it does. One of its most obvious effects is that it increases the size of the thymus gland substantially by nearly 100 per cent in some animal studies and the thymus becomes much more active. This is a very significant finding. Iscador works both by attacking the cancer cells directly and by enhancing the immune system.

Not all cancers respond well to Iscador. Leukaemia, for example, does not. It works best with carcinomas and melanomas.

Although mistletoe is poisonous, Iscador is relatively non-toxic. It is suggested that it can accompany any other anti-cancer treatment, as no negative interactions with other medications have been reported. However, it should not be taken by people with heart problems, pregnant women and people taking a prescription drug containing a monoamineoxidase (MAO) inhibitor.

It is often combined with a vegetarian diet excluding mushrooms, tomatoes, new potatoes as well as sugar, hard fats and alcohol. In addition, patients following an anthroposophical regime are encouraged to engage in artistic activities including dance as well as having heat baths, oil baths and massage.

In addition to fighting cancer it has the effect of aiding sleep, providing pain relief and stimulating weight gain. Many patients report being reinvigorated. For further details go to www.iscador.com.

Jason Winter's tea

Sir Jason Winter was a Hollywood stunt man who claims to have cured himself of cancer. His tea contains red clover and green tea extract—both of which are known to be beneficial for cancer patients—plus a secret herbal ingredient—about which nothing sensible can be said. It is available from his website at www.sirjasonwinters.com.

PC-SPES, PC-HOPE and Prostasol

First a warning. The herbal combination PC-SPES was withdrawn suddenly from the market early in 2002. This product had been aimed at men with prostate cancer (hence the 'PC' bit in the name). However, scientists who were studying it discovered that it also contained small amounts of Xanax (a brand name anti-anxiety drug), DES (an artificial estrogens) and warfarin (rat poison—also used to thin the blood to prevent clotting). The herbal combination, to the extent that it was successful (and it seemed to have been), appears to have worked as a herbal hormone therapy—and warfarin is indeed regularly prescribed to men undergoing regular hormone therapy for prostate problems, as there is a danger of blood clotting as a side effect of the treatment. Other side effects of the orthodox hormone approach are breast development, impotence and loss of sex drive.

There are two warnings to be made in this context. The first warning is that herbal combinations may contain undeclared elements that you would rather not have. The only way of defending yourself against this possibility is to take only combinations recommended by sources of information that you trust (and of course trust can be established only over time). Internet forums are useful for getting a variety of viewpoints and experiences. The second warning is that, although the Internet is a wonderful resource, it needs to be approached with care. Information on the Internet is not dated. There are still many sites recommending PC-SPES as a worthwhile herbal combination, even though it has been taken off the market.

In fact, the company that took PC-SPES off the market have returned with a new product, PC-HOPE, which has the following declared ingredients: reishi (Ganodema lucidum), Baikal scullcap (Scutellaria baicalensis), rabdosia (Rabdosia rubescens hara), dyer's woad (Isatis indigotica fortune), mum (Dendranthema morifolium tzelev), saw palmetto (Serenoa repens), San-Qi ginseng (Panax notoginseng) , and liquorice (Glycyrrhiza glabra L.). These are the same ingredients that PC-SPES had, but there are, they now claim, no hidden extras.

A similar product, and according to the forums a cheaper one, is offered by Dr Kurt Donsbach. Called Prostasol (previously PC-Plus), it has the same ingredients (more or less).

There are many testimonials in the forums as to the effectiveness of both PC-HOPE and Prostasol in lowering PSA levels speedily and also inhibiting cancer.

Dr Donsbach admits that Prostasol is loaded with phytoestrogens which will cause breast sensitivity, but he says this can be treated with progesterone cream and curcumin. He makes no mention of other side effects, but it would be worth enquiring. For more information go to www.donsbach.com.

Zyflamend

Inflammation is associated with cancer development and is promoted by an enzyme-protein complex, cycloaxygenase-2 (COX-2). When COX-2 is inhibited, inflammation and pain are reduced.

Zyflamend is a herbal combination that has shown anti-inflammatory impacts (as a COX-2 inhibitor) and additional major anti-cancer effects against prostate cancer cells in the laboratory. In one study it reduced cancer cell proliferation by 78 per cent. It contains holy basil (a COX-2 inhibitor), turmeric (contains curcumin), ginger (inhibits both COX-2 and 5-LOX), green tea, rosemary, hu zhang (contains resveratrol), Chinese gold thread and barberry (COX-2 inhibitors), oregano (contains more than 30 known anti-inflammatory compounds), and scutellaria— also known as Baikal skullcap (a COX-2 inhibitor).

Zyflamend also inhibits activation of NF-$\varkappa$B–a transcription factor that is crucial for cell division and therefore incidentally a promoter of cancer. So this is also good news.

It is widely available from Internet suppliers.

Botanic Healing Systems

Ayurvedic medicine

Ayurvedic medicine is a 6,000 year-old system of medicine with a great pedigree and many formal institutional structures: medical schools, hospitals, research facilities and so on. The key difference between Ayurvedic approaches to health and the Western approach has been nicely summarised by Dr Ron Kennedy: 'The Ayurveda holds that we are thoughts which created bodies. In Western medicine we are material (body) which creates thoughts.'

The Ayurvedic doctor does not attempt simply to heal the body. He seeks to heal the whole person including the mental part of the person. And because thoughts manifest themselves in the biochemistry of the physical body, such therapies as meditation, yoga, energy medicine and emotional healing, can all have a place in the healing work that is done. One important aspect of Ayurvedic medicine is panchakarma, which seeks to achieve a deep cleansing of the physical tissues of the body.

Panchakarma

Panchakarma is essentially a detoxification process—and is central to Ayurvedic medicine. The first step in Panchakarma is the use of herbal oils—either internally or using massage—to initiate the purification process. The second step is to heat the body using specific steam and warm oil therapies. This therapeutic heat is intended to drive toxins out of the tissues into the intestinal tract. The third step is to eliminate the toxins that have accumulated. This is accomplished by the use of gentle herbal enemas, known as bastis, and gentle cleansing of the upper respiratory tract and sinuses, known as nasya. The Panchakarma treatments are administered over a period of several consecutive days (up to 14 days), and are said to have a profound detoxifying and deeply purifying effect.

There are a growing number of Ayurvedic resources on the Internet. A good website for Ayurvedic information is www.ayurvedacancercare.com.

Ayurvedic anti-cancer herbs

Triphala

Triphala is a herbal formulation consisting of three medicinal plants: Emblica officinalis, Terminalia chebula, and Terminalia belerica. It is healing for the liver, helps strengthen the immune system and is an anti-inflammatory and anti-oxidant. Side effects can involve intestinal gas and other gastric upsets. There is evidence in animal studies that it can cause apoptosis and works against the enzymes involved in cell wall degradation. This is important because the stronger cell walls are, the more difficult it is for cancer to spread. It also helps protect against radiation damage.

Ashwagandha

This herb is a popular Ayurvedic medicinal substance derived from the root and berry of the plant. It is an anti-inflammatory and is often used to treat arthritis. It has also shown anti-cancer effects and helps support the immune system. It is also a stress-relieving herb. Ashwagandha has shown itself to be effective against breast, central nervous system, colon and lung cancer cell lines. Pregnant women should avoid this herb as it may induce abortion (always a good sign of potential anti-cancer activity).

Carctol

Carctol is a combination of Indian herbs that was formulated by an Ayurvedic doctor, Dr Nandlal Tiwari of Jaipur. It is available on the Internet from www.anticancerherb.com. Another useful website is www.carctolhome.com. The product is reported to be completely non-toxic and has been tested in both India (Institute of Medical Sciences) and London. The British newspaper, *The Daily Telegraph*, covered the story of Gwen Garner, a woman who had both a primary bladder cancer and a secondary pancreatic cancer. Being told there was nothing more the doctors could do, she went on a course of Carctol. Within six months the pancreatic cancer growth had stopped; the original bladder cancer disappeared.

Carctol is supposedly excellent when used during radiotherapy and chemotherapy, preventing patients from becoming neutropenic (i.e., there is no compromise of white cells).

Carctol is a combination of the following herbs:

Blepharis edulis	200mg
Piper cubeba linn	20mg
Smilax china linn	80mg
Ammani vesicatoria	20mg
Hemidesmus indicus	20mg
Lepidium sativum linn	20mg
Rheumemodi wall	20mg
Tribulus terrestris	20mg

Anyone taking Carctol is recommended to maintain a vegetarian diet. At a minimum, patients are advised not to eat 'acid foods' like unripe fruits, tomatoes, vinegar or oranges. Carctol works best with a good digestive system.

Normally one capsule is taken four times per day, but a maximum of eight is not unusual. Pre-boiled and cooled water is recommended, not tap water.

The effect is supposed to be slow and steady and normally a six-month period is recommended.

Maharishi Amrit Kalash

This is a herbal formulation of 44 herbs developed within the Maharishi movement. It is promoted as a general energy and health support and users have claimed powerful benefits in these areas. It is also used to protect against the side effects of chemotherapy. One study found that it provided significant support and helped reduce weight loss, vomiting, fever and pain. There was also improved outcomes in terms of remission for the people taking MAK with their chemo, compared to those who received chemo alone.

TCM: traditional Chinese medicine and herbs

The Chinese view tumours as the 'uppermost branch' of the disease not its root. They consider cancer to be caused by a wide range of external or internal excesses (i.e., an excessive dose of a cancer-causing chemical or an excessive dose of bad emotions). All forms of excess result in the 'chi', the body's living energy, becoming blocked in some way. Some Chinese doctors prefer to treat cancer with herbs alone, while others try to mix Chinese herbs with Western chemotherapy and radiation. In fact, many doctors in China are looking at Chinese herbs in an entirely Western scientific way—looking at them for their anti-cancer effects. The traditional herbalist sees cancers simply as symptoms and uses herbs to bring the body into a state of healthy balance.

Fu-zhen therapy, an immune-enhancing herbal regimen, has had very good results when compared with just chemotherapy and radiation. In one study of 76 patients with stage II liver cancer, 46 were treated with Fu-zhen herbs in combination with chemotherapy and radiation. 29 survived one year and ten survived for three years. Only six of the thirty given chemotherapy and radiation alone, survived one year. In fact, there are reports of success from using the herbs alone.

The most commonly used Fu-zhen herbs are astragalus, ligustrum, ginseng, codonopsis, atractylodes, ganoderma, actinidia and rabdosia. Actinidia is a root that contains the polysaccharide ACPS-R. In one study, when injected into mice, 90 per cent of tumours stopped growing. Another study showed a 50 per cent success rate with liver cancers.

Doctors at the Beijing Institute for Cancer Research have found that a herbal tonic usually prescribed for kidney ailments, known variously as Golden Book Tea or Six Flavour Tea had a highly significant effect when combined with chemotherapy against small cell lung cancer (SCLC). It appears that all traditional kidney tonics may have these beneficial effects.

Other commonly-used Chinese herbs and herbal combinations:

Astragalus

This is a Chinese herb used mainly for patients with heart disease or high blood pressure. It has recently been shown to have a very strong normalising effect on people with damaged immune systems. It is therefore recommended not only as a cancer prevention/cure but also as a herbal support for people undergoing chemotherapy and radiation. Dose: 1–3 400 mg capsules per day.

Canelim capsules (Ping Xiao)

Canelim capsules are a herbal mix that appears to be particularly recommended for carcinoma cancers (oral, intestinal, kidney, prostate, uterine etc.)—though may be of more general benefit. They are sufficiently highly regarded in China to be listed as a Class A, anti-cancer medicine in the National Basic Insurance register in China. It is claimed to be highly effective in 'killing cancer cells, boosting immunity, inhibiting cancer growth and metastasis, alleviating clinical symptoms and pain, prolonging life expectancy and improving life quality.' In China it is often used as an adjunctive therapy to detox the body from the effects of radiation and chemotherapy, while at the same time enhancing the sensitivity of the cells to that treatment. However, it is also suggested as a standalone treatment. Effectiveness is quoted as being between 50–80 per cent but what 'effectiveness' means in this context is not clear.

The ingredients of the herbal mix are given as: Radix curcumae, Fructus aurantii, Herba agrimoniae, Alumen, Niter, Wu Ling Zhi, Resnia toxicodendri, Herba agrimoniae, Semen strychni pulveratum.

Interestingly, and this suggests that it may very well be an effective therapy, is the fact that it is often used before surgery to shrink tumours.

Capsules can be ordered from www.canelim.com and www.herbalbooth.com.

Dong Quai (Angelica sinensis) (also known as Tang Kuei)

This is a highly reputed blood tonic and has had successful results in treating cancer either alone or in combination with other herbs. Women have used it as a douche against cervical cancer.

Imusan

This is a rather expensive but widely used combination of Chinese herbs and mushrooms specifically designed to enhance the immune system. one capsule of Imusan (300mg) contains:

Pyrola rotundifolia (wintergreen)	30mg
Xian He Cao (Agrimonia pilosa)	24mg
Yan Hu Shuo (Corydalis yanhusuo)	24mg
Ganoderma Lucidum (reishi)	24mg
Shi Suan (Lycoris radiata)	24mg
Mou hui toui (Patrinia hetrophylia)	24mg
Di bu long (Stephania delavayi)	23.7mg
Hua jian jiu teng (Stephania sinica)	23.7mg
Rabdosia rubescens	21mg
Cheng-min chou (Cistance deserti cola)	19.5mg
Liang miau zhen (Zanthoxylum nitidum)	15mg
Ginseng	12mg
Pollen	12mg
Glycyrrhiza glabra	3mg

Kanglaite (KLT)

This has been clinically trailed with very positive outcomes. Mainly used as an adjuvant therapy, alongside chemotherapy and radiation, it nevertheless has cancer retarding and immune system enhancing properties. KLT was developed using an extract of the herb known as coix seed (Semen coicis) which is a cooling herb used for supporting the spleen in Chinese medicine. For more information go to www.kanglaite.com. For details of coix seed see: www.tcmtreatment.com.

This brief discussion of these few Chinese herbs does not exhaust the subject. There are certainly many other Chinese herbs that will be beneficial.

It should be noted that traditional Chinese herbalists have an attitude to the value of a herb that is totally opposite to the way Western doctors view drugs. For a Western doctor the best kind of drug is one that has a specific effect against a specific ailment. The more generalised a drug's effects, the less it is valued. In fact any drug that claims to be a cure-all will be automatically disregarded as being valueless. In Chinese herbalism the reverse is true. For them, the most inferior herb is the one that acts against a single specific problem. The most valued is the one that has a broad spectrum of effects. Since herbalists seek first and foremost to promote total health and so aid the healing of the individual, this makes sense.

The point can also be made here that most Chinese herb books do not list cancer as a disease that herbs can fight. Instead they list the herbs that are effective in strengthening the immune system. More specific agents may be listed as anti-viral agents.

Juzentaihoto

This is sometimes known as JT-48 or JTT. It is a blood-strengthening herb and is reportedly very effective in helping chemotherapy patients recover.

Jiaogulan (Gynostemma pentaphyllum)

This is another Chinese herb with a growing reputation and is apparently known as the herb of immortality. Like other herbs it has a wide range of beneficial actions including tumour suppression.

Oldenlandia

This is one of the oldest and most widely used Chinese herbs—also called Snake Needle Grass. It is used against fevers, viruses, swellings and toxic conditions. It helps the circulation and it is a major ingredient in most Chinese anti-cancer herbal mixes.

Scutellaria

There are two different herbs from the same family, both of which have anti-cancer effects:

Scutellaria baicalensis

This is a widely-used Chinese herbal medicine that has historically been used in anti-inflammatory and anticancer therapy. It is used synergistically with Oldenlandia.

Scutellaria barbata

This appears to have multiple anti-cancer effects, helping to induce apoptosis and boosting the immune system and so retarding tumour growth.

This latter herb may also be a helpful adjunct to other herbs that directly attack cancer cells in that it is a PARP inhibitor. PARP is the acronym name for a particular enzyme that helps cells repair themselves. Inhibit the enzyme and you inhibit the ability of a cell to repair itself.

Tian Xian

This herbal combination of 30 Chinese herbs is famous throughout China—to the extent that there are many fake versions on the market. It appears to be effective against cancer, as a support for those taking chemotherapy and as a pain reliever. It was formulated by Chinese herbalist Dr Wang Zhen Guo, who describes its action in this way: 'Tian Xian liquid removes body heat, is a toxin neutralizer, purifies blood, stops pain, supplements (energy), and regenerates blood.' It is available as a liquid, capsules and as suppositories.

Unfortunately it is also very expensive. For further details see www.tian-xian.com. For testimonials go to www.cancer-central.com.

Thunder God Vine (Tripterygium wilfordii hook)

The herb, thunder god vine (lei gong teng), is a Chinese herb generally used for inflammatory conditions such as rheumatoid arthritis. But researchers from Johns Hopkins School of Medicine have found that it can also stop tumour growth. Its active ingredient is triptolide. Researcher Jun Liu, professor of pharmacology and molecular sciences found that low doses of thunder god vine blocked cell growth in 60 different types of cancer, and even killed off some cancers in laboratory conditions. (Source: *Nature Chemical Biology*, 2011; 7: 182). There are a number of negative side effects associated with this herb ranging from gastric upsets to rashes.

Miscellaneous

Chris Teo's herbal centre

Chris Teo is a retired Professor of Botany and a dedicated Christian who has, in a very short time, built up a worldwide reputation for his herbal cures for cancer. He is not an orthodox Chinese herbalist, but this seems the best place to discuss his work. Living in Penang, Malaysia, he has not had the problems that many herbalists in the West. If he had attempted to do what he has done in the USA, he would have been pilloried as a quack and a charlatan.

'I am glad that I live in the East. Here, herbal medicine is part of our oriental heritage. So I am not treading on hostile ground when I talk about and practice herbal medicine. Of course there are doctors who are against me and label me a 'quack'. But there are many other doctors who agree with my work and even refer their patients to me.'

Teo has formulated close to a hundred herbal combinations for different purposes using herbs that he grows on his own farm or which he imports from China. Malaysia is, we should remember, one of the world's richest herbal terrains. With these herbs he has treated, with a great deal of success, many hundreds of people, many of whom were considered terminal. He has had a great deal of success—though he refuses to put this success in percentage terms—not just in making tumours disappear, but in helping people become well and free from pain. He has also formulated herbal regimens for people who are still undergoing radiation or chemotherapy. This is a low-cost service. He does not charge for his consultations only for the herbs.

If you think Malaysia is too far to go for a cancer cure, the writer Bernie Siegel has revealed an interesting fact. Life expectancy for cancer patients undergoing treatment is directly proportional to how far they have to travel, and by implication how much energy they have to put into it. In short, those who travel furthest for their cancer treatments live longest.

Chris Teo may also be a useful resource for people in Europe and the USA where new laws are coming into effect the effect of which will be to reduce access to many herbs. Those interested in getting hold of any hard-to-find herb might wish to contact Chris Teo in Penang www.cacare.com.

Sho-saiko-to

Kampo is the traditional herbal medicine system of Japan. Sho-saiko-to is a kampo herbal formula for the liver. There is growing interest in these herbal formulas and their potential for cancer patients. Most research has focused on its benefits as an adjuvant therapy with chemotherapy and radiation. Studies show clear survival benefits for those taking kampo herbal combinations such as Sho-saiko-to (the largest-selling of these preparations). However, given their proven benefits for the liver, many people are taking Sho-saiko-to as part of an overall herbal anti-cancer strategy irrespective of whether or not they are having chemo.

Sho-saiko-to's ingredients are: bupleurum root (Bupleurum chinense), pinellia tuber (Pinellia tuberifera), scutellaria root (Scutellaria baicalensis–also known as Baikal skullcap), jujube fruit (Zizyphus jujuba), ginseng root (Panax ginseng), liquorice root (Glycyrrhiza uralensis), and ginger root (Zingiber officinale).

Recommended dosage: 7.5g of the formula per day.

The Japanese government regulates preparation of these formulations very tightly, and their quality is considered to be very high. For more information go to www.honsousa.com.

The European herbal tradition

We should not forget that Europe also has a strong herbal tradition that is nurtured particularly in the Germanic countries. The following herbs are proposed as being good for cancer by Maria Treben, a renowned Austrian herbalist, and Dr Vogel, an internationally renowned Swiss herbalist.

Horsetail tea (Equisetum arvense)

This is one of the most ancient of cancer cures. The horsetail can also be used in the form of a poultice. Horsetail is rich in silica.

Calendula (pot marigold)

A fresh juice of all the plant—leaves stem and flower—should be drunk regularly.

Yarrow (milfoil—Achillea millefolium)

This is especially recommended for women.

Stinging nettles

The whole plant is used. It has a great reputation for blood cleansing. Pick in May and store for winter.

Butterbur (Petasites officinalis hybridus)

This is highly recommended both as a cancer treatment and as a pain reliever. This is the basis of Vogel's herbal product, petaforce.

None of these herbs has negative side effects, and they can be taken in large quantities.

Maria Treben recommends, as a general cancer treatment, a tea made with two litres of water, 300g of calendula, 100g yarrow, 100g stinging nettles.

For leukaemia she recommends a tea consisting of St John's Wort (15g), dandelion roots (15g), speedwell (20g), wormwood (20g), bedstraw (25g), yarrow (25g), goat's beard (25g), elder shoots (30g), calendula (30g), greater celandine (30g), stinging nettle (30g).

This mixture is mixed dry, and one heaped teaspoon is placed in a cup and boiling water is poured in and left for half a minute to two minutes (longer with dried herbs, shorter time with fresh herbs). Make one to two litres for a day and put in a thermos and sip. One cup is a quarter litre.

An American farmer promotes dandelion root

Dandelion root alone has some anecdotal support as a cancer cure. A farmer by the name of George Cairns is so convinced of its merits he took out a lengthy advert in the Chicago Northwest Times extolling its merits. According to him, he was on his death bed when the idea of taking dandelion came to him. He picked some fresh roots, took off the leaves and—without washing the soil off—he put the roots out to dry. He suggests putting them in an incubator, under a hot bulb or in the hot sun for 5–6 days or longer. When they can be easily crumbled, the bulbs should be pounded to a fine dust using a mortar and pestle. Half a teaspoon of the resulting powder should be dissolved in water and taken once a day. He attributes a number of cures to this—though admits that it does not appear to be beneficial for skin or brain cancers.

Soil, incidentally, has a long association with health. Eating pesticide-free soil is good for you. A few centuries ago, a sick farmer would get a sod of soil brought into him so that he could breathe in its healthy vapours. More recently scientists have discovered that a common soil bacteria, Mycobacterium vaccae, has an effect on us equal to some brand name anti-depressants. So get out into the garden and get your hands dirty. It's good for you.

Liver-strengthening herbs

Poor liver function is considered to be a clear precursor to cancer. It is therefore considered important by many herbalists to strengthen or maintain good liver health with such herbs as: milk thistle, artichoke, dandelion, burdock and rosemary.

Anti-inflammatory herbs

Dr Michael Cutler recommends the following herbs as having anti-inflammatory qualities. Remember, many of the therapies that appear to be effective against cancer also often cure arthritis and heart disease—probably because they work against inflammation. All three are inflammatory conditions.

Alfalfa, which provides essential minerals for bone development and can either be eaten as a raw plant or taken in capsule form.

Amur corktree is an herb sold under the name Nexrutine and has anti-inflammatory properties.

Boswellia extract can help control osteoarthritis and reduce inflammation.

Devil's claw root is a pain-reliever and anti-inflammatory, and is often found in herbal combinations for arthritis.

Ginger extract can help moderately reduce osteoarthritis pain according to some studies.

Korean angelica is an herbal agent that works on the central nervous system to help fight inflammatory pain throughout the body.

Stinging nettle leaf extracts help restrain the inflammation in autoimmune conditions like those found in rheumatoid arthritis.

Willow bark contains substances with powerful anti-inflammatory properties.

He also recommends the following non-herbal supplements.

Bromelain is an enzyme extracted from pineapples that reduces inflammation.

Capsicum is also known as cayenne pepper, chilli pepper and red pepper. It contains ample amounts of capsaicin, which causes the pungent and irritating effects. Applying this herb as an ointment or cream multiple times a day can provide you with real relief from joint pain.

SAMEe (S-adenosyl-methionine) is as effective as nonsteroidal anti-inflammatory drugs (NSAIDs) in increasing joint function and decreasing pain without the side effects.

Herbs for brain cancer

Brain cancers represent a particularly problematic group because the brain is protected by the blood-brain barrier so that not everything circulating in the blood gets into the brain. The following herbal recommendations were posted on a cancer forum as being particularly suited to the treatment of brain cancers: aloe arborescens, boswellia, hypericum, curcumin, rosemary (for the betulinic acid), garlic and melissa.

Another contributor had this experience: 'Essiac tea helped to dissolve my son's brain tumour, 20 per cent every two weeks'.

Yet another suggestion was this: 'Oleander is very effective against cancer as it passes the blood brain barrier.' You can get it in liquid form from www.sutherlandiaopc.com.

Other Botanic Systems

Aromatherapy

In France, aromatherapy is widely accepted as a clinically effective therapy for a wide range of chronic illnesses. French doctors often apply it as part of a total treatment plan. There are good reasons why aromatherapy might have a useful part to play in a health restoration strategy.

First, it is well established that a large number of oils have an immune system-enhancing effect—far too many to be listed here. A number of commercial aromatherapy websites have useful information resources (e.g., www.akobiaromas.com).

Secondly, a number of oils are believed to have a broad anti-carcinogenic effect. The following have been proposed by Robert Tisserand as possibly falling into this category: cedarwood, cypress, eucalyptus, hyssop, bergamot and geranium.

There is also evidence that lavender, niaouli or tee-tree oil smeared on the skin before radiation may help prevent burning and scarring of the skin. A bath in these oils before treatment may have beneficial effects internally (3–4 drops in a full bath).

Thirdly, there are those oils that are considered to be beneficial for the liver, rosemary being one. Since the liver has been implicated by many as the source of cancer, these oils may have a general preventative role to play. Rosemary herb has also been considered useful for cancer-protection.

No discussion of aromatherapy oils should ignore what in my house we call 'magic oil'—lavender oil. Before any kind of medical intervention, lavender oil should be rubbed on or bathed in (4–6 drops in a full bath). After any surgical treatment add lavender oil to the damaged tissue. It is famous for its healing effects when it comes to burns. If I cut myself I pour lavender oil on the cut knowing that the cut will heal quickly—within half an hour—and that there will not be any septicaemia. If I have difficulty sleeping I rub some lavender oil under my nose, and then I know I will soon fall asleep. In short, lavender is a great healer and relaxant. My rule is this: when in doubt use lavender. Lavender can be applied without risk directly to the skin.

Apart from their healing potential, there are the psychological benefits of aromatherapy baths and massages that help reduce stress and enhance psychological well-being.

Important warning

Many of these essential oils are highly potent and most should not be rubbed directly on the skin in their concentrated form (exceptions are lavender, tea tree, rosemary and peppermint). Putting a few drops in a bath is a very effective way of absorbing the oils—the skin is a highly absorbent organ. Do not exceed five drops of any oil—or 15 drops in total—in any bath.

Also, the quality of oils on the market varies widely. As with food there are organic and non-organic oils. It is important to ask for oils of therapeutic quality.

Flower therapy

It is part of common folklore that some people have green fingers. They appear to have a special intuition for plants, and that plants respond to their touch. 'All flowers talk to me, and I reply,' said the chemist George Washington Carver.

One person who had such an intuition was Edward Bach, a Welsh doctor who gave up his practice to develop a healing system based on flower essences. He extracted flower essences by steeping the flowers in spring water in the sunlight. The purpose of these flower essences is to direct our individual spiritual, emotional, mental and physical development in the direction of health. According to Dr Bach: '[Disease] is the means adopted by our own souls to point out to us our faults, to prevent our making greater errors, to hinder us from doing more harm, and to bring us back to the path of Truth and Light from which we should never have strayed.'

For Dr Bach, disease does not have a physical cause but, rather, it is the result of a spiritual disharmony within the person. It was his belief that each person has a spiritual dimension which is the soul. This soul is aware of the individual's life mission, which needs to be given expression in the physical, mental and emotional life of that person. But when a person deviates from the mission, or is blind, deaf and unfeeling to the promptings of the true mission, the result is disease. The worst of all the errors is when love is not freed, but is instead denied. All virtues without love become destructive. 'Righteousness without love makes us hard. Faith without love makes us fanatical. Power without love makes us brutal. Duty without love makes us peevish. Orderliness without love makes us petty.' says an anonymous commentator.

Disharmony results in various negative emotional states. By correcting these states, a state of harmony can be restored. The flower essences work, it is argued, by radiating harmonious energy at frequencies that help to correct distortions in the energy field of the patient. The idea has been developed in Australia and America so it is now possible to choose from a range of over 100 essences. Although I have listed this among the botanical therapies, it has perhaps more in common with the vibrational therapies that I discuss Section 7: *Cancer: Energy, Mind and Emotions*.

One way of choosing which flower essence to use is simply to sniff each of the 38 essences that Edward Bach found and to see which of them the mind and body respond to. Another way is to read the list of emotional states that they are good for dealing with. A number of different 'remedies' can be taken at the same time up to a maximum of six.

For emergencies of any kind, and particularly for anxiety attacks, a ready-mixed 'Rescue Remedy' is available. I once recommended this to a highly sceptical scientist who was having a panic attack. I asked him later if it had calmed in down. Yes, he admitted, but it could have been a placebo effect. Does it matter? I replied. If it was just a placebo, maybe he needed to take the Rescue Remedy to trigger it.

For the cancer patient who is self-denying, the following remedies may be useful: agrimony, centaury, chicory, red chestnut. For those who are overly strict and rigid: rock water. Violet gives feelings of placidity, gentian dissipates depression. For those feeling depression, desperation or despair any of the following may be helpful: larch, pine, elm, sweet chestnut, star of Bethlehem, willow, oak or crab apple. For those undergoing recovery from traumatic events: walnut and willow. Three to five drops are taken four times a day with or without water.

Flower remedies are widely available in health shops. There are ranges based on the flowers of America and Australia as well as the standard Bach Flower Remedies.

Miscellaneous

Kombucha (mogu)

The kombucha is a fungus that looks like a thick, pale yellow pancake. It has the ability to transform heavily-sugared tea into a health drink over a period of a week. Kombucha produces acids similar to those made by the liver. It binds with toxins in the colon and disposes of them through normal elimination. Kombucha discourages cancer and promotes good sleep, energy and helps protect against the side effects of radiation and chemo. This is not a new discovery. On the contrary, it has been used as a health support for thousands of years. Getting a kombucha should be easy, as kombucha divide every week. The length of time it takes to produce the tea is the same time it takes to split into two plates. It's almost the ultimate in natural pyramid schemes.

To make the tea, float the kombucha in a flat ceramic or glass dish and cover it with a any kind of heavily sugared tea you like (to flavour it). You can add ginger. Leave in a warm place and after 5–7 days pour off the drink and take a glass or two a day for the following week while you brew up another week's supply. For more information contact: The Kombucha Network at www.kombu.de/suche2.htm.

It is worth mentioning here that ginger has been shown to kill cancer cells in a laboratory study involving ovarian cancer cells. It killed them in two ways: by causing apoptosis (normal cell death) and also by inducing the cancer cells to eat themselves (known as autophagy). Regular drinks of ginger tea made with fresh or dried ginger could play a useful role as part of a varied anti-cancer regimen.

Anti-viral herbs

It is now believed by some virologists that as many as 40 per cent of all cancers may have a viral cause. The problem this poses for mainstream medicine is that they have very few effective anti-viral drugs. Antibiotics work against bacterial infections but have no effect on viruses. One broad spectrum anti-viral drug, DRACO, is being developed at MIT's Lincoln Labs but when it will become available is anyone's guess.

However, there are many herbs that are known to be effective against viruses, and cancer patients would be wise to include these on a regular basis as part of their overall recovery programme. There are several different ways of taking these herbs: capsule, tea, and essential oils (either in bath or in a carrier oil massaged into the skin).

The most favoured herbs are:

Lavender—have baths at night with lavender essential oil.
Echinacea—it is suggested that you take this herb on a six week on, six week off cycle.
Astragalus
Peppermint—if bathing with peppermint oil do so in the morning as it is a good waker-upper.
Olive leaf extract
Schizandra sinensis
Liquorice root
Mullein
Green tea
Goldenseal
Others include: elderberry, dragon's blood, juniper, lemon balm, oregano (use essential oil with care), tea-tree oil and eucalyptus oil

In addition you may also consider the following:

Garlic
Ginger: chop up a good-size section of raw ginger root and steep in hot water (possibly, as the Chinese do, add chopped garlic and spring onion). Drink throughout the day.

Antifungal herbs

Given that yeast and other fungal infections appear to coincide frequently with cancer—though whether they invade weakened systems after the cancer has appeared or whether they have a causative role is much disputed. Nevertheless, their presence has a negative impact on the immune system and so steps should be taken to eliminate them if this is possible. Note that healthy bacterial flora in the gut is essential for healthy digestion so, in addition to the herbs, you would be wise to include a good quality probiotic and a good source of digestive enzymes—these are particularly indicated for anyone who has undergone chemotherapy and/or radiation.

Here is a list of the most recommended antifungal herbs.

Black walnut (hull); **barberry**; **cajeput**; **calendula** (also commonly known as marigold); **Cassia alata** (not to be confused with Senna cassia); **cedar** (leaf, berry, wood)—cedar leaves act as an antifungal, antiviral, antiseptic, expectorant, and lymphatic cleanser; **chaparral**—best taken as a salve or ointment; **cinnamon** (bark); **cloves**; **fennel** (seed); **frankincense**; **garlic**—use it raw to get the medicinal effects. One suggestion is to let it steep in warm liquid coconut oil (coconut oil is also an effective anti-viral, anti-fungal food which is solid at room temperature); **geranium**—particularly known for its supportive qualities for pancreatic, adrenal and liver functions; **goldenseal**; **guajava**; **lavender**; **lemongrass**; **myrrh**; **neem**—best taken topically through the skin. This is considered very powerful in Ayurvedic medicine; **olive leaf extract**; **oregano**—make sure you dilute for applying to the skin, it's really strong; **pau d'arco**; **peppermint**; **pine**; **ravensara**—also apparently beneficial against viral hepatitis; **rosemary**; **sage**; **spilanthes**; **tea tree**; **turmeric**; **usnea**—should be diluted before taking internally or applying to the skin, as it's very potent.

Biological Therapies

Introduction

Our bodies have enormous powers of self-healing. The following therapies work by activating the body's own immune system.

Some of these need to be done, or certainly are best done, in a clinical setting, while others, such as homeopathy, can really be done only under the supervision of a trained and experienced professional. Some of these therapies will require you to make use of the services of an alternative clinic—in Mexico or Germany or elsewhere.

Here, then, are a number of therapies that have potential against cancer.

Coley's toxins

One highly successful method of curing cancer has remained more or less sidelined for over a century. In 1888, Dr William Coley discovered accidentally that a man had undergone what seemed like a spontaneous remission from cancer after suffering from a particular bacterial infection. Coley followed this lead and developed a number of toxins that he tested out on other patients, often successfully. His toxins were the by-products of two bacteria: Streptococcus pyogenes and Serratia marcescens.

The toxins cause a transient but marked fever accompanied by chills and tremblings. Thus, Coley's toxins is a form of fever therapy (see below). A survey of 1,000 of Coley's cases showed a 45–50 per cent five-year survival rate. The best results were with giant cell bone tumours where the five-year success rate was 80 per cent or more.

Amazingly, they were then put on the list of unproven treatments by the American Cancer Society, which, as we have seen, seeks to denigrate any non-drug-based therapy.

After decades in the wilderness, it seems Coley's toxins are once again being offered as a treatment by a number of clinics: www.sdiegoclinic.com, www.hufeland-klinik.de, CHIPSA.com, and Issels.com.

For instructions on how to make your own Coley's toxins go to www.second-opinions.co.uk/coleys_instructions.html.

Fever therapy

One doctor from ancient Greece said: 'Give me the power to produce fever and I'll cure all disease.'

Fever, of course, is not a disease itself but a sign. It is a symptom that the body is fighting off some disease. It is generally a very effective defence. Many invading bodies die when the body's temperature rises. Fevers should therefore be encouraged and not artificially cooled down. Fever therapy is simply the harnessing of this knowledge for the purposes of inducing high fever under clinical conditions. As we have seen, hyperthermia is a subject about which both alternative and orthodox doctors agree—fever is good for you.

An active fever can be induced by the injection of Coley's toxins, the drug Vaccincurin, or Pyrifer. A passive fever can be induced by placing the patient inside a cylinder and subjected to ultra-short waves. Modern medicine has developed other ways of interfering with the thermostats in the brain. They can even raise the temperature of selected portions of the body without affecting other parts. The object is to bring the patient to a state where his body temperature is 105–108° F (40.5–42.2° C) for 60–90 minutes. This is the temperature at which cancer cells, but not normal cells, are damaged. During this treatment the body loses potassium and so a potassium-rich diet must be maintained: lots of bananas, rice and potatoes. Healthy cells are not damaged until temperatures rise to 109.5° F (43° C). Sometimes heat can be applied to a solid tumour through a heat probe placed inside the tumour.

This therapy can even be done at home. The patient can sit in a very hot bath and then lie in bed surrounded by blankets and hot water bottles for five or six hours at a time. Go to www.curezone.com/ Schulze/handbook/hyperthermia.asp for a detailed description of this process.

Passive fever treatments are usually done three times a week for as long as it takes. Fever can even be produced by hypnotic suggestion. Alternatively, one might stand with an onion under each armpit in the hot sun, as one early doctor instructed his patients.

Since fever is the body's mechanism for fighting off disease, it directly promotes the body's own defence mechanisms. Detoxifying enzymes and white blood cells are released into the system in higher concentrations.

Some doctors use this therapy in conjunction with chemotherapy—allowing them to lower doses by a third or a half.

It is not only cancer that responds to fever treatments. One doctor is supposed to have cured two epileptics by having them stand barely dressed for an hour in mid-winter. They were then put into a hot bed to let them sweat it out. Syphilis was also cured by fever therapy before the discovery of penicillin. The means by which the cure was effected was to infect the syphilitic patient with malaria. The result? Regular and persistent fevers that took the body's temperature to 104° F or 105° F degrees for the necessary duration. Then the malaria could be cured with quinine. For this line of reasoning Professor Julius Wagner von Jauregg won the Nobel Prize in 1927.

Kriotherapy

In juxtaposition with fever therapy, and sometimes called 'cold room therapy', is kriotherapy (spelt with a 'k' to distinguish it from the more orthodox treatment, cryotherapy, which is used to treat a number of surface cancers). It is a treatment developed in Japan (late 1970s) and in Eastern Europe (early 1980s). It consists of standing in a very cold room (temperatures are minus 110–135°C) for three minutes wearing nothing but a swimming costume (warning: do not wear contact lenses!). The impact of the cold reduces blood flow briefly but then, when you come out of the room, the blood that has been hyper-oxygenated by the lungs and heart is released. Subjecting the body to such extreme temperatures stimulates the blood circulation system, endocrine system, the immune system and the central nervous system.

Several sessions are recommended over a few days. This is a treatment for which great benefits are claimed for depression, fatigue, arthritis, back pain, asthma and sporting injuries. It is also promoted as a fat loss therapy. However, this therapy is not recommended for people with high blood pressure.

For cancer patients the potential benefits in terms of enhanced immune response, and the improvements it offers in terms of energy and mood, make this an interesting, not too expensive therapy.

It is available for £50 per session at Champneys spa centre in Tring (www.champneys.com) and at the Kriotherapy Centre in Battersea, London (www.kriotherapy.com) . It is also offered at a number of spas in the Czech and Slovak Republics as well as in Latvia and Estonia. I have been unable to find any kriotherapy treatment rooms in the States but surely they will soon become more widely available.

Individual treatment equipment is available—called cryosaunas—but the temperatures they can achieve at present are not as low as the 'cold rooms'.

Homeopathy

Everyone's Guide to Cancer Treatment, 1994 edition, says this of homeopathy: 'Around 1850 homeopathy became popular. This was based on its Law of Similia, which states that disease results from suppressed itch ('psora'). Over 3,000 drugs, each a highly distilled organic or inorganic substance, were used for cures.'

This rather bizarre description does three things very effectively. It says first of all that this is a weird and wonderful delusionary system of treatment; secondly, it gives the distinct impression that it is based on some arcane and difficult system of belief, and thirdly the use of the past tense strongly suggests that it no longer exists.

All of this is rather unfair to practising homeopaths because homeopathy as a system of treatment is alive and well.

Suspicion of homeopathy runs very deep among the orthodox scientific and medical communities. In 1986, the British Medical Association published a report entitled *Alternative Therapy*. In this report, the authors stated their commitment to scientific method in these words: 'scientific method lays … emphasis on observation, measurement and reproducibility'. They then went on to say: 'It is simply not possible, for example, for orthodox scientists to accept that a medicine so dilute that it may contain not so much as one molecule of the remedy in a given dose can have any pharmacological action.'

We can note here that the kind of medicine being described is homeopathy and that it is being rejected not on the scientific grounds of observation, measurement or reproducibility but on the ideological grounds that they can't understand it—indeed they go on to state that homeopathy is not 'consistent with natural laws as we now understand them'. There is no suggestion that the problem may be with their understanding of natural laws.

A proper scientific approach based on observation, measurement and reproducibility would approach the question differently. In my view, a true scientist would say: 'I don't understand how this works but let's observe and measure and see whether it does in fact have reproducible results.' In 1997, *The Lancet* published the results of a meta-analysis of 186 well-controlled studies into homeopathy and the results appeared to demonstrate that homeopathy was significantly more effective than a placebo response. However, alongside the study were two commentaries that criticized the results on the grounds that it conflicted with our understanding of reality. As one writer noted: '… to put it starkly, there is no place in our current scientific theories for any possible mechanism by which homeopathy might work.' (Dylan Evans, *Placebo*, p.149)—and yet, according to *What Doctors Don't Tell Us* (newsletter 25 May 2006), 'In the past 24 years there have been 180 controlled, and 118 randomized, trials into homeopathy, which were analyzed by four separate meta-analyses. In each case, the researchers concluded that the benefits of homeopathy went far beyond that which could be explained purely by the placebo effect.'

But homeopathy does in fact have a very clear theory—one that is also shared in certain circumstances by orthodox medicine—and one for which there is scientific support.

Homeopathy was developed by Samuel Hahnemann as a result of his studies into the effects of quinine. Hahnemann discovered that quinine, in a normally healthy person, creates the same symptoms as malaria. Since it was also a very effective cure for malaria, Hahnemann came to the view that symptoms did not arise from the disease—instead they arose from the body's attempts to fight the disease. So, by exaggerating the symptoms, the disease can be more successfully fought off. Applied to other areas this perception has interesting corollaries. A cough should not be suppressed, rather it should be encouraged. After all the cough arises because the body is seeking to expel something. We should help it, otherwise whatever is causing the irritation will remain in the body. Similarly, a fever should be promoted rather than cooled, the heat of the body is fighting the infection so we should encourage it to stay hot and so help it defeat the infection sooner. This is a perfectly legitimate—and indeed commonly accepted—point of view even among some orthodox doctors.

So, Hahnemann followed this logic through to its inevitable conclusion and suggested that we should use drugs that promote the same symptoms as the disease—this is the real explanation of his Law of Similars. This is a perfectly simple and reasonable theory and it goes against no laws of nature. Hahnemann made the following observation, 'Most medicines have more than one action: the first a direct action, which gradually changes into the second (which I call indirect secondary action). The latter is generally a state exactly the opposite of the former.'

We have discovered this effect in chemotherapy. It is the effect known as resistance. A drug attacks the flawed action of the body (i.e., the disease that is embedded in the cells of the body). The cells have a natural tendency to resist this action so they amplify the original effect. Eventually the drug's effects are neutralized. The doctor sees the drug no longer has an effect and withdraws it and the result is that the problem is much worse. Sometimes of course the drug is able to so overcome the cells' flawed action so that a cure is effected. The problem is in those cases where the drug is not effective. Its effects ultimately are to worsen the problem. Hahnemann therefore had the idea of reversing the process. If you reverse the action by amplifying the effect, the cells will resist this by diminishing the cause—and so working towards a cure. When the drug is removed the cells are working in the direction of health.

What causes problems for most people, however, is Hahnemann's discovery that dilute doses of drugs work better than strong doses. Now there is nothing in homeopathic theory that predicts this effect. It is the result of an observation. Why it is true is not truly known.

Hahnemann, because of his suspiciousness of drugs, wished to use very dilute forms of drugs. He wished to interfere with the body's own healing power as little as possible. It therefore made sense to experiment and see how far he could dilute the drugs before they lost effectiveness. To his surprise, even though he diluted them to a level where, theoretically, they should contain not even one molecule of the original substance—a point known as Avogadro's limit—they were still effective.

Even Hahnemann had no explanation for it except to say it was a spiritual principle. Yet, there is interesting evidence that supports Hahnemann's observation. Researchers using nuclear magnetic resonance techniques can distinguish between homeopathic dilutions and pure water. Other researchers have shown that homeopathic dilutions rotate light passed through it in a different way than pure water. But these experimental results are still contentious.

But can homeopathy help in the fight against cancer? Enid Segall, Secretary-General of the British Homeopathic Association, argues that it has.

'Homeopathy is very supportive to patients with cancer …. Certainly, there are people I talk to regularly who have been cured of cancer with the help of homeopathy ….'

Homeopathy is a whole-person approach to treatment. It deals with the disease process rather than the disease product. This distinction remains, as we have seen, the great dividing line between alternative/complementary approaches and the orthodox approach. Homeopaths ask how it is the cancer formed and what in the body's physical ecology is supporting the cancer's growth. In this, they are in agreement with naturopaths and, indeed, with almost every other practitioner of non-orthodox healing. This approach to cancer is largely ignored by the orthodox medical profession who are almost entirely focused on elimination of the disease product, in this case the tumour, but have little interest in why the tumour developed in the first place.

Most homeopaths recognise that removal of the end product—the cancerous tumour—may be a useful adjunct to their treatment. However, toxic chemotherapy is not one of the forms of treatment that they approve of.

Homeopathic treatment is generally proposed as an adjuvant therapy (i.e., one that supports other, preferably natural, therapies). Indeed, homeopaths are very cautious about their role in cancer treatment. There seems to be some resistance to the idea that homeopathy alone would be effective in curing cancer, although they would not deny it was possible. But this generally defensive attitude to homeopathy is a modern phenomenon. One hundred years ago, J Compton Burnett MD wrote a short book entitled *Curability of Tumours by Medicines*. Here he gives a number of examples of cancer cases that he cured entirely by homeopathic means.

Here is one case of breast cancer he describes successfully treating.

'(Jessie S) came on May 24th 1888 and informed me that two years previously a lump came in her left breast, which lump persists in growing, and pains. In the left mamma there was a tumour in its outer lower fourth, about the size of a lady's fist …. In three months, … the tumour was gone and thus far has not returned. Thuja 30, Acid nit. 30 and Sabina 30 were used in infrequent dose, and each given during one month by itself alone and in order named …. I ought to have added to the foregoing narrative that I forbade salt and milk, other than in very moderate quantities and recommended a partial exclusion of meat from the patient's dietary as also the ovary irritating condiment known as pepper. Pepper, salt and milk are bad in cases of mammary tumours from ovarian or uterine irritation, and many of these tumours are of such origin.'

Salt and milk have been widely implicated as nutritional no-nos, but pepper? Modern science comes to Dr Compton Burnett's support. In 1980, researchers found that mice exposed to black pepper developed significantly more tumours—mainly liver, lung and skin. 77 per cent of the pepper treated mice developed tumours compared with only 11 per cent of the controls.

Here is another case quoted by Dr Compton Burnett.

'On November 17th, 1887, I was requested to see a gentleman resident in London who was said to have a very large tumour in the abdomen and no efforts to cure it had been spared …. There seemed no chance of a cure and an operation had been declared to be impossible … the final outcome of all the deliberations was that it was cancer, or at any rate a tumour connected with the spleen which was or had become malignant in its nature, and that the result must necessarily be fatal …. I think any practical physician or surgeon will concede that a more hopeless case to cure by medicines is hardly to be found ….

'My own plan in difficult cases that seem so hopeless is to lay firmly hold of some point that may serve as a reasonable therapeutic starting point whence to carry out a cure. As a start there is here the traumatic element in the case that is positive, and my own favourite and well-tried anti-traumatic is Bellis perrenis …. Bellis perrenis as an anti-traumatic and also Ceanothus americanus as splenic, presented themselves to my mind, but which? Candidly confess, I thought the good man doomed but determined to try and save him, and not knowing which of my two remedies was the more likely to do something quickly, (for the case was urgent—patient's friends had already taken a last look at him as they thought) I gave the two in alternation, and much did I subsequently regret this double shot, for the use of two medicines at one time teaches next to nothing. Bellis o and Caenothus 1X were given in five drop doses every four hours in alternation …. The result of this medication was that after a while the patient could turn over in bed, then he could get in and out of bed by himself and in 17 days from beginning the medicine … [the] patient came to my West End rooms in a cab with his wife. [Dr Burnett then describes various changes in the case and changes of medication.] He did not need any subsequent treatment and he came to say goodbye on June 24th 1888. He had lost the tumour and the enlargement and induration of the lymphatic in the left side, and he was rapidly gaining flesh and strength …. The cure was complete and *permanent, which I know, patient turns up in my rooms every three months for his own and my satisfaction. Such a case is an oasis in the desert of a physician's hard life.'*

These anecdotal cases are quite sufficient to establish a sensible claim that homeopathy on its own can be effective in treating tumours, even at a very late stage in development.

But Burnett agrees that it is vital for the homeopathic doctor treating cases of cancer to have the full range of orthodox medical training to help the diagnosis of the ailments.

We don't, of course, know how many cancer cases Burnett failed to cure but he certainly felt that his success rate was better than anyone else's—and certainly justified greater attention being given to this medicinal approach to cancer treatment.

Laurie Monteleone, a contemporary American homeopath, explains that there are three approaches that a modern day homeopath might take when treating a cancer patient. The first is to target the tumour by selecting remedies that match the symptom picture of the tumour and these remedies may even be injected at the site of the tumour. Another approach the homeopath might take is to use remedies that improve the effectiveness of the channels of elimination: kidneys, lymph, etc., so helping to detoxify the body. Finally, there is the classical approach, which is to consider the whole constitution of the patient and prescribe remedies that strengthen the patient's mental, emotional, and physical state so allowing self-healing to occur.

One anti-cancer therapy that we may soon be hearing a lot more of is the use of homeopathic nosodes. A nosode, here, is a remedy created directly from diseased tissue—which is then diluted in the same way that other homeopathic remedies are. (Homeopathic nosodes have been prepared against nearly every epidemic and endemic disease on the planet. (So forget the flu shot and get a flu nosode.) In the case of cancer, the nosodes are made from the blood of cancer patients who have recovered from cancer or who are in a state of remission. This blood is assumed to contain as yet unidentified immune substances whose healing power can be transmitted to other cancer patients.

The best known example of a cancer-fighting homeopathic nosode is Carcinosin, created from breast cancer tissue. However, while it has clearly demonstrated to have anti-cancer activity in animal studies, it has not been as effective as had been hoped as a stand-alone cancer cure. That does not mean, however, that it is not a useful weapon to be used along with other anti-cancer therapies.

More recently a new nosode, considered to be more potent than Carcinosin, is CarcinPLUS™. This was made from the blood of a woman who had cured herself of cancer using only natural supplements and spiritual healing. (The supplements she used to cure herself were: proteolytic enzymes—pancreatin 56,000USP-units/300mg, papain 492FIP-unit/180mg, bromelain 675FIP-unit/135mg, trypsin 2,160FIP-unit/72mg, chymotrypsin 900FIP-unit/3mg, rutosid 3H2O(Rutin) 150mg; quercetin 134mg; turmeric 800mg; coenzyme Q-10 300mg; folic acid 800mg as L-5 methyl-tetrahydrofolate and omega 3 fatty acids 1.5g EPA/DHA.)

CarcinPLUS™ is available only by prescription. For more information go to www.homeopathyworks.com and www.phisinc.com.

For anyone interested in reading more about homeopathy, Dale Moss's article in the *Townsend Letter for Doctors and Patients*, June 2004 is worth reading (www.tldp.com).

Moss describes the work of Dr Ramakrishnan, born into a family of homeopathic practitioners who nevertheless had to watch two siblings die of cancer as neither responded to any of the homeopathic treatments they were given.

Dr Ramakrishnan dedicated his life to developing a homeopathic cure for cancer. He described his work in his book that he co-wrote with Catherine Coulter, *A Homoeopathic Approach to Cancer*.

Ramakrishnan's first breakthrough was to abandon the classical approach. As Moss notes, 'Classical homeopaths are taught that continued repetition of a single remedy, particularly at high potency, is unwise, because too frequent dosing might worsen symptoms being treated or induce undesirable new ones characteristic of the remedy.'

However, Dr Ramakrishnan took a very different approach, treating cancer as an acute emergency rather than a chronic disease. He chose therefore to give high potency remedies on a daily basis in multiple doses. An aggressive approach to an aggressive disease. Further, he gave his patients daily doses of one remedy for a week and then a second remedy for the following week. The first would be an organ specific remedy and the second a nosode such as Carcinosin. Using what he called his 'plussing method', he dissolved three pellets of each remedy in two small bottles each containing 11 teaspoons of distilled or spring water. The patient takes a teaspoonful of the solution every 15 minutes ten times a day over a two-hour 15-minute period. Between doses, he shakes or stirs the solution slightly. At the end of the day's dosing, one spoonful of solution remains, which becomes the basis of the next day's dose after the patient refills the bottle with water. This process goes on for one week. The next week, the patient switches to the second bottle. This therapy must be followed for eighteen months or two years until the patient is stable and cancer-free.

Does it work? Dr Ramakrishnan claims a cure rate for lung cancer of 58 per cent; for oral cavity cancer, 90 per cent; for breast cancer (and prostate cancer), 80 per cent; ovarian cancer, 69 per cent; and cervical cancer, 68 per cent. For leukaemia and Hodgkin's lymphoma, his claimed cure rates are 54 per cent and 77 per cent, and for brain lesions his cure rate is 70 per cent. These are extraordinary figures compared with what orthodox doctors achieve. Sceptics, however, have queried the reliability of these figures.

Dr Ramakrishnan practices primarily in India, where homeopathy is widely available and respected, so patients will generally seek his treatment in the first place rather than when all else has failed. As Moss says: 'Having an intact immune system greatly improves chances of successful treatment.'

Dr Ramakrishnan reports: 'I now know which cases will do well and which will not. If I take a case at Stage II, I can be pretty sure of curing it. If the patient is at Stage I and the tumour is removed, then the patient follows with homeopathic treatment, he should do well for a long time, with no shocks or surprises in the case.' Cancers at stages III and IV are more difficult to cure but Dr Ramakrishnan has cured many seemingly hopelessly advanced malignancies.

Finally, Dr Prasanta Bannerji, a homeopathic doctor who works in Calcutta, has found the combination of two widely-available homeopathic remedies have the ability to reverse glioma, a brain cancer, and is probably beneficial for many other cancers. This was demonstrated in a study led by Professor S Pathak, Department of Molecular Genetics, at MD Anderson Cancer Center. In the abstract of results he states: 'Fifteen patients diagnosed with intracranial tumours were treated with

Ruta 6 and Ca3(PO4)2. Of these 15 patients, six of the seven glioma patients showed complete regression of tumours.'

This is the protocol they used:

- Ruta 6c, in pills No.40, two pills a dose, two doses daily, morning and evening.
- Calcarea Phos 3X, in tablets, two tablets a dose, two doses daily, noon and night.

The pills/tablets can be taken on tongue just suck it or chew it. If Ruta 6c liquid is taken one dose = two drops in a spoonful of water.

For further information contact Dr Prasanta Banerji at PBH Research Foundation, 10/3/1 Elgin Road, Calcutta—700 020, India, Tel: +91 33 22472845, Fax: +91 33 22477275 pbhrf@vsnl.com.

This is a protocol that appears to be remarkably powerful. To keep abreast of discussions on this subject you can go to http://health.groups.yahoo.com/group/Ruta6.

Ruta 6 and Cal Phos can be obtained from any online homeopathic store. One easy to use site is www.abchomeopathy.com—the forums are particularly interesting and many other homeopathic combinations are discussed.

Live cell therapy

In the 1930s, a Swiss doctor, Paul Niehans, discovered that it was possible to cure people suffering from a number of conditions using intra-muscular injections containing a saline solution with a suspension of glandular cells. He became famous for offering this treatment as a rejuvenating therapy to film stars and others who could afford it.

One of his associates, Dr Wolfram W Kuhnau, adapted the technique and brought it to Mexico, where it is offered by the Centre for Holistic Life Extension, www.extendlife.com. Kuhnau has since died but his work is being carried on by Dr Luis Velazquez.

In this therapy, the foetal cells of the blue shark are injected into the cancer patient. The idea is that the stem cells will detect which area of the body is depleted of healthy cells and will work to replace them. There appears to be little danger in the procedure, which is not a standalone cancer cure. Certainly, cellular rejuvenation by means of live cell therapy has long established itself as a viable therapy.

However, anyone undergoing such treatments should be aware that German studies have linked the therapy with a number of fatal or otherwise serious allergic reactions. Dr Kuhnau, however, insisted that his therapy was totally safe—and no evidence to the contrary has come to light. Cancer patients receive only three injections, once a week, then two others at three months and six months. Dr Kuhnau is reported to have treated over 20,000 patients with this therapy over 40 years without any toxic effects greater than some fatigue.

One word of caution: it seems that the biggest therapy scams relate to rejuvenation, weight loss and other cosmetic issues. This is an area where the buyer needs to be particularly aware. A number of websites offer 'cellular therapy' or something similar in pill form. These are unlikely to be effective in themselves and are certainly not likely to be effective in relation to cancer.

Oxygen therapy

'Remember, where cells get enough oxygen, cancer will not, cannot occur.' Otto Warburg, 1966

We have already discussed the relevance of oxygen in relation to cancer. Cancers often, if not always, are generated by tissue conditions of low oxygenation. Also they tend to thrive in these conditions. Consequently, it has been proposed that cancer tumours can be effectively prevented and treated by increasing the oxygen levels of the blood and tissues.

The problem is exacerbated by poor food, poor eating practices—fast eating, overeating—lack of exercise, bad breathing techniques, rigid postures (caused by muscular tightness which in turn is the result of stress)—all of which worsen the problem. It is argued that good mental attitudes and meditation work partly because they lead to more relaxed and deeper breathing. The result is that the oxygen content of ill people is very much less than that of well people.

A number of ways of achieving higher oxygen levels in the body have been used—apparently with the sort of success that validates the theory.

Haematogenic oxidation therapy (HOT)

Also known as ultraviolet blood irradiation (UVBI), This is one option for getting higher doses of oxygen into the bloodstream. It is a simple and painless method of treatment. A quantity of blood, 100–200ml, is taken from the patient and oxygen is then bubbled through it. The blood is then irradiated with ultraviolet rays for five to ten minutes then left to settle for an hour before being returned to the patient by drip. This is a form of ozone therapy. According to Issels, who used this therapy,

'[The blood] is: sterilized, normalized, regenerated and reactivated. Defense cells regain their aggressive capacity. Returned to the host, these cells can once more attack microbes and cancer-promoting viruses which are characterised by an anaerobic metabolism—making them unable to survive in the actively oxidised environment that HOT creates.'

This treatment is generally done on a weekly basis for two to three months or for as long as it takes to achieve the desired result.

A similar treatment, called recirculatory haemo perfusion, is available in Malaysia. See www.ozonehospital.com.

Ozone is a very powerful form of sterilising and cleansing agent. The tap water in most continental European towns and cities is ozonated rather than chlorinated. Most German public swimming pools are also ozonated rather than chlorinated. Ozone is a strong anti-carcinogen while chlorine can under certain circumstances promote cancer. Ozone is a far more powerful agent than oxygen probably because it is highly unstable and releases a lot of energy as it transforms into ordinary oxygen molecules. In 1980, *Science* reported a study into the effects of ozonated air on cancer cells. The growth of the cancer cells was inhibited by 90 per cent. Ozone has also been implicated in dramatic success stories against AIDS.

Ozone can be injected directly into the muscle, or it can be taken in simply by drinking ozonated water. Some patients have an ozone shower. This involves wrapping themselves naked in a plastic bag or jump suit and blowing in ozone from an ozone generator. It is also common to have humidified ozone applied either vaginally or through the rectum in short 30 second to one minute bursts. This allows a very rich ozone concentration to be absorbed by the blood in a painless non-invasive way.

While, in America, ozone is labelled by the FDA as a toxic gas, in Germany, ozone therapy is very common. Is it dangerous? According to author Ed McCabe, in one year, 644 German therapists reported using ozone therapy on 384,775 patients, a total of 5.5 million ozone treatments, and the incidence of negative side effects was 0.0007 per cent.

Some people have claimed tumour-suppressing effects from simply drinking ozonated water. An ozonating machine costs about $175–$300 or more. There are a number of models on the market. It is a simple matter to pass ozone through water for a few minutes immediately before drinking it. A very useful site giving the whole ozone story is www.geocities.com/ojoronen/OZ.htm.

Hydrogen peroxide

Another form of hyper-oxygenation therapy is through the use of hydrogen peroxide. Intravenous H_2O_2 was first used during the 1918 influenza outbreak. It then became widely used for a wide variety of viral and bacterial illnesses, with good results. In fact it was the preferred form of treatment until antibiotics arrived on the scene. The body itself manufactures hydrogen peroxide as a first line of defence against toxins and other invaders.

Hydrogen peroxide can be taken in many ways. Doctors prefer to give it in the form of an intravenous drip, and this is probably the best way when chronic illness is being treated. However, it can be taken at home in other ways. But it is important to note that hydrogen peroxide, in strengths greater than three per cent, is dangerous. It can normally be bought in strengths of three per cent or six per cent from any chemist shop. Food grade hydrogen peroxide is 35 per cent. This is the purest form and many advocates of hydrogen peroxide therapy urge users to use food grade H_2O_2 for internal use. But it must be diluted! Undiluted H_2O_2 is extremely dangerous. A drop of food grade H_2O_2 on the skin will cause a white burn mark. Warning: anyone with children should not have it around the house!

Hydrogen peroxide can be taken orally, it can be added to a bath, it can be rubbed on the skin or it can be gargled as a mouthwash.

Suggested quantities are as follows, for oral use (either for drinking or mouthwash):

- **35 per cent food grade**: increasing daily from one drop to 25 drops in a glass of water. However, it appears that not many people can tolerate 25 drops in a glass of water.
- **6 per cent solution**: half a teaspoon to two teaspoons in an eight-ounce glass of water (5–10ml H_2O_2 in 0.22l water).
- **3 per cent solution**: should be mixed one part to five parts of water and then drunk slowly increasing from one to five ounces a day. This regimen can be increased to 5oz (142ml) three times a day for a week at a time. This all depends on whether it is being taken for

curative or maintenance reasons. A maintenance programme of 5oz a day, two days a week, is recommended.

It should be noted that not everyone agrees that it should be taken orally. There are arguments about its effects on stomach acidity and bacteria. There is also the question of whether it can be properly absorbed into the bloodstream in this way or whether it is broken down to oxygen and water in the stomach.

Everyone says that hydrogen peroxide should not be persisted with if it is uncomfortable.

Dr Donsbach of the Hospital Santa Monica argues that a preferable way of getting the peroxide effect without the discomfort is to take the same quantity of magnesium peroxide (magnesium dioxide) instead.

H_2O_2 should be taken on an empty stomach and at least an hour should separate its use and intake of vitamin C as they negate each other.

For use in baths: half a cup of food grade 35 per cent or a pint (0.6l) of three per cent can be added to half a bath of water. Soak for twenty minutes and it is claimed you will feel rejuvenated. To give an indication of how powerful the skin is as an absorbing organ, a 200 pound (91kg) person can absorb up to four pounds (1.8kg) of water from a twenty-minute soak in a bath.

Counter-indications: hydrogen peroxide should not be taken by anyone who has had a transplanted organ. Rejection of the organ may result.

There are also a number of fairly inexpensive oxygen-enhancing products on the market—the following two products combine dissolved oxygen, trace elements and other ingredients: Cellfood and Oxygen Elements Plus. Both of these are available on the Internet and come with many testimonials as to their benefits. They combine two approaches—increasing oxygen levels of the body's tissue and the provision of trace minerals—both of which appear to be highly beneficial for people with cancer.

Pharmaceutical drugs and oxygen

Synta Pharmaceuticals Corp. is currently researching a drug that they call STA-4783 which is designed to overload cancer cells with oxygen containing chemicals. It is apparently having some success in extending patient lives with minimal side effects. It is likely that other similar drugs will also come to market, and it may be worth enquiring about this approach when discussing therapies with an oncologist.

Virus therapy

It is known that certain viruses have an anti-cancer effect. People have been cured of their cancers after natural infection with measles and also with viral fowl plague, also known as Newcastle disease. In humans the only known side effect of Newcastle disease is 'pinkeye'. An Hungarian-American doctor who runs a clinic in Hungary Laszlo Csatary has studied this type of therapy with herpes and influenza viruses with exciting results. Influenza viruses have shown a strong protective effect against a cancer-like disease in experiments with chickens. Since Newcastle disease has the best effects, a live virus vaccine, called the MTH-68 vaccine, has been developed. There are reports of clinical trials in Hungary, but I have not read of any results. Side effects are not, it seems, a concern. Most patients note subjective improvements in pain relief but clear results have not yet been released.

The common mumps virus has also shown anticancer effects in Japanese research. It has been particularly helpful in reducing oedema (swelling of lymphatic system—a common result of radiation), cancerous bleeding and pain. Tumour regression was also noted.

United Cancer Research Institute, in Budapest, is run by Dr Laszlo K. Csatary and Eva Csatary. They can be reached via a Fort Lauderdale phone/fax number: 00-1-954-525-3120.

Summing up

The earth and all the plants in it that grow around us are mini-universes of bio-chemical diversity—and all of these biochemical elements have evolved to sustain and protect that plant. Animals of many species have learnt to make use of these plants too for diet, and to cure the ailments they are prone to.

There is no doubt that herbs—along with diet and a large number of supplements (see Section 6: *Cancer: Vitamins and Other Supplements*)—have enormous potential as weapons against cancer or as ways of maintaining and enhancing health and supporting the immune system. Essiac and OPC, in particular, have a large following.

Remember, most drugs start their life when one or other of these plants provides researchers with an extract that has beneficial effects. The researchers then seek to create an artificial analogue of these natural chemicals. But this artificial version is not developed because there is any improved health benefit in this new version; it is developed so that companies can make money by patenting their version. Nature cannot be patented; artificial analogues can. But nature must always be superior simply because nature is the environment in which we have evolved. Our bodies have developed to benefit from nature.

The choice of which herbs to choose is yours—and as we can see there is an enormous range of options. Some of these herbs can help directly to fight a cancer, others to enhance our immune system, others still will improve our energy and health in other ways. But do look once again at the warnings at the beginning of this section. Herbs are potent and need to be respected.

I personally arrived late to this appreciation of herbs but I am now a great devotee of them—particularly of the essential oils. Of these, lavender is by far my favourite. Not only does it help me sleep but it is a powerful healer. Its healing powers are so easy to see that I am at a loss to understand why it is not widely used in our hospitals. After every surgery, it would be so easy to spray the patient's body with lavender oil—and, if this were done, I have no doubt whatsoever that recovery would be greatly speeded and the incidence of hospital-acquired infections reduced. You can judge this effect easily in your own home. The next time you cut your finger—no matter how deeply—or burn yourself, simply pour pure lavender essential oil liberally over the wound. Within half an hour it will very likely to have healed up completely and painlessly—and there will be no risk of sepsis or infection. No antiseptic cream available at the pharmacy can boast such immediate efficacy.

God's pharmacy is a treasure house that we should do our utmost to protect and nurture.

Cancer: Vitamins and Other Supplements

Everyone knows that vitamin C is good for you—but what kind of vitamin C? In what quantities? And what about the other vitamins? The minerals? The other chemicals—both natural and man-made? There is a dizzying variety of supplements that attack cancer, stop it in its tracks, and boost the immune system. In this section I will look at the main supplements that are recommended as having anti-cancer and wellness benefits as well as those which are contra-indicated or about which there is some controversy. I will also be looking at other 'supplements' or chemical compounds that have been developed with a view to helping people with cancer to recover. You will find everything you need to know here.

Vitamins and Other Natural Supplements

The first issue to be discussed in relation to vitamin and mineral supplements is whether or not we should be taking them at all. Not everyone on the alternative side of the cancer treatment fence is in agreement. And of course it is a fundamental question. So let us now consider the arguments given on both sides.

To supplement or not to supplement

Among health conscious people there is a debate as to whether supplements are a good thing.

The arguments against taking supplements

1. We should be able to get all the nutrients we need from a healthy diet. So rather than take supplements we should concentrate on making sure we eat a properly balanced diet.
2. Supplements themselves have gone through some form of processing—and therefore suffer from the defects attributed to other processed foods. Also we cannot be sure that supplements contain the levels of vitamins that they claim to contain. If we argue that pharmaceutical companies cannot be trusted to tell us the truth about drugs, then the same arguments apply to the health supplements industry. They cannot be trusted to tell us the truth about the real value of supplements.
3. Vitamins and minerals work best when they are in organic combinations with other vitamins and minerals. In this form they work synergistically and so the resulting beneficial effect is maximized.
4. Some synthetic supplements block the body's access to natural sourced vitamins (notably vitamin E). This is just one of a number of potential dangers associated with indiscriminate intake of supplements.
5. By taking supplements in large doses we are fooling ourselves that we are getting the essential nutrients we need for good health and so we pay less attention to the overall diet—which should be almost entirely if not completely plant based.
6. Such large doses of vitamins and/or other supplements are potentially toxic.

The arguments in favour of taking supplements:

1. We need to take larger quantities of most vitamins and minerals than we can easily find in the food we eat. Vitamin C is an obvious example. An orange contains perhaps 70mg of vitamin C while Linus Pauling (of whom more later) recommended 6–18 grams per day (equivalent to between 85 and 257 oranges!)—and some people take much more.

2. There is no evidence at all that vitamin C has ever harmed anyone. In fact the number of people who are believed to have been harmed by any vitamin or mineral supplement is negligible to non-existent. Drugs, used properly and improperly, are known to cause hundreds of thousands of deaths every year. Studies that purport to show problems with vitamins—beta-carotene for example—are based on extremely low dose levels.

3. We know that the food we eat is depleted of vital nutrients by the use of artificial fertilizers and pesticides and irradiation. In fact, given the wide use of pesticides, it is likely that most vegetables are poor in minerals (pesticides leach minerals from the soils). Since the mineral content of vegetables comes from the soil, diet is unlikely to provide what we need. In the case of animal husbandry, intensive farming techniques combined with the use of antibiotics and hormones make the resulting food a poor source of wholesome nutrition.

4. Much of the food we eat has had most of the vital nutrients destroyed by heating during the cooking process.

5. Pollution depletes our body's vitamin resources. The more polluted our environment, the greater our need for higher levels of vitamin intake.

6. There is the possibility that cancer is a deficiency disease—and it may possibly be a deficiency in trace minerals. If so, we need to correct that deficiency in some way—and that means taking supplements. A vegetarian diet alone may not be sufficient because even vegetarians get cancer. In fact vegetarians, although their overall cancer risks are lower than for meat eaters, they have higher incidences of colorectal cancer, a fact that no-one really understands—though it may be caused by higher intake of soy products (the Japanese also have very high incidences of stomach, colon and liver cancers).

7. There is strong evidence that prescription drugs deplete the body of vitamins and minerals. The more prescription drugs you take the worse the problem is. If you take prescription drugs, then you really have no choice but to take supplements.

Weighing it all up

All these arguments on both sides of the dispute are good. Each of us has to weigh them up to arrive at a compromise that makes sense for us.

My own view is that we cannot rely on synthetic supplements alone—nor can we rely on fresh vegetables and fruit alone. Eating organic vegetables and fruit, preferably from a local producer, coupled with some supplements seems to me to be the necessary compromise. And although I see no way round the need to take synthetic vitamin C in large doses, I recognize that the 70mg of vitamin C in an orange is very likely equivalent to much higher quantities of synthetic vitamin C measured in terms of biological activity.

In addition, there are many other supplements that are not vitamins or minerals which should have strong claims to our attention as potent cancer fighters.

Free radicals and the need for supplements

There are many processes within the body that help us to remain healthy and resistant to disease. Attacking the body are a wide range of enemies: bacteria, viruses, fungi, many kinds of poisons, etc. In addition, the body is being damaged by the effects of free radicals.

What are these free radicals? Basically they are molecules that have been deprived of an oxygen atom and are therefore hungry for oxygen. They find this oxygen in the fats embedded in the walls of normal cells. They therefore have to attack the cell walls to get the oxygen they require. This damages and can even kill the cell. Free radicals are themselves the normal by-product of the body's chemical reactions—particularly those processes involved in eliminating potentially toxic cellular waste materials. The more toxic waste materials there are, the more free radicals are created. And although free radicals are often seen as baddies, there are circumstances when they play a useful role in combating bacterial infections.

Free radicals are being formed all the time but their impact is controlled by the body in a number of ways. One is by having the means to repair the cell wall damage. Vitamin C is important for this process.

Another way is to intercept the free radicals before they do any harm. Vitamins A, C and E and the mineral, selenium, are called antioxidants because they help the body to protect itself in this way. They neutralize the free radicals before they reach the cells walls. Vitamin E works synergistically with selenium and also works with vitamins A and C by protecting them from oxidation—hence they are referred to as anti-oxidants. Superoxide dismutase (SOD) is also an efficient free radical scavenger.

Vitamins are of extremely low toxicity. It takes months on extremely high doses before the body begins to react negatively to those that are fat soluble—which can therefore be stored—such as vitamins A and E. (Vitamin C is not fat soluble and therefore is quickly passed out of the body.) This indicates, on its own, that the body welcomes these vitamins. When the body ceases to be able to tolerate them it indicates this by creating, almost always, a sensation of nausea. This should be sufficient warning to desist. An overdose of vitamin A will not take you by surprise in the same way as an overdose of any pharmaceutical or recreational drug.

What is also interesting is that, even before physical signs detectable by blood tests appear, the mind responds to low levels of vitamins: vitamin B complex deficiency can lead to mental illnesses. Depression is also a very common response to vitamin C and B deficiency. If we accept some arguments, most cancers and many heart diseases are completely explicable as being the result of inadequate vitamin intake.

Minerals are a slightly different matter. For some there is very little if any toxicity, while for others there are known limits beyond which it would be unwise to go. Details of these are given below.

How much should we take?

Anyone reading around the subject will discover that there is very little agreement as to how much of any vitamin or mineral we should be taking. British writers tend to be quite conservative, while Americans tend to be much more aggressive. This book takes the view that a risk-benefit analysis favours taking too much rather than too little. People with cancer should be more aggressive than people wishing to provide themselves with some protection. However, very large doses should be built up slowly—and also tapered off slowly.

Measurements of what is adequate

For most vitamins and minerals there is an RDA (Recommended Daily Allowance) value. This is usually an extremely low figure set by the FDA (the US Food and Drug Administration). For example, the RDA for vitamin C was for many years 60mg. This was a measure of the amount an average person should take to ensure that he or she did not suffer from deficiency. In the US this has been replaced by the terms Reference Daily Intake (RDI) or DRI (Dietary Reference Intake). This is defined as representing 'the upper tolerable limit of vitamin and mineral intakes that the US Food and Drug Administration recommends for adults and persons 4 or more years of age,' with little change in values—for example the RDA for vitamin C is now 75–90mg. Tolerable? To whom? Do four-year olds have the same needs as 75-year olds? Since many people comfortably take several thousand milligrams of vitamin C, we clearly have a problem.

Individuals vary in their needs

Setting a measure such as RDA or DRI assumes we are all more or less equal in our needs. This apparently is not the case. The Nobel Prize-winning biochemist Linus Pauling remarked: 'Human beings differ from one another; they show a pronounced biochemical individuality.' Indeed, according to his calculations, it is extremely unlikely that anyone on Earth is 100 per cent average, that is to say, sharing characteristics with 95 per cent of the population for every biochemical process in the body.

So it may be that some people are suffering deficiencies even though they are receiving much higher than RDA/DRI intakes. Modern nutritionists now work with another term: ODA (Optimal Daily Allowance). There is some variation from nutritionist to nutritionist as to what constitutes an ODA level—but in all cases it is significantly higher than the RDA or DRI level.

Can a multi-vitamin/mineral strategy cure cancer?

There are no 100 per cent guaranteed cures for cancer. However, a study by Albert Hoffer and Linus Pauling compared two groups of cancer patients. Those who continued eating as they had done before they got cancer had an average life expectancy of 5.7 months. Those who changed their diets and took high-dose multi-vitamin and mineral supplements had an average life expectancy of six years! Women with cancers of the breast, ovaries and cervix did better, averaging ten years. So, on the basis of this result, there appears to be a very strong argument for taking supplements.

The safety of vitamins

From time to time there are scare stories implicating this or that vitamin or mineral. You should know that over the years 1983–2005 in the USA there were a combined total of exactly ten deaths associated with vitamins. More people died from eating soap. The safety record of minerals is almost as good—most fatalities coming from gross over-ingestion of iron supplements. Compared to the hundreds of thousands each year who die as a direct result of their standard medical treatment this is small beer. Even aspirin use, or abuse, causes 700 deaths a year in the USA.

Vitamins

We will now look at the evidence put forward supporting, or casting doubt on, the value of the main vitamins and minerals identified as being important in the fight against cancer. The most important vitamin is vitamin C so we will look at that first and in some detail.

Vitamin C

For anyone seeking to survive or prevent cancer, and not averse to taking supplements, large doses of vitamin C are highly recommended. However, before starting to take so-called 'megadoses' (doses of 1g and up) of vitamin C, you should read this section carefully. The forms of vitamin C found in your local supermarket or pharmacy chain are not highly regarded.

The vitamin C controversy: science and politics

The vitamin C controversy is one of the best-publicized and most fiercely-argued in the annals of non-orthodox cancer treatments. Its most famous proponent was Linus Pauling, a double Nobel Prize winner: in 1954 for chemistry and in 1962 he won the Peace Prize. It was Dr Pauling's view that daily megadoses of vitamin C could prevent cancer—and could also cure cancer, and in the worst case enabled you to live longer with better quality of life. 'Vitamin C deficiency is common in patients with advanced cancer …. Patients with low plasma concentrations of vitamin C have a shorter survival.'

The *Independent* newspaper's obituary of Linus Pauling, who died in 1994, ended with these words: 'His theories on vitamin C have now been largely discredited.' This chapter will show that this is not, in fact, the case.

Pauling wrote three books putting forward the evidence in support of vitamin C: *Vitamin C and the Common Cold*, *Vitamin C and Cancer*, and *How to Live Longer and Feel Better*. In these books he quoted extensive experimental support for his conclusion that vitamin C has a general anti-viral effect which protects against any virus including influenza, polio, hepatitis, mononucleosis, and herpes.

In addition, '[G]ood intakes of vitamin C and other vitamins can improve your general health in such a way as to increase your enjoyment of life and can help in controlling heart disease, cancer and other diseases and in slowing down the process of aging.' (Pauling, 1986)

This is a big claim to make. So what proof or evidence or theory did he put forward? First he pointed out that patients with cancer usually have very low concentrations of vitamin C in the blood plasma and in the blood leucocytes. This lack prevents the leucocytes from doing their job of engulfing and digesting bacteria and other foreign cells, including malignant cells, in the body. He felt that it was reasonable to suppose that the low level of vitamin C indicated it was being used up in the effort to control the disease. By giving patients a larger amount of vitamin C, their bodily defences should therefore be strengthened. This then was his starting point. Further evidence came from epidemiological studies that showed higher cancer incidence among people whose vegetable and vitamin C intakes were low.

He then established a professional relationship with the Scottish doctor, Ewan Cameron. Cameron had come to vitamin C by another route. His starting point was the known fact that malignant tumours produce an enzyme that attacks the intercellular cement of the surrounding healthy tissues. This weakens the cement to such an extent that the cancer is able to invade. Cameron suggested that one way of defending against the cancer might therefore be to strengthen the intercellular cement. Since vitamin C is known to be involved in the synthesis of collagen (the material of which the intercellular cement is composed), high doses of vitamin C should have the effect of strengthening these defences by allowing faster synthesis. This should protect against the spread and growth of a tumour.

Cameron and Pauling started to experiment with vitamin C on terminal cancer patients at Vale of Leven Hospital in Scotland over the next few years. The results were so exciting that when Pauling suggested they do a double-blind clinical trial, Cameron refused. He believed in the value of vitamin C. To deprive any of his patients of this treatment would therefore be unethical. So instead they carried out a controlled study, comparing the outcome of 100 patients who were randomly assigned to Dr Cameron's care to the outcome of 1,000 patients assigned to doctors who did not believe in or use vitamin C therapy. The result? The patients treated with a daily 10g of sodium ascorbate had a survival time 4.2 times longer than for patients who did not take such large doses. Some continued to survive, and survive, and survive.

A small but significant per cent of the 'terminally ill' cancer patients for whom death was considered inevitable within a matter of weeks or months went on to long-term survival. In short, for some patients, admittedly a very few, vitamin C cured their cancer. (We must remember that Pauling did not give any patients doses higher than 10 grams. What would have happened if he had given them 20 or 30 grams, the levels that most advocates now consider to be the minimum necessary if a cure is to be obtained?)

These are exciting results and one would have thought the cancer associations would have been leaping over themselves to replicate the results. Nothing could be further from the truth. Pauling took these results back to the National Cancer Institute in America. They were only interested, they said, in animal studies. But when Pauling applied for grants to conduct this animal-based research he was turned down eight times. Eventually, he made a point of what was happening by publishing an advertisement seeking private donations to help him continue his research.

In this 1976 *Wall Street Journal* advertisement, he wrote: 'Our research shows that the incidence and the severity of cancer depends on diet. We urgently want to refine that research so that it may help to decrease suffering from human cancer. The US Government has absolutely and continually refused to support Dr Pauling and his colleagues during the past four years.'

Eventually sufficient pressure built up and the Mayo Clinic was asked to conduct clinical trials of vitamin C. One of these was conducted by a Dr Moertel in 1985. His conclusion, which was widely reported in the press, was that there was no evidence that vitamin C had any beneficial effect on cancer patients. He had conducted a double-blind clinical trial that showed no difference between the survival of those who had been given vitamin C and those who had been given a placebo. Pauling was severely critical of the conduct of this trial.

'[Moertel] suppressed the fact that the vitamin C patients were not receiving vitamin C when they died and had not received any for a long time (median 10.5 months). [This misrepresentation] has done great harm. Cancer patients have informed us that they are stopping their vitamin C because of [these] 'negative results'. (Pauling 1986)

The question raises itself as to why the US National Cancer Institute was so keen to ally itself to a negative result for vitamin C and so slow to support positive findings. Critics point to the fact that the pharmaceutical industry is well represented in the committees and subcommittees of all of the leading cancer-related institutions. If it were ever found that vitamin C was indeed a powerful anticancer agent, then the pharmaceutical companies could say goodbye to their lucrative business. Simply put, there is no money to be made out of selling vitamin C.

Pauling summed up his experiences thus: 'Everyone should know the war against cancer is largely a fraud.' If you think he is alone in this view then here is the view of fellow Nobel prize winner, James Watson, discoverer of DNA, 'The war on *cancer* is a bunch of *shit*.'

Benefits of vitamin C

We should note in passing that benefits of taking large doses of vitamin C have been claimed for a wide variety of ailments ranging from wasp and snake bite, to heart disease, meningitis, shock, schizophrenia and diabetes. In fact the list is so long that it would not do any harm to take large doses of vitamin C whatever the problem. Certainly, children with Down's Syndrome, who have higher leukaemia rates, should be put on vitamin C supplements (and also green tea). People with skin cancers can make a paste by adding a few drops of water to vitamin C powder and rubbing this on exposed cancerous areas several times a day, leaving it to dry. There are anecdotal reports that this has caused surface cancers to heal over.

In 2007, researchers at Johns Hopkins found that vitamin C had an important anti-cancer effect in that it helped to diminish levels of a protein called hypoxia-induced factor (HIF-1). This protein helps oxygen-starved cells to convert sugar to energy without using oxygen, and it is also important in initiating the development of new blood vessels, which the cancer tumour needs to support its growth. Lower levels of the protein means that the growth of the cancer is impeded.

Vitamin C is also beneficial for cancer patients undergoing chemotherapy and radiotherapy. Victor Marcial, MD, an oncologist in Puerto Rico, says:

'We studied patients with advanced cancer (stage 4). Forty patients received 40–75g intravenously several times a week. These are patients that have not responded to other treatments. The initial tumour response rate was achieved in 75 per cent of patients, defined as a 50 per cent reduction or more in tumour size …. As a radiation oncologist, I also give radiation therapy. Vitamin C has two effects. It increases the beneficial effects of radiation and chemotherapy and decreases the adverse effects. But this is not a subtle effect, is not 15–20 per cent. It's a dramatic effect. Once you start using IV [intravenous] vitamin C, the effect is so dramatic that it is difficult to go back to not using it.'

How much vitamin C do we need?

Clearly vitamin C has a wide range of functions within the body and is an important nutrient. But why do we need such large quantities? The official RDA (Recommended Daily Allowance) for vitamin C is 60–90mg per day. Most people assume that the RDA is an average intake that they should aim for, or an amount which should not be exceeded by too much. In fact, this is wrong. 60–90mg a day is the quantity needed to ensure we do not get deficiency diseases like scurvy. So the RDA is a minimum amount. Vitamin C is a food substance or nutrient. Does it make sense to take in only the minimum amount of a food substance that will stave off deficiency diseases? Applied to food intake as a whole, does it make sense to take in only the amount of food that will prevent us from dying of starvation?

Once we have established that the RDA is a minimum amount, we should try to find out what the Optimum Daily Allowance (ODA) is. This will presumably be somewhere between the minimum and the maximum amount. But what is the maximum amount? The maximum amount obviously will be that amount that will lead to toxicity or ill-health. Taking this as a guideline we discover an interesting fact: there is no maximum level of vitamin C that will cause ill-health or toxicity! One suggestion that it could lead to kidney stones has never been validated.

It appears that no matter how much we take, we can never reach a dose that is toxic. There are two reasons for this. First, the body welcomes vitamin C in large quantities. Secondly, if the body gets more vitamin C than it can handle at any one time it dumps the excess vitamin C by causing diarrhoea, which stops as soon as vitamin C levels become manageable again. This diarrhoea-causing amount will vary from person to person. Known as the bowel-tolerance level, it will normally be in the region of 10–20 grams a day for a healthy adult but it will increase sharply to 30–60 grams or even more if there is a viral infection. Going back to Pauling's argument: this increased ability to tolerate higher levels of vitamin C during periods of ill-health suggests that the body is capable of using more vitamin C at times of ill-health. This leads, in turn, to the conclusion that the body is using the vitamin C to fight the illness. So one measure of ODA would be an amount slightly less than the bowel tolerance level.

We can approach this question from another angle. Humans are one of a small group of animals that don't produce vitamin C in their bodies. We share this defect with the other apes and, curiously, with that archetypal experimental animal, the guinea pig. For us, vitamin C has to be taken in from outside (i.e., in the food). Most mammals, however, manufacture vitamin C in their livers through the action of a particular enzyme. So how much vitamin C do these animals produce? It varies from species to species. A goat for example produces approximately 13 grams a day per 70kg of body weight under normal conditions, but if it gets stressed it will produce up to 100 grams or more. Mice produce 275mg of vitamin C per kilo of body weight a day under normal conditions. A mouse the size of a 70kg man would therefore be producing 19 grams a day. These amounts can increase ten-fold when the animal is under stress.

This is, for me, the clinching evidence that large quantities of vitamin C are beneficial—and are indeed the 'normal' levels we should be taking in for optimal health. First, since man is a mammal, he almost certainly needs vitamin C in quantities similar to other mammals of the same size and weight. Secondly, if animals produce more vitamin C when they are under stress then presumably, the vitamin C is useful to help the body cope with stress—and illness is a form of physical stress. Interestingly, dogs and cats, which produce relatively low amounts of vitamin C have, after man, the highest cancer rates in the animal kingdom.

This leads to an interesting question: Why is it that man doesn't create his own vitamin C? The Encyclopaedia Britannica gives one possible explanation. Our inability to produce vitamin C may be the result of some genetic disease that wiped out the enzymes that perform this task in the liver. It is simply an accident of history that we have somehow been able to overcome.

Many people in America and Australia are taking ten or more grams a day just to maintain their health. For children, one advocate recommends that they can—and should—take one gram per year of life. An eight year old could take eight grams a day. This is perhaps an extreme point of view but it is clear that a couple of grams will not cause an overdose.

Expensive urine?

Finally, to deal with the argument that large doses of vitamin C merely lead to 'expensive urine' (i.e., to wasted vitamin C), experts have made the following points:

1. The urinary system is very prone to infection and so it actually makes sense to direct an anti-viral and anti-bacterial agent like vitamin C through this system. People who don't have 'expensive urine' may be more prone to urinary infections.
2. The presence of vitamin C in the urine does not indicate tissue saturation. Tissue saturation causes diarrhoea. The amount needed to get a urine reading is very much lower than the amount needed to cause diarrhoea.
3. The level of vitamin C in the urine is a good indication of the level in the tissues. If urinary levels are low, then so too will the tissue levels be low. High levels of excreted vitamin C are indications that the body's defences are in good shape.

How to take vitamin C

Having established the credentials of vitamin C, it is now necessary to explain that there are a number of different forms of the substance and that they are not all equal. The worst possible form of vitamin C is the stuff you buy in the local chemists, the large orange tablets that make a fizzy orange-tasting drink. Do not take vitamin C in this form. The best is to buy a tub of vitamin C powder in the form of ascorbic acid or sodium ascorbate.

As straight ascorbic acid, it is slightly acidic. Usually, however, vitamin C is sold in tablet form as 'buffered' vitamin C, which means they are in a non-acidic form. This means that they are sold as a salt (i.e., as calcium ascorbate or sodium ascorbate) and so on.

Most vitamin C advocates warn that the calcium ascorbate form is not recommended when a cancer tumour is present. Unfortunately, most on-the-shelf vitamin C pills are calcium ascorbate, including the ester-C form of vitamin C. For cancer patients, L-ascorbic acid, sodium ascorbate, magnesium ascorbate, potassium ascorbate and zinc ascorbate are the preferred forms. For further information on vitamin C, the following websites are recommended www.vitamincfoundation.com, and www.orthomed.com.

Pauling does warn that anyone going on a megadose regime of vitamin C to fight a cancer should not start with large doses—there is a danger of the tumour haemorrhaging—which can be fatal. Large doses should be gradually built up over a period of weeks, starting with say three grams a day and increasing by one gram every day, continuing until the bowel tolerance level has been established. A dose slightly lower than this should then be maintained. Pauling also warned that one should never suddenly stop taking it—instead it should be tapered off. He warned that a sudden stop might result in 'rebound scurvy'. Not everyone believes that this is a danger—but it may be, and it would be wise to take precautions.

There is one final caution. If the cancer patient taking the vitamin C is in a defeated-defeatist frame of mind, the vitamin C may not be effective. This is because the vitamin C may be harnessed by the body for other purposes. (This point is discussed more fully in Section 3: *Cancer Research and Politics*) It is important that the cancer patient taking vitamin C should be encouraged and helped to take on a positively-resisting frame of mind.

Vitamin C, in a buffered form, can also be taken intravenously. This allows the intake of very high doses of vitamin C directly into the blood plasma so getting much higher blood plasma levels of the vitamin than are possible by taking it orally. In fact this can be done at home if you follow the instructions at www.canceraction.org.gg.

It is also offered by most alternative clinics. In Britain it is offered by the Dove Clinic at www.doveclinic.com. Practitioners can contact http://bioimmune.com.

Alternatively, you can dissolve the vitamin C desired in DMSO and rub it on the skin. DMSO is a powerful solvent that will take the vitamin C directly into the blood stream. I imagine this procedure would be very uncomfortable but would be perfectly safe—as long as the normal precautions associated with handling DMSO are observed—namely, very clean hands and skin and no gloves or jewellery of any sort (see below for more information about DMSO).

Taking mega-doses of vitamin C intravenously (100+g at a time) makes use of vitamin C in an entirely different way—it becomes a pro-oxidant rather than an anti-oxidant—and it is recommended that oral ingestion of vitamin C to bowel tolerance level should continue at the same time. A number of clinics are offering intravenous vitamin C therapy and it does seem as if this has a greater anti-cancer effect. For further information you can go to the following websites:

www.canceraction.org.gg
www.maryclinic.com
www.orthomed.com/cancer.htm
www.brightspot.org/cresearch/ivccancer.html

For people with brain cancers the fat-soluble form of vitamin C, ascorbyl palmitate, is recommended. Not only can it be stored in the body longer than normal water-soluble vitamin C, but it can cross the blood-brain barrier. However, in capsule form this supplement is useless. It needs to be dissolved in flax oil first.

Another, easier, way of getting vitamin C into the brain is to change it into DHA (dehydroascorbic acid—not to be confused with the other chemical DHA [docosahexaenoic acid] that is found in fish oils). One way of making this is to dissolve as far as possible say five grams of vitamin C (a teaspoonful of powder) in a small amount of water. Then add the same amount of fresh three per cent hydrogen peroxide. Wait until the foaming reaction has completed and consume. This combination is not acidic to the stomach.

Finally, a new form of vitamin C has recently hit the market. Lypo-Spheric vitamin C claims to be far more bio-available than other forms so that very little is 'wasted' in urine. For more information go to www.livonlabs.com. I have read a number of testimonials in free discussion groups of how easy this form of vitamin C is to tolerate and how quickly it has an effect. It may be that if the claims that 100 per cent of the vitamin C gets through to the cells that Lypo-Spheric vitamin C taken orally may have the same impact as vitamin C taken intravenously.

Summing up

I have nothing against Dr Moertel personally, but the chart below makes a point that cannot be made in any other way. It is not scientifically valid, it may even be considered in very bad taste, but it has a poetic immediacy that is unassailable.

Name	Age at death	Other information
Linus Pauling	93	advocate of vitamin C
Albert Szent-Györgyi	93	discovered vitamin C
Dr Charles Moertel	66	anti-vitamin C researcher, died of cancer

It is perhaps fitting that Moertel and Pauling, arch enemies in life, should die within months of each other. Linus Pauling's death has often been sniggeringly attributed to prostate cancer (and therefore by implication invalidating his vitamin C theories)—but it is my view that anyone who dies at the age of 93 actually dies of old age, no matter what the death certificate may say. Until a few months before his death, Linus Pauling was alert and in good form. Clearly, he was living proof of the value of the regime he was recommending. Pauling's own recipe for a happy, healthy, long life, which he published in 1986, is as follows:

1. Take 6–18 grams of vitamin C every day. Do not miss a single day.
2. Take 400–1,600IU of vitamin E a day.
3. Take 1–2 high-dosage vitamin B tablets a day.
4. Take 25,000IU of vitamin A per day.
5. Take a multi-mineral supplement every day which should include: calcium, iodine, copper, magnesium, manganese, zinc, molybdenum, chromium and selenium.
6. Keep intake of sugar to below 50 lbs a year.
7. Apart from sugar, eat what you want—but not too much of any one food. Don't get fat.
8. Drink plenty of water every day.
9. Keep active and do exercise but never excessively over-exert yourself.
10. Drink alcohol only in moderation.
11. Don't smoke.
12. Avoid stress. Work at a job that you like. Be happy with your family.

When it comes to living longer, I prefer to take the advice of the longer-lived.

In case anyone still has doubts about Pauling's stature as a scientist, James Watson, Nobel Prize winner and co-discoverer of the DNA double helix structure, referred to him as being an intellectual giant on a par with Einstein and Newton. Watson believed Pauling was only weeks or months away from solving the DNA problem when he himself found the solution. Francis Crick, Watson's partner in the DNA discovery, was equally certain of Pauling's statute: 'I do not think … that it is right to discuss the impact of Linus Pauling on molecular biology. Rather, he was one of the founders of molecular biology. It was not that it existed in some way, and he simply made a contribution. He was one of the founders who got the whole discipline going.'

Food sources for vitamin C: fruit—particularly citrus fruits.

ODA: for normal maintenance 3–5 grams per day. For cancer: as much as you can tolerate.

Vitamin A (and/or beta carotene)

Note that beta carotene is known as the precursor of vitamin A. Vitamin A is obtained from animal sources while beta carotene comes from vegetables. Beta carotene is changed to vitamin A in the body only when it is needed, so vitamin A is best taken in the form of beta carotene. In that way the negative effects—possible toxicity—can be eliminated.

In a controlled study with people who chew betel nut and who therefore have a higher incidence of oral cancer, the group who received vitamin A (200,000IU per week) had a pronounced remission from precancerous lesions and had fewer new lesions. One 1985 study, showed that cancer spread was much lower among mice fed with vitamin A supplements.

Another study has shown that women who take vitamin A during chemotherapy report a much lower incidence of unpleasant side effects—no doubt because of its important role for the growth of epithelial tissue.

Food Sources: Active vitamin A is found in fish oils, liver, eggs and dairy products. Yellow vegetables and fruits like mangoes contain beta carotene. In both forms it is very susceptible to oxidation and can be destroyed by heat and light—so carrot juice has to be freshly pressed and drunk quickly to be effective.

ODA: 10,000–50,000IU per day though higher amounts up 100,000IU can be taken for extended periods—three to four months—in the case of patients fighting cancer.

Dangers: Vitamin A may cause birth defects or be toxic to infants so pregnant and lactating women should keep their vitamin A intake low (5,000IU or less). Also women who wish to become pregnant should reduce their vitamin A intake well in advance of conception.

Vitamin A is stored in body fat and is not water soluble so there is the potential for toxicity. However, you must take at least 100,000IU of vitamin A daily for a period of months in order to display any signs of toxicity. Beta carotene, on the other hand, can be given for long periods of time virtually without risk of toxicity.

Signs of toxicity: Yellowing skin, fatigue and nausea, blurred vision and loss of hair.

Vitamin B complex

These vitamins are not all—or even mainly—antioxidants. However, there are some strong anti-cancer effects associated with the B vitamins.

Thiamine, vitamin B1, is recommended by some as a key component in a cancer cure as low levels of this vitamin prevent cell apoptosis (programmed cell death), and apoptosis is a process that people with cancer will want to encourage.

Riboflavin (B2) deficiencies, for example, have been shown clearly to lead to high levels of oesophageal (throat) cancer in animals. Also, niacin (B3) is known to be good for the liver. Vitamin B3 helps promote the transport of oxygen by dilating the blood vessels. More importantly, it is required for the production of NADH (Nicotinamide Adenine Dinucleotide), which is absolutely essential in a number of different ways for enabling aerobic metabolism. Since aerobic metabolism is exactly what we want to encourage if we want cancer cells to return to normal status, large doses of vitamin B3 should in theory be very helpful in the fight against cancer.

Lastly, B3, niacin, is known to have positive effects on mood, so can be taken as an anti-depressant.

It should be noted that niacin in large doses has the effect of causing a temporarily uncomfortable intense flush which is not at all pleasant but not in any way harmful. There is an alternative form of B3, niacinamide, which does not cause this sudden flush. However, since the sudden flush may be an important effect, it is not known whether non-flush vitamin B3 is as good as niacin.

Vitamin B6: High intakes of this vitamin are associated with low rates of colorectal cancers. Studies on mice have also shown that, at high doses, it can eliminate colon cancers.

Vitamin B12 appears to have a strong synergistic relationship with vitamin C. In one study in which mice were implanted with tumour cells, only two out of fifty receiving the combination developed tumours. All fifty of the controls developed tumours.

Folic acid (also known as vitamin B9) deficiency is widespread, and this lack has been shown to be associated with cervical and breast cancers. Cervical cancer will respond to treatment with high doses of folic acid. A Japanese study has shown that large intakes of folate (10–20 milligrams) in combination with 750 micrograms of B12 had a very impressive protective effect. However, that said, there is increasing concern that folic acid in the form that is found in supplements and added to food is an artificial chemical, and much that is taken in is not metabolised in the body but remains in its unmetabolised form—with worrying consequences. It is therefore much better to get folates in their natural form from foods. A cup of cranberries and blackeye beans, one and a half cups of pinto and garbanzo beans would supply a minimum day's needs. Other folate rich foods are: most beans, fruits, fruit juices and green leafy vegetables. Note that new evidence is showing cranberries to be very powerful inhibitors of cancer cell division.

Generally speaking, individual B vitamins should not be taken on their own in large doses for any length of time as this can lead to deficiencies in the other B vitamins—because they compete. The general rule of thumb is that you can take individual B vitamins up to three times their normal value in comparison with the intake of B complex as a whole. Folic acid is a possible exception to this rule.

Food Sources: widely available in dark green leafy vegetables, beans, brown rice and brewer's yeast but cooking reduces bioavailability.

ODA: B2: 50–500mg; B3: 500mg–1g; B12: 10–500µg; folic acid: 800µg–2.4mg.

Toxic effects: There are no known toxic effects for B2 and B12, but for niacin there is the potential for a hot flush or itchy effect. There has been some recent concern that high intakes of folic acid are associated themselves with higher incidences of cancer. But these concerns need to be balanced against decades of research which have shown that high intakes of folic acid have healthy consequences.

However, for people with leukaemia, folic acid must be absolutely avoided as it promotes the disease. The first chemotherapy that had any impact on leukaemia was a folate-blocker.

Vitamin D

The RDA for vitamin D is 200IU for those under the age of 50, and 400IU for those over 50. However, new research has demonstrated that these levels are laughably low. The average person gets about 10,000IU from sunbathing for about 20–30 minutes under a hot sun. And, as far as vitamin D is concerned, the more sunlight exposure you have the better. (For a more detailed discussion of sunlight see Section 7: *Cancer: Energy, Mind and Emotions*). Food sources of vitamin D are poor sources in comparison to sunlight. A teaspoon of fish oil contains about 400IU.

What are the dangers of too much vitamin D? None. If it were toxic we would start feeling ill if we spent too much time out in the sun (aside from any effects of heat). Only one person in the world has ever been found to be suffering toxicity, and he was taking in 2.5 millionIU a day (how he managed that, I have no idea). And he recovered quickly when this level of intake was stopped. In fact current research indicates that deficiency probably starts at intakes of less than 4,000IU a day. Vitamin D can be stored in the body for about 60 days.

Until recently, this vitamin was seen simply as being necessary for the absorption of calcium. But it is now known to be a potent anti-cancer weapon in its own right. It has been found that vitamin D stabilizes chromosomes, repairs DNA damage, triggers programmed cell death, and inhibits angiogenesis (the development of a blood supply that the cancer needs to grow). It has been estimated that long-term high exposure to sunlight could prevent around 60 per cent of cancers.

One scientist, Steve Martin believes that vitamin D 5,000IU mixed with 6mg of melatonin, powdered and dissolved in warm coconut oil (which itself is loaded with lauric acid, a healthy fat even if it is a 'saturated fat') and taken at night on an empty stomach is as good a cancer preventative as any, and that higher doses might even be curative.

Other research has found that a metabolite of vitamin D (i.e., one of the chemical compounds that is produced as vitamin D is broken down in the body) called calcitriol (which is available on prescription) combined with a non-steroidal anti-inflammatory drug such as ibuprofen can significantly reduce the growth of prostate cancers by 70 per cent. Both inhibit the production of prostaglandins which, among other effects, cause inflammation. Taken together they have an effect about three times greater than each taken alone.

Summer diagnosis prolongs life. Why?

I am indebted to Ian Clements for the following facts: Epidemiological studies by group led by Professor Johan Moan, Department of Physics at the University of Oslo found that, whether it be cancer of the breast, colon, prostate, lung, or a lymphoma, you live longer if your cancer is diagnosed in the summer.

What do these studies mean? Something about summer has a treatment effect on cancer. Whatever it is, you live longer if you are diagnosed in the summer but die sooner if you are diagnosed in the winter. Remember, these patients already had cancer. Whatever it is about summer, it is not a preventative effect that Professor Moan discovered, it is a treatment effect. Something about summer prolongs the life of cancer patients.

Dr Ying Zhou at the Harvard School of Public Health, looked at total vitamin D input, from both sun and diet, to see if high vitamin D intake improved the survival of cancer patients. They found that early stage lung cancer patients with the highest vitamin D input (from summer season and high intake from diet) lived almost three times longer than patients with the lowest input (winter season and low intake from diet). Three times longer is a huge treatment effect.

Marianne Berwick and her colleagues, at the New Mexico Cancer Institute, found malignant melanoma patients with evidence of continued sun exposure had a 60 per cent mortality reduction compared to patients who did not. That implies a robust treatment effect from sunlight. Remember, sunlight is often blamed as a cause of melanoma. In fact the correlation of sunlight with melanoma incidence is not very clear. If it were, we would expect melanomas to appear mostly on parts of the body most exposed to sunlight. That is not the case.

Vitamin E

Vitamin E is often touted as the vitality vitamin. It has the unique characteristic that there are no known deficiency illnesses associated with it. What we call vitamin E actually comprises two closely related chemical families: the tocopherols (alpha-, beta-, gamma-, and delta-) and the tocotrienols (alpha to delta). Some vitamin E sold in stores is actually a synthetic form of only one of the tocopherols. Natural sourced vitamin E containing both tocotrienols and tocopherols is best.

It is not at all clear what the benefits and drawbacks are of vitamin E. Some say that vitamin E can protect cancer cells. On the other hand, it appears to help people to retain their hair during chemotherapy. New research has now found that the tocotrienols are more interesting for cancer patients than the tocopherols. They appear to have a dampening effect on cell proliferation, and so can help reduce cancer's ability to spread.

A number of studies have shown low vitamin E levels in the blood of people with lung, breast, bladder, cervix, and colorectal cancers. In a study of mice exposed to cigarette smoke, those supplemented with vitamin E and selenium suffered eight per cent deaths compared with 51 per cent for the ones fed a diet deficient in these two substances. One study showed that the group of women with the lowest vitamin E levels had five times the risk of breast cancer compared with the group with the highest vitamin E levels. Some studies have also shown that vitamin E may help to reduce the side effects of chemotherapy. Having said that, there is also a body of opinion that believes that vitamin E both protects the tumour and can even promote tumour growth.

There are fears that synthetic forms of vitamin E provide little or no benefit but will block the ability of cells to absorb and make use of natural vitamin E. It is known that the body's ability to absorb one of the most important dietary forms (gamma-tocopherol) is hindered by high doses of synthetic vitamin E. Natural source vitamin E, providing a mix of tocopherols and tocotrienols, or any supplement with a high tocotrienol content is best.

Having said all this there does appear to be a man made variation of vitamin E that has a notable anti-cancer effect. This is alpha-tocopherol succinate. It has been shown to have a strong inhibitory effect on cancer cell growth with a number of different cancers. Life Extension (www.lef.org) markets a dry powder form of vitamin E alpha-tocopherol succinate.

Food Sources: vegetable fats and oils, whole grains and dark green leafy vegetables, nuts and legumes. However, food processing eliminates most of its vitamin E content. Unrefined or cold-pressed oils are best.

ODA: 200–800IU per day (some advise up to 1,600IU per day).

Toxicity: It is not advised for those with high blood pressure. However, no toxic effects have been clearly shown for doses below 3,000IU per day. Signs of toxicity include nausea, flatulence, headache and fainting.

Vitamin K

Vitamin K was discovered in 1929 by Danish scientist, Dr Henrik Dam. He called it 'K' for its 'Koagulation' properties. It is sometimes referred to as 'the forgotten vitamin'. There are three types of vitamin K, known as K1, K2 and K3. Vitamin K3 is man-made and not normally recommended by most alternative practitioners (for exception see below). Vitamin K is required in large quantities and is associated with anti-ageing and for its antioxidant qualities (it is more powerful than vitamin E).

Laboratory research into vitamin K2 has shown it to cause leukaemia cells to self destruct and to have inhibitory effects against myeloma and lymphoma cancer lines.

Vitamin K has also proven to be effective against liver cancer in human studies. In a study published in the Journal of the American Medical Association (JAMA), individuals with hepatitis C, and therefore at high risk of virally induced liver cancer, were supplemented with vitamin K2 and compared with a group that did not receive the nutrient. Less than ten per cent of the people receiving K2 developed liver cancer, compared with 47 per cent of those in the control group.

However, Dr Jonathan Wright, a highly respected American doctor who favours alternative approaches, recommends a combination of vitamin C and vitamin K3 in a ratio of 100:1—with a minimum vitamin C intake of 6g. A dietary supplement, ProsStay, developed according to this protocol is available from Life Enhancement (www.life-enhancement.com). Dr Wright is a consultant to Life Enhancement Inc. ProsStay is, as its name suggests, mainly targeted at prostate cancer, but there are reports that it is beneficial for other cancers too.

Food Sources: The richest natural source of vitamin K2 is natto, a fermented soybean product. Otherwise it is found in dark green vegetables—in sufficient quantities to interfere with anti-coagulant therapies such as warfarin.

ODA: 100μg.

Caution: It is not recommended for pregnant women or nursing mothers.

Minerals

> 'You can trace every sickness, every disease, and every ailment to a mineral deficiency.'
> *Dr Linus Pauling, twice Nobel Prize winner*

Everyone knows the importance of vitamins. But minerals, including trace minerals, are at least equally important for the healthy transfer of oxygen in and out of cells and for the other necessary bio-chemical operations required to maintain the good functioning of the body. Unfortunately, the vegetables that we depend on for our minerals are grown in increasingly mineral-depleted soils. However, as we shall see with calcium, not everything mineral is necessarily to be applauded.

Calcium

In relation to cancer, there is a big dispute over the question of calcium's potential for good or harm. There are two questions. First, is supplementing with calcium beneficial? And secondly, is it potentially dangerous?

The most famous advocate for calcium is Robert Barefoot, an American self-styled chemist, who is famous for promoting calcium from coral reefs—so-called coral calcium—as a cure all for cancer and many other conditions. His claims regarding the benefits of coral calcium are, however, heavily disputed by other leading alternative health advocates.

Ralph Moss reviewed the scientific literature and could find no support for the claims. Indeed he found that there may be a slight tendency for calcium to promote cancer —particularly prostate cancer.

In relation to prostate cancer, there is clear evidence that the calcium in dairy products inhibits the absorption of vitamin D and thereby promotes the growth of prostate cancer. Men who consume more than 600mg per day of dietary calcium had a 32 per cent higher risk of prostate cancer than those who consumed 150mg or fewer per day.

It is important for cancer patients to keep this in mind in the face of claims by coral calcium proponents that one should increase calcium intake to very high levels. An overdose of calcium can lead to hypercalcaemia, a dangerous excess of calcium in the blood. Many patients with cancer already have a disturbed calcium metabolism—caused by the tumour itself—so that they are in any case hypercalcaemic. The symptoms of this are constipation, nausea, vomiting, abdominal pain, loss of appetite, and the production of abnormally large amounts of urine. Very severe hypercalcaemia often causes brain dysfunction with confusion, emotional disturbances, delirium, hallucinations, and coma. Muscle weakness may occur, and abnormal heart rhythms and death can follow.

A number of doctors have found that calcium has seriously negative consequences for patients with advanced cancer. One, Dr Forbes Ross, reported: 'On another occasion I had reason to administer calcium salts … to cases of cancer …. I was appalled at the rate of growth of the cancers.' (Dr Forbes Ross, author of *Cancer: Its Genesis and Treatment*)

Dr Max Gerson also believed calcium to be dangerous and blamed a number of cancer deaths on his use of calcium. It is now known that intracellular calcium is higher in cancer patients than in the normal population and is associated with rapid cell division. My advice therefore remains to be cautious.

Further support for a cautious approach to calcium supplementation comes from a recent study. A 1998 Harvard School of Public Health study of 47,781 men found those consuming between 1.5g and 1.99g of calcium per day had about double the risk of being diagnosed with metastatic prostate cancer as those getting 500mg per day or less. And those taking in 2g or more had over four times the risk of developing metastatic prostate cancer as those taking in less than 500mg.

Even when calcium is desired, not everyone agrees that calcium supplements or a diet of meat and dairy products is a good way to take it. Calcium, they say, should be taken in vegetable form. Their argument is that milk and meat—the sources of calcium with which we are most familiar—make our systems acidic and the body releases calcium from our bones to neutralize this effect. The best non-meat sources of calcium are seaweeds like kelp, all leafy greens, figs, dates and prunes. In support of this view, some studies have shown that vegetarians have a significantly lower incidence of osteoporosis than meat eaters.

Milk, it should be noted, is contra-indicated for another reason. It has high concentrations of IGF-1 (Insulin Growth Factor) which has been found to promote breast and prostate cancer.

However, having said this, there is a calcium product on the market that is claimed to be beneficial. This is Calcium D-glucarate. In this case, it is not the calcium but the D-glucarate that is significant. This is a naturally occurring substance that attacks an enzyme, glucoronidase, which interferes with the body's attempts to rid itself of cancer. It is considered to be a highly effective preventative of cancer—one that anyone who has already been treated for cancer should consider. It is inexpensive and can be obtained from www.lef.com.

Finally, it should be noted that calcium has poor bioavailability without the co-presence of magnesium, boron and vitamin D (sunlight). In fact, where they exist, low calcium levels may be caused not by inadequate calcium intake, but by poor magnesium intake and lack of exposure to the sun.

Germanium

There are two forms of this mineral: organic and inorganic. Some cases of kidney failure have occurred with the latter. But water-soluble, organic germanium does not have these problems.

Indeed, it is considered to have an extremely powerful anticancer effect as well as being able to normalize the whole body's chemistry. The discoverer of organic germanium, Dr Kazuhiko Asai, a coal engineer, wrote of the organic germanium that he had synthesized: 'My organic germanium compound has proved effective against all sorts of diseases, including cancers of the lung, bladder, larynx and breast.' He believed the reason for this ability was that germanium enriched the oxygen levels in the body. 'I should say that all diseases are attributable to deficiency of oxygen. The dangers of an oxygen deficiency in the human body cannot be over-emphasized.'

Food sources: It is very high in medicinal plants, notably shelf fungus (Trametes cinnabarina) but garlic and ginseng also contain significant amounts.

ODA: None but recommended dose in case of need: 30–150mg.

Toxicity: At levels below 500mg no toxic effects have been reported. Skin rashes and stool softening have been reported for doses of over 2g a day.

Iodine

Iodine is vital for good health, but the Western diet has become depleted of food sources that contain iodine. In addition, baked goods such as bread that used to contain iodine now contain bromine, which competes with iodine within the body. The result is that we are getting inadequate supplies. Iodine is known to be antiviral, antibacterial and an important anti-cancer agent. In addition, it helps raise the pH of the body and helps to convert toxic estrogens into less toxic metabolites. This makes it particularly important for anyone with a hormone-based cancer. The low incidence of breast cancer in Japan is often attributed to the high iodine intake in the Japanese diet. It has also been noted that prostate cancer in Japan rarely goes beyond the prostate—and one can live with a cancer that doesn't spread for a very long time! This too is associated with the high iodine intake in the standard Japanese diet—though it needs to be repeated, the Japanese, in fact have very high overall incidence of cancer, and you might wonder why iodine is not protective there.

Iodine can be taken in the form of seaweed or in a more concentrated form as potassium iodide solution or Lugol's solution, both of which are available on the Internet. Iodoral is a potassium iodide formulation in the form of tablets. Atomic iodine (also called nascent iodine) is an iodine product with enhanced electrical activity—seven per cent solution is required.

Note that soy products have a tendency to leach iodine—and other minerals—from the body, which is the main reason why soy products should in general be treated with caution.

Food Sources: Seaweed, potassium iodide solution, Iodoral, Atomic Iodine

ODA: 10–200mg per day.

Toxicity: Signs of an iodine overdose can range from a persistent metallic taste in the mouth, coughing, shortness of breath, diarrhoea, thirst, fever and even shock. However, it is now known that concerns about iodine over-dosing have been exaggerated in recent decades. Dr Albert Szent-Györgi, the Nobel Prize winning biochemist who isolated vitamin C wrote: 'When I was a medical student, iodine in the form of KI (Potassium Iodide) was the universal medicine. Nobody knew what it did, but it did something and did something good.' In those days the standard dose was 1g, which contains 770mg of iodine. This level did not cause an overdose. Naturopathic doctor, Loretta Lamphier believes cancer patients should be taking 100–200mg daily.

Iron

It is now generally accepted that cancer patients should not take iron supplements. There is mounting evidence that excess iron is associated with lowered immunity and higher incidence of cancer. Also cancer cells have a high need for iron. Depriving them of this mineral will therefore impede growth of the tumour.

Anaemia, the well-known iron-deficiency symptom, may not in fact be caused by iron deficiency. It can be caused by a deficiency of vitamin B12 and/or folic acid as well as by the presence in the bloodstream of drugs or toxins. It is not therefore automatic that iron needs to be taken when anaemia is diagnosed.

However, there is an anti-cancer strategy that takes into account the cancer cell's hunger for iron. When artemisinin comes in contact with iron a reaction takes place, releasing a burst of free radicals. Although it is normally not advisable to take iron supplements in the case of cancer, when taking artemisinin, the reverse is true, as we wish to flood the cancer cells with iron. The free radicals then kill the cancer cell. For further details read Section 5: *Cancer: Herbs, Botanicals and Biological Therapies*.

Magnesium

Magnesium is a largely neglected mineral, but one that is required in fairly large quantities by the body. Over 300 enzymes that influence the metabolism of carbohydrate, amino acids, nucleic acids and proteins require magnesium. In relation to cancer, it is known that there is a direct inverse relationship between soil content of magnesium and cancer incidence. Where magnesium content is higher, cancer incidence tends to be lower.

It is also known that for most Western countries, magnesium deficiency is the norm. One recent Swedish study showed that less than 20 per cent of the 66,000 women it was following had a daily intake above 225mg (350–500mg is recommended). The study also found that colon cancer incidence was inversely proportional to the intake of magnesium.

Magnesium is an important healing agent and it helps to mediate the potassium and calcium levels of the body's tissues.

The problem is how to increase magnesium levels in the body. One difficulty is that low tissue magnesium levels reduce the ability of the body to absorb more magnesium from the diet. One solution is to take the magnesium transdermally (i.e., through the skin). One way of doing this is to spend a lot of time in the sea, which contains high levels of magnesium chloride. An oil based form of magnesium chloride that you can spray on is available from Global Light Network (www.globallight.net). Dr Mark Sircus is a strong proponent for this approach and his book *Transdermal Magnesium Therapy* is recommended (go to www.magnesiumforlife.com).

Another option is to have regular baths with Epsom salts, magnesium oxide or magnesium citrate powder which is also easily absorbed. Finally, magnesium can be taken by means of a homeopathic remedy: magnesium phos.

Substantially increased intakes of magnesium also benefit the heart, blood pressure, bowel cleansing, relaxation, back pain and sexual potency. Anyone who suffers from incapacitating back pain will also find magnesium extremely beneficial. It relaxes the muscles.

Food Sources: dark green vegetables, cereals, potatoes, beans, nuts, bananas.

ODA: 400–800mg (1+g a day if needed).

Toxicity: Toxicity is rare, as most people have the problem of too little magnesium rather than too much. However, a daily intake of 8g or more is likely to be excessive.

Potassium

Sodium and potassium tend to compete within the body. If the body's tissues are high in sodium then the tissues will not take up proper amounts of potassium. It is important to maintain a low sodium-high potassium balance in the body. Good amounts of vitamin B6 are also important to help regulate the balance.

Cells that lose their ability to regulate the proper balance of potassium and sodium quickly become unhealthy—a condition known as toxic tissue syndrome. The consequences are serious if not quickly corrected. That is why a high potassium and low sodium diet is necessary to correct many health issues including both cancer and problems associated with heart disease, high blood pressure, etc.

Potassium-rich foods are almonds, apricots, avocados, bananas, lima, mung and pinto beans, dates, dried figs, hazelnuts, raw garlic, raw horseradish, kelp*, blackstrap molasses*, raw parsley, rice bran, soybeans, full fat soybean flour, sunflower seeds and brewer's yeast*. (* These sources are extremely rich in potassium.)

While high potassium levels are generally recommended, it is very possible to have too much potassium and this can have dangerous consequences for the kidneys and can also put the body into a state of shock. Supplementation with potassium pills should therefore be avoided where possible. Potassium should be taken only in the form of food unless under close medical supervision.

Food sources: cereals, fruits (apricots, figs, bananas), potatoes and many others

ODA: 300–500mg.

Toxicity: Any intake above 1g should be carefully monitored. Anyone with kidney disease or heart problems, in particular needs to take care.

Selenium

Selenium is needed by all the tissues of the body. Selenium deficiency is quite common because in many parts of the world the soil is low in selenium and the result is that animals and vegetables grown on this land contains very little—and since this is what we eat and where we get our selenium from, we too are deficient.

There is very strong evidence that selenium deficiency is implicated in heart disease, AIDS and cancer—and that these problems can be rectified by adding selenium to the diet in the form of supplements. Vitamin E and selenium work together synergistically—that is, their combined effect is greater than the sum of their effects when taken separately. However, vitamin C interferes with selenium absorption so there should be a gap of an hour between taking one or the other.

People exposed to environmental pollution may become deficient as selenium is used up fighting the heavy metals. For our purposes, selenium is known to help protect cells from damage from free radicals. The best natural source of selenium is Brazil nuts—which have such a very high selenium content.

Also, a highly recommended selenium supplement is Se-methylselenocysteine (MSC) a naturally occurring selenium compound which has been demonstrated in animal and laboratory tests to cause apoptosis (natural cell death) in cancer cells.

On a personal note, 'Richard' has been a regular poster of comments on my blog (cancerfighter.wordpress.com) and he claims to have cured himself of cancer by taking high doses of vitamin C and selenium: 'I had no options, but to self-treat. If I had taken the RDA of selenium and avoided vitamin C, would I be still alive today? I don't think so! For the record I am taking 5ml of pure sodium selenite a day and 40–60 grams of pharmaceutical grade vitamin C (ascorbate acid) … now. I can report that I have no symptoms of myelofibrosis and my general health is excellent. Yesterday I played a 45-minute game of football (parents against their children). The game was extremely fast and I finished well and scored two goals. I maintain a daily regime of 30 grams of vitamin C per day, 3–4ml of selenium and 4 grams of pharmaceutical grade bicarb [bicarbonate of soda]. I recommend it to all myelofibrosis sufferers.'

Food sources: best food source is Brazil nuts.

ODA: 200–400µg (and for cancer 400–600µg—or do what Richard did).

Toxicity: Anyone taking in more than 2mg per day may suffer the effect of a garlicky odour in the breath, urine and sweat. Interestingly, birth defects may also occur at long-term intake at these levels. If you are not pregnant, very high levels of selenium can be taken and these will likely have a beneficial impact on tumour growth. Long-term intake of 500–750µg has not turned up any sign of toxicity in humans.

Vanadium

Vanadium is a trace element that has recently been discovered to have a powerful anti-cancer effect, causing cells to undergo apoptosis (natural cell death). Vanadium appears to be non-toxic at even high doses when taken as a supplement. It is cheaply available from a number of sources as it is marketed as a dietary aid. One good source is Rainbow Minerals at www.rainbowminerals.net.

Zinc

Zinc has acquired a good reputation as an immune system booster—particularly when accompanied by magnesium. However, high zinc supplementation (100mg/day) has also been associated with higher levels of prostate cancer. It is therefore best not to take more than 30mg per day.

That would have been all I could say about zinc had my attention not been drawn informally to a study that was apparently published in the *Medical Press* (details unknown) in 1953—and ever since largely neglected. This study showed that an injection of zinc and magnesium ascorbates in aqueous solution had a very profound effect on seven women with terminal cancer of the uterus. Five years later, four of them were still alive. In all, 200 terminal cancer patients received the substance, and 90 per cent were free from pain within ten days—the majority being free from pain within two days. Many demonstrated tumour regression. In addition to vitamin C, the patients all received a 3ml injection every other day. Each ml of the solution contained 1.5mg of zinc and 0.3mg of magnesium (both calculated as metal and both complexed with ascorbic acid). It is possible to find vitamin C in the form of zinc and magnesium ascorbates but, if taken orally, these would have to be taken in much larger quantities.

Food sources: Calf's liver, beef, lamb, spinach, asparagus, sea vegetables, seeds, miso, maple syrup.

ODA: 30–50mg.

Toxicity: Zinc toxicity only occurs when intake exceeds 1–2g per day. The result is gastric irritability and vomiting.

Trace minerals

Trace minerals in minute portions can powerfully affect health. Trace minerals are necessary for oxygen transport, energy metabolism, growth, and cell and nerve protection. They are essential for the assimilation and utilization of vitamins and other nutrients. They aid in the digestion process and provide the catalyst for many hormones, enzymes, and essential body functions and reactions. They aid in replacing electrolytes lost through heavy perspiration or diarrhoea. Trace minerals also protect against toxic reaction and heavy metal poisoning.

Unfortunately, important as they are, our plants and soils are so nutrient depleted, that even if we eat the healthiest foods, we are unlikely to be getting all the minerals we need. Evidence of mineral malnutrition range from minor health conditions such as energy loss, premature aging, diminished senses, to major conditions such as degenerative diseases like osteoporosis, heart disease, and cancer.

There are approximately 84 trace minerals—and every single one of them has some part to play in maintaining good health. In fact, there is a possibility that cancer is in part a deficiency disease—caused by a deficiency of trace minerals.

Trace minerals, as their name suggests, are required in very small doses—but fortunately there is one way we can get these trace minerals in exactly the amounts required for good health—because, no surprises here, the composition of the minerals we require happen to be exactly the composition as they occur in the sea. And one way, a very cheap way, of getting what we need is by dissolving unrefined sea salt—or Himalayan salt—in water and drinking it. Some more enterprising individuals have realised that shops that cater to tropical fish sell products for turning aquarium water into a close approximation of the sea by adding all these minerals. You can buy large tubs of this salt-based mix and either eat it or soak in it in a bath—because the skin is a very absorbent tissue and minerals may very well best be taken into the body transdermally.

Multi-mineral formulas

CAA capsules

These are multi-mineral and vitamin capsules formulated by an Australian farmer, Percy Weston, who was diagnosed with cancer at the age of 39. He was also at that time crippled with arthritis. He blamed these problems on the superphosphate fertilizers that he and other farmers had begun to use on their farms. The initial result was improved yields but gradually the mineral content of the soil became seriously degraded. 'At the end of five years [of using superphosphates] we had a plague of cancer lesions coming up on the ears of the sheep. It is the same condition that afflicts humans, and has the same cause.'

He discovered that the highly acidic chemical superphosphates also killed the soil bacteria and earthworms necessary for the healthy regeneration of the soil. The result was—and remains—that the majority of our food contains excessive phosphorus, and is deficient in calcium, magnesium, selenium, zinc, cobalt and trace minerals.

When his animals exhibited cancerous lesions, Percy Weston went back to using natural rock phosphate and salt containing the missing minerals. The result? His sheep healed. When he himself was diagnosed with cancer, he decided to mix together a mineral formula based on his experiences with his sheep. His cancer left him, as did his arthritis, and he went on to live to the age of 100—he was still farming at the age of 97. He was free of cancer, arthritis and heart disease to the end. He wrote an extremely important book, *Cancer: Cause and Cure*, that details his clear demonstration that one major cause—if not the main cause—of cancer is the way we grow our food. To test his theories, Weston found he was able to cause cancer in his animals at will, and he was also able to cure them every time, simply by giving his animals a diet without any trace mineral content—and then providing them with the missing trace minerals.

His multi-mineral mix (which does not, by the way, include vanadium, so this will need to be supplemented separately) should be accompanied by a diet that is low in phosphates. This largely means a diet of organic fruit and vegetables and no meat, eggs or dairy. Weston also produced another book, *Cancer Fighting Foods*, in which he lists the mineral content of most foods. His books and the multi-mineral mix are now marketed by a New Zealand company and can be ordered from www.zealandpublishing.co.nz

Beres Drops

Formulated by a Hungarian scientist, Dr Jozsef Beres, Beres Drops is a liquid formula containing a patented combination of the following ingredients: distilled water, glycerol, EDTA, glycogen, iron, L-tartaric acid, zinc, sodium, succinic acid, magnesium, manganese, L-ascorbic acid, potassium, copper, molybdenum, vanadium, nickel, boron, fluorine, chlorine, cobalt.

On September 15th 1991, the *Sunday Sun* carried the story of a Mrs Wendy Cook who claimed that three months on the drops had had the effect of shrinking a malignant tumour in her groin from 4 inches to one inch. Beres Drops are widely available from Internet suppliers.

Liquid mineral complex

The sea contains a perfect blend of minerals and this product is essentially 'purified sea water'. This is a liquid blend of 84 ionically-charged ocean minerals and trace elements. It is easily available from Internet suppliers.

Other Supplements

The following supplements are, generally speaking, natural products that help to maintain the body's natural state of health, and which have also been shown to have a positive effect in helping the body combat cancer—one of which is freely available in your own home.

Acidophilus and other 'friendly' bacteria

Did you know that you have more bacteria in your body than you have cells (and you have 75 trillion cells)? Most of these bacteria are in the gut. They are vital for the breaking down and digesting of food. They also keep other microbial predators at bay—specifically unfriendly bacteria, viruses and fungi. In fact, if you have any fungal or inflammatory attack of the urino-genital system then taking some capsules of lactobacillus acidophilus should go some way to solving the problem. Athlete's foot is also amenable. There is a healthy balance between bacteria and yeast (there are friendly yeasts too) but any sign of a yeast attack should be dealt with by taking acidophilus. They also have antibiotic properties that keep viruses under control. Polio viruses, for example, cannot survive in the presence of high concentrations of acidophilus.

Also, these bacteria help protect against cancer and even have an anti-tumour effect. Mice receiving acidophilus supplements showed 400 per cent greater macrophage activity. Macrophages are the blood components that attack cancer tumours. Animal studies show that acidophilus helps to slow down and even stop tumour growth.

A Bulgarian doctor, Dr Ivan Bogdanov, using a highly concentrated form of other bacteria, Lactobacillus bulgaricus, obtained a complete remission in one patient suffering from terminal multiple myeloma. In fact the patient was sinking into a terminal coma when treatment started. Six months later there was no sign of the disease. His only treatment was with the bacteria.

In the Bulgarian study similar results were obtained with people suffering from many types of cancer. The amounts they took on a daily basis were equivalent to eating 40–60kg of Bulgarian yoghurt. The bacteria-rich product used was called 'Anabol'. However, I have not been able to source this product. The recommended daily dose is 10–15g. More than this results in the possibility of tumour disintegration: a process which floods the body with toxic products and can kill the patient if detoxification procedures are not started immediately.

Products containing L. acidophilus and L. bulgaricus are widely available—Natren, for example (www.natren.com), has an L. bulgaricus powder and combination capsules, as does metabolics.com.

Other products can be found at the major vitamin warehouses (iherb and Vitacost)—but. in all cases, they should be kept refrigerated in the shop and at home. Potency of capsules is highly variable, so buying direct over the Internet from a good supplier is strongly advised.

Alpha lipoic acid (ALA) (with acetyl L-carnitine)

Alpha lipoic acid is a powerful antioxidant that promotes the effects of the other vitamins. Acetyl L-carnitine is a naturally occurring amino acid. In combination, these two chemicals have an established ability to counteract the effects of ageing in cells. Any substance that promotes healthy cells will work against cancer. It is particularly beneficial at repairing the damage caused by chemotherapy and radiation. ALA also helps to reprocess vitamin C.

Alpha lipoic acid promotes cell death (apoptosis) in human colon cancer cells. It increases respiration in the mitochondria and therefore increases the amount of oxygen in the cancer cell. Oxygen is toxic to cancer. One suggested dose is 1.8g.

Amino acids

Amino acids are the molecular building blocks from which proteins are built. The body contains something in the region of 50,000 different proteins and 20,000 different enzymes. These are all built up by combining 29 known amino acids in different combinations. Most of the amino acids are synthesised in the liver—another reason why a healthy liver is vital for good health. There are eight amino acids, however, known as essential amino acids, that must come from our diet. Amino acid supplementation is strongly indicated for any form of degenerative disease or indeed any mental or physical disorder such as heart disease, chronic fatigue syndrome, diabetes, epilepsy, anaemia or herpes. The amino acids that are known to be relevant in the fight against cancer—either in a curative or preventative way are:

L-arginine: This slows tumour growth and helps detoxify and heal the liver. It helps wounds to heal and helps to maintain the immune system. In large doses it may even be curative on its own. One healer, Jimmy Keller, had success with it before his work was rudely interrupted by the US legal authorities.

L-carnitine: This is a general all round amino acid that enhances the effects of vitamins E and C.

L-citrulline: This boosts the immune system, protects the liver against ammonia and is an energy booster.

L-cysteine: This is an antioxidant and a very useful protector against the harmful effects of smoking and alcohol, as well as the effects of radiation.

GABA: Gamma aminobutyric acid. This is good for anxiety, stress and depression. Better than Librium or Valium.

Glutamine: The most abundantly available amino acid. Evidence shows that it is important for natural killer (NK) cells. The more glutamine the more active the NK cells, the lower the ability of tumours to grow. Supplementing (0.3 gm/kilo of body weight) can be very beneficial. It is highly recommended for anyone undergoing radiation or chemotherapy as these deplete glutamine reserves. There are anecdotal reports of terminal cancer patients who 'stopped dying' after taking glutamine. It is recommended to take this in combination with another amino acid isoleucine.

Glutathione: This is an extremely important anti-oxidant which protects the body against the ravages of cigarettes, radiation, chemotherapy, heavy metal poisoning and the effects of drugs and alcohol. The best source of the precursors for glutathione is cold processed (or undenatured) whey and N-acetyl-cysteine.

L-lysine: Important for tissue repair and the production of antibodies, hormones and enzymes. It should be taken before, during and after any operation. This is possibly the most important anti-viral amino acid. It eliminates cold sores and herpes sores very quickly.

L-ornithine: Important for wound healing.

L-proline: Good for healing. Important for building of cell walls.

L-tryptophan: Mood stabiliser, antidepressant and stress reducer. Good for insomnia.

L-tyrosine: Antidepressant and anxiety reducer.

L-theanine: Effective against anxiety.

They should be taken on an empty stomach. There is no known toxicity: Excess amino acids are burnt off as energy or converted to fat.

Linus Pauling and his successor (as leading advocate of vitamin C) Matthias Rath claim that high doses of lysine and proline along with megadoses of vitamin C are virtually a cancer cure in themselves as these are the building blocks for collagen, the stuff of which cell walls are made. They also block the enzyme that dissolves collagen. They recommend that vitamin C be taken at a level just below bowel tolerance level, and that the same amount of lysine be taken along with about half that level of proline. A maintenance dose would be vitamin C (6g), lysine (6g) and proline (3g) but for treating cancer much higher doses are likely to be necessary—see the section on vitamin C.

Testimonials supporting the use of Rath's protocol can be found at:
www.stopping-cancer-naturally.org/us/testimonials.html.

Lysine and arginine in combination have also been demonstrated as having a beneficial effect on the production of hormones in the thymus gland—which are important for the maintenance of good health.

Cheap source of glutamine and other amino acid products: www.bulknutrition.com.

Caution: Jacob Schor, a naturopathic doctor has written that NAC (N-acetyl-cysteine) might in fact be dangerous for cancer patients in that it interferes with the actions of curcumin, selenium, vitamin D3, melatonin, ginseng and green tea among other common supplements.

Avemar

Dr Albert Szent-Györgyi (who won a Nobel Prize for his discovery of vitamin C) set out to discover why there seemed to be much lower rates of cancer in populations that consumed large amounts of whole grain products. His theory was that supplementing a natural compound found in wheat germ could prevent cancer cells from growing without affecting healthy cells. His early studies, published in the 1960s in the *Proceedings of the National Academy of Sciences USA*, showed that, in the lab at least, his theory was correct.

When communism fell in 1989, Dr Mate Hidvegi decided to pick up where Dr Szent-Györgyi had left off. He eventually discovered a way of fermenting wheat germ with brewer's yeast. He called the resulting product Avemar as a tribute to the Virgin Mary ('Ave' means 'hail' and 'Mar' means 'Mary').

Avemar has been the subject of more than 100 studies—in laboratory cell lines, with animals, and in human clinical trials—and its research has been published in more than 30 articles in respected medical peer-reviewed journals. Most of this has been looking at its benefits to cancer patients. The results are impressive. Avemar clearly not only reduces the severity of side effects of the chemotherapy but creates better outcomes in terms of reduced recurrence of the cancer—much better outcomes. In one study on oral cancers, after one year on the protocol, the group taking Avemar had a disease progression rate of less than ten per cent compared with over 60 per cent for the group not taking Avemar.

Avemar works in a number of ways. Firstly it radically reduces the ability of cancer cells to utilise glucose. Secondly it is a poly(ADP-ribose) polymerase (PARP) enzyme inhibitor. The PARP enzyme is needed by cancer cells to repair the cellular damage that frequent cell division causes. When PARP levels are depleted, another enzyme steps in and initiates apoptosis (normal cell death). It also helps the immune system to identify cancer cells so that they can be dealt with.

No studies have been done of Avemar's ability to fight cancer on its own. However, all the indications are that it would be a valuable support to any anti-cancer regime.

A product calling itself AveUltra promotes itself as an improved form of Avemar—but the company that makes Avemar denies any association with this product and questions its efficacy.

Bee Pollen and Propolis

Beekeepers don't get cancer! Several attempts to find beekeepers who had died of cancer came up virtually empty handed. Only one, in Hawaii, was found to have died of skin cancer. Russian Georgian peasants, who are noted for their longevity, are avid bee keepers.

Bee pollen is one of nature's most complete foods and has long been associated in India, China and even ancient Egypt with healing and energy. A number of animal studies have also shown that it has a strong ability to retard tumour growth. An ounce (28 grams) of bee pollen each day will, according to naturopath Diane Stein, prevent or delay the development of all malignant tumours and will help to reduce the size of existing tumours.

As for propolis, a resin gathered by honeybees from the buds and barks of certain trees and plants, this is known to have antibacterial, antifungal, antiviral, anti-inflammatory, and pain-killing properties.

In one study, propolis was found to significantly reduce two cancer markers in the blood.

Beta-glucans

Beta-D-glucans, usually referred to simply as beta-glucans, comprise a class of non-digestible polysaccharides widely found in nature in such sources as oats, barley, yeast, bacteria, algae and mushrooms. This is one of those supplements about which some debate is occurring.

According to those who like it, beta(1,3)D-glucan is a powerful stimulator of the immune system while at the same time being an effective antioxidant and free radical scavenger. Beta-glucans is safe and non-toxic and shows good effects against cancer. It is best taken with vitamin C as they work synergistically.

While most people agree with these statements, there is disagreement about whether taking this supplement is useful or a waste of money. There is also a lot of dispute about the quality of the products on the market. Some people suggest that the best way of taking it is to eat lots of porridge and/or mushrooms. Take up to 3g per day depending on your weight: 25mg per kilo of weight. Taking more than this does not provide additional benefits.

Immutol is the brand name of a purified beta-glucans product. see www.immutol.com

Brewer's yeast

Brewer's yeast is an inactive yeast that is the by-product of beer making. It is a very rich source of vitamins and minerals, particularly chromium, which regulates blood sugar. It has been described as a whole food on a par with chlorella and spirulina. It is also considered by some to be one of nature's cure-alls for everything from diabetes to, well, cancer.

Normally healthy people cannot take much brewer's yeast, as it induces nausea. Curiously though, people with cancers have been found to have a very high tolerance for relatively large quantities of this substance: half a cupful a day or more. According to the authors of information on www.pdrhealth.com:

> 'Supplementation with selenium-enriched brewer's yeast (delivering 200μg of selenium a day) over a period of several years was associated, in one study, with significant reduction in the incidence of lung, colorectal, prostate and total cancer, as well as a reduction in total cancer mortality.'

Interestingly there appears to be a connection between cholesterol levels, inflammation and cancer. A number of anti-cancer approaches are also beneficial against heart disease and arthritis. (The Budwig Protocol and Percy Weston's trace mineral product CAA both link their approach to fighting cancer as a way also of fighting heart disease and arthritis.) Brewer's yeast is another substance that has a wide range of beneficial effects including an ability to reduce serum cholesterol. Laboratory tests showed a rise in serum cholesterol was partially or totally prevented when yeast was added to the diet. The rate of reduction in cholesterol levels and cholesterol blockage was directly related to the amount of yeast consumed.

Baker's yeast is not the same and should be avoided. Panaktiv is a liquid form of brewer's yeast available from www.drmetz.de.

Citric acid

According to Mexican cancer doctor, Albert Halabe Bucay, 30–40g per day of pure citric acid crystals sprinkled over food and taken throughout the day is potentially curative (one standard tablespoon of citric acid powder per meal). Citric acid works by blocking glycolosis—the process by which sugars are converted to energy—and cancer cells are much more dependent on glycolosis than normal cells. Block glycolosis and you block the ability of cancer tumours to grow. Citric acid is cheap and widely available.

Wouldn't eating lemons be the same? Dr Halabe Bucay says no. 'Three pounds of lemon have more or less 3–5 grams of citric acid, not enough to fight cancer, as I proposed 30 to 40 grams a day for at least three months.'

Some people may find discomfort at taking in so much acid and they are advised to take standard antacids.

Co-enzyme Q10 (CoQ10)

The quinone family of chemical compounds is a very important one for cancer. One of the major chemotherapeutic drugs, Adriamycin, is a quinone. Other quinones are being tested in trials for effects against Alzheimer's and other ailments. Adriamycin is an oxidative quinone whose effects are very different from others, like CoQ10 which are anti-oxidative. Adriamycin is therefore dangerous for people with weak hearts. CoQ10 protects against this effect. Anyone undergoing chemotherapy with Adriamycin should therefore take large amounts of CoQ10.

Co-enzyme Q10 is a quinone which is found almost everywhere in nature—which is why it is called the ubiquitous quinone—ubiquinone for short. But it is present in extremely small quantities—too small to be medically useful. While many quinones have an improved immuno-strengthening effect at very small doses, ubiquinone is not one of these. CoQ10 has an increased effect with larger doses. However, it is known that people with cancer have reduced levels of CoQ10 suggesting that it is used up in fighting the tumour.

A Danish study, published in 1994, found that women with terminal breast cancer did very well when taking 390mg a day. This amount seemed to be sufficient to prevent further tumour growth and even to cause tumour shrinkage. A group of 32 women with advanced stage breast cancer were given, in addition to the normal treatments of surgery, radiation and chemotherapy, a programme of supplements including 390mg of CoQ10. Danish cancer specialist, Knud Lockwood said: 'I have never before seen spontaneous regression of the type of breast tumours that we were treating in this trial, or comparable regression on any conventional anti-cancer therapy.' There are no known toxic effects. Many people take 60–90mg a day as a general energising tonic.

CoQ10 is best taken as part of what has been called the Stockholm Protocol which included the following supplements (daily amounts): gamma linolenic acid (1.2 grams); omega 3 fatty acids (3.5 grams); beta carotene (58mg or 32,248IU); vitamin C (2.8 grams); vitamin E (2500IU); selenium (385μg); CoQ10 (390mg).

In addition, high-dose vitamin B complex should be added and the CoQ10 should ideally be taken in an oil base to aid absorption—dissolving in olive oil or coconut oil being best.

While the vitamin E level recommended here is very high and should probably be lowered after a few months, the vitamin C level of the Stockholm Protocol has been criticised for being too low, and no one should feel constrained from increasing this by four, five or even more times.

A new form of CoQ10—ubiquinol (CoQH)—delivers much higher benefits. And even better is liposomal ubiquinol. One study reportedly indicates that an intake of 400–500mg of this liquid liposomal ubiquinol was on its own sufficient to cause remission in a number of different cancers. For further information go to www.scientificliving.net.

Colostrum and Transfer Factor Plus

Colostrum is the pre-milk that new-born babies get from their mother's breast for the first few days they are breast fed. The colostrum available as a nutritional supplement is not sourced from human breasts, however, but from cows.

Colostrum contains many bioactive compounds. A recent study in Sweden focused on alpha-lactalbumin, an immune factor present in colostrum. This was found to cause cancer cells to 'commit suicide'. Colostrum also contains lactoferrin which is known to prevent or shrink cancers. Conjugated linoleic acid (CLA) and other fats found in colostrum also have anti-carcinogenic properties.

Knowledge of the benefits of bovine colostrum is not new. In India, Ayurvedic doctors have long known about its health benefits and it is so commonly used there that it is delivered by the milkman. As it is a food, there are no toxicity problems.

Some say that the reason colostrum is effective is that it contains transfer factors and that it is much more effective to take a concentrated dose of transfer factors, such as the branded formulation, Transfer Factor Plus.

Transfer factors are tiny molecules found in colostrum which provide information on immunity. If you take these molecules from a person who has recovered from a disease and give them to someone who hasn't, the second person will gain a significant degree of immunity and ability to fight back. Research on these transfer factors has been going on for over 50 years. One study into their potential for cancer patients looked at 20 terminal cancer patients whose average life expectancy was 3.7 months. The patients were given nine capsules per day of Transfer Factor Plus along with a number of other supplements: digestive enzymes, probiotics and vitamins. After eight months, 16 of these individuals were still living and were either in remission, improving or they had stabilized. There was clear evidence also that the immune system had been boosted by over 400 per cent, measured in terms of natural killer cell function.

Transfer Factor Plus can be obtained from www.my4life.com

Human breast milk has also been shown to have a strong anti-cancer effect in the laboratory, killing over 40 different kinds of cancer cell in test tube studies. One of the arsenal of compounds that helps achieve this is a protein called alpha-lactalbumin. So if you have a supply of fresh breast milk at hand, do make use of it!

DHEA

DHEA stands for dehydroepiandrosterone. It is a hormone produced in the adrenal glands. It is associated with fat burning, increasing libido and slowing down of the ageing process. DHEA production peaks around the age of 25 and then gradually decreases until, by age 80, the average person is only producing 10 per cent of that. Recently, studies suggest that it could have potent anti-cancer effects by enhancing the immune system and impeding cancer growth. In one animal study with rats implanted with a cancer causing agent, only one-third of the rats injected with DHEA went on to develop the cancer, compared with 96 per cent of the control group. It is also believed to be effective against stress.

The best time to take DHEA is the morning and dose levels of 25–50mg are recommended (a man of 25 will produce around 25mg per day).

DIM (diindolylmethane)

This is a compound molecule found in the brassica family of vegetables (broccoli, cabbage, Brussels sprouts etc). These are the vegetables that show the highest anti-cancer properties. DIM appears to work in multiple ways—it is immune boosting, anti-inflammatory, helps anti-angiogenesis and promotes apoptosis. It also controls hormones and has an anti-viral, anti-bacterial impact. All in all this probably should be one of the top choices when it comes to choosing supplements.

It is the fact that it controls oestrogen that makes it a very popular supplement with women. The recommended dose is 200–400mg per day.

One user made the following recommendation:

'When buying a DIM supplement, it is suggested that you read the label of the DIM product you're going to buy. Be certain that you are getting 120mg of DIM complex, which is standardized to 30mg DIM per dose. Because DIM is very hard to absorb, the products needs to be in a specialized complex that improves bioavailability. Although most women only need one dose of DIM per day, women suffering with a large amount of oestrogen dominance symptoms may find greater relief by doubling the dose and taking DIM twice a day. Because some women may have a minor stomach ache after taking DIM, taking the supplement with food will eliminate the problem. Research of DIM's safety has shown no harmful effects, even when the doses were at hundreds of times the amount provided in the supplements. A common side effect of DIM is a harmless changing of the colour of your urine. Because these changes can occur when you eat a large amount of broccoli or asparagus also, drinking 6–8 glasses of water per day will solve the problem.'

(breastcancer.org forums)

DMG

DMG (N-dimethylglycine) has been around a long time, but it is only recently that it is becoming widely known as being one of the most important health supporting supplements. It has a powerful and very fast impact on the immune system, which makes it a valuable support for people with AIDS and cancer.

One story demonstrating its anti-cancer potential was reported in *Preventive Medicine Magazine* in 1990. Hans Kugler, PhD, a researcher in Health Sciences, successfully treated his dog Foxie who had been diagnosed with a large abdominal tumour, using DMG. An ultrasound and blood tests had revealed the tumour was very large and had spread to the liver and kidneys. Kugler put Foxie on a daily regimen of 250mg of DMG daily, as the primary source of treatment. After six weeks the tumour had shrunk to half its original size, and continued to decrease until the twelfth week when it was barely noticeable. Later examination revealed the tumour was completely gone, and Foxie had returned to normal health.

To boost the immune system, it is recommended those with active cancer or HIV take 750mg–1g of DMG daily, sublingually (under the tongue), in between meals for 6–8 weeks. This should be taken as 2–3 capsules/tablets three times a day. Those in remission should consider taking 250mg–500mg DMG daily.

Ellagic acid

This is a naturally occurring polyphenolic constituent found in many different fruits and nuts—in red raspberries in particular, but also in strawberry, blueberry and walnuts. It is also, it seems, a highly potent anti-carcinogen which has the ability to inhibit mutations within a cell's DNA. In some studies cancer activity was stopped within 48 hours.

Normal cells have a life cycle which, like all life cycles, involves birth, maturity, old age and death. In the case of cells, when they die they are replaced. The process of natural cell death is known as apoptosis. Cancer cells, however, do not die. Instead they multiply, first dividing into 2 cancer cells, then 4, 8, 16, 32 and so on—and they all continue to live. Ellagic Acid has the effect of causing cancer cells to undergo normal cell death within a matter of days.

There is a lot of excitement about the potential benefits of this chemical, and even the American Cancer Society has not been able to ignore it—though it unhelpfully informs readers that it is not available as a supplement. Nevertheless, they are technically correct—any supplement claiming to contain ellagic acid is a fraud. However, supplements containing ellagitannins will provide the raw materials which are converted to ellagic acid in the body. The raspberry's seeds contain the highest concentrations of ellagitannin.

I would start my Internet search at www.ellagic.net and compare this product with others available from other sources. For skin cancer there is Raspex SPF-30 skin gel which is made from meeker raspberries and has strong ellagitannin content. See www.smdi.org/products.htm.

Enzymes (digestive)

The reason enzymes are important is this: digestive enzymes are produced by the pancreas. When there is cancer in the body, one of the ways the body reacts is to see it as a foreign protein that needs to be digested. Unfortunately, the cancer is an efficient producer of chemicals that destroy these enzymes. This forces the pancreas to work harder to produce more enzymes. The result can quickly be an exhausted pancreas, especially as the pancreas may have been weak in the first place.

To help the pancreas, you should drink green juices, cut back on eating meat, occasionally fast, and supplement your diet with pancreatic enzymes. Pancreatic enzymes should be taken when your system is most alkaline: namely, when you awake, and between 2–3pm in the afternoon.

There are a number of different kinds of proteolytic digestive enzyme: proteases digest proteins; lipases digest fats; and amylases help to digest carbohydrates.

Enzymes not only attack cancer cells directly, but also promote immune activity by helping stimulate production of a substance called tumour necrosis factor (TNF) which attacks cancer cells. They also interfere with metastatic activity, so stopping the cancer cells from spreading.

The most important source of proteolytic enzymes is the pancreas. Enzyme formulations often combine pancreatin with papain, a powerful enzyme derived from the papaya, and bromelain, an enzyme derived from the pineapple. These can also be bought individually.

Pancreatic enzymes should play an important part in any overall anti-cancer strategy and should be taken in large quantities. One highly-rated enzyme product is made by the German Wobe Mugos company and is marketed as Wobenzyme. The use of pancreatic enzymes was first proposed by Dr John Beard in 1902 and were the cornerstone of Dr William Kelley's anti-cancer program (see Section 3: *Cancer Research and Politics* for further details)—he cured his own terminal pancreatic cancer with their help. His enzyme formulation can be bought from www.2line.com/drkelleyHOT.html.

Dr Nicholas Gonzalez, who is now the leading proponent of the Kelley approach to cancer treatment, also uses enzymes as a central part of his cancer cure. He is said to favour pork pancreas made by www.nutricology.com. Serrapeptase is another enzyme that has strong anti-inflammatory properties, which may make it part of a useful package of anti-cancer enzymes.

Fulvic acid

Not all ancient deposits of vegetation turned into oil or coal. Some simply became what is known as humic deposits. Some of these deposits are very rich in a substance called fulvic acid. It has recently been discovered that fulvic acid is absolutely essential for plant health, and the same is true of animals and man. However, because of modern farming methods, the plants we eat are depleted of this acid. In addition to being necessary for the absorption of minerals and vitamins, fulvic acid has shown extremely powerful anti-viral activity as well as being a potent cancer fighter (it appears to interfere with a cancer tumour's ability to grow). Recent scientific investigations of this complex chemical appears to indicate that it is one of the finest electrolytes known to man; that it assists with human enzyme production and is also a very powerful anti-oxidant and free radical scavenger.

There are a number of products on the market claiming to contain fulvic acid—mainly colloidal mineral mixes. Vital Earth Minerals (www.vitalearth.org/index.htm) market the product with the best reputation, Fulvic Mineral Complex. On this website you will find an article discussing the benefits of fulvic acid.

Glyconutrients

Glyconutrients are the name given to eight essential saccharides (sugars). These are: mannose, glucose, galactose, xylose, N-acetylglucosamine, N-acetylgalactosamine, fucose (not to be confused with fructose), and N-acetylneuraminic acid. These are required to make glycoproteins, which in turn are essential for cellular communication—poor cellular communication leads to poor immune response and vice versa. Medicinal mushrooms and aloe vera are particularly high in these glyconutrients.

It is important to note that glyconutrients need to be taken every day for extended periods of time to be effective. While there are some expensive glyconutrient supplements available (e.g. those sold by Mannatech) many people make up their own inexpensive glyconutrient powder by mixing together the following in roughly equal parts: kelp powder, fenugreek powder, whey protein concentrate powder (with added enzymes is best), brewer's yeast, shark (or bovine) cartilage powder, psyllium powder and lecithin powder—add shiitake mushroom powder, cayenne pepper (optional). Buy one pound of each item and mix together thoroughly. Eat one full teaspoon twice a day. Another recommended mix consists simply of one table spoon of apple cider vinegar with one tablespoon of blackstrap molasses. Molasses is the syrup that remains after refined sugar is crystallised and extracted from sugar cane. It is a rich source of minerals and glyconutrients though its high iron content means it is not a perfect source for people with cancer—cancer cells need iron for cell division. Against that, it is high in potassium and is an alkali ash food which is good. Or, of course, you can simply take aloe vera, which is another excellent source all on its own.

Grapeseed extract

Laboratory studies have found that grapeseed extract causes colon cancer cells to undergo apoptosis (natural cell death). I don't think necessarily this is a unique effect only applicable to colon cancer cells. More likely the study focused on colon cancer cells and found an effect—one that very likely is applicable to many types of cancer cells. Note that grapeseed oil does not, as one might imagine, contain all the beneficial phytochemicals of grapeseed extract—as many of these phytochemicals are not soluble in oil.

Honokiol

Honokiol is a biphenolic compound that has been isolated from the bark and seed cones of the magnolia tree. This is a relatively new compound in terms of cancer research but early indications are that it is powerful anti-angiogenesis promoter for a wide range of cancers. It can also cross the blood-brain barrier so it could be used to slow or reverse the growth of brain cancers.

HonoPure is a product with 98 per cent honokiol. For more information go to www.HonoPure.com.

Recommended therapeutic dose: three grams per day in divided doses, with food.

Human growth hormone (HGH)

There is a lot of controversy about the value of HGH and it's worth doing your own research, but one report from a man called 'Dave' on a yahoo chat group told of the following experience: 'I have leukaemia, was given chemo, and seven years later, the leukaemia began to return, I discovered accidentally that if I took half a unit human growth hormone, daily, it boosted my immune system, red blood cells and platelets about forty per cent. That's been five years ago.' He later switched to low-dose-naltrexone (LDN—see below for details)—for reasons of cost and found it to be just as effective. Dave also found that HGH helped healing when he severely bruised a shoulder in a bicycle accident.

Lactoferrin

Lactoferrin is used for treating a wide range of conditions ranging from intestinal ulcers to hepatitis C. It is also used as an antioxidant and to protect against bacterial and viral infections. It promotes healthy bacteria in the intestines and is a powerful immune booster. It is also very important for the proper regulation of iron delivery to cells and bone marrow production. It also has strong anti-fungal effects and so should be taken by anyone suffering from candida.

The fact that it is a key element of mother's milk and colostrum tells us that it is an important health booster, and there are many anecdotal reports of its health benefits—and that includes cancer.

Lactoferrin can be bought as a supplement and suggested doses are anywhere from 40 to 250mg per day. Make sure it is undenatured. Alternatively you can buy colostrum powder.

Lycopene

Lycopene is a caretenoid that is found in tomatoes and a number of other vegetables/fruit: red guava, red grapefruit, red pepper, watermelon, papaya and sweet potatoes. High lycopene intake is associated with lowered incidences of prostate and colon cancer. Some studies indicate that upping intake of cooked tomatoes is beneficial. In one anecdotal case, a 62-year-old man with advanced prostate cancer experienced regression of his tumour after taking 10mg of lycopene per day and 300mg of saw palmetto three times per day.

Melatonin

Until recently, the functions of the pineal gland have remained pretty much a mystery. However, melatonin, the pineal gland's chief hormone, is now receiving a lot of attention. For one thing it is now known to regulate the circadian rhythm, the body's biological clock. It is used as an antidote to jet-lag and as a supplement that is helpful in reducing anxiety, panic attacks and migraines, in addition to being an effective sleeping pill, especially as a safe way to get insomniac children to sleep. It does not have the side effects of other sleeping pills and does not interfere with REM (rapid eye movement) dream states.

Now, new studies are suggesting that it also bolsters the immune system, keeps our cells in a good state of repair, is an powerful anti-oxidant (five times more powerful than vitamin C), protects against electromagnetic radiation and the toxicity of chemotherapy, slows the growth of tumours and cataracts and keeps heart disease at arm's length. As one cellular biologist, who takes 1mg every night, said in a *Newsweek* article 'I want to die young as late in life as possible, and I think this hormone could help.' (*Newsweek*, Aug 7, 1995)

An Italian study has shown that a nightly 10mg dose has significantly improved one-year survival rates of metastatic lung cancer.

While no one is suggesting that melatonin on its own is a cure for cancer, they are saying it is an important weapon. As we grow older we secrete less and our sleep patterns become disrupted. And sleeplessness leads in the long term to ill health. Research shows that tumours are switched on during the day and switched off at night. The longer the day (i.e., exposure to light), the longer the cancer cells are switched on. Dr David Blask, who has researched the impact of sleep on cancer, says: 'With constant light, tumours grow seven times faster and soak up incredible amounts of linoleic acid, During the day, the cancer cells are awake and linoleic acid stimulates their growth. But at night cancer cells go to sleep. When we turn on lights at night for a long time, we suppress melatonin and revert back to the daytime condition.'

This may explain why nurses who often work the night shift have higher rates of breast and colon cancer.

To be effective, melatonin must be taken at night before going to bed. Most people get good effects from doses of 1–10mg but there is no sign of any toxicity at higher doses, and some therapists are using as much as 50mg doses as part of their protocol. No scientist has yet developed a concentration capable of killing a mouse, and human volunteers who took 6g a day for a month, merely reported some stomach discomfort and residual sleepiness. As one researcher noted, 'Its nastiest side effect is sleepiness.'

Roger Coghill, a scientist who runs his own laboratory in Wales, believes that melatonin is the secret to longer lives—but he also believes that doses in the one gram and more range are not the way to take it. He believes that the best way is to take it in its natural food form: banana, super green drinks, peanuts—or, even better, in the form of Asphalia, his trade name for a food supplement made entirely from Festuca arundinacea, a meadow grass with the highest known physiological level of plant melatonin in the world. St John's Wort is another melatonin-rich botanical which aids sleep and is often used as an antidepressant.

However, Dr Steve Martin makes the point that melatonin is not very bioavailable when taken as a pill. He believes it should be dissolved in milk along with vitamin D3 and taken at night for best results. He suggests 5,000IU of vitamin D3 along with 6mg of melatonin as a breast cancer prevention regime, but for those who already have breast cancer, especially oestrogen dependent cancer, then much higher amounts of both should be taken.

Other sleep aids: tryptophan, lavender essential oil, St John's Wort herb, valerian herb, Miracle Mineral Supplement (sodium chlorite). Two writers to a health group I subscribe to raved about their sleep-promoting protocols. One claimed benefits from a combination of a calcium-magnesium tablet with a few tablets of brewer's yeast. The other protocol was 600mg of tyrosine, 200mg of tryptophan with zinc and kelp (amounts unspecified). All of these, unlike sleeping pills, promote a deep, restful, natural sleep.

Methyl jasmonate

This is a chemical found in jasmine oil—and also in grape skins. Indeed it is one of the major odour components of jasmine. Research published in *Nature*, the scientific journal, (published online 14 August 2003) determined that methyl jasmonate was a highly efficient attacker of leukaemia, breast and melanoma cancer cells. This chemical needs to be dissolved in distilled water and inhaled through a steam vapour inhaler. [**Warning**: Do not swallow it, as this is dangerous.] It is recommended that this should be done once a week for a number of months. More frequent inhalations should be avoided at first because there is a danger of overpowering the body with toxic breakdown products. This chemical is considered to be highly effective. For product and more information go to www.methyljasmonate.com.

Modified Citrus Pectin (MCP)

Scientists at Columbia University have recently published a paper showing that MCP stops the growth of prostate cancer cells in the laboratory. This effect was seen in both hormone-dependent and hormone-independent forms of the disease. Pectin is found in many fruits, including citrus fruits. It is what we use to make jam set, and is found mostly in the pips and the pith of citrus fruits. The pectin in MCP has been changed to make it easier for the body to take it in through the gut. Two newly developed forms of MCP are marketed as PectaSol and PectaSol-C.

OGF (opioid growth factor or met-enkephalin)

When required, the body naturally produces morphine-like substances known as endorphins which have numerous functions ranging from control of pain and mood, to regulation of the immune system, growth of cells and angiogenesis. One endorphin that has been studied extensively in relationship to cancer is known as 'met-enkephalin'. Because met-enkephalin has been shown to control growth of cells, it is often referred to as opioid growth factor, or OGF.

OGF does not directly destroy cancer cells and is not cytotoxic. It does, however, slow down the growth of the cells and is thought to allow immunological mechanisms (e.g. macrophages, natural killer cells) to accomplish the task of destroying the cancerous cells. Over the last 25 years a great deal of research has been done, and it seems that it has very beneficial effects against cancer, but large-scale human studies have not been done because it is a natural, non-patentable substance so there is no commercial incentive.

> 'OGF appears to be an extraordinarily promising agent in the therapy of cancer. Phase I studies have determined an excellent safety profile, which is practically unrivalled in the field of oncology therapeutics. Furthermore, OGF has been demonstrated to exert beneficial effects on the immune system, thus eliminating fears of long-term damage to the body and immunity.' (medInsight Research Institute report)

OGF is administered by injection—either intravenous or subcutaneous. It can be self-administered at home.

One source for OGF is Biofactor GMBH in Germany, where it is sold under the name LUPEX®, intended for human use in cancer, AIDS and autoimmune diseases, Biofactor Tel.: +49 5322 96 05 14; Fax: +49 5322 30 17; email info@biofactor.de.

Another source for OGF is Netzah Israel Pharmacy in Tel Aviv, Israel. Fax: +972-3-7617329; email pharmacy@medinisrael.com.

Quercetin

Quercetin is a flavonoid which is found in apples, onions, and black tea—and it may be the reason why eating two apples a day has been touted as a natural way to prevent cancer. Quercetin has demonstrated a wide range of health benefits in areas as diverse as asthma and heart disease. In relation to cancer it has also been suggested that it is a potent anti-cancer agent and should be seen, as one Mayo Clinic researcher commented, as a 'chemopreventive and/or chemotherapeutic agent for prostate cancer'. However, its benefits are not confined to prostate cancer.

For anti-cancer effects a daily intake of a minimum of 1.5g (in divided doses) is necessary, though no negative side effects are associated with intake levels three or four times more than this.

Resveratrol

Resveratrol is an antioxidant found in grape skins—particularly the skin of the red grape—raspberries, mulberries and also peanuts. It functions as an antifungal agent. It has also been found to be a very powerful anti-cancer agent promoting cell death in cancer cells. Laboratory tests have clearly demonstrated that resveratrol may help prevent both heart disease and cancer. Resveratrol is widely available as a nutritional supplement but the question of how much is needed to prevent or attack cancer is not known. When buying resveratrol, check carefully the amount per serving and choose the highest dose you can find. Longevinex is the most highly-rated brand at www.longevinex.com—note that this also contains quercetin. A good mix.

Salvestrol

Salvestrols are a class of phytonutrients that, in humans, are used by a specific enzyme specific to cancer tumours (the CYP1B1 enzyme) to initiate a cascade of processes, including apoptosis, that result in the arrest or decline of the cancer.

An article in the *Journal of Orthomolecular Medicine* ('Nutrition and Cancer: Salvestrol Case Studies', 4th quarter 2007) documents the successful use of salvestrol (a formulation developed by two UK scientists) against cancer. Patients with inoperable lung cancer, melanoma, prostate cancer, breast cancer and bladder cancer took this new product and recovered, surprising their doctors no end (as always).

Salvestrol should be supplemented with biotin, magnesium, niacin, iron and vitamin C, as well as an organic vegetarian diet and exercise.

This is certainly a supplement to consider for a period of two to three months. An average adult should take around 4,000 points (the unit of measure used) per day.

SOD

SOD (superoxide dismutase) is known to be a highly effective protector against free radicals. There is only one product on the market at present that is effective in getting SOD past the digestive barriers. This is a cantaloupe extract combined with a wheat germ extract called GlisSODin.

Urea/urine therapy

Urea is a substance found both in the blood and the urine. High urea levels are associated with good health. While urea itself can be bought cheaply, the best source is in the form of whole urine. That's right. You should drink your own pee! Urine is not dirty, as many people imagine. It is packed full of agents that help combat bacteria, viruses and fungi. Applied to burns and wounds, it speeds up healing. It's free and it's healthy.

We've probably all laughed when we read of an Indian Prime Minister or a Chinese businessman extolling the virtues of drinking their own urine. But there are good reasons to suppose that it is good medicine. Certainly, we shouldn't laugh. Morarji Desai, once Prime Minister of India, lived to the ripe old age of 99 all the while extolling the virtues of a daily glass of his own urine. Over 200,000 Japanese gargle or drink urine every day and this therapy is promoted by Japan's Miracle Cup of Life Institute. Urine drinking is also catching on in Europe, particularly in Germany. In India it goes by the name Shivambu therapy.

One proponent of urine drinking is Hong Kong businessman Lee Hak-shing, who claims to have cured himself of a number of ailments including rheumatism, headaches, bladder stones and skin allergies. A Japanese doctor, Dr Ryoichi Nakao explains this effect by noting that urine contains interferon, a natural immune substance found in the body.

Auto-urine therapy (i.e., drinking one's own urine) is a health modality that has a lot of research behind it, all indicating favourable results for a wide range of health issues. And interest in urine is not confined to China, Japan and India. In America, Dr Burzynski, who developed the antineoplaston therapy (see Section 3: *Cancer Research and Politics*), derives his peptides not from blood but from urine. He says: 'Urine is not really waste material, but probably the most complex chemical mixture in the human body, and therefore it can deliver us virtually any information about the body. So from the cybernetic point of view it is just a treasure of information.' Blood is not such a complex mixture as it contains fewer chemicals. So urine tests reveal more about the body than blood tests.

The use of chemicals derived from urine, is not new. During the Second World War, British cancer researchers tested a urine-derived product that they called H11 and used it on 243 terminal cases. Forty per cent of the cases apparently recovered. However, what exactly this product contained is not known, as the research did not receive any support, and the details that have survived are very sketchy.

One of the major constituents of urine is urea. The average adult human excretes about an ounce of urea a day. One Greek doctor, Evangelos Danapoulos, has treated cancers in and around the eye by injecting urea, with, he claims, almost complete success. Urea has no side effects. In animal studies, urea has been injected directly into tumours, particularly melanomas, with the result that they regressed or were eliminated.

While Danapoulos claims it is virtually non-toxic, American researchers suggest that the maximum concentration to be used should be 40 per cent.

Urea can also be taken orally, and this has, it is claimed, a strong beneficial effect on the liver and through that to the lungs. One way to make it more effectively distributed to other tissues and organs is to mix the urea with creatine hydrate, a chemical that also has a history of being used to fight cancer, being the supposedly active ingredient of a now much-maligned anti-cancer drug known as Krebiozen.

Directions for mixing: 28 grams of urea are dissolved in 0.9l of water. This mix is divided into seven portions. One portion is drunk every 90 minutes through the waking day. This can be taken with 3.5 grams of creatine hydrate, divided into seven doses of 0.5g. It has an unpleasant taste so you may want to have something to eat at hand.

Or you can, as many Indians, Chinese, Malays, Japanese, Germans and others do, and drink your own urine. Walter Last, an Australian natural therapist, says this: 'I also know personally of several cases of cancer cures exclusively or mainly due to urine therapy; sometimes the addition of urine therapy to a natural cancer program appeared to be responsible for the successful outcome.'

Walter Last recommends a urine fast as a great way to heal almost anything. During the fast, the only liquid taken in is one's own urine. All the urine excreted should be drunk. Non-chlorinated water should be added if necessary to bring the total liquid intake to five litres.

For those who object to drinking their own urine, there is a company in India that proclaims the virtues of cow's urine and sells a number of products derived from it: www.cowurine.com.

Methylglyoxal

Another constituent of urine is Methylglyoxal (CH_3-CO-CH=O or $C_3H_4O_2$), an organic compound found in many food items. This substance has had an interesting history as a potential cancer treatment—but each time the research has threatened to show the effectiveness of this compound, it has been sidelined.

Dr William Koch (1885–1967) was one of the first to investigate this area, and he was able to produce a 'reagent'—which he called glyoxilide—that was successful in curing a number of cancer cases—except for those that had previously been treated with radiation. The full story of his attempts to get his treatment accepted is provided at www.williamfkoch.com. His failure to do so made him so furious that he refused to provide any details of his later research. He kept his formula a secret. In short, he went into one of the great sulks of cancer history. Albert Szent-Györgi, of vitamin C fame, also appears to have isolated the substance and discovered its anti-cancer effects. However, once again nothing came of this research. More recently, it was investigated by a team of cancer researchers in Calcutta led by Prof. Manju Ray with seemingly extraordinary results.

In 2001, Indian biochemist, Prof. Manju Ray, trialled the drug on 19 patients with 'very advanced stages' of cancer. Of these, all of whom would normally have died within months, only three did in fact die; five had their cancers stabilised, and eleven were effectively cured. Further studies resulted in an overall cure rate of 70 per cent in cancer patients who were diagnosed as terminally ill. It is very likely the cure rate would higher if taken at earlier stages.

Even better, methylglyoxal, unlike other chemotherapy drugs, is virtually non-toxic for normal cells. As a cancer drug, it works by starving cancer cells of ATP (adenosine-5-triphosphate). Cancer cells require large amounts of ATP to fuel their growth.

'We have what we think magic bullet against cancer,' says Manju Ray. So far, it has been found to work against colon cancer, acute myeloid leukaemia, non-Hodgkin's lymphoma, and cancers of ovary, breast, liver, lung, bone, gall bladder, pancreas and oral cavity.

The drug was developed by the Indian Association for the Cultivation of Science (IACS), a Calcutta (Kolkata)-based research organisation. They were funded by the Department of Science and Technology and the Council of Scientific and Industrial Research. For many people, this itself is a major problem, as IACS is not a medical institute, and professional egos have been severely ruffled. This is of course not the first time that the discoveries of biochemistry have been attacked by the medical profession. Vituperative attacks were published in the Indian press, and little has appeared in print since then.

However, Prof. Ray stands by her claims. According to her, chemists have known about the methylglyoxal molecule for about four decades and its anti-cancer effects in animals have also been studied. 'But surprisingly, no one bothered to initiate further research leading to human trials,' she said. Her lack of surprise comes from the fact that methylglyoxal is not patentable. No one is interested in doing research on possible anti-cancer cures that won't make big profits.

Researchers were initially concerned about the possible dangers of methylglyoxal, but when it is taken in combination with protective agents such as ascorbic acid and vitamins, it had no major toxic effect.

The problem, however, is how to get hold of this drug and what dose levels to take it in. As yet it is not widely available. However, against this picture of a side-effect-free cure all, a less attractive image is appearing. Dr Vincent Gammill who has used methylglyoxal has this to say: 'I don't recommend methylglyoxal for general use. There is too much of a risk of formaldehyde in the manufacturing process, it is easily oxidised, and it can be toxic. It does have its uses and I occasionally use it—maybe ten per cent of the time. It is not curative, it is expensive.' He also warns of a potential for harm to eyes, pancreas and heart. 'The incautious use of methylglyoxal would certainly increase the risk of rapid ageing.' Enquiries can be made to Dr Vincent Gammill at the Center for the Study of Natural Oncology (www.natural-oncology.org).

However, a German doctor, Dr Dieter Reinstorff, has gone back to the Koch research and has prepared a homoeopathic formula that appears to be methylglyoxal-based and that he calls SSR Super Quinone. At US$300 a course of 14 vials, this is quite expensive. For more details contact Dr Dieter Reinstorff, Bruno-Lauenroth Weg 31, 22417 Hamburg, Tel.: 040/ 5 20 25 02; Fax: 040/5 20 33 10.

Two other methylglyoxal products that are available and may be useful are Koch's TMT homoeopathic remedies, and a methylglyoxal MG Concentrate, which can be bought from www.gethealthyagain.com.

Or it may be that simply drinking one's own urine will provide sufficient quantities to effect a cure.

Two recent books on the benefits of urine therapy for those who wish to follow up on this subject are *The Miracles of Urine Therapy* by Dr Beatrice Bartnett, and *Your Own Perfect Medicine* by Martha Christy.

Other Anti-Cancer Formulations

In this chapter I will be looking at a number of miscellaneous formulations and approaches many of which have been specifically developed to attack cancer directly. Some of these make use of natural products, while others will appear to be highly unnatural. Nevertheless, they all claim a significant degree of success in treating cancer. Also in this list are drugs that have been found, serendipitously, to have an anti-cancer effect although they are not normally used against cancer.

Active hexose correlated compound (AHCC)

AHCC is made from a combination of hybridized Japanese medicinal mushrooms. There are reports that a number of cancer patients suffering from breast, prostate, and other forms of cancer have experienced dramatic improvement and even full remission after taking AHCC.

Most of the research has been done in Japan where AHCC was developed. In one study of five breast cancer cases given 3g of AHCC a day, two (40 per cent) had gone to complete remission by the end of the eight- month study. It should be noted that participants in these kinds of study have usually been considered terminal. This is an astonishing result. AHCC is widely available from Internet herbal suppliers.

There are a number of other mushroom extract formulations that have shown effectiveness either alone or, more commonly, as supporting therapies for people undergoing chemotherapy. Among these are PSK (This is the Japanese name. It is also known in China as PSP), Ganoderma, MycoSoft and others. There appears to be clear evidence that these formulations make chemotherapy more bearable and at the same time improve survivability rates.

Bentonite clay

This clay has a strong healing effect and should be plastered over a malignant skin tumour. See photographs at www.silvermedicine.org/clay-cansema-silver1.html.

Beta sitosterol

Beta-sitosterol is a very common phytosterol. It is widely distributed in the plant kingdom and found in such botanicals as saw palmetto, pumpkin seed and pygeum africanum. It is specifically recommended in the case of prostate cancers. Double-blind clinical trials have demonstrated that it is highly effective on its own against prostate problems. In various studies, dose levels of 20–130mg per day have completely reversed enlarged prostates. It is also known that beta-sitosterol can reverse colon cancer and lymphocytic leukaemia. It is also a general booster of the immune-system. Athletes are using it to help reduce inflammation caused by intense physical workouts.

CanCell

The story of CanCell is one of the quirkiest in all the annals of alternative cancer cures. The original formula for CanCell was developed in 1936 by James Sheridan, a chemist. He called his discovery 'Entelev'. Later it was taken up and modified by Edward Sopcak in 1984.

It was Sopcak who called his version CanCell. Sopcak and Sheridan shared an interesting and un-American idiosyncrasy. Neither of them wished to profit from their cancer cure and so would give it away free to anyone who asked. This idealistic stance, however, could not last forever. In recent years, a number of products that are 'CanCell-like' are for sale over the Internet: Cantron, Protocel, and Entelev are three competing products. (It is also marketed as Sheridan's Formula, Jim's Juice and Crocinic Acid). The formulas of all these products are slightly different and it may be worth trying a second if the first doesn't appear to be having an effect. Cantron is apparently closer to the original formula than some of the others.

There are even competing theories as to why it works. Sheridan, himself, believed it worked by interfering with the respiration of the cancer cell, while in Sopcak's view it interfered with the cancer cell on the level of vibrational energy causing it to self-digest. Neither Sheridan nor Sopcak claimed that their product was a cancer cure-all. On the contrary, they have consistently claimed a 50–55 per cent success rate.

Side effects are apparently minimal.

The main problem with CanCell is that it conflicts with a wide range of vitamins, minerals, herbs, etc.—many of which are also recommended against cancer, chief amongst them vitamin C, CoQ10 and flaxseed oil. The full list of things to be avoided can be found at the CanCell home page at www.alternativecancer.us, but the following items top that list: CoQ10, vitamin E, vitamin C, selenium, Essiac, ozone, ellagic acid, IP-6, L-carnitine, glutathione, glutamine, sea silver, lipoic acid, creatine, taurine, acetylcysteine, L-cysteine, ginseng, 714-X, hydrogen peroxide, and colloidal silver.

Since, according to testimonies, this is such an effective way of dealing with cancer, it is probably worth choosing this option and monitoring effects closely. If it works, good; if not, then move on to something else.

Protocel is now sold simply as a dietary supplement that will rid the body of 'unwanted and unproductive cells' at www.protocel.com. They have two formulas, of which Formula 50 is considered more powerful. Cantron can be obtained at www.cantron.com.

Cansema/TumorX Salve

These powerful anti-cancer products are pastes made from the herb bloodroot (Sanguinaria canadensis)—see discussion of bloodroot in Section 5: *Cancer: Herbs, Botanicals and Biological Therapies.*

Carnivora

Carnivora is an extract from the digestive juices of the Venus Flytrap. This plant is very good at digesting animal proteins, and it caught the attention of a German oncologist by the name of Helmut Keller. Dr Keller has tested out carnivora on both animals and humans at his clinic in Germany—with good results. Carnivora contains a powerful chemical, plumbagin, which has demonstrated clear anti-viral and anti-cancer properties in independent tests. It does this by promoting the cellular production of hydrogen peroxide. It is also a powerful healer—yet it is virtually harmless, so much so that Russians have suggested it can be used as a food preservative. Self-administered venus flytrap juice is not advised, as it contains other chemicals that can cause unpleasant side effects. Keller's carnivora has been purified and is non-toxic.

All research on carnivora has been done with injectible extracts. Capsules are available on the Internet but their effectiveness is unknown. The drug can be obtained from the Carnivora Research Co., www.carnivora.com

Cesium therapy (also known as high pH therapy)

This is becoming an increasingly popular approach to the treatment of cancer. It was first promoted in the 1970s and 1980s by Dr Keith Brewer, and is therefore also referred to as Dr Brewer's high pH therapy. Brewer noted that cesium, one of the basic chemical elements, was one of the few chemicals that could enter cancer cells—indeed it was readily sucked up by cancer cells—and this uptake was further enhanced by vitamins A and C, as well as zinc and selenium salts. Inside the body it has the effect of making the cells more alkaline.

When the quantity of cesium taken up was sufficient to raise the cell pH to 8 (a very alkaline state) the cancer cells stopped dividing and soon died. In animal and human tests it has been found that large tumour masses start to shrink over a period of a few weeks. 'Also,' Brewer reported, 'all pains and effects associated with cancer disappeared within 12 to 36 hours; the more chemotherapy and morphine the patient had taken, the longer the withdrawal period.'

The basic argument of cesium therapy is the same as for the alkaline pH diet (see Section 4: *Cancer: Detox and Diet*). Cancer cells arise out of an acidic tissue environment and are cured by the simple expedient of returning the cells and their environment to a highly alkaline state.

Take 3–9 grams a day of CsCl [Cesium Chloride] or Cs2CO3 [Cesium Carbonate] along with vitamin C (4–30 grams), and any zinc and selenium salt such as zinc citrate (60–100mg) or selenium (200–800μg). These have a dramatic effect on the uptake of the cesium salt by the cancer cell. The cesium should always be taken with food. The presence of cesium salts in the body fluids helps also to neutralize the acidic and toxic material leaking from the tumour mass, and this reduces the risks of toxaemia. This is an important point as some otherwise successful regimes kill the cancer but also kill the patient with the toxic wastes that are suddenly released into the body.

However, a major drawback of cesium therapy is that it can easily cause heart problems since it uses up tissue potassium rapidly. For this reason, potassium supplementation is absolutely vital. One person who took cesium with apparently successful results reported that he took the following additional supplements: potassium (3g or more), magnesium (1g), CoQ10 (400mg), pancreatin (10g), Neprinol—a combination of nattokinase and serrapeptase enzymes (20 caps), taurine (1g).

These supplements must be continued for at least three months after use of cesium has been discontinued as it stays in the body, depleting potassium levels for that length of time.

Potassium is the problem as cesium is known to deplete the body's supplies (and we need 2–4g a day) but taking too much potassium can also be problematic.

Side effects of cesium can include tingling around the lips, diarrhoea, constant sweating and other side effects that relate to the die off of cancer cells. It also has a tendency to increase the uric acid levels of the blood which can have a harmful impact on the kidney so uric acid levels need to be monitored carefully. It is best to consult with a sympathetic doctor so that regular tests can be done to ensure all is well while on this regime. One solution is to take the pharmaceutical drug Xyloprim (allopurinol) both before and at the same time as cesium is being taken, so that excessively high values of uric acid do not develop. A natural alternative uric-acid lowering regime (recommended on www.highuricacid.org) involves drinking lots of water; eating 20–30 cherries a day; drinking two glasses of apple cider (not the vinegar, the cider itself); taking a green drink, and eating high-fibre foods.

Cesium can also be taken through the skin. One suggestion is to dampen the skin with DMSO and then spray the cesium on. Use areas of skin close to the tumour or soft areas (i.e., under the arm) where absorption can be maximised. Alternatively dissolve the cesium in the DMSO before putting on the skin.

It sounds like this should be the eureka cancer cure. Unfortunately, clinics working with advanced cancer patients report that only about 50 per cent appear to benefit (though this is exciting in its own right). It has been suggested that the benefits of cesium chloride, or alternatively, ionic cesium, can be enhanced by a low-carbohydrate diet.

Cesium chloride and ionic cesium can be bought from a number of suppliers such as www.rainbowminerals.net and www.cesium-chloride.com.

An alternative way of raising the pH is to take modified liquid silicon. This is marketed as MLS-02. This product has a pH of 14 in its concentrated form but in a two per cent solution the pH drops to 11. Other chemicals with this pH level would be highly toxic, but MLS-02 is claimed to be completely benign and can be used topically on the skin or ingested. For further information go to www.arrowheadhealthworks.com/mLs02.htm.

Yet another alternative is to take a teaspoon of sodium bicarbonate in water or mixed with blackstrap molasses. It is best to take it at night before going to bed as the alkalinity will interfere with the stomach acid needed to digest food.

Finally, it should be said that the increased alkalinity of the body in persons on a long-term treatment with cesium seems to retard the aging process. Dr Keith Brewer himself started taking CsCl at the age of 87 and at the age of 92 pronounced himself to be fitter, healthier and much more vigorous than five years previously.

There is a cesium therapy discussion group at the yahoo health groups site: http://health.groups.yahoo.com/group/cesiumtherapy.

Cimetidine

In 1979, *The Lancet* carried a letter from two doctors at Nebraska University describing the curious fact that two of their cancer patients had both had spontaneous remissions while taking the non-prescription drug cimetidine, also known as Tagamet, commonly used to treat heartburn. One had squamous cell carcinoma and the other large cell lung cancer. In August 1982, three other doctors reported in *The Lancet* that a patient with stage 4 malignant melanoma had started taking 1g of cimetidine and had had an almost instantaneous recovery, with tumours disappearing within a few weeks (Thornes R D, Lynch G, Sheehan M V. 'Cimetidine and coumarin therapy of melanoma'. *Lancet* 1982; ii: 328). Over the years there have been a number of similar anecdotes with a wide range of cancers.

This would appear to be a no-brainer. It's relatively safe though it does have the potential to interact with other drugs and in males there is the possibility of breast enlargement. Against that it could be remarkably effective. For a more extended discussion, follow this link: www.second-opinions.co.uk/cimetidine.html.

Cimetidine reactivates the immune response against cancer, (and to HIV and other diseases) while inhibiting angiogenesis and the growth of cancer cells. The standard daily dose is 800mg a day (200mg four times a day).

Colloidal silver

Colloidal silver is a powerful antibiotic and anti-viral agent and so is a useful preventative against almost any kind of infection. It disables the enzyme that one-celled bacteria, viruses and fungi need for their oxygen metabolism while in no way harming normal cells.

It is also possible that colloidal silver might have a beneficial effect on cancerous tissues, forcing the cancer cells to return to their undifferentiated state. An orthopaedic surgeon Robert O Becker found that a low current (high currents promote cancer growth) passed between two pure silver electrodes had the side effect, in one of his patients that he was treating, of curing his cancer.

Whether or not colloidal silver has the same effect has not absolutely been demonstrated. Indeed the problem would be to ensure that the colloidal silver reached the site of the tumour.

There are two main issues relating to the use of silver. The first is whether colloidal silver—a solution containing microscopically small particles of silver—or ionic silver, a solution of silver ions, is best. One head-to-head test came out firmly on the side of ionic silver. However, most solutions are likely to contain both colloidal and ionic silver.

The other question is that of side effects. Silver is generally recognised to be wholly non-toxic. However, the intake of silver salts can lead to a cosmetic condition called argyria, in which the skin becomes silvery grey in colour. It must be stressed that there is absolutely no evidence that the intake of pure colloidal or ionic silver will result in argyria.

In any case, argyria can be treated both by lasers and/or with a self-administered vitamin and mineral chelation therapy (for details see: eytonsearth.org/forum/about7.html).

Many people make their own colloidal silver using simple and fairly inexpensive equipment which can be bought on the Internet. However, machines that use thin strips of silver wire should be avoided—silver rods are best. Store bought colloidal silver solution can be very variable in quality. It may be better to buy a colloidal silver concentrate and dilute it with distilled water. In this way you have control over the concentration required. For more information about colloidal silver makers go to the Transformation Technologies at www.braintuner.com.

The question of delivery of colloidal silver within the body is usually assumed to be by ingestion. However, if the problem relates to infected lungs then delivering the colloidal silver via a nebuliser—a device used mainly by asthmatics that converts liquid medicine into an aerosol mist —may be preferred. However, if the lung condition is serious make sure you have qualified medical personnel at hand as the impact may be very quick and the immediate response of the body may be negative.

Dichloroacetate (DCA)

In January 2007, an article in *New Scientist* magazine alerted the world to what may be a cheap, out of patent, cure for cancer. In lab. tests conducted at the University of Alberta, the drug, DCA, which has been used for many years to treat a number of rare metabolic disorders, was found to kill cancer cells in vitro and also in animal studies.

In cancer cells, the mitochondria, which in normal healthy cells are the energy factories, have been switched off. The cancer cell, instead, gets its energy through an inefficient process of glycolysis which requires large amounts of glucose. The mitochondria also control the process of apoptosis (normal programmed cell death). DCA appears to reawaken the mitochondria—and this in turn switches on apoptosis—causing the cancer cells to die. The drug is taken orally in water and is fairly safe though there are some uncomfortable side effects including pain or numbness. Nevertheless, it does appear to be a true cure for cancer. However, I am not holding my breath against the day it will be a standard treatment.

For leukaemia, Steve Martin recommends a daily intake of the following combination: DCA (12mg per kilo of body weight), caffeine (600mg), sodium selenite 1g (5 × 200mg), and vitamin B1 (2–4g). This is a standalone formula and must not, he says, be accompanied by any anti-oxidant supplements.

Digitalis

Digitalis is a well-known extract from the foxglove and is used for certain heart conditions. A number of cancer researchers have discovered that it also has a very potent anti-cancer effect for a wide variety of cancers. It appears to work by inducing apoptosis (natural cell death). It is currently available in two forms, one of which has no anti-cancer effect. Digitoxin (from Digitalis purpurea) is effective; the similarly named, and now more commonly used, Digoxin (from Digitalis lanata) has no anti-cancer effect.

In 1974, Dr Bjorn Stenkvist of University Hospital, Uppsala, Sweden, started a long-term study on digitalis. He discovered that of the 44 patients (all of whom had breast cancer) who were on digitalis there was only one recurrence after five years compared with almost 25 per cent of the control group who did not take digitalis (21 patients out of a group of 88). The digitalis had reduced recurrence of cancer by 90 per cent. Twenty-two years later Stenkvist revisited his patients and discovered that of his digitalis group only six per cent had died from breast cancer compared with almost fifty per cent of the control group. Details of this and other research supporting the use of Digitoxin can be found at www.second-opinions.co.uk/ heart_drugs.html. As Dr Wayne Martin has commented, 'Digitalis is the right drug being used to treat the wrong disease.'

Dipyridamole and anticoagulant drugs

A cancer that doesn't spread to other sites does not kill the host. If we can impede metastasis to other sites then we have a good way of attacking cancer. The drugs that I will now discuss, which are currently used for various heart conditions, all appear to have the additional effect of impeding metastasis.

Dipyridamole is a drug widely-used in treating patients who have survived an episode of coronary thrombosis. It has very few if any side effects. In *The Lancet* (March 23, 1985, p. 693), E H Rhodes et al. of St Hilaire and Kingman Hospital in Surrey, reported that for the previous 11 years they had been maintaining 30 grade III and IV melanoma patients on dipyridamole (300mg a day). The five-year survival rate for the whole group was 77 per cent. None of the level III patients had died. Compare this with an expected five-year survival for level IV melanoma of 32 per cent.

Dipyridamole works by preventing free floating cancer cells from attaching themselves to the sides of blood vessels at distant sites.

Anticoagulant drugs, which are normally used to dissolve blood clots in patients who have had or who are in danger of having a heart attack, also appear to have an ability to interfere with metastatic developments.

Barry Groves explains the mode of action: 'It was demonstrated as long ago as 1903 that distant metastases from cancer cells circulating in the bloodstream couldn't end up just anywhere; that for a distant tumour to form, it needed a thrombus (clot) at the site of the metastasis .... In 1958, Professor O'Meara of Trinity College, Dublin, showed that dividing cancer cells were surrounded by fibrils which gave off clotting factors causing the deposition of fibrin.' This fibrin has the dual effect of allowing the cancer cells to form a clot at a distant site and at the same time to protect the colony of cancer cells from attack. Any chemical that attacks this fibrin will impact on the ability of the cancer to spread. Drugs that are used for this purpose are warfarin, heparin and streptokinase.

Support for this theory was found in a retroactive study of 1,500 patients (Michaels L. 'Cancer incidence and mortality in patients having anticoagulant therapy'. *Lancet* 1964; ii: 832–5). This study found that the patients who had been on long-term anticoagulant therapy had only one-eighth of the expected number of cancer deaths.

In one anecdotal report, a woman who had a widely metastasised endometrial cancer suffered a heart attack and was given streptokinase. An unexpected result was that her cancer went into immediate remission, though for how long is not recorded, except that it lasted for several months. For further details of the anti-cancer effects of these drugs go to www.second-opinions.co.uk.

DMSO and MSM

Dimethyl sulphoxide (DMSO) is an organic sulphur compound. It is a clear, colourless and largely odourless liquid that has demonstrated clear anti-tumour qualities. Over 6,000 articles in scientific journals establish a very solid claim for it to be recognised as an anti-cancer weapon. Vets use it freely when treating cancer in animals. It is available on the Internet from www.dmso.com and www.dmso.org (two distinct companies—and from veterinary suppliers.

DMSO can be taken by intravenous injection, orally, or it can be rubbed on. It is absorbed very rapidly through the skin and this is a very efficient way of getting it to the intended site. Patients who wish to undergo radiation and chemotherapy should take DMSO as it also reduces both the pain and the side effects caused by these treatments.

DMSO has a wide range of biological activities. One reason given for this is that it creates very powerful bonds with water molecules. This allows it to penetrate membranes and to pass from one organ or tissue to another with great ease. It has a wider range of biochemical actions than any other known chemical agent. One Chilean study showed that DMSO in conjunction with low doses of a chemotherapeutic drug was able to obtain remissions in 44 out of 65 cancer patients. This result was even more amazing because these patients had all previously had chemotherapy without success. Twenty-six of the cases involved women with metastatic breast cancer. Twenty-three obtained remission. Whether the remission was permanent is not known. It is also not known what effect DMSO on its own, without the chemotherapy, would have had.

DMSO, in a 12.5 per cent solution, shows long-term growth inhibitory action on cancer tumours in laboratory settings.

One dramatic case of a DMSO-implicated cancer cure (mentioned in Richard Walters book, *Options*) occurred in 1970, when the mother of 3-year-old Clyde Robert Lindsey of Pasadena, Texas took her son to see Dr Eli Tucker of Houston. Clyde had a very deadly cancer known as Letterer-Siwe disease. The cancer had spread throughout his body and orthodox doctors considered the case to be hopeless. Dr Tucker gave the boy a dilute mixture of DMSO mixed with haematoxylon, a chemical normally used as a dye to trace the location of pathological animal cells. The haematoxylon-DMSO combination therefore had a special affinity for tumour cells. Inside the cells the haematoxylon oxidises and this has the effect of causing the cancer cells to die. Five drops of this substance in a glass of distilled water every morning from then till now, has completely eliminated all signs of Clyde's cancer and he is, by all accounts, alive today.

It is believed by some that DMSO works by re-establishing aerobic metabolic processes in the anaerobic cancer cell. This in effect forces the cancer cell to revert to a healthy state, and then undergo apoptosis, healthy programmed cell death. A full description of this process can be found at David Gregg's site: www.krysalis.net/cancer.htm. (This is an extremely detailed but clear analysis of a number of anti-cancer approaches by a biochemist. Highly recommended!)

Are there any side effects to taking DMSO? A garlicky taste in the mouth and bad smell on the breath. Some people suffer from headaches, dizziness and mild nausea. A localised skin rash or burning feeling can occur on the skin.

Warning: DMSO is an extremely powerful solvent. It will dissolve anything, including latex gloves and plastic. Obviously no one wants anything poisonous to be dissolved and taken into the body so all jewellery should be taken off and the skin's surface should be cleaned thoroughly before DMSO is used (According to some, 99.99 per cent pharmaceutical grade DMSO is advised. This can be easily tested as pure DMSO will crystallise at 68°F—in the main part of the fridge for example. If it doesn't crystallise in the fridge it is not pure). DMSO should never come in contact with plastic—only glass and a high quality stainless steel spoon. A dose level of 1–2 teaspoons a day should be sufficient. DMSO is also effective against brain tumours. It has been suggested that a good way of getting cesium chloride into the body is to dissolve it first in DMSO.

MSM supplements are made from DMSO and are thought to have many of DMSO's advantages without negative smell or toxicity. MSM appears to inhibit pain and improve blood flow. It is important for collagen, needed for cell walls and helps the body maintain a good pH level. And there is evidence that it slows the growth of cancer tumours, and may even turn malignant tumours into benign tumours. Some people have combined DMSO and MSM to good effect. MSM is widely and cheaply available and is used as a treatment for arthritis.

Transdermal anticancer therapy using emu oil

More and more people are looking at the transdermal approach (getting herbs, vitamins, minerals etc directly to the site of a cancer by applying them to the skin nearest the tumour)—the key problem is how to get them to penetrate the skin—and the usual answer is to mix with DMSO. But Emu oil is now being touted as a possible alternative. Here is one person's report:

'I've been using a mixture of 50 per cent DMSO/50 per cent emu oil, plus about 6 drops of lavender oil. My skin is sensitive and I've reacted to DMSO when applied anywhere above the waist —mostly itching/some mild burning feelings and dry skin. This mixture has only given me a very brief and very slight itching. The skin has not dried at all and actually feels very smooth and soft afterwards. I've used it on my neck and back and have been pleased with the results. The Emu oil is a carrier oil and penetrates the skin quickly so it doesn't stay greasy. And the lavender smell is lovely and completely masks the DMSO odour.'

Another report on how to deal with the unpleasant after effects of DMSO: 'An holistic MD told me to put sesame or coconut oil onto the area where DMSO is applied. It pretty much stops the burn/itch, and leave it on, do not wash off.'

Epicor

This is a fermented yeast product that was discovered to have a powerful beneficial impact on the immune system. Used in the process of making animal feed products, it was noted that people working with this product had substantially fewer days off work than workers in other areas of the company. It is now being used by athletes whose immune systems are negatively affected by their low levels of body fat to help them stay unaffected by the colds and flus that are common in top level athletics.

Escozul

Escozul is the name given to the Cuban blue scorpion venom that has acquired a reputation in Spanish speaking countries for its anti-cancer effects. Some testimonies suggest that it is curative, while others suggest that it has a beneficial impact in stopping cancer growth and even reducing the size of tumours in a wide range of cancers. Apparently, the real Escozul is in short supply and is only available from a few organisations in Cuba. However, there are a number of websites claiming to be able to supply Escozul for varying sums of money—these should be avoided at all costs. A website set up by patients who have used it successfully is www.escozul-cancer.com.

Haelan 951

Haelan is a fermented soy drink which appears to have powerful effects on cancer. One credible witness is Ross Pelton PhD (pharmacist, clinical nutritionist and author of *How to Prevent Breast Cancer*) who was the administrator at an alternative cancer clinic, Hospital Santa Monica. He used Haelan to treat a group of six cancer patients who were suffering the symptoms of cachexia common to late-stage terminal cancer patients. These patients were not expected to live long, in some cases only days.

The six patients drank an eight-ounce bottle per day, and within two days four of them were out of their beds and walking, and within a week they all were. Pelton says Haelan works because of its 'high concentration of anti-cancer agents, [and] phenomenal concentration of nutrients, phytochemicals and protein.'

In another case, a Texan by the name of Sherman Sanders claims that Haelan enabled him to cure himself of terminal stage liver cancer (cholangiocarcinoma) and to undergo chemotherapy with little discomfort.

A bottle a day is the recommended dose.

A cheaper and, according to some, better-tasting alternative to Haelan is Soy Essence (www.jarrow.com/products/fermentedsoy.htm).

Hydrazine sulfate

How does cancer kill people? Mainly through causing extreme weight loss and debilitation. This is a process known to doctors as cachexia. Dr Joseph Gold decided that one way to approach the cancer question was to interfere with this cachexic process. If he could do this then cancer tumours might grow but they wouldn't generally speaking kill the person who had them. Cancer might then be seen in the same way as diabetes: a disease which—if it couldn't be cured—could at least be controlled. At the time Gold was writing, no one knew what caused cachexia.

Gold investigated this question and came to the conclusion that cancer imposes a waste recycling system on the liver and kidneys. The process works like this: cancer uses glucose as its fuel. The waste product that emerges is lactic acid which is excreted into the blood system and is taken up by the liver and kidneys. The lactic acid is then reconverted back into glucose by a process that requires a great deal of energy. The more glucose that is created, the more fuel the cancer has to feed on and the more waste products that return to the liver for reconversion. This process depletes the body and energises the cancer. When the body cannot keep up, the result is cachexia.

Gold looked for a drug that would interfere with this process. He found it: hydrazine sulfate (or more commonly 'sulfate'). His experiments showed that hydrazine sulfate did indeed have an effect on the cancer-energising process by deactivating a key enzyme in the liver. He also found that it had very few side effects. That is to say it was not a very toxic substance in its own right.

His first human guinea pig was a woman who was expected to die within a matter of days from Hodgkin's disease. She was completely bed-ridden and not having eaten much for some time was 'paper thin'. Administration of the drug resulted in very quick improvement. Within a week she was shopping, within five weeks she was pottering about her garden. Dr Dean Burke, a leading scientist at the US National Cancer Institute who took the side of the alternative approaches to cancer and who attacked the focus on chemotherapy, once declared: '(hydrazine sulfate is) the most remarkable anti-cancer agent I have come across in my forty-five years of experience of cancer.'

That was in August 1973. So, why isn't everyone now taking hydrazine sulfate? Because it eventually wound up on the American Cancer Society's list of unproven therapies. This was despite the evidence that Gold put forward to support the value of hydrazine sulfate.

Gold claimed that out of 84 patients with advanced stage cancer treated by other doctors with hydrazine sulfate, 70 per cent showed subjective improvements (i.e., lessened pain, improved appetite) and that 17 per cent had had objective improvements (tumour regression, disappearance of cancer related disorders). These are very good figures given that all the patients were considered terminal and the success rate should therefore have been close to zero per cent.

Russian scientists at the N N Petrov Research Institute of Oncology in St. Petersburg have replicated these results. In 1974, they used hydrazine sulfate on 48 patients who were considered terminal. They found that almost 60 per cent felt subjectively much better, indeed euphoric! Their appetites improved and the pain lessened or disappeared. Over half of these had clear signs of tumour control. In March 1979 another Russian study followed 225 patients. They found that 65 per cent had an anti-cachexia response and 44 per cent had an anti-tumour response.

Subsequent studies show that it works against every kind of tumour at every stage.

In 1985, Tim Hansen, an eleven year old boy with three inoperable brain tumours was given one week to live. A few weeks later he was put on hydrazine sulfate. When last recorded, he was still taking the hydrazine sulfate as the tumours were still in evidence ten years later—but he was still alive and the tumours had not grown.

Gold's own history of his research and the obstacles that have been put in his way by the National Cancer Institute is published at www.hydrazinesulfate.org.

Gold's recommended dosage for adults weighing over 45kg (100lb) is 60mg per day for the first three days, then 60mg twice a day for the next three days, and 60mg three times a day thereafter. This treatment must continue for as long as there is evidence of a tumour in the body. No dose higher than 60mg is to be tried as this can cause nerve damage. For patients weighing under 45kg, the dosage should be halved. Doses should be taken about two hours before next meal (i.e., on a very empty stomach).

There are, however, a number of cautions that need to be taken on board by anyone taking this route.

One minor side effect that appears to affect a very small percentage of patients undergoing hydrazine sulfate therapy—and is associated only with high doses for lengthy periods—is a slight pain or temporary numbness in the patient's extremities. This condition is, however, quickly controlled by reducing the dosage.

A much more important concern is that hydrazine sulfate is a monoamine oxidase inhibitor (MAOI) and the following should not be used during hydrazine therapy: tranquillisers or sedatives in doses greater than 100mg per day (especially benzodiazepines and phenothiazines) should be avoided, also antihistamines, alcohol and other agents that depress the central nervous system such as morphine. Also vitamin B6 should not be taken. Foods high in tyramine must also be avoided. These tend to be aged and fermented products such as most cheeses, cured meats or fish, sour cream and yoghurt, tofu and tempeh, bouillon cubes, sauerkraut, pickles and yeast extracts. Also restricted are broad beans, avocados, bananas, raisins, figs, dates and dried fruit in general as well as overripe fruit.

The result of mixing tyramine containing foods with hydrazine sulfate can be severe headaches and high blood pressure.

Dr Gold, developer of hydrazine sulfate, specifically warns: 'Central nervous system depressants — such as barbiturates, tranquilizers and alcohol — are incompatible with MAO inhibitors and use of the two together could result in extremely dangerous effects.' One other reported problem is that it has a tendency to lower blood sugar levels. This needs to be monitored. See the website www.hydrazinesulfate.org for further information. Hydrazine sulfate is cheap and available on the Internet.

Immunocal/undenatured whey (glutathione)

Glutathione is a small protein which is noted for its ability to detoxify the body, binding to such toxins as heavy metals, solvents, and pesticides in a way that allows them to be easily excreted. Glutathione is also an important antioxidant. In relation to cancer, it has been shown to inhibit cancer growth. In general, higher glutathione levels are associated with good health.

Immunocal is the brand name of a product that boosts glutathione levels in the body. Undenatured whey isolate products are also highly recommended as a way of boosting normal cellular glutathione levels while at the same time depleting glutathione levels in cancer cells. Recommended dose is 30–60g a day.

Inositol hexaphosphate (IP-6 or phytic acid)

Inositol hexaphosphate is found naturally in high-fibre foods such as beans, brown rice and wheat bran. A number of animal studies, but as yet no human studies, indicate that it is extremely effective against a wide range of cancers. It appears to work against all cancer cells by normalising them—turning them back into normal cells. Interestingly, it has been found to work against every kind of cancer cell studied in animals, and there is no known toxicity.

According to Dr Abdul Kalam Shamsuddin, Professor of Pathology at the University of Maryland School of Medicine in Baltimore, who developed IP-6, someone with cancer should be taking 4.8–7.2g of IP-6 and 1.2–1.8g of inositol. One reputable brand is Cell Forte. It is available in powder form from www.totaldiscountvitamins.com, and Dr Shamsuddin recommends two scoops (supplied) in the morning and two in the evening.

Interestingly, IP-6 has a very broad range of health supporting effects. It boosts the immune system, helps lower cholesterol, prevents kidney stones as well as the complications of diabetes and sickle cell anaemia, and reduces the risk of cardiovascular disease, including heart attack and stroke.

Iridodial

This is an extract of a family of substances found in ants which has very powerful DNA repairing capabilities. Iridodial operates as a natural genetic repair kit and has been shown to have a powerful effect on cancer tumours causing regression, even in cancers such as lung cancer that are generally resistant to treatment. Apparently, iridodial is needed by ants that live in areas of strong geomagnetic radiation. There are a number of suppliers on the Internet.

Dr Hans Nieper, the well-known German alternative doctor, considered iridodial to be potentially the most exciting anti-cancer chemical worth researching at the end of the last century. A liquid extract is available from www.arrowheadhealthworks.com.

Laetrile

Laetrile is the litmus test of all litmus tests. If you find a book on cancer and you wish to know where on the intellectual spectrum the writer is sitting, the quickest and easiest way is to look up 'laetrile' in the index and read what they have to say on the subject. If the writer is against it, then they are most likely writing from an orthodox position (though some natural therapists are also anti-laetrilists). If, on the other hand, the writer writes with great approval of this substance, then they are talking from an alternative view point. That's all you need to know to make your decision. What you do then is up to you.

Laetrile is the name given by one of its early promoters, Ernest Krebs, to a substance found in concentrated form in apricot kernels and almonds. Also known as amygdalin, nitriloside and vitamin B17, it is found in varying quantities in up to two and a half thousand other plants, many, indeed the vast majority, of which are edible.

In the early seventies, Dr Harold Manner of the Biology Department at Loyola University, Chicago conducted a study on a strain of mice genetically engineered to produce females that develop spontaneous mammary tumours. Using a combination of enzymes, vitamin A and laetrile he reported in his book, *The Death of Cancer*:

'After 6–8 days an ulceration appeared at the tumour site. Within the ulceration was a pus like fluid. An examination of this fluid revealed dead malignant cells. The tumour gradually underwent complete regression in 75 of the experimental animals. This represented 89.3 per cent of the total group.' (quoted in Moss, *The Cancer Industry*, 1982)

Further tests on 550 mice, comparing enzymes, vitamin A and laetrile alone and in combinations of two, and in combination of all three together showed that the enzymes alone or in combination with either laetrile or vitamin A, produced regression in 52–54 per cent of the mice. Laetrile on its own had no visible effect. But when all three were in combination, there was total regression in 36 out of 50 cases (i.e., 72 per cent).

So laetrile needs to be taken with vitamin A and enzymes to be really effective.

Pure laetrile, however, has very recently been taken off the shelves in Britain and it has been illegal in much of the USA for decades. Opponents of laetrile argue that it is potentially toxic and can lead to cyanide poisoning. However, this can happen only if pure laetrile is taken orally— because any cyanide that is released does so as a result of the action of the digestive enzymes—and is in any case a largely theoretical fear—very few if any actual deaths have been nailed emphatically to laetrile's door. In the late 1970s an estimated 50,000–100,000 cancer patients were taking over 1 million grams a month (in total—not individually!). Only two or possibly three deaths from an accidental overdose of this substance have been reported—and even these cases are contentious (i.e., there is the distinct possibility that no one has died of laetrile poisoning). Based on these facts, laetrile does not seem to be particularly dangerous or toxic.

Indeed, laetrile-rich foods can be eaten more or less with impunity: bitter almonds and apricots—particularly apricot kernel oil—are eaten in large quantities in the Hunza valley in northern Pakistan. Until modern diets started to impact on their way of life, cancer was unknown.

Anecdotal evidence from a number of doctors supports the use of laetrile therapy. Leon Chaitow, in his book *An End to Cancer?* (1983), quotes the Dutch doctor, H. Moolenburgh:

'I have been treating cancer patients for twenty-five years and introduced laetrile four years ago (i.e., in 1973). That was a turning point. For the first time I saw people who stayed alive in the late stages of cancer, against all expectations.' And again: '… a lot of patients with hopeless cancer feel better, have less pain and live longer than I would have expected. And some cases live on and on and on, which could not be expected at all. I did not see that sort of patient before laetrile.'

How does laetrile work? There have been two theories. The first is that it is a vitamin and that its deficiency has led to the vitamin-deficiency disease of cancer. For that reason it is sometimes called vitamin B17. However, it is the second theory that carries more respectability.

According to this theory, laetrile is a parcel that contains poisons. When the parcel is unwrapped the poisons are released. Normal cells do not have the power to unwrap the parcel. Only cancer cells have that power. Laetrile is a substance that can be separated (by certain enzymes, in the presence of water) into glucose, benzaldehyde and hydrocyanic acid. The last two substances are each, individually, a poison but together they work synergistically (i.e., they are more powerful together, in combination, than they are separately). The enzyme that unwraps this package is beta-glucoronidase. This enzyme appears in great quantities in and around cancer cells—but not normal cells.

Laetrile apparently works best on slow-growing cancers in the early stages of malignancy. Late-stage malignancies need to be slowed down. One way of achieving this is through copper replacement therapy—copper is a vital mineral that is eliminated by cancer cells. Copper supplements help to slow down the respiration rate of the cancer cell and this improves the chances of laetrile working.

Proponents of laetrile therapy insist that tumour regression is only one possible result of laetrile therapy. Pain relief and improved subjective feelings of well-being also result. This well-being is the result of the benzaldehyde, which is a known pain-killer.

The question of tumour regression is sometimes brought up as evidence that laetrile is ineffective. Laetrile, it appears, does not make tumours grow smaller. Certainly, at first sight, it seems to make sense that if laetrile does not cause tumours to grow smaller then this is a clear sign that it is an ineffective anticancer agent. This raises an important question about the nature of cancer and tumours.

Laetrilists argue that tumour size is not in fact a good indicator of anti-cancer activity. Their reasoning is as follows. A tumour does not just consist of malignant cells. It also contains a large proportion of normal cells. Chemotherapy attacks all cells so it is not unusual to see significant short-term tumour regression with chemotherapeutic drugs: they kill the malignant and the normal cells together. However, the long-term result may be, in fact, to make the tumour even more aggressive by increasing the proportion of malignant cells. Laetrile, on the other hand, does not affect the normal cells—only the malignant ones. Therefore the tumour will not decrease very much in size. It will simply have been made non-malignant. The body of the cancer may remain, but without the engine.

Laetrilists are almost universal in saying that laetrile therapy must be accompanied by dietary measures—a raw vegetable diet is generally recommended. In fact, such a diet will contain a large amount of dietary laetrile. Indeed, one of the things that makes the laetrile controversy so bizarre is that laetrile is a very common component of food. Between 1,200 and 2,500 plants contain laetrile: most cereals and fruits and many vegetables. Such ubiquity must have a purpose, and surely is evidence of its safety when taken nutritionally. However, laetrile remains isolated in an intellectual no-go area by the medical establishment.

A diet that contains good quantities of the following would be high in laetrile: chick peas, bean sprouts, nuts, mung beans, blackberries, raspberries and the seeds of apples, apricots, cherries, plums and pears. However, bitter almonds are the easiest source: 50–60 a day are recommended.

Laetrile can be injected or taken orally. Treatment generally consists of one to two grams taken orally every day with meals (not more than one gram at any time). Some doctors supplement this with intravenous injections ranging from 3g a week to 9g a day (for a short period of a few weeks only).

Those who still need to be convinced of laetrile's safety can take heart from an experiment with mice undertaken at a leading US cancer research centre (Sloan-Kettering). For thirty months, mice were injected daily with 2g per kilogram body weight, of laetrile (equivalent to giving a human a quarter of a pound or 0.1kg, a day). At the end of the period, these mice were healthier and exhibited better well-being than the control group who did not get any laetrile.

How this experiment and other laetrile supporting research got suppressed takes up a fascinating chapter in Ralph Moss's book *The Cancer Industry*, the best book on the history of cancer and orthodox medicine in the 20th century.

Laetrile is also known as amygdalin or vitamin B17 by those who advocate its use. Note that it deteriorates very fast and so only fresh laetrile should be used. Many people prefer simply to eat whole apricot kernels. However, larger doses can be taken intravenously—if you can find a doctor who will do this. This is a therapy that is available at some Mexican clinics.

Laetrile is widely available on the Internet. One reputable source is cytopharma.com. Also look at www.laetrile.info. It has also been suggested that laetrile should be taken with zinc and vitamin C to be properly effective.

Low-dose naltrexone (LDN)

Naltrexone (branded under the name: Revia) is an FDA-approved drug originally designed to help wean addicts off heroin. However, in 1985, Bernard Bihari, MD, a New York City doctor, discovered that very low doses of this drug had a very powerful stimulating effect on the immune system. In addition to stabilizing AIDS, he found that this treatment also had a powerful, beneficial impact on many cancers including cancers such as neuroblastoma, multiple myeloma, and pancreatic cancer, which are normally considered incurable.

Interestingly, this treatment has the effect not of curing cancer but, in many cases where all other treatments have failed, of stopping it in its tracks. This is not 100 per cent assured but seems to be a very high frequency effect. However, the LDN needs to be taken permanently, as the cancer will start growing again when the LDN is discontinued.

It is safe, cheap and has no side effects (apart from possible sleeplessness in the first week or two of starting) For further details go to www.lowdosenaltrexone.org or www.ldn4cancer.com. It is also effective for a wide range of auto-immune diseases. However, there is a caution. Naltrexone is also known as Antibuse—for those with long memories this was a drug developed to help alcoholics and heroin addicts kick their habit. Normally, if you drink or abuse opiate drugs while taking naltrexone you will feel ill. However, I am assured that the levels involved here with LDN therapy do not interfere with the enjoyment of alcohol—though one self-described connoisseur of wine says she simply, for no obvious reason, doesn't need to drink as much as she once did.

For those who have a problem obtaining LDN—for the reason that the normal dose is in 50mg tablets while the therapeutic dose is 1.75–4.5mg (taken once a day at bedtime)—prescriptions can be sent to one of a number of pharmacies in the USA that specialize in LDN. For those without a computer one is Irmat Pharmacy in New York (tel.: 1-(212) 685–0500 or 1-(800) 975-2809). A list of other pharmacies is provided on the above websites. Do not take the slow release form.

However, it is much cheaper and easier to dissolve a 50mg tablet in 50 ml of distilled water and use a dropper to get the amount required (4ml of water will contain 4mg of LDN).

A word of warning: high doses of naltrexone appear to promote cancer so do not take more than the recommended doses above.

Lymphotonic PF2

This is a formulation based on a plant extract from calendula, isolated by a top-level Russian team headed by Prof. Doctor Eugenii Severin, President of the Russian Research Center of Molecular Diagnostics and Therapy, Moscow.

One 72-year-old patient with prostate cancer that had metastasized to the bone had a complete remission after using lymphotonic PF2, according to one of the personal testimonials supporting this product. This and other case reports can be found at www.goodbyecancer.com where you can also order the tonic. It is also claimed to be effective in helping reduce the side effects of radiation and chemotherapy.

On a critical note, none of the case reports follow the patients beyond noting their complete remission at the end of a few months of treatment, which took place more than a few years ago. How many had relapses? What other studies have been done since then? I have asked the company for further details but none were provided. This may be a case where the buyer should be cautious.

Alternatively, you can take this as support for the anti-cancer effects of calendula herb.

Mebendazole

Mebendazole is a drug used against worms and other parasites—and appears to have a strong anti-tumour effect. This drug is called a spindle poison because it interrupts the formation of microtubules, cellular filaments that separate newly-made DNA. Chemo drugs such as Taxol and alkylating agents are also spindle poisons, but they have toxicities that mebendazole does not have. Mebendazole does not harm normal cells. In the last few years, a number of studies have found that mebendazole is a powerful inducer of apoptosis in a wide variety of cancer cells, both in culture dishes and mouse models. Microtubule inhibitors are a major target of interest for chemo drugs. In this case, a simple anti-worm drug inhibits microtubule functioning at low non-toxic concentrations. In a culture dish and in mice, mebendazole induces apoptosis in a diversity of cancer cells at extremely low concentrations.

Cimetidine, the generic version of the anti-ulcer drug Tagamet, promotes the toxicity of Mebendazole by inhibiting its degradation in the liver. Mebendazole is usually sold as a chewable tablet. When chewed and allowed to remain in the mouth for a short period, the Mebendazole can enter the blood through the mucosal membranes of the mouth. Of course, it can also enter the blood via the gastro-intestinal tract. This drug is extremely non-toxic, even in doses of 4.5g a day.

Fortunately, if you have a friendly doctor, you may be able to persuade them to prescribe this drug. If you need scientific support ask them to do a search for 'mebendazole cancer' on PubMed—a website for research professionals. Alternatively, you can tell them you need it for a bad case of worms.

MGN-3 (BioBran, Noxylane)

This supplement was developed by Dr Mamdooh Ghoneum, an Egyptian immunologist at Charles Drew University of Medicine and Science, Los Angeles. (I have not been able to find any information as to why it is called MGN-3, but I guess that the first two letters are Dr Ghoneum's initials). Dr Ghoneum has said that MGN-3 is, 'the most powerful immune complex I have ever tested'.

This supplement appears to have a marked effect in increasing natural killer cell activity as well as natural interferon and tumour necrosis factors. It is a potent immune system booster. MGN-3 can also be used to lessen the toxic side effects of conventional cancer treatment.

MGN-3 is made from the outer shell of rice bran which has been enzymatically treated with extracts from three different medicinal mushrooms: Shiitake, Kawaratake and Suehirotake. In Japan, these mushroom extracts have become the leading prescription treatments for cancer.

Articles on MGN-3 quote the story of a 58-year old multiple myeloma patient diagnosed in 1990. He underwent several months of chemotherapy following his diagnosis. Although his condition seemed to stabilize, his blood still showed markers for multiple myeloma eight months after chemotherapy. He then began taking MGN-3, and in less than six months, follow-up laboratory work showed no indication of cancer. In 1998, eight years after his initial diagnosis, he was still alive and cancer-free. He is the first patient known to have survived multiple myeloma, according to Dr Ghoneum. *Everyone's Guide to Cancer Therapy* certainly concurs that surviving multiple myeloma is not common: 'Almost all patients with multiple myeloma who do respond to chemotherapy will eventually relapse if they do not die of some other disease in the meantime.'

However, the benefits of MGN-3 are not restricted to any particular cancer, nor to cancer alone. Dr Ghoneum believes it is of immense benefit for a wide range of conditions—particularly for AIDS. Unlike other forms of cancer treatment, MGN-3 is a totally harmless substance and has no known side effects.

How much should one take? Normal capsule dose is 250mg. To maintain normal good health two capsules a day are recommended but for people with cancer the dose should be 12 capsules a day—1g with each meal for the first two weeks, reducing to 1g a day thereafter. MGN-3 has been shown to be safe to use for long periods of time.

At the time of writing, the US distributor of MGN-3 was having difficulties with the FDA. However, this product is widely available from its Japanese source under the BioBran name. It is also available under the name Noxylane.

Microhydrin (Active H)

Microhydrin (also marketed in Europe as Active H) is a formulated chemical known technically as Flanagan hydrogen enhanced silica. Patrick Flanagan, its creator, who is credited with over 300 inventions, says his inspiration was the fact that people living in northern Pakistan, who are renowned for their longevity and robust good health, benefit from drinking the glacier melt water that comes off the Himalayas. This water, loaded with hydrogen ions, is a powerful health product in its own right. Standard tap water, by comparison, robs the body of hydrogen ions and this results in disease. Microhydrin was developed specifically to provide a ready source of hydrogen ions. It is a mineral composed of silica, potassium and magnesium that has been saturated with hydrogen in such a way that, when consumed, it floods the body with electrons in the form of hydrogen ions. Albert Szent-Györgi, discoverer of vitamin C, called electrons 'the fuel of life'.

Microhydrin has shown a number of very powerful effects:

- It makes the body more alkaline.
- It is very effective at neutralizing free radicals.
- It assists the oxygenation of cells
- It helps remove toxic wastes from cells.
- It increases the electrical conductivity of the body's fluids.

Microhydrin's antioxidant properties have been used by athletes for its ability to increase substantially the oxygen levels of cells. It has been used by mountaineers to climb Everest without oxygen tanks. Anything that increases oxygen levels in cells is good for health and bad for cancer.

A new very much more powerful formula, Microhydrin Plus, is also available. Another product, Hydrogen Boost, appears to be the same but much cheaper.

MMS (sodium chlorite)

Serendipity is the word we use when we meet something entirely unexpectedly. You will remember that increasing oxygen to tissues is one way of impeding or even reversing cancer. One product that claims to deliver oxygen to the body is stabilised oxygen—which is, in fact a very dilute solution of sodium chlorite (not sodium chloride which is table salt). Now it is contentious whether or not this product actually does deliver oxygen in a way that is usable by the body. However, that does not mean that stabilised oxygen is useless. In fact it could, if utilised in the correct way, be one of the most powerful anti-cancer weapons in our arsenal.

What happens is that when you mix a few drops of sodium chlorite with vinegar or lemon juice, it releases chlorine dioxide — and, according to a 1999 statement by the American Society of Analytical Chemists, chlorine dioxide is the most powerful pathogen killer known to man!

Jim Humble, a mining engineer, discovered the powerful healing effects of stabilized oxygen while working in Guyana. He has since developed a more concentrated solution—which he calls, perhaps a little unwisely, Miracle Mineral Supplement (he has since decided that MMS stands for Master Mineral Supplement! But at the same time he appears to be trying to protect his use by creating a church around the substance and calling himself Bishop (why not Archbishop?)—this is an approach that a number of people have used to protect their use of various alternative therapies in the face of FDA hostility—who are attacking its use by saying people taking it are doing no more than ingesting 'bleach'—however, any Internet search will come up with enthusiastic testimonials from users. As I write this I am myself taking it as one of my weapons to control a cellulosis infection in my leg, an extremely dangerous condition, but which I appear so far to be on top of—watch the obituary columns!).

Humble's full story can be found at www.miraclemineral.org/part1.php. This is an interesting read. The first half of the book is free, the second costs a few dollars (and you must read both parts because there are cautions that you need to know about—especially in relation to the dangers associated with the rapid unblocking of arteries). What emerges is that this substance is not only fast acting against malarial parasites and viruses—it also appears, in some cases at least, to help eliminate cancer. What its mode of action is, is not clearly understood. It may be that it attacks a viral or fungal cause of cancer, or it may be that it reacts explosively in contact with cancerous cells, while remaining completely safe to normal cells.

MMS is inexpensive and available from Internet suppliers. Humble recommends starting with a few drops and then slowly increasing by one drop a day until there is a feeling of nausea. This dose level should then be maintained until the nausea (a Herxheimer reaction caused by the body being temporarily overcome by toxins released by the healing or curative process) is no longer felt. It is then possible to continue increasing the dose.

MMS2

The original MMS (see above) is now known as MMS1 and Humble has now come up with a second chlorine-associated chemical which he is marketing as MMS2—which comes in capsule form. The capsules contain calcium hypochlorite—which is the stuff you put in swimming pools to disinfect them—since swimming pool water is not poisonous, this is safe to ingest. The chemical converts into hypochlorous acid on contact with water—and you must drink a lot of water with the capsules, at least two glasses. Humble claims to have anecdotal evidence that MMS1 and MMS2 each separately but both together if possible have cured individuals of HIV virus and prostate cancer.

Humble's recommended protocol is: 'For cancer, take four capsules a day (one every two hours), plus MMS1 every hour.'

'Overnight cure for cancer'

The so-called OCC—Overnight cure for cancer—is an attempt to turn cancerous cells back into normal cells by infusing a solution composed of MMS1 added to lemon juice (or citric acid crystals). After 3 minutes you add DMSO and MSM and wait another three minutes. You then rub the solution onto the skin. There appears to be a great deal of experimentation as to quantities. One person used 80 drops of MMS1 with 400 drops of citric acid and 400 drops of DMSO and then rubbed it all over his body and left it on for an hour. He said he suffered no ill-effects. Does it work? Watch this space.

For more information on the protocol and theory behind it go to Webster Kehr's site at www.cancertutor.com.

My only comment on this suggestion, based on my experience, is that MMS1 is powerful stuff and if you have any fungal or parasitic problem the MMS is going to kill it in a way that leaves blisters on the surface of the skin—you can almost hear the scream of agony as they screech to the skin's surface and die—within minutes of rubbing the stuff on (with DMSO). This can be extremely uncomfortable. What it does to a cancer tumour I can't say but too sudden a toxic breakdown can be very harmful. Cancers do not need to be eliminated overnight. This protocol may be more usefully done over two to three weeks by focusing on specific areas of the body and then gradually shifting this focus until all parts of the body have been covered. However, this concern may be unnecessary as the MMS is supposed to cause normal cell death rather than death by toxic necrosis.

Oncotox

Oncotox is a proprietary formulation that is well-known among anti-cancer therapists. Formulated by Dr Donsbach, a well-known alternative cancer therapist who works at the Hospital Santa Monica in Tijuana, Oncotox is a liquid concentrate of five known anti-cancer agents: resveratrol, IP6, lactoferrin, arginine and curcumin. It can be bought from www.donsbach.com/cancer.htm.

Phycotene

Phycotene is a complex of 17 different carotenoids and micro-nutrients extracted from Spirulina and Dunaliella algae. It was developed by Dr Christopher and in research conducted at Harvard university on hamsters, it demonstrated powerful anti-cancer effects—so powerful that one of the researchers, Dr Joel Schwartz, believes it to be a 100 per cent cure for oral cancers in hamsters. No human studies have been done. It is also available as a cream. Source: www.rbclifesciences.com.

Poly-MVA

Poly-MVA (the initials stand for Minerals, vitamins and Amino acids) is a patented formulation consisting of the element palladium which has been complexed with alpha lipoic acid and a number of other vitamins and minerals. It is claimed that this substance is a powerful re-energiser of cells, immune stimulant, chelator of heavy metals, detoxifier, and helps maintain alkaline pH levels. There are a number of convincing testimonials relating the benefits of Poly-MVA for a wide range of cancers, both on its own or as part of a parcel of alternative therapies. There is a big buzz about this product and the only problem with Poly-MVA is the price. It is fairly expensive. For further information go to www.polymva.org.

Seanol

Seanol is the registered trade name for an extract of marine algae that acts as a powerful anti-oxidant and anti-inflammatory agent. In animal studies, it has shown marked benefits for circulatory problems from blood pressure and arthritis to sexual dysfunction. It is also showing huge potential cancer benefits—it slows down tumour cell division. Testimonials support claims that it is a natural energy booster and that it clears brain-fog. It is sold under the trade name of Fibronol and Fibroboost. See www.fibronol.com and www.lifesvigor.com/78100.html.

Shark (and bovine) cartilage

It is not quite true that sharks don't get cancer—but it is almost true. Cancer is, it appears, very rare in sharks, skates, rays and other members of the elasmobranch family—which includes the dogfish. Why is this the case? According to Dr William Lane, who has almost single-handedly pushed shark cartilage as a cancer cure, the answer lies in the fact that sharks do not have bones. Instead their skeleton is composed of cartilage which has no blood vessels or nerves. The cartilage contains a substance that inhibits the development of blood cells. Cancer tumours cannot grow without a network of blood vessels to nourish them. The development of a blood supply is known as angiogenesis. In normal adults the blood network is already well developed. Angiogenesis therefore occurs in adults for specific purposes— ovulation and pregnancy, healing of wounds and fractures— and the development of cancer tumours.

Others argue that if shark cartilage works it does so for other reasons. So the question is does it work? One well known experiment conducted in Cuba but followed by the documentary programme '60 Minutes' had the following results. Of the original 29 terminally-ill cancer patients, nine died of their cancer within the first 17 weeks of the start of the trial and a further six died of other causes. Fourteen (48 per cent) were alive and cancer free three years later. The protocol they were on was 60g/day for the first 16 weeks and then 20g/day thereafter. Apparently, taking 60g orally is not easy and some prefer to take it as a suppository.

One cheaper recommendation is to eat shark steaks, according to one source, these are 90 per cent cartilage

Claims are also made for the anti-cancer effects of Bovine cartilage. Though why bovine cartilage is supposed to work it is hard to say—cows, after all, do get cancer.

The Chinese have been eating shark cartilage for centuries in the form of shark's fin soup. No Chinese wedding is complete without the shark's fin soup served half-way through the banquet. It is considered to be a rejuvenator and aphrodisiac. One billion Chinese can't be wrong—or can they? An unfortunate side effect of China's growing prosperity is therefore the likely extinction of the shark. In fact this potential impact on shark populations has provoked a great deal of anger against those promoting shark cartilage. However, a more powerful anti-angiogenesis agent appears to be the herb bindweed (see Section 5: *Cancer: Herbs, Botanicals and Biological Therapies*).

Shark liver oil and squalamine

Squalamine is the first known example of a class of compounds called aminosterols, steroids chemically linked to an amino acid. It is found in high concentrations in the livers of dogfish and sharks. It has shown significant anti-cancer activity and is currently being studied at Johns Hopkins School of Medicine. Squalamine can be taken as a capsule. It remains unscathed through the digestive tract and appears to be able to cross the blood brain barrier, making it potentially effective against brain tumours. It works as an anti-angiogenesis agent as well as being an immune system booster. Unfortunately, mercury pollution appears to be a problem with shark liver oil, and squalamine products and some investigation may be required to obtain a pure product.

Summing up

If there is a key difference between conventional medicine on the one side and the so-called 'alternatives' it is this: Conventional research is focusing harder and harder on the specifics of each different cancer cell, on the genes and enzymes that control these cells—looking for ways to block the actions that drive the cancer cell. This can seem enormously heroic. And is certainly an extraordinary intellectual enterprise. Unfortunately, as I have said elsewhere. It rather misses the point. I have likened it to trying to understand a game of tennis by deconstructing a tennis ball.

On the other hand, people who use the alternative therapies, generally speaking, seek to work with the whole body—the environment in which all cells move—in a painless and non-damaging way, believing that the body as a whole is infinitely wiser than the scientists who prod and poke at increasingly infinitesimal landscapes that keep changing.

Siddhartha Mukherjee, oncologist and author of the book *The Emperor of All Maladies*, admits that science will most likely never come up with a cure for cancer. He visualizes that in 2050, the cancer patient following a conventional regime will take one pill for a while, but when the cancer changes, they will switch to another pill—going from one to another as the cancer mutates to resist the effects of each pill that is thrown at them. Meanwhile, he thinks, for most cancers, the only option will be to persevere with chemotherapy, causing great pain and damage in order to achieve relatively small gains in life span.

And yet, as the stories in Section 8 (*Cancer Survivors' Stories*) testify, cancer can be beaten by combining—in multiple ways—diet, herbs, supplements and a variety of energy-based and/or mind-body therapies. The result is health, not sickness; extended life, not reduced possibilities.

We know that cancer is best viewed as a systemic illness and not just as a problem of 'evil' cells. The tissue environments of all cells require and respond to the complex biochemistry of vitamins, minerals and many other extracts of the natural world. When we take in vitamin C we cannot know to what purposes the body will direct it. But we do know that when the body is ill it needs vitamin C in very much larger quantities that it can take in. It is the same with the minerals that are needed also for the enzymatic actions necessary for health.

As I collated the supplements that have one way or another been proposed as having benefits for people with cancer, I was stunned by their variety—and the possibilities they carried within them for returning illness back to health.

Which ones you find persuasive is of course your decision.

Cancer: Energy, Mind and Emotions

'Wellness—a happy mind in a happy body.'

Jonathan Chamberlain

This section covers a wide range of ideas from electrical and magnetic devices, sunlight, energy healing, prayer, exercise and the extraordinary interplay of our physical and emotional lives. I will look at the interplay of mind, emotions and physical health and how we can harness psychological forces to help us reach a place of good health.

Energy Medicine

Introduction

We have become so used to thinking of medicine in terms of pills, capsules, tonics, injections and so on, that it may come as something of a shock (to make a rather obvious pun) to learn that there is a growing interest in the use of magnetism, electricity, colour spectrum radiation and other forms of more subtle vibrational energy as tools for healing—specifically for cancer.

While some of these ideas may be uncomfortably new-agey, others are grounded in good old electrical engineering and electromagnetic science. It is a highly controversial area and has a long way to go before it gains popular, let alone professional, acceptance.

Let's start at the beginning. It is generally accepted that 'radiation', which is another way of saying energy emitted from an external source, can positively or negatively affect the body. Radiation may manifest different wavelengths and wave patterns—e.g., sine (smoothly varying), saw-tooth and square waves. These have different biological effects, with the more natural, constant sine wave radiation being the least effective for medical purposes—possibly because it is too smooth—but it becomes more interesting for this purpose when pulsed (i.e., the underlying wave has a pattern of change (e.g., in its frequency or its energy). These vibrations vary in force from extremely weak energies, such as those that emanate from a lump of salt crystal, to powerful penetrative energies such as X-rays. Light is electromagnetic energy: light and X-rays are distinguished from each other simply by having different wavelengths on the same electromagnetic spectrum. All electromagnetic radiation has a constant speed, so we sometimes speak of frequency (waves per second) rather than wavelength.

The second fact we need to understand is that everything, every single thing—from sub-atomic particle to a system as complex as the human body—has a vibrational (electromagnetic or EM) signature.

Given that every atom contains positively charged protons and negatively charged electrons in dynamic movement, we see that even single molecules must emanate an EM field. The same is true at the cellular level and beyond. The body itself has an electromagnetic field, which is the combined field of every single living cell in the body.

The world we live on—the planet earth—as a whole has a magnetic field. Physicist Bruce Harvey has put the importance of magnetism in these words: 'magnetism is as fundamental to the structure of matter as the electric force which binds the negative electrons to their positive nuclei. As we delve into the inner mechanisms of nature, magnetism becomes ever more significant. It is the regulator of processes. The phenomena we observe in the macro world are by-products of the inner workings of matter.'

In this chapter we are going to explore how energy has been used in healing.

Nicola Tesla and the Tesla coil

Whilst therapy with magnets and electricity goes back thousands of years, electromagnetic devices are more recent. One of the best-known inventors in this area is Nicola Tesla, and although he didn't set out to invent a therapeutic device, he did note the potential. Others went on to use his technology to do so. Tesla was born in Smijlan, Croatia in 1856 and immigrated to the United States in 1884. He worked for a time as Thomas Edison's assistant but then, after falling out with his boss, became Edison's greatest rival.

Tesla was a true genius, many of whose inventions have wrongly been attributed to others. Perhaps the most important of his intellectual bequests was the fact that he invented a means of producing alternating current (AC) electricity. To him also we owe neon lights, speedometers for cars and even the world's first hydro-electric plant, located at Niagara Falls.

But our interest in Tesla here lies in a device that he developed —the so-called Tesla Coil. This transformer generates high-frequency currents and it occurred to Tesla that, '[some of] these currents might lend themselves to electrotherapeutic uses.' He experimented on himself—once, having been hit by a taxi, he aided his recovery by exposing himself to these fields. He had also found that the energy waves had the effect of energizing him and helping him to work long hours without getting tired. He persuaded his friend Mark Twain to experience it, and he too enjoyed the benefits—until apparently he found himself afflicted with a sudden bout of diarrhoea.

As with the Rife machine (see below), a little goes a long way. He found that an hour in front of the machine was too long.

He was not alone in thinking he had invented something with a useful side-effect. This was a time when the controlling bodies of American science had not built up their political muscle to the extent they have today. Doctors and inventors felt free to experiment and to comment honestly on what they saw. On September 6, 1932, at a seminar presented by the American Congress of Physical Therapy, held in New York, a Dr Gustave Kolischer announced: 'Tesla's high-frequency electrical currents are bringing about highly beneficial results in dealing with cancer, surpassing anything that could be accomplished with ordinary surgery.'

A number of other pieces of equipment that are claimed to be developments from Tesla's work and which are available for health purposes are offered by the following website: www.myholistichealthshop.com. These include a high-frequency violet ray and a 'molecular enhancer'—www.altered-states.net is another interesting site that sells a wide range of devices.

Since Tesla, there has been a strong tradition of developing electromagnetic devices including Lakhovsky's multiple wave oscillator, the Rife generator, the Tesla photon machine, the Pappas pulsed magnetic induction device, the light beam generator and the V.I.B.E. (vibrational integration bio-phonic energizer).

Lakhovsky's multi-wave oscillator (MWO)

Georges Lakhovsky was a Russian émigré scientist living in France in the years immediately after the first world war. He knew of Tesla's work and developed these ideas going on to publish an article entitled 'Curing Cancer with Ultra Radio Frequencies' (Radio News, February, 1925).

Lakhovsky invented the Multi-Wave Oscillator (MWO) which produced a wide range of radio frequencies from very low to very high, with many 'extremely short harmonics'. The MWO consists of two antennae with a number of concentric rings—the high voltage discharges move from one ring to the next and in the process create complex multiple wavelength electrostatic fields. Anyone using the MWO sits between these circular antennae while the high voltage, multiple frequency electrostatic fields are received and absorbed by the tissues. A very interesting website that contains a translation of Lakhovsky's article is www.altered-states.net.

His explanation for why it worked was that: 'The cell with very weak vibrations, when placed in the field of multiple vibrations, finds its own frequency and starts again to oscillate normally through the phenomenon of resonance.'

The MWO produces a broad range of high frequency pulsed signals that radiate energy into patient via two resonators: one resonator acting as a transmitter and the other as a receiver. The patient sits on a wooden stool in between the two resonators and is exposed to these energies for about 15 minutes. According to Lakhovsky, these energies increased the resonance of healthy cells and created disequilibrium in disease organisms.

Bob Beck (about whom more below) popularised this machine in the States in the 1960s and has published designs. These are available on the web. However, attempts to market the machine in the USA have met with severe FDA disapproval. However, I did find one US site of interest at www.zephyrtechnology.com.

Another convert to the MWO, Ralph Bergstresser, decided that the best way to resist FDA pressure was to seek protection for medical freedom under the freedom for religion laws. He founded a church that worshipped the machine. For a couple of years, he and his followers were able to go to church, sit around the MWO—which was placed on an altar with resonator antennas glowing—and receive the 'blessed waves' from the Sacred Oscillator. However, he was eventually thrown in jail. But he emerged a year or so later undeterred and continued to manufacture and sell the machines along with other electromagnetic devices (see www.purpleharmonyplates.com).

The Rife square-wave frequency generator

Round about the same time that Lakhovsky was working in France, a San Diego inventor by the name of Royal Raymond Rife was inventing perhaps the most famous of all the healing machines: the Rife frequency generator.

Before inventing the Rife generator, he built an extraordinarily powerful light microscope with a magnification of 60,000×, which made it possible to study living bacteria and viruses—unlike the standard microscopes then and now that required tissue to be dead before it can be viewed.

As a result of watching living bacteria he claimed to see something very interesting—the bacteria could change their forms from bacillus to a fungus to a virus. In all he identified four forms, one of which—the monococcoid—he found in 90 per cent of cancer patients. Another form (the BX form) was, he claimed, the form in which it caused cancer. Any of the forms could change into a BX form within 36 hours.

The idea that relatively harmless bacteria can change into cancer-causing viruses is utterly rejected by most scientists—but Rife is not alone in his belief. We have already seen that Gaston Naessens, who himself, independently, developed a similar microscope, saw similar events unfolding through the lens and, as a result, developed his anti-cancer substance 714-X.

Having discovered them, Rife experimented by passing energy frequencies through the microbes. He found that each microbe had a fundamental frequency that would cause it to resonate and then explode (just as a fine wine glass explodes when a sound of the right pitch hits it).

Rife then built a generator that emitted radiation of various frequencies that destroyed the microbe he had identified as the one that causes cancer—which he called the BX virus. It was tested at the University of Southern California in the early 1930s. Rife reported the results: '16 cases were treated at the clinic for many types of malignancy. After three months, 14 of these so-called hopeless cases were signed off as clinically cured.'

The patients were treated every three days—this was found to be more effective than daily treatment, the reason being that the lymphatic system had to deal with the toxicity created by the dead particles of the BX virus. In fact all the patients in the study eventually recovered. The machine had a 100 per cent cure rate in cases of terminal cancer. If there are cures for cancer this is certainly one of them.

There is no doubt about the authenticity of the research—nor of the high quality of the scientists who participated in the study: it included a university president, a director of a major medical school, Northwestern Medical School, and other eminent doctors. The study was run under the auspices of the American Medical Association of Los Angeles, personally facilitated by the President, Dr Milbank Johnson. So what happened?

The story is that Morris Fishbein, who (despite a complete lack of medical qualifications) headed the American Medical Association, was also a front man for the pharmaceutical industry. Through his efforts pressure was exerted on everyone involved to distance themselves from the machine. Some key supporters were bought off with large grants to allow them to retire in peace—and silence. Others, it is claimed, were killed. At least two unnatural deaths occurred among key supporters of Rife. One was poisoned and another was burnt to death when his laboratory burnt down. Equipment was stolen or tampered with. The manufacturers of the equipment were forced by various means into bankruptcy. It was, by all accounts, a mean and nasty war.

However, some doctors continued to use the machine. In 1940, Dr Arthur Yale reported the results he had obtained using Rife's generator. He reported on four cases that would have been fatal within 90 days. One was a 53-year-old man with a grapefruit-sized tumour in the rectum. Within a week, the pain had gone and within sixty days the entire tumour had disappeared. Pain relief, it should be noted, is a possible sign that the cancerous stage of cachexia has ceased.

The AMA reacted to all of this work by threatening doctors who used the machine with loss of license and even jail terms. Rife himself was taken to court. A laboratory that was investigating Rife's claims was burnt to the ground in 1939, killing the key researcher. Rife continued his work despite this pressure. However, harassment also continued. In 1961, one of his partners, Jim Crane, was sent to jail for three years. He was not allowed to defend himself with evidence showing the machine's effectiveness.

As for the machine, there appears to be absolutely no doubt that it worked then and works now. The underlying principle is that every living organism has an internal vibratory frequency. If this frequency is altered, or if the power of the frequency is amplified, then the organism can be destroyed. So the objective of the Rife generator is to tune into the natural resonance of disease-causing microbes and then to increase the intensity of the frequency until they disintegrate.

The Rife generator then, is a machine that is capable of producing frequencies and directing these frequencies through the body. Note that Rife used square-wave frequencies, not the normal smooth sine-wave form. Usually, the machine is used to send frequencies throughout the whole body—but it is also possible to direct the waves to specific parts of the body.

Proponents of the Rife frequency generator say that any illness—from athlete's foot to yellow fever—can be treated effectively using this machine.

Contemporary 'Rife' machines

Most of the 'Rife machines' on the market today are developments of the original idea—details of the original devices have largely been lost. You can also buy software that claims to convert your own computer into a Rife generator.

One issue with these machines is whether analogue is better than digital. In my view analogue is best.

Another issue that buyers need to consider is whether to have a machine that goes through a pre-set program of frequencies—or whether to take a machine that is programmable to specific frequencies specified for the particular disease.

It seems at first sight that a programmable machine capable of targeting specific disease would be best. Most of these machines will come with a protocol of which frequencies should be used for which health condition. The problem is that there is no general agreement as to which frequencies are specific to cancer. One researcher, Gary Wade, has solved this problem by creating a machine that has a 45-minute program that covers all ultrasound frequencies within the relevant range. Gary Wade will make a machine specifically upon request (current cost around US$2,000). He can be contacted at: Transformation Technologies www.rifeenergymedicine.com There are many other machines on the market with prices starting at around US$1,500.

People undergoing therapy with this machine must make sure they drink plenty of water before and after using the machine—and they should expect to feel tired afterwards.

Also, it should be noted that the Wade generator produces ultrasound frequencies which tend to dissolve blood clots. Therefore, the unit should not be used within several weeks after major or minor surgery, nor on anyone who has phlebitis, who has had a stroke or who is pregnant. For more information also see: www.rifetechnology.com

The Rife Bare machine

Developed by an American chiropractor, James Bare, in 1995, this uses resonant light frequencies to target bacteria, viruses and fungi. It is a non-contact machine which apparently has good results in these areas and in the area of pain relief. Bare makes no comment about any benefits for cancer patients because any such claim would immediately make him a target of abuse on the grounds of quackery—not to mention lawsuits. However he does refer to beneficial 'physiological effects'.

The original Rife machine had a plasma tube that is missing in most contemporary 'Rife machines' which focus more on the radio frequency side of things. But it is Bare's contention that the plasma tube that converted radio frequencies to pulsed light was a necessary component. To read a more technical description of the device, go to www.rt66.com/~rifetech/.

Prioré

The next important figure in the history of healing machines was an Italian who settled in France and who invented a machine that appeared to cure not only cancer but parasite infections. It did this not by directly attacking the tumour or the parasite, but by stimulating the host's cells to eliminate the source of disease. This was witnessed over the years by a number of eminent scientists.

In 1953, Antoine Prioré began treating human patients whose cancers had been judged hopeless—and many were cured. His medical colleague maintained a huge file of these cases, but the file later was mysteriously lost. But Prioré faced enormous hurdles in his attempt to get recognition for his work. Given the fact that he was a simple electrical repairman living in Bordeaux and had no academic status at all, this was an uphill task and he was to die in the early 1980s a broken man.

Part of the problem was that he was utilizing concepts that had at that time no theoretical framework. There is nothing a scientist hates more than something that works but which appears to be meaningless gobbledy-gook according to the current theory. It appears that Prioré found a method of using a fixed magnetic field in combination with electromagnetic radiation.

It may be relevant that his initial inspiration came from seeing that a piece of fruit that had fallen near a machine that gave out electromagnetic radiation did not go rotten for a long time.

Everyone who worked with him at various institutions was convinced that he was able to cure cancer, first in animals and then in humans. And it must be the case that his first equipment must have been cheap to make and portable. Over the years his dream was to make bigger and stronger machines, but sadly these never materialized.

There are organizations in France seeking to replicate his work. Sadly, little is known about the exact specifications but it is surmised that Prioré is unlikely to have used a finely-tuned machine. It is likely to have produced frequencies across a broad range and the strength of the magnetic field also does not appear to be critical. Two attempts at duplicating his machine have used magnetic fields of 620G and 1,240G.

There does not appear to be any Prioré-type machine in use at this time. A machine that appears to be in some ways similar to Prioré's has been invented by American physicist, Abraham Liboff of Oakland University, California. His 'Method and Apparatus for the Treatment of Cancer'

(US Patent #5,211,622) produces an alternating magnetic field superimposed on a static magnetic field. Again, as with the Prioré machine, this appears to have caused cancer tumours to die. Again, while the machine has been patented, I have no information as to whether it is in use.

Contemporary electrical approaches

I am not suggesting that you go out to deliberately to get struck by lightning, but an early report of lightning and its effects on cancer were reported in *The Lancet* (January 10, 1880) by a surgeon named Allison. He reported that 30 years previously he had known of a case of a farm labourer suffering from a mouth cancer who had been struck by lightning. This had nearly killed him, but he recovered and the tumour also disappeared. It may be relevant that shock therapy of a similar kind is commonly used in the Amazon basin of Brazil—and is known to be very effective in dealing with poisonous snake-bites. Five or six hits with a standard stun gun have not only neutralized the poison but also eliminated the pain of the bite. No one knows how it manages this feat yet it is well attested to. Could this be the answer to cancer?

The idea that electricity can be curative was developed in Germany and Austria under the name galvanotherapy.

Dr Rudolph Pekar and galvanotherapy

Dr Rudolph Pekar (1912–2004), an Austrian medical doctor and inventor, originated a way of treating cancer using an electrical current which he called galvanotherapy and which is now widely used in Germany and in China where it is, apparently, producing an overall cure rate of 30–40 per cent for all types of cancer including advanced cases of malignant cancer—and much higher cure rates with less advanced cancers. Galvanotherapy is sometimes also known as percutaneous bio-electrotherapy

In this treatment electrodes are clipped to needles inserted in the skin near the malignant tumour. A low current is passed through the electrodes. This creates an electromagnetic field in which charged ions cause the inside of the cancer cells to 'melt' and then implode. The resulting waste material is eliminated through detoxification.

Only very weak DC currents not exceeding ten volts are used. There is little pain involved in the procedure which is done under local anaesthetic. More than 70,000 people have undergone the procedure which is done at a number of European clinics and Chinese hospitals.

For further information contact the International Association for Electromedicine at Onkologische Schwerpunktpraxis, Frauengasse four (Villa Gisela), zip code A-4820 Bad Ischl, Austria. An Internet search will also find clinics that offer this therapy.

Bob Beck's blood purifier and magnetic pulse generator

Bob Beck was an American inventor who played an important role in promoting the use of inexpensive electro-therapy machines. He invented two machines that are relatively inexpensive but claim to eliminate all harmful microbes from the body.

The first machine he called a blood purifier. This is an electronic device that uses two small electrodes that are placed over major blood arteries (not veins) on the wrists or ankles, and held in place with a strap. Both electrodes are placed on the same wrist or ankle about an inch apart. With most models it is possible to modify the strength of the electrical charge.

This small electric current electrifies the blood as it circulates past the electrodes. It takes about ten minutes for blood to circulate throughout the body. It is recommended to use the machine anywhere from 20 minutes to two hours a day.

The basic premise of the blood purifier is that microbes and other disease causing organisms have a far lower tolerance to electrical currents than normal cells. However, it is important to note that one side effect of this procedure is to make cells highly porous and so any chemicals—such as alcohol—in the bloodstream are absorbed at a far greater rate. It is recommended that no drugs or alcohol be taken into the body at least 48 hours prior to using the blood purifier.

Bob Beck was also a strong advocate of colloidal silver and most Beck blood purifiers double up as cheap colloidal silver-makers. In my experience these machines are better than most in the quality of the silver rods they use.

Bob Beck also invented a magnetic pulse generator that uses a high intensity, short duration magnetic pulse of approximately 43,000 gauss (current normal background magnetic fields are approximately 0.5 gauss) as its means of killing or immobilizing parasites. The coil produces pulses every 5–8 seconds and can be placed anywhere on the body including the head. There are many suppliers of this machine on the Internet.

A number of research institutes are experimenting with 'nanopulses' of electricity with cancer cells in Petri dishes with exciting results (as reported by the BBC (5 Feb, 2004). This seems to support the use of machines such as Bob Beck's. Interestingly, these researchers say the same effect of promoting cell death is also seen in cells associated with obesity. It is worth noting that Bob Beck himself lost an immense amount of weight through the use of his machine.

Hulda Clark's zapper

This is a small, inexpensive, hand-held device that operates on the same principles as the Rife ultrasound frequency generator, but is limited in the range of frequencies that it addresses. It is also limited in its ability to penetrate deep into the body. It appears to be beneficial for the muscle tissues. One recent experiment into its effectiveness compared the spoiling rate of a chicken leg with and without being exposed to a zapper. This informal experiment found that it takes about three days for normal fresh chicken legs to spoil. After 'zapping' for an hour each day the chicken legs will last up to seventeen days before spoiling.

All three devices—Beck's blood purifier, his magnetic pulse generator and Clark's zapper—are attempting a similar thing, namely, to use either small electrical currents or high intensity magnetic pulses to kill living organisms that are in your body that shouldn't be there. This includes organisms such as viruses, bacteria, mould, fungi, and the larger parasites such as tapeworms, ringworms, roundworms, flukes, etc.

GEIPE

GEIPE is a very specific anti-cancer device that has as its aim the de-activation of an enzyme by means of an electric current. The American independent cancer researcher, Jay Kulsh believes the answer to curing cancer lies in deactivating the enzyme ribonucleotide reductase (RR) Without this enzyme the cancer tumour simply cannot grow. Concentrations of the enzyme are much higher in cancer tumours than in normal tissue. There have been previous attempts to deactivate the enzyme using chemotherapeutic drugs—so far without success. Kulsh took the view that the best way of de-activating it was to focus on the fact that at the 'core' of this enzyme is a free radical (an atom or group of atoms with an unpaired electron) which is essential for its activity. As he writes: 'Such free radicals can be neutralized or disabled by passing [a] mild direct electric current through the tissue. Since the concentration of the target enzyme RR is much higher in cancerous cells, as compared to healthy resting cells, the gentle DC electrotherapy would act selectively on malignant growth.'

Kulsh was not the first to make this suggestion. He cites a previous experiment using this approach that reported 98 per cent reduction in the tumour mass of lab animals—representing, in his words, 'a virtual cure'.

Kulsh has two devices that he is willing to sell. One is an invasive device that requires an electrode to be inserted surgically into a tumour. However, he has another non-invasive device that he says can easily be used at home. It needs to be used at least eight hours a day for up to eight weeks.

Kulsh claims that the cancers most likely to respond to his approach are solid tumour cancers of bladder, bone, brain, breast, cervix, colon, oesophagus, kidney, liver, lung, ovary, pancreas, prostate, rectum, skin, stomach, testicles, throat and uterus.

GEIPE stands for gentle electrotherapy to inhibit pivotal enzyme (ribonucleotide reductase). For further information: www.cancer-treatment.net.

Electro-carcinoma therapy

This form of treatment was developed at The Institute for Natural Health Methods in Marburg Germany, and has also been used in China. It involves passing a weak direct current (DC) through the tumours, which can shrink, as a direct consequence and even disappear completely.

A large-scale Chinese study covering 10,000 patients from 1987–2000 found that it had a 30 per cent effectiveness in bringing about the complete dissolution of the tumour, and that in a further 40 per cent of cases there was reduction in the size of tumours.

Chinese medical professionals use platinum wire needles to apply the DC current directly into tumours. The Marburg Institute approach is to pass the current from plates placed on the skin near the tumour. There does not appear to be any difference in effectiveness.

The electro-carcinoma therapy is a local procedure that can be done on an outpatient basis. It has few side effects. Each treatment lasts two to three hours and some patients only need two or three sessions before the tumour 'melts', others need more. With the help of a special computer monitor program and controls, the physician controls the treatment and observes the procedures in the body and the growth.

Simple magnet-based therapy

Some doctors are experimenting with magnets as a healing device in cases of cancer. Dr William Philpott of Choctaw, Oklahoma treated a 20-year-old patient with an inoperable glioblastoma—a form of brain cancer. He placed the north-pole of a ceramic magnet on the back of the patient's head at the point where the tumour had initially started to grow. The magnet was left in this position 24 hours a day.

At the beginning of the treatment at the American Biologics (now International BioCare) hospital in Tijuana, Mexico, this patient was incapable of making any response to his environment. After three days of continuous treatment, he was able to wiggle his fingers in response to questions. Three weeks later, he walked out of the hospital with the assistance of only a walker. The patient continued magnetic-field exposure of the brain five hours a day and was reported to be well six months later except for a residual imbalance problem.

Obviously a normal bar magnet is of no use for this kind of treatment as both north and south poles appear on the same side. What is needed is a flat magnet, magnetised so that opposite poles are on opposing flat sides.

It is also possible to buy magnetic beds to sleep on. However, one needs to distinguish between beds that are based on static magnets and those that have alternating current generated fields. These can give temporary benefits but for long-term benefits a bed that gives a steady state magnetic field is required. One, developed by Dr Dean Bronlie, marketed by Magnetico, has a force field nearly ten times stronger than that we currently experience emanating from the earth. See www.magneticosleep.com for further information.

The flow of this magnetic energy through the body for the eight hours of sleep has, Bronlie claims, a remarkable effect on healing. He focuses particularly on its benefits for people with arthritis, but more interestingly for our purposes, it has a demonstrable and powerful effect on the oxygen levels in the blood and the efficiency of the body's biochemical reactions. What is the evidence? Most athletes find it very difficult to improve their VO_2 max readings—this is a measure of the maximum amount of oxygen they can use. However, over a matter of months, Canadian athletes lying on his magnetic bed were able to improve this by 30 per cent—an amazing finding. Also the amount of oxygen in the bloodstream increased. This ability to hyper-oxygenate the body suggests that the magnetic bed could have a powerful beneficial effect against cancer.

Gary Null is an American writer. His website, www.garynull.com, contains a lot of valuable information on the subject of magnets, the research behind their use, controversies and sources for magnets. He notes that strong magnetic fields can help the body protect itself against viruses, bacteria, and fungi by hyper-oxygenating the blood. Magnetic fields also reduce the acidity of the body's tissues making them more alkaline and therefore healthier and less attractive to these invading microbes.

In relation to cancer he notes that cells depolarise (i.e., they lose their magnetic character) before becoming metastatic. He gives the following advice: 'When using magnets for cancer, remember the following rules of thumb: the magnetic pole used must be negative ['south']. The field should be larger than the primary lesion and the gauss greater than 25. Success rate increases if both the gauss and duration are increased. A minimal duration of 20 hours per day for no less than three months is required in most cases.'

Experiments with cancer cells in Petri dishes have shown clear evidence that north (negative) polarity fields retard growth while there is some slight evidence that positive polarity may have the opposite effect and promote cellular growth. Because of these impacts, pregnant women should avoid strong magnetic fields for any length of time.

Null notes also that the use of magnets both improved success when used as an adjuvant therapy by those opting for radiotherapy and/or chemotherapy while at the same time reducing the side effects. Null also takes the view that magnets are more effective when used with herbs and supplements.

Complex Electromagnetic Therapy Machines

Ion magnetic induction therapy machine

The ion magnetic induction therapy machine, developed by Professor Panos T Pappas, also claims to kill cancer cells. For specifications for the building of this machine, see www.portalmarket.com/specifications.html.

Here the general theory behind all these machines, restated time and time again by each new inventor is expressed simply: 'All of the many types of living cells that make up the tissues and organs of the body are tiny electrochemical units. They are powered by a 'battery' that is continually recharged by the cells' metabolic chemistry in a closed loop of biological energy. When a cell is poisoned, damaged, deprived of nutrients or infected, energy is lost in fighting the problem and the [electrical charge] falls to a level where the cell loses its vitality and either struggles to heal itself or dies …. [T]he induction of tiny currents of electricity is remarkably effective in healing, regenerating and revitalizing cells damaged by trauma.'

This machine produces continuous harmonic radiation of between 0.3–250MHz. For further information see www.papimi.gr and www.papimi.com. A number of clinics offer this therapy but the machine itself does not appear to be commercially available to the general public.

Magnetic field therapy

Swedish engineer Ivan Troeng developed a magnetic bench that has a static electromagnetic field of 650 gauss. Patients lie on the bench for 1–2 hours per day. This treatment appears to be only available at one of Europe's leading alternative cancer centres, the Humlegaarden Clinic in Denmark see: www.humlegaarden.com). As with all forms of magnetic therapy, the therapy is not focused on producing a cure, rather, it focuses on putting the body into a state where it heals itself.

Pulsed electro-magnetic field therapy

These machines produce a pulsed magnetic field and are marketed as tools for pain relief and for bone healing—however their effects are broader, and as with other magnetic devices they claim to significantly increase the oxygenation of tissues and to have broad wellness and anti-ageing benefits. The therapeutic strength of any EM field should be in the frequency range of 1–300Hz. One site that reviews a number of machines is www.pemft.org—one machine this site doesn't review is the Curatron—www.curatronic.com.

Quantronic resonance system (QRS)

This is the name of a machine developed in Germany. It consists of a pad that you lie on and a pillow for the head. These are plugged into a normal socket. The result is a very low level pulsed (saw-tooth wave) magnetic field. In fact, the field produced is so weak that it is lower than the prevailing background magnetic field of the earth. Originally it was thought that such a low field would have zero impact on the body but it has been demonstrated that even a very short period of time (five minutes say) spent lying on this pad will have an impact in improving blood flow. The normal recommended treatment, however, is to lie on the machine for two sessions a day, each lasting only eight minutes and to persist for at least six weeks. This has for many people with a wide range of severe symptoms been effective in about 40 per cent of cases of providing a 'complete relief of symptoms' (a rather euphemistic way of saying 'cure').

This machine has been intensively studied by university researchers and was even used by the Russians in the MIR space station. The QRS was installed to counter the problems of calcium wasting from cosmonauts' bones, to increase their circulation and to provide additional energy. Dr William Pawluk, co-author of the book *Magnetic Therapy in Eastern Europe*, described his experience of the machine: 'I was very surprised the first time I laid on it that I could actually feel it. I could feel changes in my body. I could feel heat, the sensation of a vibration and deep relaxation. Physical aches improved on the large pad as the treatment progressed.' His extremely interesting article on this machine can be found at www.quantronmedicine.com.

With cancer, it is known that the cell membrane tension voltage is only 20mV compared with 50mV for a sick cell and 70–110mV for a healthy cell. Background EM fields can help push the cancerous cell's membrane tension voltage up—but if the EM field is too strong, this may damage the cell. This explains why a very weak field—a gentle breeze rather than a storm, as Pawluk describes it—may be better.

Pawluk also notes that the level of the QRS radiation is on the same level as the delta brain waves and that part of its benefits may be that it simulates a short period of deep sleep.

Testimonials covering a very wide spectrum of ailments—including cancer—can be read at www.hightechhealth.net/QRS/testimonials.htm. Many have commented on its powerful overall healing help for those undergoing surgery and radiation along with pain relief. It is also seen as a powerful anti-ageing tool. Many note that increased blood oxygenation levels have resulted.

The machine is commercially available at around US$2,600.

SCENAR

This is a device developed by the Russians and is now widely used in Russia. It looks somewhat like a TV remote control. It is placed on the body where it picks up electromagnetic signals. It processes and responds to these signals—so it is engaging in a kind of energetic conversation with the body. It is claimed to be very successful in treating a wide range of ailments including circulatory, muscular-skeletal, and those relating to the digestive or genitor-urinary systems. Whether or not it can itself cure cancer no one is saying. Such a claim would get it banned in short order. But, nevertheless, for the person with cancer, SCENAR can support and help the healing processes.

Zoetron system

The war against 'quacks' and 'charlatans' resulted (February 2003) in the US Federal Trade Commission (FTC) suing the promoters of a magnetic pulse system for curing cancer called the Zoetron system. The case never came to court as the originators of the Zoetron system mounted a fierce defence. The case has now been settled out of court and the Zoetron system, renamed Nanopulse therapy, is seeking to establish its scientific credibility through small-scale double-blind clinical trials.

The basic theory behind the Zoetron system is as follows. Cancer cells are known to have many more receptors for iron on their external surfaces than normal cells do. Cancer cells have a great need for iron (the reason why supplements containing iron should not be taken by cancer patients). In the Zoetron approach, very small particles—nanoparticles—of iron are introduced to the body. The iron particles will then tend to accumulate disproportionately on the surface of cancerous cells compared to non-cancerous cells. The body is then exposed to an externally-generated pulsed magnetic field strong enough to reach the area of the tumour. The nanoparticles of iron are excited by the magnetic fields and this agitation creates heat. This is really a form of hyperthermia as the objective is to raise the intracellular temperature of cancer cells to 110°F, which is the temperature at which they die. This system, the creators said, has no effect on normal cells, which have low levels of iron.

Until it can prove its value, the therapy is not currently available but, in a personal email to me, Michael Reynolds, one of the developers, said he fervently hopes that one day it will be widely available at a cost of about US$3,000 per course of treatment (including all the associated tests)—but when that will be no one knows.

The V.I.B.E. machine

The V.I.B.E. (vibrational integration bio-photonic energizer) is a machine developed by Gene Koonce, an electronics technician. This machine is clearly a direct descendent of the Tesla coil and Lakhovsky's multi-wave oscillator.

Koonce believes that 'disease is a state of non-vibrating, non-charged or non-energized cells.' The V.I.B.E. machine puts out an electromagnetic field with a high voltage pulse. This recharges the cells bringing about a state of high cellular energy. People stand or sit a few feet away from the machine for only a few minutes at a time. People have said they experience a great energizing effect from this. This energizing effect does seem to lessen with time. One suggestion is that you don't feel it so much when your cells are charged up. There is also anecdotal evidence that people with high PSA scores suggesting prostate cancer have experienced sharp drops in this cancer marker. One other anecdote told by Bill Henderson in one of his cancer newsletters testified to a man with lung cancer expelling cancerous matter after having been exposed to a VIBE machine's rays.

For more information go to www.vibemachine.com where you will find testimonials. At the time of writing the machine costs US$17,500.

Essentially identical but rather cheaper machines can be obtained from a number of other companies. It seems that the founders of these various companies once worked together. Something happened along the way and they each ended up developing their own equipment based on the same concepts. Compare the Evenstar and SEAD machines at:

www.bels-tech.com, www.energizeforhealth.com/sead-units-products.html, www.evenstar-tech.com.

Miscellaneous Healing Machines and Therapies

The light beam generator

This is a newly-developed piece of equipment manufactured by ELF Laboratories, Inc., which claims to have a wide range of healing potentials (www.lightbeamgenerator.com). Cancer is not listed on their website but there are anecdotal claims that it is beneficial. The company literature says this about the machine: 'The LBG® works by helping to rebalance the charge of the cells' electromagnetic fields. Using cold-gas light photons and extremely low-energy electromagnetic frequency patterns, the LBG® helps separate these cells from each other and their accumulated inflammation, swelling, abnormal growths, and other lymph blockages.' Of course anything that works against inflammation is likely to work against cancer cells.

Microwave resonance therapy (MRT)

This is a high-intensity, low-frequency treatment applied to acupuncture points to treat entire acupuncture meridians and in this way to encourage the body to return to physiological equilibrium— known as homeostasis. This has been developed by Professor Sergei Sitko in Russia. He has used this on over 8,000 patients suffering from a wide range of illnesses. Unfortunately, outside Russia, it is difficult to find anyone offering access to this approach so it remains at this stage theoretical.

Light therapy

A machine called an Eichoterm Solarium is in use at the Humlegaarden Clinic in Denmark (www.humlegaarden.com). It radiates light combining UVB and UVC rays with an intensity typical of a nice hot day in the tropics along with 'orange collared heat rays'. Typically a patient will receive the therapy for up to an hour, equivalent to a whole day sunbathing in the tropics. According to the clinic's brochure: 'This causes photo-chemical processes to be activated in the skin, the result being a strong detoxification of the body. Excellent results have been seen for cancer, disseminated sclerosis, skin diseases, arthritic diseases, circulatory diseases and many other chronic diseases.'

Ultraviolet blood irradiation (UBI)

UBI—also referred to as UVB therapy—has been around a long time and it appears to have a broad range of health benefits including circulatory improvement, killing bacteria and viruses, improving immune system. It also appears to be beneficial for cancer and for auto-immune diseases but no-one is shouting about this too loudly to avoid the inevitable repercussions. Essentially it works in this way: doctors extract blood from the patient and irradiate it. The blood is then pumped back into the body. It costs US$100–200 a go to have this procedure done, and patients are advised to have up to eight treatments. It is completely non-toxic. A list of doctors offering this therapy can be found at http://altmedangel.com/1a.html.

Dr Gorgun's GEMM therapy

Dr Seckiner Gorgun is a Turkish medical researcher who has developed a radio-wave generator, which he refers to as a GEMM device. This sends 'precisely calculated therapeutic radio waves' that interfere with the ATP production which cancers need to fuel their rapid cell division. When the ATP production is halted the cancer cells are killed. He has apparently had good success treating terminally-ill patients with brain tumours, bone cancers, breast cancers and others. For more information email info@gemm-therapy.com.

Sono photo-dynamic therapy

This is a combination of sound and light therapies. In both cases a substance sensitive to light and/or sound is injected into the body and is activated by light or sound waves. The object is to create free radicals specifically to attack the cancer cells. This therapy appears to be most effective with cancer tumours close to the surface. For more information contact the Hope4Cancer clinic in Tijuana www.hope4cancer.com.

Subtle energy therapies

Most of the machines/therapies discussed so far have made use of electricity or magnetism in an easy to conceptualize manner. There is an enemy (a microbe or parasite) that is attacked by a weapon—or there is a cell whose vibrational frequencies are enhanced.

However, to consider 'energy medicine' to be simply an additional area of medicine on the fringes of other areas of medicine is a misunderstanding. The truth is, energy medicine is a new paradigm, a new way of understanding the body and healing processes that includes all other medicines, including the allopathic tradition that in this section I have referred to as orthodox medicine.

The idea that the body is a pulsing energy system is one familiar to anyone interested in Eastern healing traditions. The Chinese have long used the concept of qi (pronounced 'chee') energy, which they see as a life force that flows through certain 'meridians' or vertical channels. Indian Ayurvedic medicine similarly is based on a concept of prana energy that relates to certain energy centres they call chakras. However, in this chapter, we are going to look far beyond these traditional ideas.

Underlying all the therapies that will be discussed below is the idea that the universe, the world and our bodies are systems of energy that interconnect: light, electricity, magnetism and other subtle energies are all at play within these interconnecting systems. The science that underlies this understanding of the world is described by quantum physics rather than classical, Newtonian, mechanical physics. It should also be noted that most of what we call orthodox medicine is virulently hostile to this new concept. This is a major battleground. Readers are invited to make up their own minds.

The old way of looking at the universe and our bodies is to see them as a system of solid physical parts that relate to each other in a way governed by fixed mechanical laws. Our bodies are therefore machines.

The new way of looking at our bodies is to see them as intercommunicating systems of energy—and there are many different forms of energy.

The primary or fundamental form of energy is electromagnetic energy. It is present in and around everything. To say that we are wrapped in an envelope of electromagnetic energy, however, seriously understates the complexity of what is going on in our bodies. Every part of our body—and every micro-part of each and every part (down to the level of electrons and beyond) is pulsing and vibrating and so creating micro-electromagnetic fields The interplay of all these myriads of vibrating patterns helps both to establish coherence within the whole system and at the same time is a network of communication from one part to another (or rather between each part and every other part). When there are injuries or imbalances in a specific location within the system this will have an effect on the local vibration which will communicate itself to the rest of the system.

And interestingly, when we look at the body as a system (or systems) of energy, we see that our individuality does not stop at the physical boundary of our skin but flows into the space around the physical body and therefore comes into contact with the energy systems of other living beings around us.

Many, probably most, medical doctors and scientists are extremely uneasy with this kind of talk—but research has established without a shadow of doubt that strange things are going on that simply cannot be explained by a macro molecular-chemical concept of the body. Acupuncture is one therapy, for example, that has clearly demonstrable and repeatable effects. It is commonly used even in hospitals as a pain-relieving procedure. Yet, to the scientist who cannot escape the confines of the old, mechanical view of the body, the theory of acupuncture is bizarre and indeed meaningless. It is simply 'wrong'. And yet it works. One doctor has suggested that the reason therapies like acupuncture work is that patients are experiencing a placebo effect (without explaining the nature of placebo). Either that 'or the whole of physics and chemistry as we know them are wrong,' as more than one scientist has put it.

It is not possible to even begin a summary of some of the complex ideas suggested by this new paradigm of medicine. For further discussion of the science behind energy medicine you should consult the following books: *Vibrational Medicine* by Richard Gerber, MD; *Energy Medicine: the Scientific Basis* by James L Oschman, *The Body Electric* by Robert O Becker and *Perfect Health* by Deepak Chopra.

However, what we can say is that extremely exciting results have been reported from the use of therapies or equipment that interface with the body's bio-energetic system.

Acupuncture

Acupuncturists seek to promote the flow of healing energy through vertical channels that run down the body. They make use of needles to stimulate positive energy or to retard negative energy flows. No one has claimed that acupuncture on its own is effective against cancer (but then again it would be illegal for any non-qualified doctor to make such a claim!). One British veterinary surgeon, John Carter, has used acupuncture successfully as part of a general protocol against cancer in animals. Acupuncture has also been used to help reduce the side effects of chemotherapy and radiation.

AIM (all inclusive method) program

The AIM Program is at the most extreme fringes of energy medicine. The starting point is simple enough. We are all energy systems and our health is impacted by energy disharmonies—but these disharmonies are detectable and by focusing a balancing energy to counter the disharmony, the original disharmony can be eliminated. Particular disharmonies have been associated with specific diseases—though the AIM Program makes it very clear that they don't try to 'cure cancer', instead they seek to eliminate the disharmonic energy pattern that they have learnt to associate with cancer.

So far so good. However, to understand where the AIM people are coming from we need to have some understanding of hologram theory. Holograms are three dimensional images created by a complex interaction of lasers. The interesting thing about a hologram is that you can't cut it in two. If you try, you do not end up with two halves but with two wholes. Each part of a hologram contains the whole. This has got some scientists excited because the universe as a whole appears to share some of the characteristics of a hologram. One of these characteristics is that information can be shared instantaneously by two particles irrespective of the distance between them. This has been demonstrated by a French physicist, Alain Aspect. There are many websites dedicated to discussing this issue far beyond my own ability to follow them and for those of you who wish to learn more may I suggest you do a Google search of 'hologram theory'.

But the key point we need to keep in mind is that if something impacts one part of a hologram, the effects are instantly felt by all parts of the hologram. Now, each living entity is a system of energy and is surrounded by an invisible energy matrix. The next conceptual leap—if we are to go along with their thinking (in my opinion a big if)—that we must make is to accept that the energy matrix that surrounds each person is also present in any photograph of that person.

Following hologram theory, we can surmise that the photograph can be the recipient of balancing energy therapy and the person in the photograph will benefit from this energetic input—even though they may be thousands of miles away. This is precisely what the AIM program does.

The promoters of the AIM Program make a big point of calling their approach 'spiritual healing'. Their website explains their concept: 'Our Spiritual Technology delivers thousands of balancing energies for both gross and subtle (e.g., karmic) energetic imbalances. Among the additional energies are special activating frequencies that enable your higher self to select automatically, via your photograph, those frequencies you need at any given time. In addition, there are enhancing energies that help increase your Life Force and ability to respond to energetic crises. The AIM energies cover a wide range of issues for realizing wholeness in living beings.'

In practice, those taking part in the AIM Program submit a whole-body photograph which is placed on a tray that is permanently irradiated with subtle energies. Currently, a year's therapy costs US$1,000 per person (US$2,000 per family group of five). For further information see www.energeticmatrix.com.

Is this science or is it a scam? Those who argue that it is science say that the science that underlies the AIM Program is quantum physics and as even Nobel prize winner Richard Feynman commented: 'I think I can safely say that nobody understands quantum mechanics.' Lynne McTaggart's recent book, *The Field*, is as good an introduction as any to some of the concepts. However, since this technology does seem to be fantastical—almost in the realm of the magical—it is worth pondering a few thoughts:

'Miracles happen, not in opposition to nature, but in opposition to what we know of nature.'

St Augustine.

'Any technology which is sufficiently advanced is indistinguishable from magic.'

Robert Heinlein.

'Those who are not shocked when they first come across quantum theory cannot possibly have understood it.'

Niels Bohr.

Nevertheless, choosing this approach does involve a huge leap of faith, even suspension of reason—and I, like anyone with a rational, scientific bent, would dearly love to see a double-blind controlled trial. But I do see the problem: who could we trust to carry out this trial? How do we know this is not a load of hooey. The truth, in the sense that nothing is certain, is that we don't. So how can we choose this approach without the fear that we are being taken advantage of? Perhaps it comes down to money. If you have the cash and you're prepared to take the risk (who knows, maybe it does everything they say it does). Then why not? Otherwise, this can be safely set aside.

Bio-energetic healing

Some healers appear to have the ability to work in a subtle way with the energy fields of the body. They have differing understandings of what they are doing but the end result is a patient who is demonstrably healthier. This healing can go under a number of names, with differing philosophies. One such school of healing calls itself pranic healing, another is psychic or spiritual healing. I talked to John Eastman, a naturopath and bio-energetic healer. I asked him about his healing work and how he explained it. This was his response:

'Healing is a universal phenomenon. It is not restricted to any one religion, group, country or culture. Sometimes healing takes place instantly after just one session. More often it works gradually and progressively over time. It certainly doesn't require any belief on the part of the person receiving the healing as witnessed by the fact that babies, children and even people who are unconscious have recovered from ill-health as a result of healing energy.

'There are different levels of energy. On one level, the level of the physical body, there is the energy that flows through us. This is often referred to as 'qi' (or chi) energy (East Asia), or prana energy (South Asia). But there is another energy which we can say both precedes and at the same time transcends chi or prana. Whatever name we use to call it we can say that this energy is spiritual or divine energy.

'It is this spiritual energy that we use to heal with. When I am healing, it is this energy that flows through me. I am not using my own qi energy. I am channelling universal divine energy. That is why instead of feeling tired after healing I feel very clear, extremely energized and even, I can say, spiritually uplifted. Spiritual healing, complementary medicine and orthodox medicine are not mutually exclusive. Certainly spiritual healing can support and improve the outcome of other forms of medicine and healing.'

John Eastman can be contacted at www.johneastman.com. There are many such healers.

A case of such healing caused quite a stir in Victorian England. Harriet Martineau was an early nineteenth-century novelist, journalist, social reformer, educator, children's writer, philosopher of naturalism, environmentalist, social scientist and pioneering feminist who published over fifty books and almost two thousand articles and newspaper columns. She became a chronic invalid. The best efforts of all the leading doctors did nothing for her. For five years she suffered until, in 1844, a travelling healer—who interestingly referred to himself as a 'magnetizer'—by the name of Pencer Hall treated her. His treatment consisted of giving her 'magnetic passes'. After three days she was able to eat and sleep comfortably for the first time in five years. Thereafter the treatment was continued by her maid.

Interestingly, John Eastman refers to his own healing technique—which he evolved entirely independently—as bio-energetic alignment: this involves moving the hands over the body without physical contact. Such an action might very well be described as a magnetic pass.

The suggestion that electromagnetic fields are involved is supported experimentally. Dr John Zimmerman (a leading US researcher in the field of magnetic therapy and who works at the Colorado School of Medicine) using sensitive electromagnetic sensing equipment found that healers are capable of producing very strong electromagnetic fields from their hands—so strong it went off the scale of his magnetometer. Clearly if it can be measured then it's real.

Other healers, such as those using the Chinese qigong technique are doing something different. Qigung therapists are able to transmit heating energy from their palms. They are also, for different purposes, able to absorb infrared energy from the environment.

One organisation that provides free energy healing is the Johrei Foundation. For further information go to www.johrei.com.

Throughout the world there are energy healers—many of whom have arrived at their calling by circuitous routes. One way to find one near you is to look for spiritualist churches. See also the discussion on psychic surgeons below.

Colour therapy

Colour therapy involves irradiating the body—or specific parts of the body—with light of a particular, designated colour which is determined by the therapist after diagnosis of the problem. Sometimes it is called spectro-chrome therapy.

Colours are, like X-rays and radio band frequencies, forms of electromagnetic radiation. They inhabit a very narrow stretch of the Spectrum of Electromagnetic Radiation. But just as microwaves, X-rays and ultraviolet rays have an effect on the body, so too, it is argued, do the different colours— both combined in the form of full-spectrum white light or separately.

Research has shown that the average light bulb and neon strip, such as provide the lighting in most homes and offices is not healthy as they do not provide full-spectrum white light. Full-spectrum lights are available. John Ott, who is one of the pioneers in the field of light and its effects on health discovered that full-spectrum lighting helped reduce hyperactivity among children. It was his view that conventional lighting and televisions that leak radiation can cause hyperactivity. The beneficial effects of sunlight are dealt with separately. Here we will look at how colour therapy works.

The colour therapist works with a projector that has five coloured plates—red, yellow, green, blue, violet—that can be used separately or in combination to produce any of the following colours: the primary light colours: red, green and violet; the secondary light colours: yellow, blue and magenta; and the tertiary colours: lemon, orange, turquoise, indigo, purple and scarlet.

Green is the colour that harmonizes and maintains the natural physical balance, so this is the colour most often used. Disease and illness cause the body to shift to one side or the other. If it moves more to the yellow this means the body will be feverish or inflamed. This needs to be corrected with a dose of blue light. If the movement is the other way, towards the blue, then the patient will feel dull and sedated and will need a dose of yellow, perhaps.

Each colour has a range of qualities and effects on the body. Red, for example, stimulates the liver and helps build haemoglobin; green stimulates the pituitary and acts as a general purifier and disinfectant of the body; scarlet is aphrodisiac and stimulates the kidneys; orange is for those with weak lungs and who need to stimulate the thyroid. The colours are light colours—not pigment colours.

So far, we have been in the realm of the easily understood. But colour therapists make two claims that are less easily accepted. The first is that water poured into a glass of the correct colour will become energised with the qualities of the colour and can then be drunk as medicine. Secondly, the colour need not be applied directly on the individual's body. In fact the person can be absent, as long as some 'witness' of the patient's presence can be used to receive the treatment. The 'witness' can be a drop of blood, a piece of hair or even the person's own handwritten name and address on an envelope. An explanation of these claims is given below under vibrational medicine.

And what is it like to receive colour therapy? One patient described her feelings during a session. First the therapist bathed her in a lemon colour. 'At first I felt nothing but as time progressed there was a feeling of fullness and tightness in the area. By the end … I was feeling just slightly nauseous.' Then the therapist changed the light to a dark red filter. 'I was immediately relieved of the slight discomforts and became aware of a new sensation farther down, a fullness and yet somehow a relaxing and soothing vibration [and after 15 minutes] I was on the verge of being asleep.' The therapist changed the coloured light to green. '… the moment he did I was wide awake. My whole body started to tingle. My breath came fast and my heart was pounding. … It was most similar to the excitement that builds up just before orgasm.'

In subsequent treatments this women did not respond so strongly to the sensations—in fact called them mild. This woman was, it is claimed, cured of fibroids and cancer.

A course of colour therapy treatments may consist of only 4–6 sessions. In fact few colour therapists use the whole room colour projection described above—instead many use phials of coloured waters. For further information and referral to colour therapists, contact the International Association for Colour Therapy at www.iac-colour.co.uk.

Crystal therapy

Recently, crystals have been promoted as having healing properties that vary with the material, colour and shape of the crystal. Crystal healers take as their starting point the belief that all matter is made of nothing but vibrating energies that are aligned with the universal energies, and that crystals are forms that unify and focus these energies. During a crystal healing any number and variety of crystals may be used and placed on the body— particularly on and around the chakra points, which lie on the central line of the head, body and pelvis.

A crystal healer bases all decisions about placement and arrangement of stones on his/her intuition. In fact, as with many other vibrational practices, the psychic sensitivity of the therapists is considered to be an important healing element in itself. Since the universe is a single energy field, it is argued, then each and every person is a locus for this universal energy. By aligning the healer's energies with the patient's, healing is aided.

Crystals are believed to have the ability to magnify energies and they are generally placed on chakra points. Crystals can also be placed in water to create an energised gem elixir which works along the same principles as the flower essence elixirs—though the latter are generally considered to be more wide-ranging in their effects. Crystals help to align mental and emotional energies.

Crystal healing devotee, Katrina Raphael strongly recommends the crystal luvulite. 'Luvulite is the pressure release valve that can bring peace and understanding to a mind and body that have lost their source of strength ….' It helps the mind focus its own healing energies. 'This healing force if properly used, has the power to heal any dis-ease and restore complete mental and physical health.'

Luvulite, unfortunately, is a fairly rare and expensive stone. However, other stones (e.g., quartz) do have healing qualities attributed to them.

Is this airy-fairy new age nonsense? James Oschman, author of *Energy Medicine: the Scientific Basis* (2003), is not willing to dismiss crystal healing. He notes that all living tissues are essentially crystalline in nature: 'Crystalline arrangements are the rule and not the exception in living systems'—but the crystals that comprise muscles, connective tissue and the other organs consist of soft, flexible, liquid crystals. Oschman hypothesises that these crystals enhance the energy exchange between two individuals—that the crystals function not so much on their own but as a vehicle for the healer's own healing energies. 'Crystalline molecular arrays found throughout the body are exceedingly sensitive to energy fields in the environment.'

Healing sounds

Primal sound therapy, as taught by the Maharishi Ayurveda Health Centres, is based on the idea that all matters of health originate at the 'quantum level' of the body—which is in tune with the energy web of the universe. Ill-health comes when this energy connection is blocked for some reason. It is therefore necessary to open up the energy channels so that we can get back in touch with the primal energy vibrations, which always work in the direction of health. One method of achieving this is to use vibrating sound.

There are a number of sound therapies. Perhaps the simplest to access is that put forward by Jonathan Goldman in his book *Healing Sounds*. He suggests that an harmonic meditation heals by 'balancing the chakras'. To do this is simple. You place yourself in a comfortable meditation pose and breathe from the abdomen. Then you focus on each of the seven chakras in turn starting from:

1. the base of the spine (close to the anus)
2. a point a few centimetres below the navel
3. the navel
4. the heart: this point is in the centre of the chest between the two nipples
5. the throat
6. the brow: the position of the third eye
7. the crown: the top of the head.

While focusing on each point make an open throated vowel humming sound as full of vibrations as is possible, starting with a low tone and an 'uh' or 'ooo' sound. At each chakra point the tone should shift up a notch and the vowel sound should change like this: uh-ooo-oh-ah-eye-ih-eee.

The more one does this the more proficient one will become, even without previous experience of singing. One doesn't have to be a 'good singer' to get benefit from this. Jonathan Goldman also claims that healers can use sounds to heal their patients.

There is in fact laboratory-based experimental support for the idea that sound can directly kill cancer cells. Researcher, Fabien Maman, played the Ionian scale on a xylophone note by note: C-D-E-F-G-A-B and then C and D of the next octave, next to a Petri dish containing a cancer cell (one of the HeLa line). After fourteen minutes of this, the cancer cell exploded. His explanation was this: 'Healthy cells seem to breathe in a way that allows them to absorb and integrate the sound without resistance. They did not appear to keep the power of the sound frequency inside of themselves like the cancer cells did. The healthy cells appeared supple and able to freely receive, absorb and return the sound energy. In contrast the cancer cells appeared inflexible and immutable in their structure.'

For more information contact:

- Maharishi Ayurvedic sound healing: www.theraj.com
- Sound Healers Association: www.healingsounds.com

Music as a whole is also health-promoting—but not all music. Experiments with plants have shown that percussive rock music has a negative impact. Mozart, on the other hand, is life affirming. As is Bach and the intricate choral harmonies of Monteverdi and Schutz. Black music from early honky-tonk and gospel to Motown similarly makes you want to sing along. Strauss's waltzes make you want to twirl and dance. The life affirming qualities of music should not be under-estimated. Many years ago I was persuaded to go to a concert of Indian dulcimer music, about which I knew nothing at all. If I had known it was going to last three hours and that the seats we would be allocated were going to be so uncomfortable I wouldn't have gone. As it was I had had a long day and was feeling tired and irritable. But Shiv Kumar Sharma, one of India's leading traditional instrumentalists, slowly wove a web of sound around the hall and then suddenly it was over. I couldn't believe I had been listening for three hours. I emerged from that concert hall utterly refreshed.

Lakhovsky's cosmic energy cure

Georges Lakhovsky, whose multi-wave oscillator we have already discussed, had come to the conclusion that all life radiates vibrations—these radiations emanate from the oscillation of minute cellular magnetic fields. Every cell is essentially an electrical circuit with its own electromagnetic field. Ill-health occurs, then, when there is a disequilibrium caused by a war of radiations between the natural healthy cells and the radiations emanating from viruses or other invading pathogens. If the invading microbial radiation is stronger, the cells' healthy radiations are affected and are unable to maintain their own proper level of radiation. On the other hand, if the cells' healthy radiations are stronger, the microbe is killed.

From this, it follows, that if the body can be flooded with oscillations of the same frequency as that of a healthy cell, then the cells should be able to return to their healthy frequencies and so be able to fight of the disease. For this purpose he developed his multi-wave oscillator described above.

However, he did not stop there. Thinking about the source of the energy needed to charge the cells in the first place, he came to the conclusion that it was the energy that streams through the cosmos. It should therefore be possible, he thought, to focus this energy without the help of any artificial machinery.

He made a copper circlet, thirty centimetres in diameter, and attached it to a support made of ebonite, a material made of black vulcanized rubber, which he stuck into the flower pot. He then took two groups of geraniums. Half he injected with a bacteria that causes cancer—the other half were his controls. When the cancerous growths had developed, he placed the coil round one cancerous plant. After several weeks he found that all the cancer infected plants had died—with one exception. The plant in the coil was not only alive, it was not only cancer-free, but it had grown twice as large as the normal plants.

Subsequently, a number of experiments have been done both with copper circlets in the form of collars, bracelets and belts. These appear to have a profound normalizing effect—so making them beneficial for a wide range of illnesses. Even cancer patients have, it seems, experienced remissions. Any length of copper wire can be used—apparently even standard insulated cable.

Some people swear to the beneficial effects of placing copper circlets round the neck, waist, arms above the elbow and legs above the knee. Secure them in place in any way you can. Since the effect is to normalize the body's natural healthy state by eliminating poisons some early discomfort may be experienced—occasional pains, headaches and even flu-like symptoms—and a lot of water should be drunk to help this elimination. Doctors have used these copper circlets in many countries for many problems and no long-term toxic effects have been noted.

For those who may be cynical about the supposed effects of radiation from outer space, I would urge you to read Lyall Watson's book *Supernature*. Watson is a scientist who demonstrates very clearly the evidence supporting the view that radiation from the sun, moon, planets and indeed the entire firmament of stars have powerful impacts on our physical bodies.

Psychic surgery and psychic healers

Psychic surgery is practiced widely in Brazil and the Philippines, and despite investigations that expose the frauds, practitioners are claimed to have a good record of healing.

In Brazil, a healer by the name of John of God (Joao de Deus) has attracted thousands of visitors to his centre in Goias in Brazil. One visitor commented to me: 'I visited him twice. On both occasions there was healing but no cure.' Others, however, claim to have been cured of all manner of illness. For further information see www.friendsofthecasa.org.

In the Philippines, psychic surgeons appear to perform surgery with their bare hands or with rusty knives without any anaesthesia and without any pain. The hand appears to delve into the flesh and a bloody lump of flesh appears in the psychic surgeon's palm.

Hocus pocus? Some investigators say they are all out-and-out frauds who use magic sleight-of-hand to pluck what appear to be cancerous tumours, but which are in fact concealed lumps of chicken or cow flesh. But they do have one potent weapon that the modern medical doctor generally does not avail him/herself of: the 'psychic surgeon' is working with the placebo effect and not against it.

In Britain, a psychic surgeon called Stephen Turoff has made a name for himself as a healer and a guide. He sees people for a modest fee at his Danbury Healing Clinic in Chelmsford, England and also in Coin, near Malaga in Spain. Contact: The Danbury Healing Clinic, The Miami Hotel, Princes Road, Chelmsford, Essex CM2 9AJ, England, Telephone +44 (0)1245-348325. However, it is worth reading the readers' reviews of a book about his work: *Stephen Turoff: Psychic Surgeon*, on www.amazon.co.uk. Most of the reviewers had personal experience of his healing work, but not all were positive about their experiences.

Biologist Lyall Watson studied a psychic healer in the Philippines. The man would point his finger about an inch from the patient's skin and an incision would appear. Watson himself received such an incision from which a scar remained (see *Personal Spirituality*, D Benor, 2006, p.146).

A final anecdotal note: My otherwise cynical physiotherapist aunt had a friend who had breast cancer. My aunt accompanied her to the Philippines to visit one of these healers. Shortly after the visit the friend noticed her tumour had disappeared.

Psychic healers are also an enigma. One famous Brazilian healer worked without touching his patients he would write down prescriptions as patients filed past. In one test, 1,000 patients filed past. Later, his diagnoses were, according to the report, found to be phenomenally accurate.

This ability should not be easily dismissed as impossible. In 1985, an American doctor by the name of Norman Shealy began to work with a journalist, Caroline Myss, who claimed she had always had an intuitive ability to 'know' things. They lived more than 1,000 miles apart. He would phone her and ask her to help him diagnose the state of health of the patient in his room. Once she was comfortable with this procedure and was able to relax, she would intuitively 'enter' the patient's body, travelling through it to assess the health of each specific organ. According to Shealy, her diagnoses were 93 per cent accurate.

Radiation hormesis

The word 'hormesis' is Greek for 'rapid motion' and is used to describe a phenomenon where low doses of toxins or other stress-causing effects have a beneficial impact on biological systems. Radiation hormesis is when that effect is created by very low level ionizing radiation (just a little higher than normal background radiation).

It is known that some stones do give off slightly higher than average radiation and these appear to have healing properties that may be beneficial to those suffering pain or who have cancer. One company selling stones that are claimed to have healing effects is Night Hawk Minerals: www.nighthawkminerals.com On their website you will also find stories of people who have used the stones. Jay Gutierrez who runs the company makes big claims for its curative powers in relation to cancer. But, as usual, it is a case of 'suck it and see'.

Bill Henderson, whose Healing Cancer Gently newsletter is a useful source of information discussed his own use of one of these stones. 'Within about four hours of taping one of the rocks to my upper left arm, pain I had experienced there for five years disappeared. I originally pulled a muscle there in the gym. But after the muscle tear healed, I had 'neuro-toxins' in the muscle which just would not go away …. It has been so sore for the five years that I could not sleep on my left side. If I rolled over during the night, the pain would wake me up. Well, that pain is gone now, since I taped Jay's stone to my arm.'

Reflexology

Foot massages have been known to have a beneficial relaxing effect since time began. The present day system of reflexology arose as a result first of Dr William Fitzgerald in 1913. He came to the view that there were ten vertical energy zones running down the body. After further experimentation, he found that by putting pressure on a specific area of the body he could anaesthetize related areas along the zone. This early work was developed by Eunace Ingham in the 1930s. She found that working on the feet alone was the same as working the whole body. It should be noted that acupuncturists also recognize that the foot, hand, ears and other places are microsystems that mirror the workings of the entire body—as a result, some acupuncturists only work on the ear, no matter what or where the ailment is.

Modern reflexologists have mapped out very precise points on the soles and sides of the feet that correspond to the different organs of the body. If there is any problem in any of the organs small crystalline deposits can be felt in the related areas in the feet. The massage eliminates these crystal deposits and this has a healing effect on the organ concerned. As with acupuncture, one way to find areas where there might be a health concern is to test for sensitivity. Any sensitivity is a sign that attention is needed (i.e., rub the spot that hurts or is sensitive)—later you will find it is not so sensitive.

Reflexologists will never diagnose specific illnesses though they will say which tissues or organs are in need of attention.

Clearly, reflexology, while not being an anti-cancer therapy specifically, can play a useful role as part of a bundle of therapies aimed at improving overall health.

Reiki and therapeutic touch

Reiki is both a contact and a non-contact therapy in which the Reiki healer focuses healing energy from the palms of his/her hands to the area of an illness or to places on the meridians of the body. As with all Chinese-based healing systems, the body is viewed as being filled with channels, known as meridians, of living energy, qi [pronounced 'chee']. It is the healer's job to invigorate the flow of this energy and to remove blockages in the meridians.

The positions of these meridians is very precisely known to Chinese healers but Western doctors are bemused by them as there is nothing in their knowledge that conforms to these meridians—they do not follow the circulatory or nervous system. However, recently, French researchers injecting radioactive isotopes into human subjects found that they travelled along the lines of the meridians. Also, researchers in bio-magnetism say that the energy flow along the meridians is the way in which the bodily magnetic system completes its cycle. The brain pulses a negative magnetic impulse which travels down the spine and then returns to the brain, along the meridians, through the flesh and organs of the body, in order to complete the circuit.

Reiki is not the only name given to this form of healing: qigong masters also use it and in America there is a technique known as therapeutic touch, which despite its name does not involve physical contact.

One clinical test to assess the effectiveness of therapeutic touch was conducted by New York University researcher, Daniel Wirth. In a double blind study involving 44 patients with full-skin-thickness surgical wounds cut deliberately for the purposes of the study. The subjects inserted the arm with the wound through a hole in a wall. They could not see what was happening on the other side. They were told that their bio-potential was being measured by a non-contact device, a procedure lasting five minutes each time. Half the patients received non-contact therapeutic touch treatment and half the patients held their arm into an empty room. A doctor who did not know which patients were receiving the treatment was delegated to measure the wounds with a special digital and highly accurate device. There was no placebo effect involved because there was no suggestion that any healing was taking place. By day 16, more than half of the treated group had completely healed (wound-size zero) while none of the untreated group had healed. Something clearly is going on.

In another case demonstrating the healing powers of what is known as 'laying on of hands', a Lutheran nun in Darmstadt, Germany was helping to build a chapel when she had a bad fall which resulted in a compound pelvic fracture. The nuns maintained an all night all day vigil for two days and then, against the doctor's advice took her out. They prayed and performed laying on of hands. Immediately after the laying on of hands she stood up and announced that she was free of pain. After two weeks the nun presented herself back at the hospital and the doctors had to agree that she was cured.

A friend of mine took her son to see John Eastman, an energy healer who is extremely uncomfortable being called that. Her son had had an injury playing ice hockey and his knee was swollen. His mother reported to me that during the energy healing session she could see the swelling visibly reduce. She was very impressed.

It is known that healers appear to have developed an ability to radiate electromagnetic energy, these forms of healing appear to be other manifestations of the same effect.

Sunlight and sunbathing

Sunlight has been getting a very bad press in recent years. Certainly, there is some evidence to suggest that excess sunlight causes non-fatal forms of skin cancer (but only, some say, in those whose skin is fair and whose diet contains too much animal fat). But to conclude from this that the best thing to do is to stay indoors would be counter-productive. The fact is that there is also a very good correlation between high exposure to sunlight and low incidence of internal cancers. This beneficial effect is far more important than any negative effect.

In one study, rabbits were exposed to different levels of natural light. The rabbits exposed to the most light, developed the fewest tumours, had fewer metastases and fewer deaths. In a Russian study, animals exposed to sunlight had only half the number of malignant growths compared with controls not exposed to sunlight. A US Navy study of cancer incidence amongst sailors found that there was a relatively high incidence of skin cancer, but a substantially reduced incidence of all other cancers (two and a half times lower than the average). The incidence of breast cancer in mice has been cut in half by exposing them to ultraviolet light.

In one anecdotal case described by Dr Kime, author of a book entitled simply, *Sunlight*, a 41-year-old patient of his had a breast removed because of cancer and had been given chemotherapy treatments, because the cancer had moved into her lungs and bones. However, the doctors treating her were not hopeful of success. She approached Kime who felt there was nothing he could do for her cancer but that he could perhaps help her improve her overall health. He removed the refined polyunsaturated oils and fats—particularly margarine which is known to lower the immune system—from her diet and asked her to eat only whole foods, nothing refined. He also told her about some of the research that had been done with sunlight and cancer. She acted on his advice and started to spend a great deal of time out of doors in the sunlight.

Before starting the sunbathing she had been losing weight, but after several weeks of sunbathing and good dietary practice, her weight levelled off and she began to notice she had more energy. She eventually went back to see her doctors and they could find no apparent symptoms of her widespread cancer.

It is natural for us to visualize the warm rays of the sun as life-enhancing. We feel better out of doors in the sun. This is not an imaginary effect. The immune system responds positively to sunlight, and sunlight has been shown to increase the amount of oxygen in the body's tissues. High blood pressure is also correlated with high cancer incidence and sunlight has a very strong lowering effect on blood pressure—and so reduces the otherwise higher cancer incidence. So, all in all, a day pottering about on a beach or in a garden on a warm summer's day is a day well spent.

Sunlight of course is very important for vitamin D production. Foods supplemented with vitamin D are a poor substitute. In this context, it should be noted that sun creams and sunblocks are to be avoided, as they prevent the intake of the ultra-violet light needed by the body to make vitamin D. The suggestion that sunscreens should not be used is highly controversial and appears to fly in the face of good sense. However, in relation to cancer, the evidence in favour of the protective effects of sunscreens has not been clearly demonstrated in epidemiological studies. For example, in 1998, Dr Marianne Berwick, an epidemiologist at Memorial Sloan-Kettering Cancer Center in New York, presented an analysis of sunscreen use and skin cancer at the annual meeting of the American Association for the Advancement of Science (AAAS). Her conclusion: 'We don't really know whether sunscreens prevent skin cancer.'

To deal with all these factors, different strategies have been suggested. One is to spend an amount of time unprotected and then, when there is a danger of being burnt, to add a sunscreen. Others suggest using sunscreen only on the most exposed surfaces. Others still suggest that you should gradually increase exposure without using a sunscreen to prevent burning. There are a number of organic sunscreens coming on to the market and green tea is strongly protective—so keep the kettle on and keep pouring it over you (having waited for it to cool down!). Life Extension Foundation offers a Total Sun Protection Cream SPF-30 that helps protect also against free radical damage www.lef.org. Another suggestion is to use coconut oil. This is a healthy oil and it appears to prevent burning.

For those who do suffer non-melanoma skin cancers, BEC5 curaderm cream is reported to be very effective.

Some people are very sensitive to exposure to sunlight. They should increase their intake of carotene by drinking fresh carrot juice. This will help them become more tolerant. Others, particularly those of African extraction, have dark skins that block absorption of vitamin D. The darker your skin naturally is, the longer you need to be out in the sun to get its benefits. Sadly, whether it is lack of sunlight or down to diet, African Americans have a far higher incidence of cancer than people with white skin, and they also succumb faster to the disease.

One of the ways in which sunlight is supposed to work is that it electrically charges the air as it passes through the atmosphere. For good health and sense of well-being, we need the right balance of negative and positive ions and of the right kind. Heating and air-conditioning systems, electrical equipment and synthetic materials all tend to increase the positive ions and take out smaller negative ions. The result is ill-health. Negatively charged ions increase one's feelings of health and increased energy and mental and emotional exhilaration. Experiments with rats show that cancers grow faster if they breathe common indoor air as opposed to normal outdoor air.

And of course sunlight is relaxing and so makes the body better able to tolerate physical and mental stress. It also helps make the body's tissues alkaline, the importance of which needs no stressing.

Further evidence that sunlight is beneficial comes from a study that shows that New Yorkers who retire to Florida have lower cancer levels than New Yorkers who stay in New York.

In another study, researchers found that the time of year in which a cancer operation took place had a significant influence on the likelihood of the malignancy recurring. Patients who had a high intake of vitamin D in their diet, and who also had their surgery in the summer were more than twice as likely to be alive five years after cancer surgery compared to those patients who had low vitamin D intake and whose operations took place in the winter.

Earlier, we discussed the advisability of avoiding sunscreen as far as possible, you are also advised to avoid sunglasses, or indeed any form of eye wear, while in the sun.

According to Dr Joseph Meites, an endocrinologist at Michigan State University, light entering the eyes causes nerve impulses which influence the pituitary and the pineal glands to trigger a release of various hormones. 'We have no idea how many diseases are linked with hormone problems, but we do know that several diseases such as diabetes, infertility, cancer and thyroid disorders are involved with hormone imbalance'. The pineal gland is the source of melatonin, a potent free-radical scavenger.

The man who did most to raise our awareness of the value of natural full-spectrum sunlight was John Ott, author of a number of books, his first being *Health & Light: the effects of natural & artificial light on man & other living things.* He once found himself talking to the daughter of Albert Schweitzer. He asked if they had found much cancer among the local Africans at his Lambarene clinic. She told him there was no cancer when they first arrived but that it had become a significant problem. Ott casually asked whether the local people were wearing sunglasses. She told him that sunglasses had become the latest sign of status. Everyone had to have a pair.

In another case, cancer researcher, Dr Jane C. Wright, decided to test Ott's ideas. On his advice, Dr Wright instructed fifteen cancer patients to stay outdoors as much as possible that summer in natural sunlight without wearing their glasses, and particularly without sunglasses. By that autumn, the tumours of 14 of the 15 patients had either stabilised or gone into remission. But why had the fifteenth person not also benefited? Ott discovered that this woman had not followed his instructions—although she had not worn sunglasses, she had continued to wear her prescription glasses. This blocked the UV light from entering her eyes and so prevented her from getting the full benefit of the sunlight.

In 1961, Ott's attention was drawn to a curious fact. An elementary school in Niles, Illinois, was found to have the highest rate of leukaemia of any school in the USA, with five times the national incidence. Engineer and health activist Barry Groves tells the story: 'Because of the intense glare from the sun, in the newly-constructed building in which glass had been used extensively, the teachers in two of the classrooms kept the blinds drawn and the children were exposed all day only to 'warm-white' fluorescent light. All of the children with leukaemia were being taught in these two classrooms. After several years of keeping the blinds drawn and the fluorescent lights on, the teachers in these two classrooms left and were replaced with teachers who preferred to let the sunlight in. At the same time, the warm-white fluorescents were replaced with cool-white lights. From 1964, the time of Ott's last visit, there were no further cases of leukaemia reported in that school.' (www.second-opinions.co.uk)

In addition to getting as much natural sunlight as possible, you should consider replacing all light bulbs in the home with full spectrum light bulbs.

Geopathic stress

This is a cause, not a therapy, but one you need to be aware of. Just as electromagnetic fields can bring healing, so they can bring harm. Even natural fields, caused by underground streams or stresses in rocks, or from the 'grids' of earth energy can cause illness (hence geopathic, or ground disease). This is a big subject in itself, and you are recommended to explore it, since even changing where you sleep can remove causes of illness.

Early stimulus to study of this field—occupied largely by earth-energy dowsers and (for example) the German profession of 'Bau-biologie' (biology of buildings)—came from the identification of 'Krebs (cancer) houses' in Germany. Here, cases of cancer and multiple sclerosis were determined as being associated with the unhealthy coincidence of earth energy 'lines' in the habitual sleeping places of these people. This kind of ground-source electromagnetic energy must not be confused with outgassing of radon from radioactive rocks such as granite, which is easily tested for and a required survey in known areas.

Man-made electromagnetic stress

It naturally follows that since man-made electromagnetic fields now occupy the entire electromagnetic spectrum (rather than a very small proportion of it from nature), and at levels millions of times higher than nature, our electromagnetic environment is effectively very highly polluted indeed. Our bodies evolved over millions of years within a very subtle electromagnetic environment, but in tune with what there was. We are electromagnetic organisms, now suddenly swamped by man-made fields and out of synch with the faint natural frequencies of the planet. And yet we are almost completely unaware of it.

A minority have what is called 'electromagnetic hypersensitivity', which means they react instantly and at times severely, to certain ranges of frequencies, and at very low levels. Electronic circuits need protection from this kind of interference, but there is nothing to protect people, despite research increasingly showing correlation of brain cancers with mobile phones, leukaemias from power lines, degradation of dairy herds from stay ground currents (alternating current leaks to earth from transmission lines) etc. The insidiousness lies in our being normally completely unable to feel or sense electromagnetic fields—with the exception of infra-red heat and the visible spectrum of light.

If you have wi-fi in your house or wireless telephone handsets (digital cordless or DECT phones) wireless baby monitors or intruder alarms, then there is high-frequency radio-transmission going on in your house for as long as they are switched on. And if you haven't, maybe your neighbours have: a typical transmission range is 300m.

When electricity flows through the wiring in your house, it creates electro-magnetic fields (EMFs). If your house is situated near an electricity pylon or a cell-phone transmitting mast then you are being exposed to harmful radiation. If you make lots of calls on your mobile phone then you are exposing your brain to harmful radiation. If your bed is situated close to electrical sockets or to meters, then you are being exposed to harmful radiation.

There are many things you can do to protect yourself, by avoiding these devices, checking what there is around your home, shielding at least sleeping areas in your home, or having a geopathic energy specialist around to check where you live. Useful sources to begin with are: www.royriggs.co.uk and www.powerwatch.org.uk.

Cancer: the Mind and the Emotions

Introduction

Is there a connection between cancer and the mind, the way we view ourselves and our emotional states, both conscious and unconscious? Are there ways that we can harness the mind to improve our likelihood of recovering from cancer? These are some of the issues I will be looking at in this chapter.

Psychological impact of low-oxygen state

We have, in previous pages, frequently mentioned the fact that a low-oxygen state is held to be the key cause of cancer. It is easy, but a mistake, to see this as simply a fact that relates only to the state of the body's physical tissues. The truth is a state of low oxygenation has an impact on the whole person. Ingrid Naiman, author of *Cancer Salves: A Botanical Approach to Treatment*, describes the following impacts on the person suffering from low oxygenation: 'The symptoms of poor oxygenation include pallor and fatigue, poor circulation to the extremities (cold hands and feet), and sometimes dizziness or mental fuzziness. The psychological symptoms are subtle: lack of fortitude, an easy sense of defeat, conviction that the effort needed to do something cannot be made, vulnerability, and perhaps even some disorientation.' (www.cancerchecklist.com)

I had a friend, Pauline, who died of colon cancer. She refused to accept any of the suggestions that I sent her. She was totally passive in the face of her disease. Not everyone with cancer feels this way but it is clearly a common enough syndrome. Dr Shultze, the herbalist, believes that only a small per cent of the people who start on his 30-day dietary program will make it to the end. The rest do not want enough to live—or are not convinced enough in the merits of the diet perhaps—and so cannot force themselves to make the effort.

If you, the reader, have cancer yourself, I would like to suggest to you that you form a personal 'Get Well Again Committee' of say one to three friends whose job it is to read this book with you and to discuss and ultimately advise you on what to do. These friends can also facilitate the getting of whatever it is you need to get. They can force you to do, perhaps, what you may not feel you have the energy to do. But that's what friends are for. And not all of the approaches in this book require effort—but they may require hope and a desire to live. You may not even have that: such is the impact of the body on the mind.

Psychotherapy and cancer-prone personalities

One of the first investigators into the field of psychology and cancer was Dr Lawrence LeShan, an experimental psychologist and therapist. Starting in the 1950s, he undertook research into whether or not there were psychological predisposing characteristics that might make explain why some people got cancer—and whether or not this could be used to help people to recover. This research spanned three decades and his conclusions were 'yes' to both questions.

He quotes the case of 'John' who had a massive, inoperable brain tumour. After working with LeShan using a special form of psychotherapy—which LeShan characterizes as 'crisis therapy'—John recovered without medication, even though his doctors had told him he had only months to live. John's psychological state before he met LeShan was one of hopelessness. After going through psychotherapy, he developed a much more positive frame of mind. His attitude to life turned around and his terminal cancer disappeared.

In his book *You Can Fight for Your Life*, LeShan described the process by which John and a number of other patients underwent complete remission. He also argued that even those he worked with who didn't undergo remission, who indeed did die from their cancers, nevertheless had the quality of their lives dramatically transformed for the better through his work with them.

LeShan's work started when he and a co-worker discovered that there seemed to be startling similarities in the personality configurations and in the life histories of people who subsequently died of cancer. A personality configuration very similar to that of people with a predisposition to suicide. LeShan believed that if there was such a configuration, it should be tracked down.

In the first stage of his research, he interviewed 250 patients—spending between two and eight hours with each one. Another 200 cancer patients were interviewed on the side for specific concerns. Close relatives of over 50 patients were interviewed for between one and three hours, and another 40 close relatives were seen from between 20 and 50 hours. This was over a period of 14 years. In addition, he undertook intensive psychotherapy with 71 patients.

As a result of his study, he came to the following conclusions:

i)   that 'there is a general type of personality configuration among the majority of cancer patients', and
ii)   that 'people whose personality or life history conforms to this pattern of susceptibility can take steps to protect themselves against the possibility of cancer.'

What LeShan discovered was that for a significant majority of cancer cases there had been, prior to the onset of cancer, a loss of a crucial relationship. This loss may have been a physical or, more frequently, an emotional loss—for instance, a failure of a marriage, or a marriage from which the heart had gone, or an attachment to a way of life or activity that promised happiness but which was denied to the person involved for some reason. From this perception he predicted that age-corrected cancer rates for women would be highest for widows, next highest for divorced women, then for married women without children, followed by married women with children and lowest for single women. Epidemiological statistics from various sources appear to support this conclusion.

Secondly, he found that for a large majority of cancer patients there is a clear inability to express hostility, anger or resentment. He went on to discover that cancers developed in people who were in despair because they frustrated their own creative potential. They denied themselves. They felt that they had to be other than themselves to be accepted, and conversely that they would be rejected by others if they were themselves.

His patient, John, had become a lawyer and joined his father's firm as a result of strong parental suggestion, and he had married a woman chosen by his parents who enjoyed being the wife of a lawyer. However, he was deeply dissatisfied. As a child John had shown a great deal of interest in music and he had dreamt of being a pianist. As a result of his therapy, John came to accept that it was possible that he could be a pianist if he really wanted to and that he had a right to fight for what he wanted. He quit his job, divorced his wife, took up the piano seriously and eventually became a pianist with a symphony orchestra. His terminal brain cancer disappeared.

While many people feel despair, LeShan discovered, the despair of the cancer patient has unique features:

The patient in despair is absolutely alone. At the deepest emotional level he cannot relate, since he does not believe himself worthy of love. He does not despair over "something", as would the usual depressed patient—rather, he despairs over "nothing".

Trapped in this alone-ness, the cancer patient is in an emotional place where it is impossible to be reached by love, where any kind of fulfilling or satisfying relationship becomes impossible. The cancer patient is even divorced from such negative emotions as anger, resentment and jealousy. As one of his patients said to him: "You don't understand, doctor. It's not that I've been or done anything. It's that I've done nothing and been nothing."

The cancer patient's own desires and wishes had been so completely repressed ... that when at the start of the therapy I asked the question, "What do you really want out of life?" the response would be a blank and astonished stare. That question had never been seen as valid.'

This despair was evident in 68 out of the 71 patients he worked with. LeShan believed strongly that patients feeling this level of despair could be helped, and his case studies showed that he succeeded. He does not give any statistics in his book regarding the number of remissions that resulted among the 71 patients—but in addition to John, he mentions four other patients who recovered, without medication, from terminal cancer.

Spontaneous remission of cancer among terminal cases is considered to be extremely rare. One estimate has been one in 100,000. Yet LeShan is implicitly claiming to have achieved an inconceivably higher success rate. One of the reasons LeShan gives no statistics is because he does not want remission of cancer to be the only yardstick of value. Indeed LeShan believes that many of those he worked with rediscovered themselves and led lives that were worth living—after decades of failing to do that. As one of his patients said: 'Death is nothing. It is inevitable. Everyone has to die. What matters is how you live and die.'

And it wasn't just the patient who was affected by the course of the patient's psychotherapy. The daughter of one patient wrote to LeShan after her mother had died:

'I know that every day she grew in courage and understanding … and was learning to fight the fears that surrounded her …. My father and I are changed … and I think it influenced her friends who visited her …. Mother's last months were filled with hope and thoughts of the future ….'

For this reason, LeShan is not concerned to boast about success rates on a simple cure-death ratio. Success can be measured qualitatively. It was the objective of his therapy to 'reawaken the inner life of the individual, and to liberate those forces which can enable the person to experience as completely as possible both himself and the meaning of his life and death.'

The crisis therapy that LeShan developed is very different from orthodox psychotherapy. First it dispenses with the view that unconscious forces rigidly control a helpless ego. He believes that the individual can be freed from constrictions to create his or her own world and to express his or her own true feelings. He also believes that this demands absolute honesty and openness from the therapist—the therapist does not allow him/herself to have an unexpressed commentary flowing in parallel to the therapy session. Everything must be made explicit. The therapist is not kind or careful. Time is short and the past needs to be confronted if the therapy is to succeed. This honesty must permeate the relationship and it precludes kindness—which LeShan sees as being a protective device for the therapist and implies a superior position. The crisis therapist must be in full personal contact with the patient, otherwise he is simply conspiring to avoid the key issues that underlie the cancer. 'Death, the figure in the background, asks the questions, and the therapist must join in the search for answers that are meaningful to the patient.'

The crisis therapist also talks to the family to prepare them for change—because they are certainly a constraining factor whether or not they intend to be. This requires a great deal of support and cooperation from the family.

And what is the goal of this therapy? To make patients confront their true selves, to become aware of their true desires and to make them feel important to themselves. In the mirror of death, some patients feel free to explore this question.

Anyone seeking psychotherapy because of cancer should discuss LeShan's ideas with the therapist at the first meeting. This will establish the foundations of the relationship.

LeShan favours the idea of psychological self-help and suggests two useful techniques: one to confront the past, the other the future. To confront the past, he suggests the following technique. In the darkness of the imagination, we can enter a time machine and return as adults to the critical times in our pasts, the times that can still cause us pain, the times when the seeds of the present—perhaps the self's self-denial—were sown, and to face the child that was ourselves then. And when we are there, adult and child, face to face, we should think what we would like to say to that child. This kind of self-confronting journey has a very powerful potential to heal psychic wounds.

For those who feel helpless in the face of the future, LeShan suggests a second technique: the person should focus on the impossible ambition and then to ask himself: 'What is the first thing that has to be done, the very first thing, to achieve this goal?' Every journey starts with a single step. If that first step is taken, there is a good chance the journey will be completed. Without that step, there is no journey.

People who are self-determining, LeShan argues, do not get cancer (or are very much less likely to). People who discover and embrace a purpose can cure themselves of cancer, even when medical science has done everything it can do and failed. If they aren't cured, at least every minute of life left to them is enhanced in value.

Key text: Lawrence LeShan, *You Can Fight for Your Life*, M Evans & Co., New York, 1976. His website is www.cancerasaturningpoint.org.

A self-help approach called Emotional Freedom Technique (EFT) claims to be beneficial for a wide range of health concerns. A free 79-page booklet explaining the approach can be obtained at: www.emofree.com/downloadeftmanual.htm.

LeShan's approach has been mirrored in Germany by Dr Ryke Geerd Hamer. Both Hamer and his wife were diagnosed with cancer shortly after their son was murdered. Hamer subsequently developed a complex understanding of cancer. In his view, cancer is a natural process that gets triggered by an overwhelming emotional shock for which the body is totally unprepared. This shock registers itself physically in the brain. Healing, in his view, cannot occur until there is first an emotional healing. Bizarrely, Hamer has been imprisoned in France for his cancer views. In earlier centuries, heretics got tortured and burned, today non-mainstream cancer researchers get pilloried in the press and arrested. For further details of Hamer's complex views on cancer go to the official English-language website of Dr Hamer is at www.newmedicine.ca.

Emotional healing

Pattie, whose story is in Section 8: *Cancer Survivors' Stories*, tells of how cancer made her re-evaluate her life 'I changed my diet, quit my stressful job, sold my too-big house, rid myself of all negative friends, and divorced my alcoholic hubby.' The result? 'I had no idea what real happiness was until 2002.'

Another woman writing in a cancer chat group wrote: 'It was not until I got away from him that I really realized how stressed I have been, especially the last two years since the diagnosis.'

Emotional healing is important. It almost always involves making hard decisions but the result can be liberating. The body has enough obstacles to healing as it is. It can do without the stress of unhappy relationships. It is also about letting go of anger.

We think of stress as being caused mainly by anxieties when faced with problematic situations but, as Mike Goldberg tellingly writes:

> *'Stress is also caused by holding onto the painful past and having negative and impulsive reaction to stress factors. It is important to rest, get away from negative and toxic people and environments, avoid conflict and drama, stop watching the news, smile, listen to soothing music and focus on blessings and not lack. Love is a beautiful energy that reduces inner stress and helps bring inner peace and peace of mind.'*

As another cancer patient wrote: 'I had lung cancer plus metastasis to the intestines and brain. Once there was metastasis my doctor gave up giving me medicine …. I decided to forgive many people because I believed I was heading for an early death. Forgiving is a very strong factor in why I am still alive today.'

Magnetism and depression

In 2004, a study at Boston's McLean Hospital to evaluate a particular anti-depression regime, required depressed participants to have a 45-minute MRI scan so that the researchers could evaluate the effects of the drugs in question on brain functions. But there was a surprising result. Almost all the people who had been severely depressed emerged from their session in a good mood, some even cracked jokes. So one of the side effects of the electro-therapy machines discussed earlier might be their beneficial effects on mood.

Importance of reducing stress when fighting cancer

It is known that stress promotes cancer. One sign of stress is 'brain fog'—the inability to think clearly. It has been shown that stress causes higher than desired levels of cortisol in the body. So how can we reduce these cortisol levels? Here are some suggestions:

1. Vitamin B complex
2. Passionflower herb tincture
3. Omega 3 oils—i.e., fish oils or flaxseed oils. If you have a compromised liver then follow the Budwig protocol (see Section 4: *Cancer: Detox and Diet*)
4. Have a massage
5. Laugh

All of these will help reduce stress and strengthen your ability to fight cancer.

Mind-body interaction

One of the imponderable facts of cancer is that some are aggressive, developing very quickly, while others are slow and steady in their development. LeShan believes the aggressiveness is a direct reflection of the speed at which the cancer occurs after the loss of life's meaning as embodied in a central relationship. That is to say, the cause of an aggressive cancer is to be found shortly before the cancer develops, while the cause of a slow growing cancer is to be found further back in the past. The psychologist, Dr Bruno Klopfer, claimed to be able to predict with 80 per cent accuracy which patients had slow growing cancers, and which fast growing, on the basis of personality tests alone. Those with the more acutely felt despair had the more aggressive cancers.

LeShan and Klopfer seem to be saying that cancer is an accurate measure of despair. This can be true only if the mind and body are inextricably entwined as entities—or indeed if there is no separation of mind and body.

This question is a very contentious one. Since Descartes, Western philosophy and science have largely been based on the assumption that mind and body are distinct and separate. The mind is seen as distinct from the brain, the physical organ that is associated with it. If they are distinct and separate how can one affect the other? If a doctor says, 'It's psychosomatic. It's all in the mind,' he is saying it isn't real, it isn't true, it exists only as a thought, not as a fact. Against this view is the one—widely accepted in ancient times—and also today by many other non-Western cultures—that mind and body are one inextricable whole. What affects the body affects the mind and vice versa.

The idea that emotions can cause cancer is a common one and indeed for most of the last two thousand years—with the sole exception of the twentieth century—it was the standard view. At the end of the nineteenth century, Sir James Paget, one of the leading medical figures of his time reflected the orthodox view when he wrote: 'The cases are so frequent in which deep anxiety, deferred hope and disappointment are quickly followed by the growth and increase of cancer, that we can hardly doubt that mental depression is a weighty additive to the other influences favouring the development of the cancerous constitution.'

It is only in this century with its over-emphasis on the mechanical features of the body, that the individual's self and his values, beliefs and feelings have been more or less totally ignored. Modern medicine deals with the body as if it were a machine. Each bit and piece can be taken out, replaced, tinkered with and so on. People don't die of broken hearts or despair anymore; they die of cerebral haemorrhage or cancer of the cervix. The result is that doctors believe it is for them—the mechanics of the body—to decide what repair is needed. And if excision of the rectum appears to be necessary for the further functioning of the body-machine so be it—out with the rectum.

There is little concern for whether the patient wishes to live with the continuing pain, inconvenience, and indignity that such an operation bequeaths.

But the great things in life: love, laughter, beauty, courage as well as the negative things such as fear, worry, danger and so on, belong as much to the mind as to the chemistry of the body. If mind and body are so separate, then why do we cry when we are sad or in pain, why do we feel a physical thrill at the sight of great beauty? Why do we jump immediately we sense danger? Laugh when something is funny? In each of these cases the physical response does not wait for the conscious message, it occurs absolutely in synch with the mental message. Mental and physical responses are two sides of a coin that cannot be separated from each other.

We can conclude from this that all thoughts are facts. If our mind and body are one then our body is intelligent and our thoughts are physical. Similarly, if the body is diseased in some way, then we cannot say that we have the disease but rather that the disease is part us, part of our identity. We are the disease.

This at least is the position of Deepak Chopra. The point of contact between the mind and body are the neuro-peptide transmitters—the body's 'messenger molecules' as Chopra calls them.

'A neuro-peptide springs into existence at the touch of a thought, but where does it spring from? A thought of fear and the neuro-chemical that it turns into are somehow connected to a hidden process, a transformation of non-matter into matter.'

Chopra calls the zone where this occurs the '? zone'. This question mark zone is a place below the visible. It is a world where quantum rules dictate reality—and one of the rules is that things can happen suddenly, absolutely and inexplicably—the so called quantum leap where A can become B instantaneously. He gives an example of such a quantum cure taking place. A patient of his, a woman in her fifties went to see him complaining of severe abdominal pains and jaundice. He thought at first that she was suffering from gallstones and arranged for surgery, but when she was opened up, it was found that she had a large malignant tumour that had spread to her liver, with scattered pockets of cancer throughout her abdominal cavity. The surgeons considered the cancer to be inoperable and closed the incision without taking further action. Chopra spoke to the woman's daughter first. She pleaded with him not to tell her mother the truth and Chopra agreed to go along with this deceit. He informed the woman that the gallstone operation had been completely successful. He expected her to die within a few months but some time later she appeared before him for a routine examination that revealed no signs of cancer. Much later the woman said to him: 'Doctor, I was so sure I had cancer two years ago that when it turned out to be just gallstones, I told myself I would never be sick another day in my life.'

We can call an event like this a miracle, a spontaneous remission, a placebo cure. But the fact is, whatever words we give it, it happens.

Placebos (and nocebos)

'They can conquer who believe they can.'—Dryden

A three-year-old boy with a severe case of whooping cough was seen by the doctor. The doctor appeared before the boy in great robes. He sat on the boy's bed and peeled a peach. Then he sugared it and cut it into small pieces. He fed each piece slowly to the boy. As he did so he told the boy that he was going to be fine, as the peaches would make him well again. He made the boy feel his health was inevitable. However, on leaving the room he told the father that he did not hold out much hope for the boy. The whooping cough was so serious it was almost certain to be fatal. However, the next day the boy was still alive and the doctor came again. As before he made sure he was wearing his impressive medical robes. As before, he fed the boy personally with some fruit. After 40 days and 40 visits the boy was well again. The doctor was the famous Sir William Osler and the boy was the brother of Dr Patrick Mallam who published the story in the *Journal of the American Medical Association* (December 22, 1969). Osler, incidentally, is famous for his comment: 'In today's system of medicine a patient has to recover twice: once from the disease and once from the treatment.'

Just believing that a pill is a powerful pain-reliever can be enough to get rid of the pain in 30–60 per cent of the people given the placebo. We can therefore conclude that the level of faith in a therapy helps to determine how successful that therapy is. Curiously, it is not the least educated and those who are of lower intelligence who are most susceptible to this effect, rather the reverse. Placebos have a higher tendency to work with the more intelligent and educated. And it doesn't appear to be a conscious decision, placebos don't work because we consciously want them to work. The basis of the placebo's action lies deeper in the mind.

One study showed placebos to be 35 per cent effective. Other studies support the view that 30–40 per cent of people respond to placebos. That the placebo effect may be even stronger is indicated by a number of studies. One showed that valium was more effective than a placebo for the first week of therapy only. After that they had equal effectiveness. This contradicts the prevalent view that placebo cures are short-lasting. Another study substituted saline solution for morphine with morphine-addicted patients who were being withdrawn from their addiction. No withdrawal symptoms appeared until the saline injections were stopped. The placebo effect is clearly reinforced when the attitude of the doctor is positive. And it doesn't make much difference if you *know* a placebo is just a placebo. According to a recent Harvard Medical School study, placebos worked even when the recipients were told that's what they were: (www.newscientist.com/article/dn19904-placebos-can-work-even-when-you-know-theyre-fakes.html)

If we can believe a disease or a pain away, then we can believe it into existence—not consciously perhaps, but at some level of awareness. If the body is intelligent then it is intelligent in every part of the body, every organ is intelligent, every cell is intelligent.

Is this really true—or is it just poetic over-statement? Consider the famous case of a child named Timmy, whose story is quoted by Deepak Chopra. Timmy suffers from multiple personality disorder. Nearly a dozen personalities contend within his physical frame. One of these personalities is allergic to orange juice but the allergic reaction stops as soon as another personality takes over.

For this fact to make sense we have to accept that the cells of the antibodies that trigger the allergic reaction have to make a choice as to whether to react or not. This choice is dependent on the choice the mind has made about which personality it is at any moment. This means the mind is capable of choosing to be allergic or not allergic. If it can choose to have an allergy it can also choose to have cancer. If the disease is something we have unconsciously chosen, then the cure too is capable of being chosen.

Given the obvious benefits of placebos, one would think that more would be done with them. But most hospitals seem more concerned to make patients feel depressed and dissociated. Cold, bare, white corridors; the smell of antiseptic floor wash; cold, plastic-tiled floors. Let's face it, hospitals seem to be creating problems for themselves before they even start. Hospitals and doctors seem to be working against placebos rather than with them. The wise patient will create his or her own placebo-enhancing mental environment.

The reverse process is true. Many patients, told their cancer is incurable, promptly fulfil their doctor's expectations by dying. This was the case with my own wife. She was told on January 17th that she had three months to live and died on April 16th. How's that for a prediction? Or was it a curse? We call this negative response the nocebo effect.

But the case of tuberculosis (TB) is instructive. A century ago, TB had the same fearful prognosis as cancer today—but then a cure was found and suddenly death rates from TB dropped sharply—even though most of those who recovered had not yet received the new antibiotic.

The power of expectations is so strong that there are good reasons for not pursuing any form of treatment towards which you have a negative attitude. The Simontons, a husband and wife team, conducted an 18-month study with 152 patients into the importance of attitude in determining the outcome of treatment with radiation. The results were clear. Patients with positive attitudes had a better response to the radiation treatment than those with negative attitudes. In fact, of the 152 patients, only two who had shown a negative attitude had a good response to treatment. Patients who had a good attitude and a more developed cancer generally did better than patients with a negative attitude but less advanced cancer. This leads to a very important conclusion. Cancer patients should only undertake treatments that they have positive attitudes towards. If you feel that the best place to deal with cancer is the hospital, and that the best weapons are radiation and chemotherapy, then concentrate positive thoughts towards these forms of treatment. If you feel they will not help then don't do them.

One of the classic cases of placebo cure was reported by Dr Bruno Klopfer. One of his patients took a drug called Krebiozen and his growths 'melted like snowballs'. A few months later, newspapers reported that the drug was worthless and the patient's tumours promptly recurred. Suspecting that the patient had a powerful belief system, Klopfer announced that he would give him a more active form of the drug. In fact he injected his patient with nothing more than distilled water, yet once again the tumours melted away. After a few more months, there were further reports announcing that Krebiozen was worthless. The patient accepted the truth of these reports, his tumours soon reappeared, and he quickly died.

A fighting attitude

A study at King's College Hospital looked at the impact of a fighting spirit on the survival of women who had mastectomies for early stage breast cancer. Ten years later, 55 per cent of the group who had the strongest fighting spirit—or whose levels of denial were so strong that they refused to believe they had the disease—had survived, compared with only 22 per cent of the group who felt hopeless and helpless, or who stoically accepted their fate.

What is a 'fighting attitude'? This is complex and sometimes controversial question. Possibly the best way of defining it is to say it is having a positive acceptance of the disease and its implications, combined with an active desire to get well again.

In another study, having a 'hopeful attitude' was the key that allowed researchers to predict which women out of 68 who came to a hospital for a cervical biopsy had cancer and who did not. Before the results of the biopsy were known, the women were interviewed and assessed for personality factors. The researchers then predicted who would have and who would not have cancer. Of the 68 women, 28 had cancer. The researchers correctly predicted 68 per cent of the cancer victims, and 77 per cent of the cancer-free women simply on the basis of their relative hopefulness or hopelessness.

In other studies, the degree of hope, faith and trust in a surgeon has been shown to correlate highly with speedier recovery. Curiously, people who avoid thinking about the outcome of an operation recover faster than those who are eternally vigilant. This is further demonstration, perhaps, of a simple truth: that the unconscious is more powerful than the conscious.

Clearly the mind is capable of unleashing very powerful forces that can lead to both health and illness. People can will themselves to death and they can will themselves to health. How can we harness these powers? Some methods will already have suggested themselves. Hypnosis, visualization, and meditation are some of the ways people have recommended. These approaches have been treated separately in the last section of this book.

Spiritual consciousness

Some cancer patients go beyond an earth-bound mind-body nexus. For them the disease is the key they needed to unlock the secret of themselves. They embrace their disease and take responsibility for their response to it. Like a smack over the head from a Zen master, the diagnosis of cancer has changed their awareness of—and attitude to—life. One such ex-cancer patient is Petrea King.

> *'Clearly I didn't sit down consciously to figure out ways of making my body sick to achieve some underlying aim. Later in my life, I didn't think, "Ah yes, a good dose of leukemia with a short prognosis is just what I need right now." Yet I firmly believe, at some more subtle level, that the particular disease and prognosis were precisely tailor made for me .... It's often said "People don't change." I believe that statement is made only by people who don't welcome change in themselves .... When we make a firm commitment to life and to experiencing our connection with the flow of power and love in the universe, extraordinary and unexpected events begin to unfold. Greater peace, equanimity and joy are experienced even in the midst of disease, and the experience of these states creates the perfect environment for physical healing to take place .... Leukemia was the best thing that ever came my way because I learned much more about myself much more quickly than I ever could have without it.'*
>
> *(Petrea King, Quest for Life, 1992)*

The spiritually awakened patient may in the end die of the cancer, but nevertheless, they may be grateful—even in the face of their own self-extinction—that they have woken to a more profound consciousness of existence and of their own lives.

It may seem strange that anyone could love their disease or feel immense gratitude to something that is seeking their own extinction. But this surprise derives ultimately from a refusal to see something very obvious and very simple: we are all going to die. The spiritually-awakened person sees this. Quite simply, he or she no longer fears death. What is there to fear? Death is natural and it is inevitable. It cannot be run away from. Those men and women who embrace the inevitability of death are freed and this freedom feels like a cosmic joke. They can thrill with the streaming energy of the universe and thrill to their awareness of the cosmic dance when the atoms of their physical bodies are dispersed to the universe—then where does the mind's energy go? Die now or die later. What does it matter?

And the curious thing is this: the energy released by this awareness can put the cancer into remission. And it makes the remaining life that is given a life that is more intensely felt, and so more profoundly lived.

It is also true that this acceptance of illness is one way in which the patient demonstrates that they have accepted themselves. This acceptance can transform the patient's entire subjective world, and this in turn can lead to the healing of disease.

A Japanese study into patients who went home to die from cancer and instead got well showed that a complete acceptance of God's will—or the will of fate—was a constant theme through all their stories. We can see what this means in more personal terms when we consider the following words of an AIDS patient:

I deal with this disease by looking at it as one of the best teachers I've ever had. I treat it with respect. I try to love it. I talk to it. I'll say: 'You are safe with me. Do not worry. I do not hate you.'
(Young person with AIDS, quoted by Dr Larry Dossey, 1993)

And another patient, the actor Mandy Patinkin, had this to say:

The greatest thing in my life was getting cancer, because it taught me how much I love my life, my family, my friends and my work. And it taught me that I must find some peace and calm every day. I never could sit still long enough to meditate, but I do it every day. I'm like a little baby Zen Buddhist.

Body-mind therapies

There are a number of healing activities, behaviours and therapies that make sense once we understand there is a dynamic of interaction between mind and body–that mind is an aspect of body and the body is an aspect of mind.

Bodywork and posture therapies

There are hundreds of schools of practitioners who offer some form of bodywork. applied kinesiology, Alexander technique, chiropractic and osteopathy, yoga, Rolfing, Lowen bioenergetics, structural integration, and many other forms of working with the body to promote health, share a basic understanding: *mens sana in corpore sano* as the Latin motto on many coats of arms expresses it: a sound mind in a healthy body. You can't have one without the other. And rather than start with the mind, they propose that it makes sense to start with the body.

If we accept that mind and body are one, then it makes sense to see the body as a memory system of the mind. Negative thoughts affect the way the muscles are used, the more the muscles are used in a certain way, certain postures result that can lead to postural imbalances which themselves will have other negative effects on the health of the person. Physical traumas too are, it seems, retained in the body long after the original 'insult' (to use the medical term) appears to have been healed.

It is helpful to understand that the entire interiors of our bodies—stomach, heart, liver, intestine and all the rest of it—are interlinked by a sheath of connective tissue— the fascia— which interconnects with every part of the body. An important element of this fascia is the diaphragm. This is not just useful for breathing but also for massaging all the internal organs. Imbalances in one area of the fascia are therefore felt throughout the system. A slight negative pull in one area can have major long-term impacts elsewhere in the body. If these, as is likely, negatively affect our breathing, this will in turn affect the amount of oxygen in our blood and tissues.

All the schools of bodywork take this as their starting point and all seek to correct any problems that they identify. Tai chi and qigong exercises may also be beneficial for the same reason—that they correct imbalances, even though this is not their primary objective.

Kinesiotherapy is one of a number of postural retraining therapies. It involves training the patient in the proper use of the body in posture movement and repose in order to achieve healing. The principle behind kinesiotherapy is that mental as well as physical energy is tied up in wrong postures and actions.

Poor posture and lack of proper exercise puts a strain on the body. However, by using the body properly we can relieve this stress. Swinging and swaying can loosen up the joints. Jarring and jolting movements need to be avoided. To straighten the spine using simple traction, you can hang your head over the end of your bed. Movements should, where possible, be slow and harmonious.

The Alexander technique was developed by the Australian Frederick Alexander. According to him 'use affects function', so ill-use distorts and misshapes the body and interferes with free functioning. When Professor Tinbergen gave his Nobel prize speech in 1973 (he won the prize for medicine) he used this forum to praise Alexander's work.

American **Ida Rolf** developed a system known today as 'Rolfing'. Her system is more concerned with structure and bodily mechanics than with posture and movement. This is one of many schools that collectively refer to their work as 'structural integration'. They work with the fascia, or connective tissue, that holds the internal body together. The objective is to free it up.

'When the body is out of alignment it creates inefficiency and imbalance resulting in stiffness, discomfort and loss of energy. When a body is aligned and balanced it moves with greater ease. It requires less energy to function. Good posture is effortless and breathing is easier. The body becomes more flexible, more coordinated and athletic performance improves.'

(www.rolfguild.org)

Osteopathy was developed by Dr Andrew Taylor Still (1828–1917), a physician from Missouri who developed a drugless system of treatment. He believed that ill health was the result of blockages to the circulatory and nervous systems. All the doctor has to do is to make sure these are cleared and Mother Nature will do the rest. Surprisingly, to the modern reader, he was very effective in curing infectious diseases.

Many modern osteopaths have retreated from this system, so that the fact that a doctor is a Doctor of Osteopathy is no guarantee that he uses a drugless medicine based on manipulation.

Anyone seeking an osteopath should first ascertain whether or not they use cranial therapy. Cranial therapists believe that through cranial manipulation they can release blockages that impede the flow of living energy that is the essential feature of health and life. Dr Andrew Weil, in his book: *Spontaneous Healing*, described his observations of an osteopath working in this way. Originally sceptical, he came away from the experience with the belief that everyone the man had 'fixed' had indeed been fixed.

The title of Weil's book is interesting and refers to healing that occurs without any treatment having been taken. Some cancers do just disappear and these are referred to as spontaneous healings. For an interesting discussion of this subject with case histories go to www.noetic.org/ research/sr/r_biblio.html.

Chiropractic is a more muscular and no-nonsense approach to fixing the joints in the spine and neck. Nevertheless it too can claim its share of success in fixing problems arising from physical trauma. It has been shown to help cure cholera.

It seems very clear that manipulating the body is an effective way of dealing with a wide range of ills, and the surprise is that it has not been taken up in any way by orthodox practitioners of medicine.

Rebounding is a useful exercise for those who cannot walk far—get a small trampoline and gently bounce up and down. This activity not only gives the internal and external muscles a mild workout but also stimulates the hypothalamus with the up and down movements. This is important for blood pressure, sleep and much else.

Bioenergetics, the healing therapy developed by Alexander Lowen, a former associate of Wilhelm Reich, is perhaps the most radical of all these approaches. Lowen believed that unconscious childhood emotional trauma became embedded in the body, and that manipulation of the body during a process that has much in common with some forms of psychotherapy is a way in which these embedded traumas can be released.

Breathing

Since stress is a major cause and stimulator of cancer, it is helpful if we can learn to relax. But breathing exercises are not just stress-busters, they are fundamental to good health and energy.

In his book, *Spontaneous Healing*, Dr Andrew Weil describes five breathing practices that will lead to improved health and vigour if practised every day.

1. Just observe your inhalations and exhalations for a few minutes. Don't try to influence them. Do this while in a comfortable position with your eyes closed.
2. Repeat the above but mentally view the cycle of breath as starting with the exhalation. This actually increases the amount of air inhaled.
3. While seated, or better while lying down, imagine that the breaths that go out and in do not start with you but originate with the universe itself. You are in the way of the cosmic breath. The universe is breathing itself through you. Feel this universal breath permeating every part of your body.

4. Stimulating breath: Sit comfortably with back straight and eyes closed. Place the tip of the tongue on the flesh just above the back of the top teeth: the so-called yogic position. Now breathe in and out rapidly through the nose, keeping the mouth lightly closed. The rhythm of in and out breaths should be rapid, even and audible. Increase duration from 15 seconds to start with to a minute. This is an energy booster if done regularly and can be done whenever you feel sleepy and want to wake up (i.e., in the morning or in the evening while driving).

5. Relaxing breath: This can be done sitting or lying down with the tongue in the yogic position as with the previous exercise. Breathe out with an audible sound completely emptying the lungs to a count of eight. Then close the mouth and inhale quietly for a count of four. Then hold the breath for a count of seven. Do this for four building up to eight cycles after a month. Speed is not important but slow is better than fast.

Weil emphasizes that these breathing exercises are genuine spiritual practices aimed at bringing mind and body to a single focus—a focus of energy. Going on from breathing, one can, in the mind's eye, let the breath escape from the nostril and follow it up the nose the face, follow it as it explores the cheeks, the skull and the locus of nerves at the back of the neck. Let it flow down the arms, down the back, round the buttocks, the legs, the feet, the toes, then back up the leg, the thighs the pelvic area. Let it rest in the solar plexus for a while then let it move up over the belly and chest and back up the neck to the nose. While your mind is following this route, let it sift the impressions that arise: was there a twinge or pain anywhere. This is a way of listening to the body.

The quality of breathing has a direct influence on the levels of oxygen in the blood and tissues—and this has a direct influence on whether the body's tissues are a good seedbed for the development of cancer tumours.

Good breathing practices also exercise the entire connective tissue of the body to which all the organs are connected. Good breathing therefore moves the diaphragm, and in so doing, massages the lungs, stomach and heart all of which are necessary for good health.

Exercise

Studies have shown that a 1–2 mile walk 3–4 times a week helps enormously in stabilizing the disease process—and sometimes reversing it. A walk like this helps the appetite, sleep cycle and energy level. Exercise is always helpful and immune enhancing—as long as one doesn't go past the point of being tired—and you allow sufficient time for recovery between sessions.

And how can exercise help? By increasing the blood's oxygen levels, releasing tension from the muscles and the spine and improving the sense of mental well-being.

One study published in the May 2005 *Journal of the American Medical Association* followed 3,000 women who had previously been diagnosed with breast cancer. They found that exercise had an enormous impact on their health and longevity. Even as little as three to five hours per week of normal walking exercise reduced their risk of dying by half.

Qigong (Chi Kung)

Qigong is a traditional form of Chinese health exercise which combines breathing, movement and meditation. There are many different schools and they may all have some benefit for cancer patients—but there is a form of qigong that was specifically developed to benefit people with cancer.

Ms Guo Lin, a Chinese traditional painter, was originally diagnosed with cancer of the uterus in 1949 and she had it removed by surgery in Shanghai. However, the cancer recurred in 1960, and despite further treatment she was eventually told that her condition was terminal. At this point she remembered that her grandfather had taught her as a child to practice qigong. She studied his books and created her own system of qigong exercise. She practiced this form of qigong for two hours every day, and six months later tests showed that her cancer had shrunk.

She continued her practice and eventually, in 1970, she started giving lessons in a Beijing park in what she called New Qigong Therapy. By 1977 she felt she had demonstrated clearly that qigong had been beneficial for many cancer patients and she announced publicly that Qigong could cure cancer. Her fame spread and soon, everyday, she was leading three to four hundred people through their qigong paces. She became a national celebrity, travelling around China to demonstrate her system. Although she died in 1984, her system of qigong is still widely practised.

Guo Lin qigong combines the following:

1. Deep and forceful breathing. Two inhalations followed by one exhalation. This is based on the idea of taking in more qi (pronounced 'chee') and releasing less to nourish the practitioner's own inner qi reserves.
2. A brisk walk to increase the blood circulation to generate more qi.
3. Producing a high pitch healing sound to attack the tumour and to stop it from spreading

According to traditional Chinese medicine, when qi (vital energy) and blood are flowing freely, the body will maintain the balance of yin and yang and disease will disappear. By practicing qigong, qi-energy and blood circulation are improved, the balance of yin and yang is restored. From a Western point of view it can be seen that practicing qigong in such an intensive way, the oxygenation of the tissues will be enhanced—and cancers do not like surrounding tissues to be highly oxygenated. In fact the need a low oxygen level to thrive.

Another important benefit is the impact on the emotions. By working out so intensively, the body is brought into a state of relaxation and the mental and emotional strength of the practitioner is enhanced.

There is also the potential healing benefit from doing these exercises in groups with other cancer patients. The diagnosis of cancer has great power to create a feeling of psychological isolation. By joining a qigong group, one can overcome this sense of aloneness. This in turn can help transform the feeling that you are a victim of circumstance to one where you are in charge. This is itself immensely energising.

There are many anecdotal reports of people who have been cured of their cancer through qigong, and a number of research studies show that in addition to reported cures, there is evidence of increased longevity, improved quality of life and better pain management.

Classes continue to run in a number of Beijing parks but you may be able to find a teacher closer to home. Alternatively a form of qigong—'Spring Forest qigong'—can be self-taught using a DVD/CD package obtainable from www.learningstrategies.com/qigong.

Mind-body therapies

Enthusiasm and eccentricity

The idea of healing through healthy mindedness is of ancient origin. In modern times it was systematised as a system of healing by a self-taught healer by the name of Phineas Quimby (1802–66). Among his followers was Mrs Mary Baker Eddy, the founder of Christian Science.

Quimby preached that the universe was filled with the divine, infinite God. We are part of that infinite universe and so have a divine element in us. Wrong thinking can shut this flow of divine healing influence. Disease is therefore the result of evil or bad thinking. A good thought is worth a dozen drugs. The mind is our very basis. We must therefore fill our mind with good, generous thoughts and shut out mean, evil thoughts. We are who we think we are. Similarly, we need to banish unhealthy emotions: fear, anxiety, worry, hatred, anger, lack of faith, complaint, contempt and so on … yes, and lust. We should even wipe these words from our vocabulary. We should fill our hearts with curative thoughts: love, courage, confidence, generosity. We need to relax and let God take over and flow through us (even if we don't believe in God).

And enthusiasm can be developed. Here is a true story. Many years ago a woman was diagnosed as having incurable TB. One doctor she consulted said that he could remove the left lung but he could in any case only give her another six months of life. A second opinion was sought and this second doctor more or less agreed. He might remove the right lung but he could only give her six more months of life. Left lung? Right lung? She lay in the hospital bed in despair. A friend of hers charged into the ward and got her out of bed. 'Don't listen to this nonsense. What do doctors know? You're coming with me.' Her friend took her to a Christian Science meeting. The woman became a Christian Scientist and lived another twenty years—and indeed lived to go to the funeral of her doctor. This is a true story. That woman was my grandmother. I put this story here because I believe my grandmother's survival depended on a shift in thinking away from the disease towards health—on finding some basis for feeling, once again enthusiastic about life.

Hypnosis

Hypnosis isn't a 'state' of mind like dream-sleep. It is a condition of mind in which all other mental states can be suggested externally.

It is well-known that people in a hypnotic trance can turn their hands warm and cold simply by focusing their attention to achieving these changes. Hypnotic suggestion can create even blisters and rashes on the skin.

The mind's brain waves have different frequencies while it is occupying different states. During wakefulness the brain waves are in the beta range (14 cycles per second or more). In sleep they are in the alpha range (7–14 cycles per second) occasionally dipping into the delta and theta ranges. Through hypnosis, we are taken into the alpha range while still in a state of wakefulness.

In the alpha state, the subconscious mind is open to suggestive input. Hypnotist, William Hewitt refers to the subconscious as 'an obedient slave' that doesn't think or reason.

'It just responds to what it is told. Herein lies the value and power of hypnosis. By hypnosis you can pump powerful suggestions directly into your subconscious. Your subconscious accepts them and causes them to become reality … it is extremely important that all suggestions given are positive, constructive and beneficial.' (William Hewitt, 1994)

In his book, *Hypnosis*, Hewitt discounts some myths. He says that people cannot be hypnotised against their will because one of the preconditions is 100 per cent cooperation. Secondly, the hypnotised person is always aware of what suggestions are being made and any suggestion that was upsetting would cause the subject to come out of the hypnotic state immediately of their own choice. According to Hewitt, almost everybody can be hypnotised. In fact, you don't need to go to a hypnotist to be hypnotised—you can hypnotise yourself. However, he suggests that it is easier to do this once you have first been hypnotised by someone else.

To hypnotise anyone, you must first induce in them a state of deep relaxation. This requires that their eyes be closed and that they focus their complete attention on a story or a set of actions. It is important to remove possible distractions such as telephones. Once in a comfortable position and in a quiet place, Hewitt advises that you slowly begin to relax the body progressively by focusing on the feet and telling them to relax, then the calves, the knees, the upper legs. You should breathe evenly using the stomach while slowly taking consciousness up to the neck and the head, telling each part to relax. Finally you tell the mind to relax. At this point the entire body is in a state of deep relaxation. You are in a state where you can start self-hypnosis by making suggestions to your subconscious.

Once the deep state has been reached, the key message can be implanted. The message should be something like: 'I am getting well'; or 'Soon, this cancer will be gone and I will be well again'; or 'Every day, I am getting better and better'. This key message needs to be repeated slowly and often so that it can sink into the depths of the subconscious. If stress and tension are the problems then the message should simply be: Relax. I want to relax. The mind should focus entirely on the message and follow it into the depths of the mind.

Richard Feynman, the Nobel-prize winning physicist, once underwent hypnosis to see how it felt. His experience of it was that he felt that nothing was happening, he could simply stop co-operating with the hypnotist at any time he felt like it—but somehow he just didn't feel like it!

However, anyone considering hypnosis should be very aware of the dangers. One girl was reportedly seriously injured when told to walk off the edge of a stage by a performing hypnotist. She did so and broke her back. Another girl was told to imagine she had been hit by a 10,000 volt charge. Shortly afterwards she went home, lay down and died. Anyone visiting a hypnotherapist should specify in advance exactly what messages are to be uttered. It may be advisable to take a sympathetic companion along to ensure this.

Hypnosis works, as the BBC discovered. In a test in 1946, a televised professional hypnotist put a number of his viewers into a hypnotic trance. Since then all professional hypnotists have been banned from the screen.

Under hypnosis, people can be made to be insensible to pain and to be induced to carry out tasks that would otherwise be considered impossible. Post-hypnotic suggestions can be implanted so that a person will carry out a task at some time after emerging from the hypnotic state. Hypnotic states will normally be slept off.

In some subjects, hypnosis is so deep that deep tissue surgery can be performed without anaesthetic. This was first demonstrated in the mid-nineteenth century by a surgeon in Calcutta, James Esdaile.

Laughter

Laughter is one means by which the body's entire chemistry can be shifted from a state of ill-health to one of health. This was the view of Norman Cousins, who in 1964 found himself in hospital with a profoundly crippling disease which involved the disintegration of the connective tissue of the body. The doctors weren't sure what it was or what to do about it—all they knew was that it was very serious. They could measure how serious it was by testing the sedimentation rate of the red blood cells. The speed with which these cells settle at the bottom of a test-tube measured in millimetres per hour is a sign of health or ill-health. A minor illness will have a sedimentation rate of 30–40. Over 60 is serious. Norman Cousins had a sedimentation rate of over 80, reaching up to 115.

Being very ill he naturally soon found himself in hospital. But Cousins quickly decided that hospital was not the right place for him. '[A] hospital is no place for a person who is seriously ill. The surprising lack of respect for basic sanitation, the rapidity with which staphylococci and other pathogenic organisms can run around an entire hospital, the extensive and sometimes promiscuous use of X-ray equipment …'

Cousins decided that, in his case, the reason he had fallen ill was that his adrenal glands had become exhausted. It is known that stress and emotional tension, frustration, rage, etc. can reduce the functioning of the adrenal glands and the endocrine system to the point where they cannot effectively deal with the toxins in the body caused by these same negative emotions.

'The inevitable question arose in my mind: what about the positive emotions? If negative emotions produce negative chemical changes in the body, wouldn't the positive emotions produce positive chemical changes? Is it possible that love, hope, faith, laughter, confidence, and the will to live have therapeutic value?'

So Cousins took the brave step of refusing any more pain-killing injections and booking himself out of hospital into a hotel where he arranged for a movie projector to be installed. He then set about watching every comic film and television program he could lay his hands on. When he wasn't watching films he was reading cartoons.

Although his pain was initially all but crippling, he found that laughter gave him real relief. Ten minutes of laughter allowed him two hours of pain-free sleep. It also led to a drop of five points on the sedimentation scale—and this improvement was cumulative.

He supplemented the programme of laughter with large doses of vitamin C, which he took by intravenous drip. He started at ten grams and decided to build up from there to 25 grams. Again, it had a measurable effect on the sedimentation rate.

Cousins went on to recover, though the after-effects of his illness stayed with him for years. He wrote up the full story in his book: *An Anatomy of an Illness as Perceived by the Patient.*

Although Cousins did not have cancer, we should note that the very factors that led to his illness are the very same ones that are implicated in cancer: stress, anxiety and so on leading to a state of adrenal exhaustion. Also, the blood sedimentation rate is a measure of general health—and general health in Cousins case led to specific improvements relating to a specific disease. If it can work with one disease it can work with all diseases.

There is however support for the beneficial impact of laughter in relation to cancer. Japanese researchers, Kazue Takayanagi and Satoru Noji reported on this case of an 88 year old woman with advance gastric cancer.

'Considering the patient's age and her desire not to receive cancer treatment, we prescribed laughter therapy as recommended by the Society for Healing Environment. The program was implemented in a laughter-inducing environment and consisted of five stages: (1) making the patient feel safe, (2) relaxing the patient, (3) increasing the effectiveness, (4) improving her condition and (5) increasing her joy of living. One year and seven months later, an endoscopy of the lesser curvature of the middle stomach body indicated that the lesions clearly improved .... The suspected lesion was localized to a limited area near the stomach wall .... Now, five years after the initial diagnosis, she maintains a good condition. Laughter, one of our casual behaviors, has the effect of reducing the stress experienced by the human body. Laughter is expected to become alternative medicine in the future, and we hope to see more reports and evidence on soothing therapies using laughter.'

Maharishi Ayurvedic therapy

Maharishi Mahesh Yogi gained instant fame in the West from his association with the Beatles and other pop icons of the sixties. He was already famous in India having launched the Transcendental Meditation movement. He has also established a number of Maharishi Ayurvedic Health Centres. Anyone seeking help from these centres will be put on a gentle regime involving a change of diet, Ayurvedic herbs, a daily routine of exercises and instruction in Transcendental Meditation.

As Dr Deepak Chopra, who used to work at the Maharishi Ayurveda Health Center in Lancaster, Massachusetts, says 'In Ayurveda, a level of total, deep relaxation is the most important precondition for curing any disorder ... the body knows how to maintain balance unless thrown off by disease; therefore, if one wants to restore the body's own healing ability, everything should be done to bring it back into balance.'

The Ayurvedic approach to healing also includes two other techniques which Chopra reports but does not describe. One is primordial sound therapy and the other is the bliss technique.

The primordial sound therapy assumes that underlying all matter there are vibrations of energy which can be heard when the meditating person is still and the mind is quiet.

'The theory behind primordial sound treatment is that the mind can return to the quantum level, introduce certain sounds that may have become distorted along the way, and thus have a profound healing influence in the body.' (It seems that when Chopra uses the word 'quantum' he is using the term as a metaphor and not as a statement relating to quantum physics.)

The bliss technique is a method for allowing the flow of joyful energy by the use of what he calls a 'faint mental impulse' which helps the mind come into contact with 'the vibrations of bliss that subtly pervade every cell of the body.'

'In and of itself, this feeling is extremely pleasant, but it also indicates that quantum healing is taking place, that disrupted channels of inner intelligence are being repaired. When these channels are closed, bliss cannot flow. When they are open, contact with the quantum mechanical body is restored.'

Dr Chopra is no longer connected with Maharishi Centres. To learn more of these techniques, you should visit www.maharishi.co.uk, www.theraj.com, or www.ayurveda-germany.com.

Meditation

Most people think of meditating as a way of relaxing and emptying the mind. Meditation masters laugh at this way of describing meditation. For them it is a way of entering a state of consciousness where other energy fields can be experienced. And these can be experienced only in the silence of the mind.

It is now known that meditation is a state of consciousness that is different from being awake, from being asleep and from dreaming. This fourth state is a measurable one. Machines designed to measure brain waves can distinguish the state of meditation from the other three states.

The tradition of meditation originated in India where it is known as dhyana, a term meaning to bring the mind to rest in the silence of the fourth state. Chopra describes it like this: 'The whole phenomenon is an immediate experience, like recognising the fragrance of lilacs or the sound of a friend's voice. It is immediate, non-verbal, and, unlike a flower's fragrance, totally transforming.'

In meditation, the meditator feels a heightened sense of awareness and inner silence. Robert Keith Wallace at UCLA found that people who meditate regularly become physiologically younger than those who don't. For the first five years, each year of meditation has the effect of making the meditator grow approximately one year younger. After that the rejuvenating process appears to speed up.

A 1986 study by the Blue Cross Blue Shield insurance company found that people who meditate have less than half the number of tumours than non-meditators. A 1979 Israeli study found that meditation helps people with abnormally high cholesterol levels to lower these levels and so reduce their risk of heart attack.

How can one learn to meditate? There are a number of different forms of meditation, and many people find that they can meditate perfectly well by following a few basic steps. The first principle of all meditation is to sit quietly in a chair with eyes closed. Then the object is to a stillness or state of vacant mental awareness. Some people use a special word or phrase which they repeat silently. Others simply focus on certain aspects of the body or breath.

One guide to good meditation practice recommends these steps:

1. Choose a quiet spot where you will not be disturbed. Make sure you will not be disturbed.
2. Sit in a comfortable position with straight back. Some people like to cross their ankles.
3. Close your eyes.
4. Relax your muscles from head to feet by focusing the mind on the tip of the nose. Then let the mind travel up the nose, round the face and skull to the back of the neck. Then slowly round the shoulders and arms, then the back, the buttocks, the legs and the feet. Become aware of any tensions and with the help of the mind induce relaxation in these places.
5. Become aware of the breathing, watching it go in and out without any desire to control it.
6. Repeat the word you have chosen as your focus word or mantra.
7. If you become aware that your thoughts have drifted. Stop the thoughts and return to your mantra.
8. Practise every day for 15–20 minutes.
9. Do not judge your performance. Do not judge anything about the performance. In meditation things just happen. It is important to be aware of them happening and to accept that they are happening but do not be in any way critical or judgmental about what happened.

Neuro-linguistic programming (NLP)

This is a method for helping people who find themselves constrained by depressive or otherwise negative belief systems and behaviours. As we have seen, this is a feature of many people who have cancer. A practitioner who has been trained in the method uses a number of specific techniques to help 're-program' people's views about themselves and the world and in doing so helps them take more responsibility for their own healing.

For many people this could be a useful, short-term tool to kick start attitudinal change.

Prayer

In one study, investigators asked people who had undergone remarkable recovery which activities they believed had most helped. 68 per cent said prayer, followed by meditation and exercise (64 per cent), visualisation (59 per cent), walking (52 per cent) music/singing (50 per cent) other forms of stress reduction (50 per cent)—prayer came out top.

We can consider prayer's possible effects in a number of ways. It may be effective psychologically for the praying person to pray for himself. By praying, the person can release thoughts and feelings within himself. Or, if faith is great, there may be a conviction that the divine being will intercede and so there may be a placebo effect. Most people will accept that prayer can be very beneficial under these circumstances.

However, according to Dr Larry Dossey, prayers are more likely to be beneficial if they are undirected and are accompanied by complete acceptance of the situation. 'Do with me what you will' is more likely to be effective than 'Dear God please cure me of my cancer in my left breast'. Certainly, it is a fact that can be immediately subjectively confirmed, that the mind is more deeply and more wholly at peace when it utters the former prayer than when it utters the latter. It seems almost as if a different, deeper, more pleasure-related part of the mind is engaged.

Is prayer at a distance effective? Larry Dossey argues that some studies do seem to indicate that prayer at a distance (i.e., my prayer for your health) may have an effect.

One man known for his healing abilities was approached by a friend to pray for healing as he had an extremely painful condition that required intensive surgery. The healer promised to do the healing and the following day the friend woke up miraculously cured. The doctors were astounded. This apparently clear cut case would have been a powerful demonstration of prayer's potential to heal at a distance. The healer in this case was Dr Lawrence LeShan, who we have already met in the discussion of cancer personalities. However, there was a problem.

'It would have been the psychic healing case of the century except for one small detail. In the press of overwork, I had forgotten to do the healing. If I had only remembered, it would have been a famous demonstration of what can be accomplished by this method.'

Dossey suggests that LeShan may indeed have prayed but unconsciously. This raises another set of questions. Does this mean that our hidden thoughts and feelings about other people have the power to harm or heal unconsciously? Dossey thinks so. If this is the case are patients affected by their doctors' belief systems? If the doctor is thinking: this woman will die in three months' time, will that affect the outcome? Again, many people are convinced that the doctor's negative thoughts will have a very negative effect on the prognosis.

And of course, in the above case, it may have been the man's faith that LeShan could indeed work a distance healing that provoked the cure. The man had handed the matter over to someone he trusted and the consequent relief resulted in the cure.

Taking good care of yourself in times of trouble

It is known that physical and, more importantly, emotional trauma can lead to cancer. It therefore makes strong sense, if you have experienced a traumatic event: the break-up of a marriage, the death of someone close or a business collapse, for example, to consider yourself to be in danger. At times like these it pays to pamper your health needs. Book yourself into a health farm, have those colonics and aromatherapy massages you've always wanted but never plucked up the courage to do. Go to a naturopath and have a general health assessment done. Ease up in other areas. Allow yourself to be taken care of by others. Decide that you are important enough to pay this attention to yourself. Let's face it, as the advertisement says, you're worth it!

Thinking of three good things that happened today

One happiness-boosting exercise is this: every evening think of three good things that happened during the day. Think about why they happened. That's it. People who have tried this exercise say that it has a subtle but positive effect on their attitudes (they focus more on the good stuff rather than the bad stuff). Others say that the exercise has improved their sleep—and their happiness.

Visualisation

The purpose of visualisation is to tell the mind what to think and therefore to tell the mind what to do in the body. The idea is to let thoughts and messages filter from the conscious to the subconscious zones of the mind. Many athletes improve their performances through mental gymnastics, or mental tennis, and so on. The mind becomes its thoughts—and so too does the body. By actively guiding the imagination, the body can be led to a state of health. If you want something enough, then simply imagine it over and over again while you are in a deeply relaxed frame of mind.

Some people may find this a difficult idea to accept. The story of psychiatrist Milton Erickson shows what can be achieved through thought alone. Erickson was paralyzed by polio as a young boy and forced to spend a lot of time on his front porch in a rocking chair watching the world go by. One day, left at home strapped to a rocking chair he found he was too far from the window to look out. Suddenly he became aware that his obsession with getting to the window was causing his chair to rock. He started to concentrate his thoughts on getting to the window. The more he did so the more the rocking increased. He soon found that he could direct the movement of the chair by working on his thoughts. It took him all afternoon but he managed to reach the window. This experience led him to the idea that he could influence other movements by concentrating his thoughts. He was eventually able to overcome the paralysis completely and begin to walk again.

How can we use this visualisation to help us stay healthy? By letting ourselves dwell inwardly on a healthy positive image. With eyes closed, for example, imagine the following: imagine your very favourite place. Maybe this is near where you live or a place that you remember from your youth or a place that you have visited on your holidays, it may even be a totally imaginary place—wherever it is it is a place where you are happy. Reflect on the happiness you feel being there. Feel the warmth of the sunlight. Feel the glow of the sun on your body. How comfortable you feel with the warm living rays of the sun permeating your whole body. It is filling your body with health and happiness, energy and love. It suffuses through all the limbs and through the whole of your being. With each breath the warmth and the light grow stronger and lighter. You release yourself into the heart of this feeling and you sit and feel this and let your mind sense these sensations. Then, when you're ready, you can return to normal consciousness.

This is just an example of the kind of creative visualisation that can, it is claimed, restore or maintain the body's health.

Some people visualise the cancer and watch as, in their minds, their body's immune defence system attacks it and slowly destroys it. Some people focus their visualisation on the chemotherapy drug or the radiation they are receiving. They imagine the drug eating up the tumour. They imagine the radiation rays like the healing rays of the sun dissolving the tumour. Or, as one patient did, as golden bullets.

There was a man who had a nearly-always fatal form of throat cancer at a late stage of development, his weight having dropped from 130 to 98lb, and he was barely able to swallow. He was given radiation treatment but was not expected to benefit greatly from it—perhaps some short-lived comfort from a temporarily radiation-shrunk tumour. In addition to the radiation treatment he was asked to visualise the radiation as millions of little bullets bombarding the cancer tumour. He also imagined the cancer cells as being weak and unable to repair themselves—while he imagined the normal cells as being strong and repairing themselves quickly. He visualised the white blood cells swarming over the dead and dying cancer cells and carrying them out of the body through the liver and kidney. He did this three or four times a day. The result? He not only recovered but suffered very little associated radiation damage.

His doctor, O Carl Simonton, had similar success with a large number of patients who were considered incurable. Of a group of 156 people with 'incurable cancers', 63 were still alive four years later, and in 43 of these the cancer had either disappeared, was regressing or had stabilised.

Some visualisation experiments have shown that volunteers can influence the numbers of various types of cell in the blood. This study conducted by Dr Jean Achterberg found that students who visualised having more neutrophils, did indeed have higher counts of neutrophils by the end of the experiment, while those who focused on increasing the number of T-cells increased T-cell counts but not neutrophils. This shows how powerful belief can be.

On the negative side, we can make ourselves ill by visualising the worst. Joan Borysenko calls this process 'awfulizing': the tendency to imagine the worst possible consequence of any event. This tendency is often obsessive and habitual, a result of past conditioning: 'Awareness of our conditioning is the first step toward unlearning attitudes that have outlived their usefulness. Such awareness opens our ability to respond to what is happening now rather than reacting out of a conditioned history that may be archaic.' (Borysenko, 1987)

It is very important to dwell on good thoughts and to stop negative thoughts from invading the inner mental space of our minds.

If we see visualisation as the right brain imagination at work, suggestion is the intellectual-verbal partner. By letting them work together we can harness powerful mental forces. Dr David Sobel, co-author of *The Healing Brain*, recalled how he was plagued by warts on his hand when he was young. The warts had resisted all standard medical treatments. One day his mother passed him an article from the newspaper. The headline was 'Warts Cured by Suggestion'. His curiosity aroused, he read on. In the article he was told that hypnosis and suggestion could get rid of warts. He decided to try it out but, as they didn't explain in the article how to go about it, he had to invent his own method.

'I decided … that I must concentrate intensely on the warts while repeating ten times (it had to be exactly ten times) the phrase: 'Warts go away. Warts go away.' I did this faithfully every day for about four weeks, at the end of which time … [they] had all vanished.'

Dr Bruno Bloch, known as the 'famous wart doctor of Zurich' built a machine that had a noisy motor and flashing lights. He told patients to put their hands in the machine until they were told the warts were dead. He would then add a pink vegetable dye to the wart and tell the patients not to wash or touch the wart until it was gone. Roughly 30 per cent of his patients were cured after one session. The relevance of this to cancer is this: warts are very similar to tumours. They are benign growths caused, like some cancers, by a viral infection. Anything that can work for warts has a good chance of working for cancer tumours.

Visualisation works. Cancer patients should make it work for them. The greater the visual, auditory and sensory involvement of all the senses they can bring to bear in the act of the visualisation the more likely success will follow.

Affirmation

Affirmation is another technique that many people have found helpful in changing unhealthy, or undesirable thought patterns and attitudes, or inculcating new positive, health-promoting thoughts, attitudes and goals. The promise of what can be achieved through this promise is stated here: 'affirmations … reprogram your thought patterns, they change the way you think and feel about things, and because you have replaced dysfunctional beliefs with your own new positive beliefs, positive change comes easily and naturally. This will start to reflect in your external life, you will start to experience seismic changes for the better in many aspects of your life.' (www.vitalaffirmations.com —an excellent site for exploring this subject in some depth.)

The key to making positive affirmations is to create a short, succinct statement and to repeat it to yourself regularly with mindfulness and commitment to the meaning of the affirmation. The above website suggests the following messages might be helpful for healing:

- Every cell in my body vibrates with energy and health.
- Loving myself heals my life. I nourish my mind, body and soul.
- My body heals quickly and easily.

Or you may want to create affirmations that change your attitudes in other areas of life, such as:

- My life is a joy, filled with love, fun and friendship: all I need do is stop all criticism, forgive, relax and be open.

You may feel that such an affirmation is not 'true' initially but the idea is that it will become true the more you repeat the affirmation. After all, the way we feel negatively about ourselves is no more than an attitude of mind. We might think of it as 'realistic', but in fact it is all an interpretation, and we often have a propensity for the dramatic and negative. Think of affirmations as creating our own placebos rather than nocebos (see above). How we think about ourselves is a choice we make.

Ten ways of reducing stress

Since stress is such an important factor in exacerbating, if not actually causing, cancer, it is worth looking at a number of ways by which stress can be reduced.

1. Progressive relaxation technique: Taking each part of the body one at a time from head and neck down to fingers and toes alternately tense and relax each muscle group.
2. Exercise: Go for a walk, run, swim or bounce on a mini-trampoline. Do Tai Chi or yoga. Take up dancing.
3. Meditate: sit in a straight-back chair and close your eyes. Imagine your breath emerging from the nostrils and travelling up your forehead, around the skull to the back of the neck—then shoulders, arms, fingers, down the back, round the buttocks, legs, feet, toes then back up, legs, groin, stomach, chest, throat, chin and back into the mouth. If you feel a tingle then that's a sign of relaxation.
4. Laugh: watch comedies on TV, video, You Tube.
5. Listen to Mozart, Indian sitar music, blues, jazz, Tamla Motown (but not heavy metal!)
6. Have a nice warm bath with lavender essential oil—also geranium, bergamot, rosemary, chamomile, lemon balm, ylang ylang essential oils.
7. Go to church and pray.
8. Hug and/or kiss someone. This releases chemicals that reduce the levels of stress hormones. Have sex. Ditto
9. Have a massage—make it a two-hour whole-body oil massage.
10. Do an art project—whether it is painting or sculpture, jewellery-making or writing.

Group support

It is useful in this context to consider what part, if any, group support should play in the fight against cancer. There appears to be strong evidence that those who live within a network of strong social relationships live longer and healthier lives. Loneliness kills. Group support should therefore help the healing process. But this is a general statement that does not necessarily apply to many particular people.

Almost every new cancer patient is faced with the problem of who to tell and what to say about the disease. Some people bottle it up and keep it to themselves. Generally speaking this is not a good idea, as it prevents people from giving support or providing information or other help that may be important: the name of a good naturopath, someone who is happy to do some research on the Internet and so on. If you have good friends, they will rally round and make a point of giving some kind of support. If you are a good friend you will rally round. The best strategy of all is to tell everyone everything. It really does get a lot of nonsense out of the way.

If group therapy is desired, your doctor should be able to point you in the right direction. However, care should be taken to find the right kind of support group. A group of women who have all had mastectomies, for example, would be very good support for any new member who had also had a mastectomy—but not necessarily for a woman who had refused a mastectomy. It depends on their attitude to not having a mastectomy. If they support the plan, that's good. If they try to get the woman in question to get used to the idea of the necessity of mastectomy, then that woman should find another group—fast.

The emphasis of group support should be on helping people to live as fully as possible, to help communication with family members and friends, to help ease the fears of death and dying and to help, where desired, with the release of emotion.

One possibly negative feature of group therapy may be that it will gradually accustom members to the idea of dying, and so place imperceptible obstacles in the way of seeking a cure.

While many people will be able to put together their own support groups made up of friends, others will want to meet and talk to others who have had, or who are undergoing, the same experience. Many forums on the Internet are informal support groups of this kind. More formal groups are often organised in such a way that the members can meet up in person.

Annette Crisswell, herself a cancer survivor and who has facilitated a support group for seven years, provided me with the following guidelines on the subject. What follows is her commentary:

'It has been found that people attending a support group do far better in terms of recovery than those who choose not to. However, not everyone flourishes in groups and I believe it is important that they are not made to feel that their chances of recovery are in any way impeded by going it alone. Each person must find the best way back to "wellness" for themselves, with confidence.'

What is a support group?

a)   A gathering of people who have experienced a trauma of some kind, either a life threatening illness, a traumatic loss, a situation that is out of control, etc. In fact, an experience that has created chaos in their lives.

b)   The group may or may not be run by an experienced counsellor. With a counsellor the group may be based more on actual group therapy, otherwise a support group is exactly what it says: a group that gives support. It is not there to advise people what they should do, condemn what they have done or to criticize or change how they are.

What are the purposes of a support group?

The purposes of a support group are:

a)   to provide as much information about the various and the latest treatments (allopathic, complementary, alternative, etc.) that are available and relevant to the objects of the group. A source of books, articles, etc.

b)   to provide a safe place for people to discuss their feelings and fears with people who have, or have had similar experiences, without fear of criticism or negation.

c)   to empower people and to revitalize their belief in themselves.

d)   to provide specialist speakers who are able to clarify and give information about all types of treatment available, so that people in the group are able to make informed choices for themselves and have their misunderstandings and doubts clarified.

Depending on the needs and desires of its members, a support group can:

a)   be simply a group of people who get together at regular intervals just to chat, exchange information, become friends, etc.
b)   be a regular gathering of people for the purpose of experiencing complementary therapies aimed at empowering the body, mind and spirit. This may include counselling sessions. The underlying principle will be a concern for the whole person of each member of the group.
c)   be a structured series of meetings, say once a week for ten weeks, in which different specialists or practitioners can be invited to give a talk or presentation. This can be combined with counselling and group sharing sessions.
d)   organise themselves—as often, but by no means always, happens with cancer support groups—round the different cancers that the individual members have, e.g., breast cancer group, lung cancer group, etc.

The basic rule of all these groups is to empower people so that each person is helped to define for him/herself positive action and attitude goals.

What a support group is not

a)   A support group is not there to advise anyone what is the right thing to do. What is right for one person is not necessarily right for another. Whatever someone chooses to do is right for them and they should be supported in their choice and empowered to realize their chosen goals.
b)   A support group is not there to counsel people unless there is an experienced, trained counsellor present.
c)   A support group is not there to coerce anyone to do or feel anything. Too often empowering people is seen simply as telling people to 'be positive' and in this way attempting to negate fear, anger and sadness. I challenge anyone who has been told that they are going to have a double mastectomy to feel cheerful and positive. There is such loss and fear and pain involved that to be told you must be 'positive' shows a total lack of empathy, bordering on cruelty. If the major focus of a group is on such a rigidly defined attitude then the result will be that members will not admit to their true feelings and so they will feel even more lonely than before. Being positive does not mean blinding oneself to all the negative aspects and possibilities inherent in the situation, replacing them with a thin brittle veneer of grit-your-teeth-and-get-on-with-it cheerfulness. Being positive, in its proper and helpful sense, is having an attitude that recognizes the feelings of sadness and inadequacy, the

fears and terrors and all the other complex emotions that are commonly experienced—but knows also that there are options and alternatives—that the future ultimately is not hopeless, that it is not meaningless, that recovery is not impossible, that change for the better will come in its own time and the burdens of the present must be borne until that better time comes.

What people who have attended a support group have said

1. I felt so alone until I joined the group. People who have not had this experience just do not understand.
2. It was such a relief to know that how I was reacting was quite normal.
3. It was good to hear what other people had done to come to terms with what had happened to them. It helped me to feel I could once more be in control of my life.
4. I discovered so many ways I could help myself overcome the disease, or the side effects of my treatment in the complementary field. It opened up a whole new fascinating area in my life.
5. It's good to be able to meet people who have been through what I'm going through and have recovered. There is life after cancer.

Summing up

This is the last of the chapters discussing the range of options available to you. Section 8 tells the stories of people who have made various, differing choices available to them and who have become cancer-free again. I hope you too have found options that make sense for you and that you too are soon (or, indeed already) on the path to recovery.

To re-iterate a point I have made several times already, each of us is different. Some of you will be drawn to prayer while others to a regular, very brisk five-mile walk. Some of you will want to meditate, while others will want to watch Buster Keaton comedies.

Nowhere is the interface of science and the so-called 'new age' more fraught than in the area of energy medicine. However, if magnetic devices do no more than raise the tissue oxygen levels (which they do, or athletes would not be making use of this technology—nor would they make use of magnets to speed up healing of bone fractures—but again they do), then they are worth it. Clearly there is something profoundly health-supporting in increased and pulsed magnetism. Again the body does create its own electro-magnetic field, and our energetic self does extend outwards, creating an aura if you will. This aura has been photographed, and for some sensitive people it may indeed be visible in daily life. This energy cloud may also contain energy that can be accessed by psychics. I have a neighbour, a professional fortune-teller, who one day, when I consulted her for experimental purposes, told me that a male friend would arrive unexpectedly and she was picking up 'Sri Lanka' but she couldn't say in what context. The very next day I bumped into someone I hadn't seen for years—someone who happened to live part of the year in Sri Lanka. What was the statistical likelihood of that?

There is no doubt that Indian yogis can achieve a great deal through long years of meditational practice—but at the same time, some yogis get cancer.

Do I believe in spiritual healing? Hard to say. Yet, if and when I myself am diagnosed with cancer, I most definitely would look for some. As always I invoke the risk-cost-benefit analysis. The risk and cost are negligible, the potential benefit is great. The need to believe sometimes just gets in the way, imposing obstacles to doing. Good teams continue playing hard even though they know they will lose a game—and I suggest to you that that attitude is one you should take on board too. Strive, strive, strive with all your might, goes the song.

And then there are the fraught questions of whether holographic theory and quantum physics have any applicability in the gross world of everyday. Do subtle energies affect the course of disease? Everyone has to make up their own mind about that.

Nevertheless, there is no doubt that exercise, physiotherapy, music and emotional involvement in artistic performance can have powerful effects on mood. I once walked a depression off by exhausting myself with an eight-hour clamber up and down hills. The next day I felt wonderfully renewed psychologically. And mood makes all the difference. Joy and depression both have their bio-chemistry—both as cause and effect. And laughter, as Norman Cousins proved, is healing.

As to whether membership of a group is beneficial, only you can say. Some of you will want that support, others will find it a distraction. In any case, I believe that cancer patients should strong-arm a close friend or two into a personal support group, and that reading should be shared and discussed.

I do believe that your own intuition will guide you in choosing the bundle of therapies you eventually do decide to undertake—and that this is as good a way of proceeding as any. If you simply feel lost and don't have any intuitions, you may find some way to your hidden self through art or writing or meditating, or camping out on a cold windy night in some remote spot.

If you are scientifically educated you may have found some of my explanations simplistic, confusing or just plain wrong. If so, I apologise; but these are complex areas and any attempt to grapple with, say, electro-magnetism in any depth would quickly leave the average reader (among whom I place myself) brain-addled. This book is a guide to what is available, as you will find it described, and you are invited to do your own further research. As always, the phrase 'buyer beware' should be kept at the forefront of your mind.

It remains for me to wish you luck on your own journey and I hope this book has been helpful to you in directing you on your journey to health.

Cancer Survivors' Stories

They did it. You can too!

In this section you will find the stories of 25 people who have cured themselves of cancer—some by combining conventional and alternative therapies, but the vast majority by means of alternative therapies alone. These stories demonstrate the important role complementary and alternative medicine (CAM) can play in helping people with cancer recover fully and completely from this terrible disease—the incidence of which is rising year on year.

Introduction

Do complementary/alternative approaches to cancer recovery work?

In the previous sections of this book I have argued that there is a great deal to be wary of in the conventional approaches to cancer treatment. While surgery, in the short term, appears to be a fifty-fifty proposition, the same cannot be said of radiation and, with a very few exceptions, chemotherapy. The dangers associated with these treatments are not simply that they are painful. They can result in life-long damage to health and quality of life, and what is less often recognised, they often significantly shorten life. One statistician has calculated that the average person with the average cancer will live four times longer if he/she does nothing than if she/he does something (i.e. undergoes conventional treatment).

On the other hand, I have argued that there are enormous numbers of other approaches—diets, herbs, supplements, along with therapies that engage the body, mind and emotions in a health-promoting, cancer-defeating way.

But the key question is this: Is all of this just nice-sounding theory, or do they really work? Can these alternative or complementary approaches really cure cancer?

How do we measure effectiveness?

The problem we face is that of measuring effectiveness. We have seen in the discussion of research and politics (see Section 3: *Cancer Research and Politics*), that the people who control the validating process, the people who control medical and cancer research, have very little incentive to find cures that don't make money. The enormous profits that pharmaceutical companies make on drugs cannot be made from selling diets, herbs, supplements or meditation and visualisation strategies. In the absence of a real commitment to do scientific research on these alternative approaches, how then can we judge whether or not something works?

The answer has to be empirical—are people following alternative approaches and succeeding in extending their lives, improving the quality of their lives and even becoming cancer-free again? The answer is a resounding *yes*.

This section

In this section you will read the stories of over two dozen people who have indeed recovered from cancer either by a combination of conventional and alternative approaches—or more commonly by means of the alternative approaches alone.

In preparing this section, I set out to find people who had cured their cancers and invited them to contribute their stories. Many were happy to provide their stories and I would like to thank them for their generosity. In some cases, however, there was suspicion that I was seeking to profit from other people's work (a quite understandable concern) which I hope to avoid by circulating this section as widely as possible free of charge in pdf format. If you have this version, please send it to all your friends and ask them to send it on to all their friends. If you want to download a free pdf version, then please go to my website at www.fightingcancer.com.

The more people are made aware of the real potential of alternative approaches to cancer, the less frightening a diagnosis will become. Let us remind ourselves: This is a disease that currently fifty per cent of us will face in our lifetimes—and it will strike perhaps three-quarters of our children's generation (if incidence rates continue to climb as they are expected to do). So it makes sense to be prepared.

And then there was one case, a well-known exponent of alternative approaches, who refused to have her story appear in this book because she disagreed with much of what I had written. In her view there was only one way to deal with cancer—her way, which had been revealed to her by God. Ah well! You can't win them all.

Many cures already exist

The idea that there is only one way to deal with cancer is not one that I agree with, and not one supported by these stories. The people whose stories appear in this section have done very many different approaches. So I think it is clear that the search for a cure for cancer is misplaced. There are already many cures. None of these cures may be 100 per cent effective on their own (though of course some may be pretty close) but in combination with other therapies their potential increases.

Do the maths

The mathematics is simple. If approaches A, B, C and D each have a fifty per cent chance of working—and if they have different curative mechanisms, and if they don't interfere with each other—then if you do one of these approaches you have a fifty per cent chance of curing your cancer; if you do two, the probability will increase to seventy-five per cent; do three and it rises to eighty-seven per cent; do all four and the result is close to ninety-four per cent. And then of course there are approaches E,F, G and so on.

And what if each of them has an eighty per cent likelihood of curing your cancer? (The answer for four approaches is 99.84 per cent!)

You may find this simplistic, but we can see that there isn't a lot of difference between the combined effects of four approaches despite the apparent difference between fifty and eighty per cent. And what comes out of these stories very clearly is the power of diet and herbs and supplements to rid the body of cancer.

But let's make a very pessimistic assumption. Let us assume that each of our alternative approaches has a very low probability of success—say 20 per cent. Then combining four such approaches will give you a 60 per cent survival probability, and you can take that up to 80 per cent by doing another four.

Clearly the more you do, the greater your chances of beating cancer.

Be your own guinea pig

Another issue that we should remind ourselves of is that we are all unique—no-one else on earth has a physiology exactly the same as mine or yours. Every single one of us has bio-chemical processes going on in our bodies that place us at the extremes of the normal distribution curve. This is a statistical certainty. That means that what works for you may not necessarily work for me. There is a good chance it will but there is no guarantee. Or it may have a different effect, maybe stronger, maybe weaker, maybe completely different.

This in turn means that each of us has to be our own guinea pig. Trial and assessment is the only way to proceed. We need to try things out for ourselves. If we like it, continue. If we don't like it, set it aside and do something else. We need to take responsibility for ourselves. But how are we going to know where to start? For some the answer will be glaringly obvious, for others a matter of grave uncertainty and consequent anxiety.

I believe very strongly in the subconscious. I believe it knows what is good for us—and it will tell us in its own way. If one approach seems very attractive for some not very clear reason, this may be because our subconscious is prompting us, or we may wake up at three in the morning with an image of a particular approach. Trust this intuition, it is almost certainly our subconscious talking to us. Or maybe just plunge in, make random choices and see where they lead you. If you really can't decide draft in some friends to help you talk it through—but remember, all decisions have to be your own decisions. You are the one who will suffer the consequences so you must do the choosing.

It is now time to let the stories do their own talking.

The stories

The stories on the following pages are by people who have taken the step to stand up and tell the world. They are doing so because they want to help others. Some of them have written books, others have websites and in most cases they have said they are willing to be contacted directly. These are not anonymous, faceless anecdotes. These are stories by people who are not afraid to stand up and tell the truth as they see it, as they have experienced it.

The collective weight of this testimony allows only one conclusion: Alternative therapies do work and are vastly preferable to the conventional 'weapons'. They offer health and happiness, not damage and pain.

I urge you to read these stories and take note for yourself. If you have cancer you can apply these lessons immediately. If you don't (at present) have cancer at least these stories will help you prepare yourself for that possibility.

The Stories of Two Children

Children with cancer present a heart-searing problem. We want to do the very best for them—and it seems sensible therefore to put them in the hands of the best doctors at the best oncology units specialising in children's cancers.

Although this seems at first sight to be unarguably the best course of action, by doing so we know that we will be subjecting them to immense pain, that they will inevitably suffer some form of brain damage—and their long-term health will almost certainly suffer grievously. If you want to see the list of possible 'late effects' of chemotherapy and radiation go to the American Cancer Society website and do a search for 'childhood cancers late effects'—the description makes for sobering reading. And remember, these late effects are not possibilities, they are much closer to certainties.

The problem for parents is that if they attempt to extract their children from such punitive courses of treatment they are likely to find that the medical system, child protection agencies and courts will require them to proceed.

For any parent wishing to explore the area of alternative therapies, therefore, the options are limited and you may need to go for a long trip abroad.

Is there any evidence that alternative approaches can be healing? These two stories suggest there is.

Cash Hyde

Cash Hyde, a young boy from Missoula Montana, was only 20 months old when he was diagnosed with a highly aggressive stage 4 brain tumour surrounding his optic nerve. The doctors gave him very little hope of survival.

They gave him seven different chemotherapy drugs and among other impacts this caused Cash to suffer septic shock, a stroke and heavy haemorrhaging of his lungs. He was given the highest possible doses of chemotherapy for two months. Cash was so sick that he didn't eat anything for 40 days. In the end the sight of his son's suffering was more than he could take and his father, Mike, asked them to stop the treatment.

Without telling them what he planned, Mike decided to try out something on his own. He didn't tell the doctors because he knew they would oppose it. Mike bought some marijuana and boiled it in olive oil. He then added this in small doses of around half a teaspoon each time to his son's feeding tube. His father reported the impact in these words: 'Not only was it helpful, it was a godsend. Within two weeks he was weaned off all the nausea drugs and he was eating again and sitting up in bed and laughing.' When he admitted what he had done the doctors continued to prescribe the cannabis—for his nausea. In February 2011, news reports announced that young Cash was still in remission. If he recovers the doctors will of course claim that the chemo. did the trick. But although the cannabis is being prescribed as an anti-nausea medication, it has a strong anti-cancer effect of its own (see discussion of cannabis in Section 5: *Cancer: Herbs, Botanicals and Biological Therapies*).

Mike Hyde has set up the Cash Hyde Foundation to promote the medical use of cannabis, which remains such a contentious subject.

Connah Broom

On 10 February 2009, *The Daily Mail* newspaper (UK) reported the following story. In August 2006 Connah was diagnosed with stage 4 neuroblastoma, an aggressive childhood cancer. He was given intensive chemotherapy for seven months but in the end was sent home by the doctors so that he could die at home. He had at this time eleven tumours in his body, mainly in the neck area. The doctors said there was nothing more they could do and told his parents that they should enjoy Connah's final months of life as best they could. That was in 2007. The Broom family decided differently. They put him on an organic vegetarian diet and a daily sauna. They also did Reiki and went to a Mexican clinic where they were able to undergo sono photo-dynamic therapy. They also give him an ultrasound treatment (unspecified) but likely from the photograph accompanying the story to be SCENAR (see Section 7: *Cancer Energy, Mind and Emotions* for details). In 2011, Connah was doing well, and all but one of the tumours were in retreat.

The doctors admitted this was unusual but denied that the alternative therapies had had any impact. You can lead a horse to water but you can't make a doctor accept that a diet is more powerful than chemotherapy drugs.

I have no doubt that one day, hopefully one day soon, doctors will eventually recognise the benefits of approaches that they currently ignore—and that a truly integrative medicine will result. I believe the pressure to do so will come from patients who, taking responsibility for themselves, inform themselves of all the options and make their own judgements as to the value of diets, herbs, vitamins and so on. By doing so, they will force doctors to recognise that there is, in fact, a great deal of scientific support for these non-conventional approaches to cancer recovery.

Both these stories are very positive and clearly support the idea that complementary or alternative approaches can be health promoting in the short term and potentially curative in the long term. How these two boys will continue to respond to their new therapies no-one can say but how many stories like these do you need before you say: 'Maybe there is something in these alternative ways of dealing with cancer.'

It is now time to look at stories of adults who have chosen alternative and complementary ways and who have, in many cases, survived cancer-free for decades as a result.

Personal Stories

The following stories are of people who cured their cancers using alternative therapies—although in one or two cases they also used conventional therapies. I use the word 'cured' without the usual apologies because no other word will do. People like Beata and Percy (read below) lived and have lived for decades free of cancer. That is what 'cured' means. Others, it is true, did succumb to their cancers, but only after having lived for years without any sign of cancer. Others in this list will not assert that they are 'cured'. They will simply say that they are fighting a battle against cancer and up till now they appear to be winning! Here then are some remarkable stories.

Beata Bishop

In the early 1980s, while working as a writer at the BBC, Beata Bishop discovered that a mole on her leg was a malignant melanoma, one of the fastest-spreading and most lethal of all cancers. She underwent painful and disfiguring surgery, but within a year it was found that the cancer had spread into the lymphatic system and was appearing elsewhere on her body. She was told by her doctors that she had a matter of weeks or months to live, and that there was nothing they could do about it.

Fortunately for her, a friend had heard of the Gerson Institute and not having any other options she chose to follow this diet developed by an eminent German physician, Dr Max Gerson (see Section 4: *Cancer: Detox and Diet* for further details). Taking her fate in her hands, she spent two months at the world's only Gerson clinic in Mexico where she learnt the theory and practice of the intensive therapy which she then pursued for a further eighteen months in London.

After two years on the Gerson Therapy, which transformed her both physically and psychologically, Beata Bishop made a full recovery.

Today she is still alive, in her 70s, extremely active and free of her cancer. She wrote her story in a book, *My Triumph Over Cancer*, first published in 1985. Beata hated this title and later had the book re-published as *A Time to Heal*. She has also collaborated with Charlotte Gerson, who now runs the Gerson Institute, in writing an updated introduction to the Gerson Diet called *Healing The Gerson Way*.

I have interviewed Beata for Conscious TV and you can find a link to this interview at www.cancerfighter.wordpress.com). Hers is a truly remarkable story. Not many people live thirty years having received a diagnosis of untreatable terminal stage melanoma.

Michael Gearin-Tosh

Michael Gearin-Tosh was, for 35 years, tutor in English at St Catherine's College, Oxford. In 1994 he was diagnosed with myeloma, a cancer of the bone marrow which is normally considered to be untreatable. Although urged to take chemotherapy, he discovered that this would give him only a four per cent possibility of a cure. His conclusion: 'Touch it [chemotherapy], and you're a goner'.

He embarked on a series of alternative treatments consisting of 12 freshly-made vegetable juices a day, high-dose vitamin injections, acupuncture, raw garlic, coffee enemas, and Chinese breathing exercises. He also used visualisation techniques in which he imagined his immune cells attacking the tumour. The result was that his cancer went into remission. He was still cancer-free 11 years later when he died in 2005 from an untreated blood infection.

Gearin-Tosh described his battle with cancer in his book, *Living Proof—A Medical Mutiny* (Scribner, 2002).

Christopher Sheppard

In November 1999, Christopher Sheppard, a film producer, was diagnosed with 'locally advanced' rectal cancer and his doctors recommended surgery—as did the homoeopathic doctors and acupuncturist that he approached to help him. However, Sheppard refused surgery and chemo. but eventually, after a lot of soul searching, did decide to accept radiation treatment. He also decided to go on what he called a healing journey. It was his view that each cancer victim, not their doctor, should be the authority on what they should do for their cancer. And they should make their decisions on the basis of their own self-knowledge, intuition and sense of the world.

For himself, he selected a modified version of the Gerson diet, developed by his nutritionist, heavily supplemented with vitamins, minerals and herbs—at one point he was taking over 100 pills a day.

He also decided to visit a Brazilian spiritual healer, Joao Texeira, also known to his followers as 'John of God'. He felt strongly that there was a spiritual dimension—that his cancer was a sign of a spiritual malaise. This led him to Tibetan Buddhism and he studied a special form of meditation at a Buddhist community. Another self-devised therapy was to join an emotional counselling group.

Within a year he was cancer-free, and remains so to this day. Radiation on its own is not generally considered curative for rectal cancers.

Christopher describes his journey in great detail at his website at www.christopher-sheppard.com.

Anne Frahm

At the age of 34 Anne Frahm found a tiny lump in her breast but, having been assured it was not malignant, she did nothing. By the time the cancer was diagnosed a year later, it had spread throughout her body. 'I will never forget seeing that light board with my skeleton displayed on it. It had tumours covering my body. The tumours covered my skull, my ribs and shoulders. Quarter-size holes had eaten through all my pelvic bones and the report showed that virtually every vertebra of my spine had tumours grown right through it. At that point, the doctor said that he thought he could keep me alive for a while. He told me straight out, "I can't cure you."'

Despite this she underwent a mastectomy, chemotherapy, radiation, hormone therapy and a bone marrow transplant. During this latter procedure she was in isolation for 52 days during which she very nearly died. 'My kidneys shut down, my lungs shut down, I got pneumonia, I was covered with fungus rashes from head to toe, my fingernails and toenails fell off. I was a wreck! [Then] toward the end of the 52 days, they did tests and came in and said they were very sorry but "it just didn't work for you". I found out that I had a lot of cancer still growing in my body so they basically sent me home to die.'

But Anne refused to give up. She decided to follow a strict nutrition plan (which I have described in Section 4: *Cancer Detox and Diet*) and five weeks later her astounded doctors could find no trace of the cancer at all.

Anne Frahm, with the help of her husband Dave, wrote her story up in a book called *The Cancer Battle Plan*.

Sadly, Anne did eventually die ten years later from cancer, but to live nearly ten years cancer-free after being given weeks to live is surely a great achievement.

Felicity Corbin-Wheeler

Felicity Corbin-Wheeler is a Reader in the Church of England and also has an international bible-based health ministry. She is also a Hippocrates Health Educator, Hallelujah Acres Health minister, and she teaches around the world. She is currently based in Portugal.

Her own cancer story started in September 2003 when she was diagnosed with untreatable pancreatic cancer. Having already lost a daughter to cancer, despite what she refers to as '"the best" of orthodox medicine' she began to research the importance of nutrition in cancer. The conclusion she came to was that a nutritional therapy should be firmly based on 'what God tells us to eat in Genesis 1:29 and 30'.

Although a diagnosis of pancreatic cancer is one of the worst diagnoses anyone can receive, she did not give up hope but put her faith in 'the living enzymes in the seeds that God tells us to eat … and the seed of the apricot has natural cancer cure qualities of hydrocyanic acid. This is also known as amygdalin or laetrile, which has been given vitamin B17 status because the seeds are vital for health.'

However, she found that she could not eat as many almonds as she felt she needed so she underwent 13 intravenous treatments in Jersey, Channel Islands, of laetrile (vitamin B17) under the direction of Dr Contreras of Oasis of Hope Christian Cancer Hospital in Mexico, with mega doses of vitamin C and DMSO (dimethyl sulphoxide) in the intravenous bag. She then continued to take B17 tablets for two years.

In addition, she also did the Gerson coffee enemas five times a day which she continues to do. 'I also went on a diet of living foods, fresh vegetable juices including wheat and barley grass and detoxed from animal protein, dairy, fats and flour.' Within four months of starting this regime, scans showed the tumours shrinking, and within a year all that was left was a scar. In a recent email to me she said this:

'Actually at [the age of] 70, I am fitter now than I have ever been! Yesterday I won the Christmas golf competition, and also the December Medals in my two different golf clubs here in Portugal, which is my daily source of vital oxygen, exercise, friendship, laughter (!) and sunlight …. In my opinion, the answer to *all* disease: cancer, diabetes, heart disease, arthritis, digestive disease, is in correcting acidity in the body and building the immune system. We are what we drink, eat, breathe and also think. The psychological and spiritual side of healing is also vital.'

Her story has been reported by the BBC (August 2004) and she has written the book *God's Healing Word*, which recounts her story. For further details go to www.felicitycorbinwheeler.org

Glynn Williams

In 1995, at the age of 28, Glynn Williams was diagnosed with Hodgkin's type Lymphoma. 'I went to see the doctor because of swelling on both sides of the groin area which came on within about a week …. I was totally exhausted, lethargic, did not have the energy to get up, had no appetite and was losing weight and I was having chills.'

He started taking Essiac tea (brand name Flor Essence)—two ounces in the morning before eating and two ounces at night. The swelling grew larger and then hardened up and the discomfort went away. By this time test results confirmed that he had advanced stage Hodgkin's. He was put on a course of 16 chemotherapy treatments but after experiencing severe side effects he quit the course of treatments after the fifth chemo. session. Throughout this treatment he had continued with the Essiac tea which he supplemented with vitamins and herbs, one 400 IU vitamin E, one 10,000 IU beta carotene, two ginseng, one shark cartilage, one 1,000 mg vitamin C, drops of liquid echinacea on the tongue every three hours, and then capsules of echinacea 380 mg. He also took a parasite elimination programme using black walnut tinctures, and wormwood capsules. He drank kombucha mushroom tea three times a day. Finally he did yoga with a strong focus on diaphragm breathing.

His doctors were amazed when he was eventually found to be cancer-free as five doses of chemo. was not considered curative. In December 2007, he confirmed that he was still cancer-free twelve years later.

Elonna McKibben

In 1989, having taken fertility treatment, Elonna found herself pregnant with quins. However, as the pregnancy progressed, Elonna began feeling deep-seated pains. It was eventually discovered, after the birth of her children, that the pains were not a side effect of her pregnancy—the exceptional nature of which had camouflaged the fact that she had a tumour on her spine.

This was diagnosed as stage 4 glioblastoma multiforme (GBM), a very rare and always fatal cancer. 'As mine was in the spinal cord,' Elonna wrote later, 'it made it even more rare, more aggressive and faster killing. I was told I would not survive long enough to see my children's first birthday.'

If that was not bad enough, the combined effect of the surgery and cancer had left her paralysed from the waist down. The doctors recommended radiation but were not hopeful that it would do more than delay the inevitable.

Fortunately, someone who read about her situation in the newspaper contacted her husband, Rob, and told him about CanCell. Elonna was naturally very sceptical: 'If there was a cure for cancer, don't you think they would be using it instead of letting thousands of people die.'

However, she started taking it on the basis that she had nothing to lose and everything to gain. Its effects were quickly obvious. 'I began to eliminate the cancer waste product about 18 hours after my first dose. It literally poured out of me: I threw it up; my bowel movements were extremely loose, stringy and frequent throughout the day; I lost it in my urine; my nose ran so much I had to keep a tissue with me at all times; I sweated it out profusely; I had hot/cold flashes and night sweats. When the nurses would give me a sponge bath after a night sweat, the water would be a golden brown colour with what they referred to as 'tapioca balls' floating in it.'

Despite these side-effects she persevered with the CanCell. After several weeks she found she was feeling much better. Christmas came and went and she started to do physical therapy to help her mobility. Then, in February 1990 she had scans to see what was happening. The radiologist was stunned to find no trace of the cancer. Despite being cancer-free, Elonna continued the CanCell treatment for a further two years. As of September 2011, Elonna McKibben is still alive, and her full story can be read on her website at www.elonnamckibben.com. She can be contacted through her protocol support group at www.elonnascorner.com

You can read more about CanCell in Section 6: *Cancer: Vitamins and Other Supplements*.

Mark Olsztyn

In March 1991, Mark experienced a major epileptic seizure which led to him being hospitalized. There, a CAT scan revealed a darkened area in the right frontal lobe of his brain. He was operated on and the tumour removed. It was found to be a low-grade astrocytoma. No further treatment was recommended, though frequent repeat scans would, he was told, be necessary.

Mark ignored this recommendation and for the next six years led a normal, hectic life. 'This was my denial phase,' he recalls. When eventually he did go for a scan in 1997, he was shocked to learn that the tumour had returned and was now stage 4. In addition to surgery he would require chemotherapy and radiation. He was also told by one of his doctors that he had better settle his affairs. But Mark insisted in thinking positively that a cure was possible.

He followed doctors' orders and underwent all these treatments even though he knew that at best they would be palliative. Fortunately, his father was a doctor of alternative medicine. 'My father immediately sent me a case of a foul-tasting liquid called PolyMVA which a colleague of his was using successfully on brain tumour patients. Because PolyMVA can be used as an adjunct to conventional therapy, I embraced it. I felt then that any nonconventional therapy that came my way, so long as it didn't interfere with what the doctors wanted me to do, was what God wanted me to do and would give me the edge that I needed to survive.

Among many other things, I became an ascetic, practiced Qi Gong, drank Essiac and Chinese herbs, joined various support groups, received acupuncture, ohmed and prayed and was prayed for, drank shark cartilage, ate macrobiotic, practiced visualization and, after four out of six rounds, quit chemotherapy. That last one was not what the doctors wanted me to do, however I felt I had enough poisoning. Over the years I gradually let go of each of the aforementioned life-saving practices except for PolyMVA and eating organic. Doctors now tell me to keep on doing whatever it is that I'm doing because it seems to be working.'

In August 2011, Mark is still very much alive and cancer-free. He can be contacted at mark.olsztyn@googlemail.com.

Shirley Lipschutz-Robinson

In 1982, doctors recommended a mastectomy on Shirley's left breast. She had suffered recurring cyst lumps which no medication could control. Up until this time Shirley was, as she calls herself, a prescription drug junkie—she was depressed, overweight and suffering from a seemingly endless parade of ailments—and the drugs seemed to only make matters worse. Her overall health was steadily declining.

But Shirley baulked at having her breast removed. She decided she needed to change her approach. She consulted a naturopathic/homoeopathic doctor who put her on a dietary regime—'a wholesome diet of fresh, organically grown fruits, vegetables, and nuts, mostly in their raw form'—supplemented with homoeopathic remedies. The results were, in her own words, 'dramatic'.

Within six weeks the lumps were gone. Within 12 weeks she had lost 60lbs. 'My energy level and stamina improved dramatically. I was able to function better overall. I became calmer, centred and focused, and generally I felt happier. My overall resistance to infections became excellent.'

In the 1990s, she experienced a lump the size of a pea in her left nipple. It grew to be the size of a small grape. She refused to see the doctor, instead self-treating it with extra flaxseed oil, herbal extracts and homoeopathy. Within two weeks her body had reabsorbed the lump and it never came back.

These experiences sparked her to study a wide range of alternative therapies. Her full story, and the story of how she treated her husband through a series of heart attacks, is told on her excellent website: www.shirleys-wellness-cafe.com. This website is a storehouse of useful information.

Pattie McDonald

In May 2002, Pattie, 58, was diagnosed with breast cancer 'the size of a quarter'. She believes now that contributing factors included being on HRT (Premarin) for six years, long-term antibiotic use and a very poor diet ('I was a fast food freak') coupled with a negative outlook on life. Her doctors recommended surgery and radiation.

However, Pattie had a close and trusted friend who had survived ovarian cancer by using bloodroot. She used both bloodroot paste and tonic. The effects of the bloodroot quickly revealed that the cancer had already spread to the neck and three lymph nodes.

The Cansema bloodroot paste was applied to the biopsy site on her breast. It took ten days to expel the tumour from her body. As the neck tumours also began to be expelled, Pattie took the tonic and applied paste against the neck. The whole process of treatment took about a month. She experienced excruciating pain and two days of no sleep. (She later found out you should take pain killers.)

In August 2002 she had an MRI scan that confirmed she was cancer-free, and four years later she has remained cancer-free.

'This experience changed my entire life—body, soul and spirit. I am a new woman. I changed my diet, quit my stressful job, sold my too-big house, rid myself of all negative friends, and divorced my alcoholic hubby. I had no idea what real happiness was until 2002.'

Pattie can be contacted at pjmacblondie@yahoo.com.

Bob Davis

In April 1996, Bob Davis discovered he had a massive cancer tumour—a foot wide and several inches thick—in his abdomen and several other tumours in his chest, some 'the size of soft balls'. The cancer had also spread to his bone marrow.

He was immediately started on a very heavy chemotherapy program over the next three months. This had very little effect: 'It [the tumour] seemed to thrive on the stuff.'

The doctor told him that the chemo. wasn't working. 'He later told me that another treatment would kill me. I knew that this was true because my body was ravaged by the chemo. I was curled up in a foetal position unable to sleep or eat. I was emaciated and had excruciating pain all through my body.'

At this time he received a call from a woman who had been selling his wife pills made of dried green barley leaves for her arthritis. During the conversation he mentioned his fight with cancer. 'Don't you know that cancer and arthritis can't grow in an alkaline body?' she said. The same barley leaves that his wife was taking for her arthritis would, she told him, also help in his fight against cancer. He started taking the pills—20 tablets of dried barley green (340mg each)—and 'in ten days my cancer was 95 per cent gone!' A number of tests including a CAT scan showed that scar tissue remained but the cancer had been killed. 'I was incredibly lucky. I know most people wouldn't be cured so simply. In fact I only know one other person who had the same response.'

A few years later, even though he had maintained his intake of dried barley leaves, Bob was diagnosed with a probable prostate cancer on the basis of a lump and high PSA levels. Resisting pressure to have surgery, Bob went on the Dr Shulze's Incurable's programme—involving juice fasting and colon cleansing. Three weeks later he demanded a PSA re-test. His PSA levels were now normal.

In 2011 he was still cancer-free. He still takes 20 tablets of dried green barley every day. 'It costs me a whopping 95 cents or so.' He has adopted a 95 per cent vegan diet 'I really like it. I feel better than I have in 40 years. People say I look younger. I have "lotsa" energy.'

Bob Davis, now aged 90, can be contacted through his website at www.cancer-success.com.

'Rompin' Ronnie Hawkins

Ronnie Hawkins is a famous Canadian rockabilly musician, reportedly one of Bill Clinton's favourites. In 2002 he was diagnosed with pancreatic cancer and given no hope of recovery. When the news was announced that he had only three or four months left to live, a film director by the name of Anne Pick started documenting the last days of his life. There was a tearful tribute concert in Toronto to bid farewell to 'The Hawk'.

But Hawkins didn't lie down and die. Instead he went on a regimen of nutritional supplements and pot. Seventeen months later, a gifted, 17-year-old named Adam McLeod, heard of Hawkins plight and offered his services. Adam was what he calls a Medical Intuitive Healer. Hawkins accepted the offer. A short time later Hawkins reported for his regular check-up and the doctors were stunned to discover that his tumour had completely disappeared.

This caused problems for the film makers documenting his last months (already they must have been a little irritated that he was taking so long dying!). They solved the problem by changing the film's title to *Ronnie Hawkins. Still Alive and Kickin'*.

Hawkins attributes his recovery to the psychic healer Adam. Ten years later Hawkins is still alive.

The healer Adam McLeod has since written a number of books and is a figure of controversy in Canada. He uses the professional name of Adam Dreamhealer.

Bruce Guilmette

In November 2004, Bruce discovered that both his kidneys had large cancerous masses inside them. Kidney cancer is known to be highly resistant to treatment and he was given only a matter of months to live unless he had both kidneys removed. Bruce refused this option, turned to a combination of diet, supplements and the use of a Rife machine. Bruce's research led him to the conclusion that cancer needs to be attacked from many different angles to be successfully put into remission. He eventually put together a complex regimen which he followed rigorously. Much of his food intake is in the form of juiced fresh vegetables. He reduced his meat consumption to no more than ten percent of his total intake and eliminated pork altogether.

Bruce died in November 2007—but he did not die of cancer. At the time of his death his regular blood tests all confirmed that the cancer was no longer active. His full story is told at www.survivecancerfoundation.org.

Ian Gawler

In 1975, Ian Gawler, a 24-year old Australian veterinarian, was diagnosed with bone cancer. He underwent surgery and had his right leg amputated. He was told that he had only a five per cent chance of surviving for five years and that if the tumours returned he would only have a few months. The cancer did return later that year.

Deciding to take a proactive approach, Ian went to the Philippines with his wife, and received treatment from several folk healers (psychic surgeons). On his return to Australia, he decided to follow a diet, take up meditation and explore a wide range of natural therapies, He believed the secret lay in stimulating the immune system and to letting go of stress and anxiety.

He won his battle and the cancer went away. To this day he remains healthy and cancer-free. He wrote a book, *You Can Conquer Cancer*, and set up The Gawler Foundation, based in Melbourne, to provide cancer support programs for anyone seeking to follow the alternative path.

He attributes his success to the fact that he took responsibility for his condition and recognized that he had been responsible for causing it. By taking responsibility, he felt in control and believed that he had the power to reverse it.

In an interview with the journalist Beryl Rule he said: 'Psychologically, the big need is to change. If we recognize that a particular pattern has aided in creating the disease, then obviously a new pattern is required …. The disease creates the excuse for change. It produces a new situation or insight that allows the patient the space to change their rigid patterns.' For more information go to www.gawler.org.

Fred Eichhorn

In 1976, Fred was found to have islet cell carcinoma, and was given a maximum life expectancy of three years though most of the doctors he consulted believed he would be dead within a year. He underwent surgery in which 90 percent of his pancreas was removed along with his spleen and part of his stomach. However, this was not expected to provide a cure. Fred decided to define the problem. He felt that in every case ill health follows like a domino effect from a first cause. The solution is to find that first cause in terms of the body's biochemistry and correct it. Then a good domino effect will result in the elimination of the disease.

He decided good nutrition—a return to pre-1900s standards (i.e., completely organic)—along with exercise and a positive mental framework, were the key cornerstones of good health.

In 1980 Fred enrolled in medical college and studied for four years followed by a further three years research.

Fred Eichhorn is cancer-free today 30 years later and so committed is he to spreading the word that he has set up the National Cancer Research Foundation (www.ncrf.org). He provides a number of testimonials on his site of people who have benefited from following his regime. For further information contact fred@ncrf.org.

June Black

June Black was first diagnosed with cancer (stage 1) in November 2000. She eventually had a mastectomy but no radiation or chemotherapy. She was put on tamoxifen but reacted badly to it and 'threw it down the toilet'. In 2005, June noticed a lump growing on the mastectomy scar and had it biopsied. The tests came back positive. The cancer had returned. She underwent two further operations but it was clear the cancer had spread. By this time she had read a lot of books and had come round to the natural approach to treating cancer. So, when her third oncologist (she had dumped two) told her: 'I recommend the whole gamut; chemo., radiation and adjuvant hormone therapy.' She found the courage to refuse, saying: 'I am sixty years old, I have lived a good life, and I have other plans.'

But at first the natural path did not appear to be doing her any good. 'After spending a month of a very strict diet and enough vitamins and supplements to fill a small shop, I realized I was losing the war against this cancer. I was losing weight, I had sweats, I was really weak and it was so bad that I thought death would be a wonderful alternative to the hell I was going through.'

Then someone suggested the supplement PolyMVA. She went on it and within four days felt better. This was in October 2005. In June 2006 she had a full array of tests and they all came back clear. She was cancer-free.

Her regime was eight teaspoons of PolyMVA a day for six 1/2 months. She then went to six teaspoons a day for about two months and since then has been taking four teaspoons a day. She also takes CoQ10, artemisinin, pancreatic enzymes and IP6 (inositol hexakisphosphate).

'This is just the tip of the iceberg of what I am taking. I also take different mushrooms, EpiCor, Lugol's iodine, DIM (diindolylmethane), and calcium-D-glucarate. If anyone is interested in my complete list please feel free to contact me at june1@mesquiteweb.com. I just had my 62nd birthday March 1, 2007 in Hawaii and gained more weight and feel fantastic. As of now, no signs of illness. I have excellent health and work full time and care for 11 cats.'

June's story is one of many testimonials that can be found at www.polymvasurvivors.com.

Percy Weston

Percy Weston was an Australian farmer who, despite being diagnosed with terminal cancer in his late thirties, went on to live till he was 100.

His story is a remarkable one. At school his favourite subject was chemistry, a fact that was to stand him in good stead when as a farmer he began to wonder why his sheep were going down with an arthritic condition affecting their knees, and manifesting cancerous lesions on their ears. Plants grown in the soil which had been heavily treated with superphosphate fertilizer also exhibited strange mutations. Thinking it through he wondered if the superphosphate fertilizer that he had been using for the previous five years was the cause. He moved the sheep onto pasture which had not been treated with superphosphates and fed them the mineral salts that the superphosphates had leached from the land. They recovered. He moved some of them back onto the treated paddock and they developed the same problems again. He moved them off it and again they recovered.

Sometime later Weston himself was afflicted with arthritis and a cancerous tumour which developed on his hand. Remembering his experiences with the sheep, Weston decided to reduce his own intake of phosphorus and started taking in minerals—particularly magnesium and potassium. The arthritis went away and the cancer tumour dried up and finally broke away from his hand.

Later he treated his wife with the same low phosphate diet and mineral supplements when she had been diagnosed with cancer of the uterus. The top gynaecologist in their state (Victoria, Australia) had advised an immediate hysterectomy. Her cancer too disappeared and she went on to have two healthy children. The specialist, when he was told of these events, commented that he had never known a woman in the condition Mrs Weston had been in when he had examined her to survive for twelve months, let alone have children.

Percy wrote his story in his book *Cancer: Cause and Cure* and has also written a book entitled *Cancer Fighting Foods*. The mineral supplements that he used can also be bought from various online suppliers.

Cliff Beckwith

Cliff Beckwith was a retired educationalist living near Knoxville, Tennessee. He was one of the founders of the Yahoo health groups information resource on flaxseed oil: http://health.groups.yahoo.com/group/FlaxSeedOil2/files (requires Yahoo Groups membership).

Here he tells his own story.

'In January 1991 I was diagnosed with advanced prostate cancer. Bone scans and other tests indicated no spread so it was decided to operate. During the operation it was discovered that the cancer had spread to the lymph glands making it stage 4. The operation was not completed as that would not be the answer. The only treatment used was Lupron (leuprolide) and Eulexin (flutamide) to cancel the male hormones. I was told the male hormone does not cause cancer, but if cancer is present, it is like throwing kerosene on a fire.

At the time of the attempted operation my PSA count was 75. It was six months before I had the second PSA. When the call came from the doctor's office I was told 'Mr. Beckwith! Your count is completely normal!' It was 0.1 and 0.1 to 0.4 is normal.

The reason it was normal was because, in addition to the hormone drugs, I had started taking flaxseed oil mixed with cottage cheese. I had read a number of books recommending this approach, which was first formulated by Dr Johanna Budwig and is commonly known as the Budwig protocol.

I quit Lupron after four years and seven months in October of 1995 as it was no longer useful. I thought I was cured but not so. In roughly two years the PSA was again rising. I began changing the amounts I took of flaxseed oil/cottage cheese which led to a series of ups and downs with the PSA results.

I learned that there are 30 strains of prostate cancer. They are all different and any man may have any combination of strains. This makes the problem different from individual to individual. Mine is a medium aggressive cancer.

In January 2004 my PSA was 6.7 which is very close to normal for a man of 85. I thought I had it beaten. It had now been 13 years since diagnosis. Most men with advanced prostate cancer do not live nearly that long. The doctor told me after a couple of years that I was one of the lucky ones. Most men with the condition I had did not make it six months.

In Jan 2004, I decided to try ellagic acid, which has proved effective in many cases. However, my PSA went up instead of further down. Then I added lycopene. I had been told that it needed to be used heavily to be effective; three 12 ounce glasses of tomato juice a day. I did that for four months.

Then I learned two things a couple of days apart. One was that Dr Budwig had said in 1956 that if one is using flaxseed oil one must not use heavy amounts of antioxidants, as it would neutralize the effect of the flaxseed oil. The other was that both ellagic acid and lycopene are powerful antioxidants.

For over a year I was hurting the effect of the flaxseed oil/cottage cheese and for four months I was cancelling it completely.

The result was that the cancer again began to develop and by the time I woke up to this fact, the PSA had gone to 131.

I know that cancer in the prostate does not kill. What kills is the cancer in the tissues to which it spreads. Flaxseed oil pretty much stops the spread. Until I went the antioxidant route it hadn't spread in 13 years. Now there are signs it has spread to the bone.

So I immediately increased the flaxseed oil to six tablespoons a day and am using my rebounder (small trampoline). The result appears to be beneficial. I had been aware of an enlargement in the prostate gland and now it is getting smaller and urination is easier. I do not believe I am in danger anymore.' (February 2006)

Cliff Beckwith died from his cancer, aged 85, in late 2007.

Chris Wark

Chris Wark's story in his own words:

It was 2003. I was having some abdominal pain on and off for the better part of the year, and being the typical male, I put it off. I was thinking it might be an ulcer and that it would get better, but it didn't. It was like Groundhog Day. Every morning I would wake up feeling good, but several times a day I would get these brief flashes of pain in the afternoon and evening. Sometimes in the middle of the night. It wasn't a constant pain and didn't interfere with my life, but I was concerned. The next morning I would wake up feeling good again. Eventually the pain became so intense that I found myself balled up on the couch every night after dinner. Time to see a doctor.

After a series of inconclusive tests, I was sent to a gastroenterologist for a colonoscopy. Turns out there was a golf ball-sized tumour in my large intestine. Great. They did a biopsy and told me I had colon cancer. It was two weeks before Christmas and I was 26 years old.

I was in shock. I couldn't believe this was my life. How did I end up with an old person's disease? I felt weak and pathetic. I was embarrassed and I shut down mentally and emotionally.

Three weeks later, on New Year's Eve, I had surgery. They removed the tumour and a third of my colon. More good news, the cancer had spread to my lymph nodes. It was stage 3. They brought an oncologist into my room and he informed me that I would need nine months of chemotherapy after I recovered from surgery.

The first meal they served me in the hospital after removing a third of my large intestine was a sloppy joe. I was starving. I hadn't eaten in three days, but I couldn't get down more than a few bites. I was relatively clueless about nutrition, but I knew that a sloppy joe was the last thing my body needed.

Before I checked out of the hospital I asked the surgeon, 'Are there any foods I need to avoid?' He said, 'Nah, just don't lift anything heavier than a beer.' Not the advice I was expecting.

When we got home, my wife and I prayed and asked God that if there was another way besides chemotherapy that He would reveal it to us. Two days later, a book arrived on my doorstep, sent to me from a man in Alaska who I'd never met. He was a business acquaintance of my father's.

That book was called *God's Way to Ultimate Health* by George Malkmus, and it detailed how he beat colon cancer nearly 30 years earlier using natural methods including the raw vegan diet and juicing, and without surgery or chemotherapy. I knew it was an answer to prayer. I realized that my diet of processed food, fast food, junk food, and factory farmed animal products was killing me.

I started to do more research on the harmful nature of cancer therapies. I discovered that chemotherapy destroyed your immune system and killed healthy cells; that it could make me infertile. And that it caused secondary cancers. That was when I decided against chemotherapy.

This decision was not well received by my wife and many family members. After intense family pressure I agreed to meet with an oncologist to hear what he had to say. He told me I had a 60 per cent chance of living five years with conventional therapies. To me that wasn't much better than a coin toss. I asked him about alternative therapies. He looked me dead in the eye and said, 'There are none. If you don't do chemo, you are insane. And I'm not saying this because I need your business.' My wife and I left the clinic terrified. We sat in the car, held hands, cried and prayed.

I knew I wasn't taking care of myself and that there were massive changes I could make to my diet and lifestyle. I decided to take control of my health, and if that didn't work, chemo would be my last resort. I radically changed my diet to 100 per cent raw vegan, eating only fruits and vegetables, and drank eight glasses of vegetable juice every day. I did every alternative holistic therapy I could find including: fasting, vitamin C IVs, rebounding, natural immune boosting and detox supplements, herbal teas, acupuncture, structural integration, hydrotherapy, saunas, and more.

I found a local naturopath who was a tremendous ally and guided me along my health journey, and I continued to research, reading all the information I could find about natural cancer therapies. Within one year of my diagnosis I was cancer free.

Now in 2011, eight years later, my wife and I have two beautiful daughters aged 3 and 6, and I am still cancer free. As I write this I am reminded of how good God is; how much He loves us and cares for us. I put my trust in Him, not in modern medicine. He led me in the path of healing and He will lead you too if you let Him.

Psalm 34.4: 'I sought the Lord and He answered me, and delivered me from all my fears.'

Chris Wark, Memphis, TN: www.chrisbeatcancer.com

Polly Noble

This is Polly's story in her own words.

I was 24, living the 'citygirl' life in London working as a personal assistant to the vice president of Sony Playstation. From the outside looking in, I appeared to have a pretty good life. I had a good job, a lovely boyfriend, a nice house—but it wasn't enough, I still wasn't happy. I always felt a bit lost and at that time I was fed up and constantly felt that 'there had to be more' to life. I just felt like something was missing. In the back of my mind, I hoped that one day I would just wake up and know what I wanted to do and how I could make my life meaningful. I had a very strong desire to know my real self and the difference I could make in the world. I had no clue that my purpose would involve me being diagnosed with cancer aged 24.

I had been feeling a bit run down, seemed to be sleeping from 8pm in the evening straight through to 8am the following morning, was suffering with some backache and had put on a few pounds. I put the weight gain down to being out on the party circuit a little too much and it was only at a check up with my gynaecologist that it became apparent that something wasn't right. In fact it was something quite scary and sinister. After more tests, I was told that I had a 3cm tumour on my cervix which had spread to several infected malignant lymph nodes in and around my pelvis. I had already mentally prepared myself for the worst and my reaction to being told I had cancer was simply, 'Okay, what do we do now? Let's get on and deal with it.' Obviously on some level I was upset but it felt natural for me to take a pragmatic approach and I refused to throw myself a pity party. That's just the kind of person I am—I was strong for everyone else to make it easier for them to deal with. Falling apart at the seams was going to be unhelpful for everyone. At the time I didn't see the point in getting upset about it, I was just keen to 'get it dealt with'. So within a week or two of my diagnosis I was rushed into hospital for keyhole surgery to remove as many of the infected lymph nodes they could reach followed by six weeks of simultaneous chemotherapy and radiotherapy, followed by what was at the time, a pioneering treatment known as brachytherapy.

During chemo. and radiotherapy I had very little appetite and shrunk to an unhealthy-looking size six, with sullen cheek bones and huge black circles under my eyes. I was exhausted, weak and grew weary of the constant prodding and poking from doctors plying me with drugs. The whole experience made me feel very disempowered and consequently I spent the majority of my day either asleep or bent over worshipping the porcelain god!

I wasn't given any information on how I could help myself or what I could do to lessen the side-effects I was experiencing so I began to conduct my own research as to what I could do. I began juicing fruits and vegetables and began eating more living foods in the form of salads. I grew up in a household where a piece of fish or meat would hold centre stage with the vegetables making a small token appearance, but gradually I began to educate myself of how I could best support my body and boost my immune system to help keep me well. Up until that point, I had never really made the connection between the foods I was eating and my level of health. Of course I knew I needed to get my 'five-a-day' but I didn't realise just how important they were or the detrimental effect some of the other everyday foods I was eating like meat, bread, sugar, cheese and alcohol were having on my body. I had always considered myself 'healthy' but soon came to realise that my idea of healthy was very different from true health.

Soon after I finished my treatment, I developed lymphoedema in my right leg making it swell to twice the size of my left leg which was unsightly, painful and almost impossible to walk on. I was told there wasn't much that I could do and that I would have to 'learn to live with it'. I told the lymphoedema nurse that that was unacceptable and took it upon myself to heal it. (I'm sure she thought I was a pompous Madam but I was 24 and I wanted a normal leg thank you very much!)

I researched and did everything I could; I had manual lymphatic drainage once a week, wore lymphoedema stockings, dry skin brushed, drank fresh juices made from anti-inflammatory foods and visualised on a daily basis that my leg had returned to its normal size. Approximately three months later, my leg was back to normal and walking on it wasn't a problem. The lymphoedema nurse would always be surprised how much it had reduced each time she measured it and would ask me what I had been doing!

On agreeing to subject my body to such harsh treatment in the form of chemo. and radiotherapy, I was made aware that there was a possibility of developing severe side-effects. Some were worse than others and thankfully it would appear I have come away fairly unscathed in the grand scheme of things. But I have suffered some nerve damage in my fingers and to this day still have problems with them. When I get cold or when I touch something cold, even for just a split second, the tips of my fingers go numb and they turn white. Eventually, the blood comes flows back to them but it can be quite painful, especially in winter. And then of course, having had such severe treatment I was told that I have been left infertile. Despite still having my reproductive organs, the treatment has had an extremely negative effect on my monthly cycle which I am currently working on getting to function once again using alternative methods.

I was also left with a compromised immune system, which left me vulnerable to contracting severe pneumonia twice in as many years. During my second stay in hospital for pneumonia in December 2009, I found a lump near my collar bone which turned out to be the cervical cancer that had metastasized to my lymph nodes around my neck. As the cancer was systemic throughout my lymph system, I was told that the cancer was now deemed 'incurable'.

I was offered surgery and radiotherapy which I was told may not make any difference to helping to cure me and having experienced awful side effects from it previously, decided it was now my opportunity to do it my way and so I politely declined.

I had read a lot about health and healing in the years between my two diagnoses, and had come to the conclusion that if the body had created something then it should be able to 'un-create' it. I had tried the conventional route and the cancer came back, so I decided now was my opportunity to explore an alternative path to healing. I began researching how to support my body and the things I could do to 'switch on' my body's healing mechanism, which has led to the most amazing journey of my life.

I converted to a plant-based raw food diet overnight, with plenty of fresh juices, meditation, visualisation and yoga making the foundations of my healing plan. I made it my full-time job to create a sacred space to aid healing on a physical, mental, emotional and spiritual level. This is my journey and it is no coincidence that I feel happier and healthier than ever before.

Three months after embarking on my healing journey, a scan showed that the cancer had reduced by 1mm although my oncologist was reticent to admit this could be down to my approach, instead suggesting that the scan may have been measured inaccurately. A scan four months later showed a little growth and although I felt some disappointment realised that cancer has been in my body for at least ten years and that it is going to take time to heal completely. I don't put a lot of emphasis on scans as I don't believe that a lump is a clear indication of my level of internal health. The lump is a mere manifestation of a problem that I am working on resolving, but just because the lump is still there doesn't mean that healing isn't already taking place on a cellular level.

I decided to take a break from having scans for a while seeing as they have to inject glucose into my blood to measure the cancer in my body which in effect promotes the cancer's growth! It all just seemed a bit counter-productive. So now, I have my blood tests and I am told they 'look good'. I don't take too much notice of tests because I feel well and I know that I am doing everything I can to aid my healing.

I certainly don't intend to have cancer forever, but I do intend to live my life with health and happiness. I commit every day to being an active participant in my health and give my body the best possible environment in which to create health by eating, drinking and thinking consciously.

We so often feel like a passenger on a runaway cancer train and I want to use my journey to empower others to take back the reins on their health and live consciously. Some foods will actually promote the cancer to grow, some will promote the cancer cells to spontaneously commit suicide, and knowing what these foods are and how to boost your immune system are crucial not only to your health but to feeling empowered and in control of your own experience.

I am passionate about helping others to help themselves get healthy and prevent a 'health crisis' before it's too late.

I now work as an holistic health coach and raw food coach, educating others on how to adopt an anti-inflammatory, alkaline diet. I work with people one-on-one, in groups, hold talks, workshops and retreats as well as provide stacks of free health information via my website www.pollynoble.com. I am also being filmed for a documentary due out in 2012 which is following my healing journey.

I have co-authored a book called *The Cancer Journey* to help navigate people through what can be an extremely frightening experience. It's the go-to handbook for anyone affected by cancer, and deals with everything from diagnosis to diet to self-help techniques, to dealing with friends and family.

Ruth Heidrich

Known as the 'other Dr Ruth', Ruth Heidrich is a six-time Ironman Triathlon finisher, has held age-group records in distances from 100-metre dashes to ultramarathons, pentathlons, and triathlons. She has completed 67 marathons including Boston, New York, Moscow, Honolulu, has held three world fitness records at the famed Cooper Clinic in Dallas, Texas, named one of the 'Ten Fittest Women in North America.' A graduate of UCLA, she holds a Master's degree in Psychology, and a doctorate in Health Education. She has also lectured in this field at the University of Hawaii, Stanford University, and Cornell University. Author of *Senior Fitness*, *A Race For Life*, *The CHEF Cook/Rawbook*, she has an 'Ask Dr Ruth' column on her website, www.ruthheidrich.com. Here is her story in her own words.

I was 47 years old and believed I was as healthy as I could possibly be! Talk about being positive, I thought I had it all! My career was taking off, my kids were successfully launched, and I loved all the travel that my job provided. I'd studied nutrition in college and ate what I was told was a very healthy diet, lots of chicken and fish and low-fat dairy. I was in the best physical shape of my life except for a little arthritis which I was told everybody gets by the time they're 30. I'd starting daily running at the age of 33 and found I loved it! So, at this time, I'd been a runner for 14 years and had even run a bunch of marathons.

What I didn't know was that my life was about to be dumped upside down. While in the shower that morning, I found a lump in my breast. I got right in to see a doctor, but he just remarked, 'Oh, you're too young for breast cancer.' He did, however, order a mammogram, 'just to be sure', he said. The results were negative—a false negative as it turned out—because of my dense breasts, it didn't pick up any abnormality. I was told to come back for yearly checks. The next year, the same result. The third year, however, the lump was now golf-ball sized and very visible! The doctor looked shocked and ordered an immediate biopsy. The diagnosis: infiltrating ductal cancer, an invasive cancer that had already spread, indicated by 'hot spots' in my bones, a lung tumour, and elevated liver enzymes!

I was so stunned and disbelieving that I got second, third and even fourth opinions. Each doctor confirmed the findings, and as for my prognosis, none could tell me whether I had three months, three years or what, just that it was 'not good.' They all recommended the standard chemo., radiation and tamoxifen. I could not believe my body betrayed me in such a manner! I was doing everything I was told were all the right things to be healthy.

I was slated for chemotherapy but dreaded going down that path—but terrified not to. I started searching for alternatives, any kind of help, anything—I did not want to die! That was when I found a tiny three-line newspaper item, 'Wanted, women with breast cancer to participate in cancer/diet research study.' I was sure that my 'healthy' diet (and I'd been told by the oncologist that my diet had nothing to do with my breast cancer), so I thought this would help prove it one way or the other. I ran to the phone and was put right through to Dr John McDougall. I was so shocked to get him in person that I was sputtering, trying to tell him that I'd just been diagnosed with breast cancer. He said, 'Get your medical records and come down to my office right away.'

After I got there, he was looking over my lab results. 'Hmmm,' he said. 'What now?' I was thinking. Another shock when he said, 'You know, with cholesterol of 236, you are at as high a risk of dying of a heart attack as you are the cancer.'

I was literally stunned by the deception of my body and what was happening—cancer, arthritis, and, now, heart disease? I was a marathoner, for goodness sake! These things don't happen to people like me! What is going on? Dr McDougall said, 'Don't worry, all of this can be reversed and avoided. Change your diet, and you'll lower your cholesterol, lower your risk of heart disease, and reverse the cancer. And, in order to show that it's the diet that's responsible for these changes, you must not have any chemo. or radiation.' Wait a minute, I thought, undergo chemo. and radiation *or* change my diet? If Dr McDougall is right, and I saw the research that supported his claim, I'd be crazy not to go with the diet! 'OK, what do I do?' Dr McDougall said: 'It's very simple—eliminate all animal foods and oils from your diet. Your diet will consist of plant foods: fruits, vegetables, whole grains and legumes.'

No 'transitioning' for me—in less than two hours, I was vegan! I found the diet amazingly easy to follow. I already loved brown rice, whole grain breads and oatmeal; I just had to replace the chicken, fish and dairy with vegetables and fruit, and throw out all the oils.

My body responded immediately. The next morning I discovered I'd been constipated all my life but never knew it. I now know what 'normal' is, thank goodness!

When I returned to the oncologist, I told him what I was doing. He responded by saying that diet had nothing to do with my getting breast cancer and I couldn't possibly get enough protein, calcium, and essential fatty acids. I made a mental note to check that out with Dr McDougall. In addition to the hot spots in my bones, I was having serious bone pain that medication could not relieve. A month later, those hot spots had significantly receded, and within three months, they were gone, as was the bone pain. The chest X-rays, however, to this day, still show an encapsulated tumour in my left lung. It hasn't grown in 29 years, and my liver enzymes are now normal.

The oncologist had no explanation for the findings and told me further that my new diet couldn't have any effect on the cancer, and that I was taking a risk in continuing to refuse chemo., radiation, and tamoxifen. Back to Dr McDougall I went! I was reassured when he again showed me the dismal results of chemo. and radiation plus data indicating I'd get plenty of all the needed nutrients.

It was during all this turmoil that I happened to see the Ironman Triathlon on TV. I was awe-struck and thought, 'I've *got* to do that!' I saw the 2.4-mile swim, the 112-mile bike, and then the 26-mile marathon. I knew I could handle the marathon and thought just adding swimming and biking would be a piece of cake! Then it hit me, I've got *cancer* and, besides, looking at all the young bodies, at 47 I'm way too old to do this. I then realized what an opportunity I was being given: diet *does* affect cancer and I can show people that you can do one of the toughest races in the world on a vegan diet and, at a relatively advanced age to boot! I got excited at the possibilities and joined two running clubs, got a swim coach, took a bicycle repair course, and was obsessed with training in all three sports. Training daily, I could see amazing progress in my speed and endurance. What's more, I was enjoying my workouts, gaining confidence that I could attain one of the most ambitious goals I'd ever set for myself—to be an 'Ironman'!

I did have to dig deep, however, as I was challenged like I'd never been before! Crossing that finish line of my first Ironman, I experienced indescribable feelings—a mix of joy, empowerment, exhilaration, and total fatigue! I could not have gone another step!

Since my diagnosis in 1982, I have completed the Ironman six times, run 67 marathons, have won nearly 1,000 gold medals including eight gold medals in the Senior Olympics, won the title of 'One of the Ten Fittest Women in North America,' and have a fitness age of 32, although chronologically, I am 76.

Because of the history of osteoporosis on both sides of my family, I tracked my bone density and found significant increases with each test. I was obviously getting enough calcium on this diet. I was also very pleasantly surprised to discover that my arthritis disappeared and I could stop taking Naprosyn, (Aleve, or naproxen), the drug prescribed for my arthritis that I was told I would need to take the rest of my life. My joints today not only are not arthritic, but I actually do my own little daily triathlon as part of my regular training! How about that? A 76-year-old triathlete! I never thought my life could take such a positive turn and am thankful that I found out, in time, the dramatic impact diet has on our health!

Regarding the rationale for avoiding any kind of oil, the healthiest foods are whole foods with little or no refinement or processing. Taking a whole food like corn, olives, etc. and extracting and concentrating the natural oils from them, represent the extreme in processing, leaving 100 per cent calories from fat and is certainly not helping in the battle of epidemic obesity in this country. As for the touted omega 3s in fish oils, it's far better to get them from the source. Fish do not make omega 3s; they get them from the sea greens, and we can do the same, either from sea greens or any of the many other sources such as leafy greens, walnuts, and flax seeds.

We also know that a low-fat (ten per cent calories from fat) diet lowers our risk of heart disease, most cancers but especially breast cancer, stroke, diabetes, and many other of the common Western afflictions. The substantiating citations for all this is in my book, *Senior Fitness*. Here's what I now eat.

Breakfast

Served in a large bowl, lots of greens for the base: mixed organic greens, 1 stalk kale, 10 or so sprigs of parsley or cilantro, half a mango, 1 large banana, and half dozen large, seeded globe grapes. Top off with 1 rounded tablespoon of B12-fortified nutritional yeast, and 1–2 tablespoons of blackstrap molasses.

Because I eat this after my daily workout, this is served late and I eat no midday meal.

Supper

Lots more greens for the base: mixed organic greens, 3–4 broccoli florettes, 1 stalk of kale, 1 stalk of celery, a quarter head of green or red cabbage, 1 large carrot, half a red (or orange, green, or yellow) bell pepper, half a large field tomato, half a sliced yam or sweet potato, raw. On top of this, add to taste, prepared salsa (mild, medium or hot), 1 tablespoon of regular mustard, 1 tablespoon of flax seed, freshly ground, a general sprinkle of curry powder, and lots of freshly ground black pepper.

Dessert

A base of blueberries (fresh or frozen, depending on availability and season)—usually 1 cup, plus about 8–9 prunes, topped with a handful of walnuts, and a liberal sprinkle of ground cinnamon.

Snacks

For those times when the hunger pangs strike, I eat carrot or celery sticks, grapes, dates, and in the evening, plain air-popped popcorn.

You'll see that my diet consists mainly of raw foods. Raw is better than cooking as cooking does reduce the vitamin content of the food but this is not absolutely essential—the essential thing is to cut out the oils and to go to a plant based diet. For me it is just more convenient to eat the foods raw—and actually I prefer it.

Ian Clements

I first met Ian when he contacted me having read my cancer books and discovered that we lived in the same town. Here is his story in his own words.

My professional background: I am by profession an electronics engineer and worked in Germany and Holland before training to be a college lecturer. I have degrees in electronics, industrial design, and research to PhD level in education, so I am very capable of reading and evaluating research papers. I worked latterly as a lecturer in further and higher education, ending my academic career as assistant principal in charge of technology. This is the story of my ongoing battle with cancer. I don't believe that you ever can say that you have cured your cancer but I am currently, as best as I can tell, cancer-free.

I first became aware of general health issues in 1966 when I noticed that I had the start of a pot belly. I started to take an interest in the subject and from then on I became increasingly knowledgeable on health issues and implemented them. One thing I have learnt over the years is that not everything you read is true and, in a number of cases, things I once believed to be true turned out later to be 180 degrees wrong, and I will admit that I have done several reversals over the years. Being a scientist, I tend to follow reported research—it is not possible to do all the research oneself.

Nevertheless, I seemed to be fit and healthy—jogging regularly, eating mainly good nutrition, not drinking too much, and I stopped smoking more than 30 years ago. I thus seemed on course to live at least to 100, and perhaps more. In fact I was just about to sit down to write a book called—rather hubristically—'How to live to 150 years', when I was diagnosed with cancer.

In October 2007, I had some tests which revealed I had cancer and this quickly led to the surgical removal of a tumour from my bladder. Unfortunately, further tests resulted and I was told that I had metastatic terminal bladder cancer. I was informed by the urologist, and by the next two oncologists that I consulted for second (and third!) opinions, that I had only weeks to live, maybe a year at most (so my expected death-by-date was October 2008; it is now, as I write this, summer 2011).

I was told by these specialists that there was nothing orthodox medicine could do—additional surgery was not possible; radiation was no use (as I was metastatic); chemotherapy would only be palliative and make my life miserable, and would not result in sufficient extra time to make it worthwhile.

This diagnosis traumatised me—I am terrified of death. Over the next few weeks I would find myself curling up on the floor, crying, trembling, terrified. I didn't know it at the time, but my wife was similarly affected; and my eldest son nearly quit his degree.

Luckily, I had recently been reading up on CAM approaches to cancer and emailing one of the CAM experts (Dr Peskin, *The Hidden Story of Cancer*), who then put me on to the nutritionist, Dr Bernado Majalca. Majalca was very positive and gave me hope (where the orthodox medicos had given me none), promising that he'd cure my cancer, no problem, if I did all he said—specific diet, juicing, and specific supplements that he sent me monthly. I followed this regime for a couple of months but it did not stop my tumour from re-growing. His protocol (most of which I think is valid, but not all) did however strengthen my immune system so that, or so I believe, when I did eventually do chemo. it was both more effective than expected and I suffered less than I might have done.

After about ten weeks on Majalca's regime—during most of which time I had been feeling quite well—my health suddenly plummeted. I had a severely infected testicle and became feverish. The doctors told me I was entering the last weeks of my life and that we should make preparations for that eventuality. I was admitted to a hospice and the general expectation was that I would die there.

However, shortly before this I had consulted with a fourth oncologist who told me that while he agreed in the main with what I had been told previously by the other oncologists, in his view there was a very slight chance that chemotherapy might be curative. He said there was a five per cent chance. Since I was dying anyway and the Majalca regime wasn't working, I decided to give it a go.

I started a regime of two chemo. drugs, cisplatin and gemcitabine. The impact was not directly bad—I just sat in a chair whilst it was poured into me, along with saline solutions. But an hour or so afterwards I was initially very violently sick, several times. But eventually a correct anti-nausea dosage was found that overcame that. But for about three months I was effectively bed-ridden. I also had to take morphine for pain-relief and this caused panics, constant drowsiness, constipation. I suppose one reason I was able to tolerate all this was that I was feeling so bad anyway.

After about three weeks I was able to book myself out of the hospice and go home. Although the hospice was very caring and supportive, the food was completely wrong for my needs. They provided tasty comfort food—full of sugar and sweet things—that was totally contrary to what a cancer patient should be eating. Back at home I was able to resume my variation of Majalca's protocol, and start exercising again. And, amazingly, gradually, I started to get better.

As soon as I could, I was back on the Internet, combing it for info; asking questions on forums; buying books; getting supplements; exchanging info. I gradually built up a huge amount of cancer-related information. From all this I created my own anti-cancer programme—exercise, lots of fresh fruit (I eventually realised berries were the best) and vegetables (especially broccoli and Brussels sprouts), no sugar, little alcohol; and lots of curcumin and black pepper, vitamin D3, and fish oil— were the major components. Luckily I had a good juicer that I had bought some time before so I was juicing vegetables three times a day to start with.

I also tried many 'cures'. None of them worked for me, or at least that was my conclusion in relation to myself. Maybe they work for other people.

Instead, I have myself evolved a programme that distils all I have learnt over a lifetime, both as an engineer, scientist and cancer patient, and which I think rests on solid scientific medical evidence too. I would like to share it with you.

This programme is based on the well-known engineering rule 'Knowledge of results improves performance'. The first step is to measure your state of health. The second is to analyse the results and the third step is to feed the body whatever it is that will correct the situation if it appears that there are problems. Then six or eight weeks later you repeat the cycle and see if anything has changed.

In fact, I work on two separate cycles. The first is an assessment of my cancerousness, the second is an assessment of my wellness. I make a distinction between these two cycles and for both these cycles I have a number of tests.

To test for my state of cancerousness I do regular testing for specific cancer markers—in my case I test for a specific urine marker for bladder cancer—the NMP22 BladderChek Test that detects elevated levels of NMP22 protein. I should warn you that the use of these blood markers is contentious. My first oncologist claimed he didn't know what cancer markers were! However, these are well understood, if not well used, by the medical profession [Note: I have discussed cancer markers in Section 2: *Cancer: Diagnosis and Conventional Treatments: The Pros and Cons of Cancer Tests, Surgery, Radiation and Chemotherapy*—J.C.] If your doctors won't co-operate, then you will have to get them done privately.

The second set of tests is those that, in my opinion, provide a good insight into the state of overall wellness. I assess my wellness by measuring my levels of vitamin D3, homocysteine, and essential fatty acids (EFAs). These are simple tests that your doctor should be prepared to arrange. Vitamin D3 levels should be high (not just normal)—above 200mmol/l; homocysteine levels should be low and as for the essential fatty acids I am aiming for and AA/EPA ratio of 1.5.

You probably won't understand that last bit so I will quote from one of the doctors I currently use as a source of good quality information, Dr Al Sears:

'There are only three fatty acids that can made into eicosanoids (the hormones that control inflammation). These are arachidonic acid (AA), dihomo gamma linolenic acid (DGLA), and eicosapentaenoic acid (EPA). From AA comes all the pro-inflammatory eicosanoids that in excess accelerate chronic disease. From DGLA come very powerful anti-inflammatory eicosanoids that accelerate cellular rejuvenation. Finally, from EPA comes very neutral eicosanoids, but its presence can help inhibit the formation of AA as well as dilute out its presence in the cell membrane thus making it more difficult to make pro-inflammatory eicosanoids. The balance of these three fatty acids in the blood will tell your future with laser-like precision. What you are looking for are the following levels:*

*AA less than 9 per cent of the total fatty acids
DGLA greater than 3 per cent of the total fatty acids
EPA greater than 4 per cent of the total fatty acids*

But it is the ratio of these fatty acids to each other that tells the full story. The true marker of silent inflammation is the AA/EPA ratio. If it is greater than 10 then you have it regardless of how good you look in a swimsuit. A good ratio would be 3, and the ideal ratio is about 1.5. You might ask where I get those numbers? If you ask who are the longest-lived people in the world today, the answer is the Japanese. If you ask who are people with the longest health span (longevity minus years of disability), the answer is again the Japanese. If you ask who have the lowest levels of heart disease in the world, the answer again is the Japanese. And you wouldn't be too surprised to find out that the Japanese have the lowest rates of depression in the world today. When you look at the blood of the Japanese population, the

AA:EPA ratio ranges from 1.5 to 3. If you have your AA levels at 9 per cent and your EPA levels at 4 per cent, then your AA:EPA would be 2.2 which is mid-range for controlling silent inflammation. For comparison the average 'healthy' American has an AA:EPA ratio greater than 12. This means Americans are not only the fattest people in the world today, but also the most inflamed. If you have chronic disease, then it likely that your AA:EPA ratio is greater than 20.'

In addition to these tests I also have a regular c-reactive protein (CRP) test. This indicates in a non-specific way the level of inflammation in the body—and cancer is about inflammation (as are arthritis, heart disease and pregnancy).

So that is my baseline for assessing what it is I need to do. I test my cancer and wellness markers on a regular basis and I tinker with my diet and exercise based on the results of these tests.

My current (July 2011) situation is this: my urologist has failed to find any evidence of cancer, though suspects it is still lurking around. My cancer markers are all down, though one or two are still above the normal threshold. I am fit. I feel healthy. In short I am winning. I am still alive.

My present diet is as follows:

Breakfast

is generally a whey powder, soya milk shake, with walnuts, freshly milled flaxseeds, and an apple; or porridge twice a week.

Lunch

is a big salad—some tinned fish with mixed leaves, bell peppers (chopped), mixed bean sprouts, spring onion, mushroom with fish; dressing of olive oil, cider vinegar, chilli pepper, mustard seed powder, curcumin and black pepper.

Dinner

is protein (fish, white meat, lamb), greens (some of: broccoli, string beans, cauliflower, Brussels sprouts, peas, tomatoes). Followed by berries.

During the day

I drink white tea and herb tea. Little or no alcohol. No sugar. Little or no dairy. Little or no carbohydrates.

I also take the following supplements: a high quality multi-vitamin and multi-mineral (Uni-Vite), several tablespoons of pure fish oil, vitamin D3 (5,000IU), zinc, magnesium, folic acid, and TMG (tri-methyl-glycine—good for reducing homocysteine levels*).*

I have prepared a paper on my full anti-cancer programme, which is available on Jonathan's website at www.cancerfighter.wordpress.com. It is available only on the understanding that it is for information only and represents my thinking at the time of writing. But I do tinker with this and if anyone wants to get my latest version they can email me at ianclements@hotmail.com.

Nuro Weidemann

Here is Nuro's story in her own words.

In January 2009 I noticed a tiny lump in my right breast. I went to my local GP. She eventually transferred me to the breast clinic where a couple of fine needle aspirations were made. I then had an ultrasound scan and a biopsy of the lump. The result was an aggressive (meaning fast spreading) form of non-Hodgkin's lymphoma with a tumour in my right breast. I was devastated!

I had worked for almost 20 years in the field of complementary health. I was of the opinion that I was of very robust health. I had quite a solid understanding of nutrition, was never really ill, had hardly any colds, went running regularly, did a very dynamic form of yoga and my busy work as a remedial massage therapist provided the necessary muscle strength training.

Admittedly, my daily coffees and teas had become more regular and also the occasional glass of wine had become more frequent. On top of my physically demanding job, the commuting between Brighton and London was stressful and every so often I wondered how much more my body could take …. However, as I never really felt ill I had no real reason to worry, I thought. So, I felt like I'd been hit by a hammer when the consultant told me. It was a terrible shock, but in a way I could see it coming. I was pretty stressed and running on adrenalin. Outside work I went running regularly and had a very busy social life … which tired me out even more. I remember driving home from London on the motorway one day and thinking 'I wonder when my body will crack?'

So getting a diagnosis of cancer completely threw me. I felt betrayed by my body. I simply could not believe it, as I didn't feel ill in the first place. For days I was in shock and kind of numb. Lots of pictures of people with cancer came up, I remembered my mum, who had died of cancer ten years previously. I was in an awful state.

The consultant told me that the form of cancer that I had was aggressive and would spread through the lymphatic system quickly. Chemotherapy was essential and possibly radiotherapy later. When I heard this I knew I couldn't face the treatment. Your hair falls out, you go into immediate menopause, your immune system is utterly shattered. I just couldn't do it.

Through this emotional fog I remembered an old friend of mine who had had cancer as a child. She overcame the illness by a purely natural approach and then a second time around 30 years later when she had cancer again, she also cured herself with alternative methods. I called her up and she encouraged me to embark on a similar route.

All the things she suggested weren't new to me. To apply them and believe in them when doctors were of the opinion that the only answer to my health problem was chemotherapy, was a huge challenge and a step I didn't know if I could make. On the other hand, I wanted to live! I didn't want to get poisoned. So I felt I didn't have anything to lose really.

So despite all the fear of the possible consequences of not doing chemotherapy, I wanted to give myself and my body a chance to heal itself.

I wanted, I needed, to try it out—at least for the next couple of weeks to see how I would do on a very clean diet, eliminating all possible sources of toxins, meditating, generally giving myself time and space to decide about my route of healing from a place where I wasn't terrified.

I gave up my job and with the help of my husband started some serious research on the 'net. I realised that this was about rebalancing my whole system—although there's this tumour, the illness is really in the whole of the body.

The first step I decided to take was to go on a diet to cut out acid-forming foods. Cancer loves an acidic environment. Stress creates a lot of acid, but so do some foods. So I cut out dairy, wheat, alcohol, meat, sugar and learnt about juicing and raw food. I also took up daily dry brushing and weekly colonics which became daily coffee enemas. I needed a way to eliminate the 'die-off ' of the cancer cells—it can be toxic enough to kill you. A coffee enema literally squeezes the toxins out of the liver. I also listened to a meditation tape every day, took hot and cold showers to stimulate the immune system, sunbathed for vitamin D, and walked along the coast near where I live. To get to the beach there is a 186-step cliff stairway. This was my way of gauging myself. How could I be that ill with cancer if I managed to climb all those steps? I surrounded myself with people who believed in me and read inspirational books. That was the hardest part, sticking to my guns when many people thought it was crazy.

But I could soon feel the whole-body approach was working. I began to feel fantastic after a couple of months. I woke up every morning and said, 'I have cancer, but I feel good.'

Here is a more detailed description of what I did. I hope it will be helpful to others who have the courage to treat their cancer using natural methods.

The first stage of my health regime looked something like this.

Phase 1

Diet

I went onto a mainly alkaline diet and cut out: dairy, meat, alcohol, sweets (including fruits, honey, any form of sweetener), gluten, salt, no nightshade vegetables (potatoes, tomatoes, aubergines). Instead I upped my organic vegetables, mainly raw as salads and juices, mostly made out of green vegetables, which I had before breakfast and dinner, supplemented by wheat grass juice. I also increased my daily water intake, trying to sip about one and a half to two litres throughout the day. My daily diet then became:

Breakfast

gluten-free porridge with a few raisins (that was my only sweet treat!)

Lunch

salad, lettuce, cucumbers, sprouts, few carrots, few beetroots, zucchinis, olive oil, lemon with a bit of quinoa or brown rice on the side and occasionally tofu.

Supper

were much the same vegetables as for lunch but steamed or as a stew with some added quinoa or brown rice.

I was on this diet for about eight weeks and it was roughly based on the book: *The pH Miracle* by Dr Robert and Shelly Young. During this time I didn't take any supplements, as I wasn't sure what would benefit me.

Additional healing approaches

In addition to the change of my diet, I had weekly colonic hydrotherapy, did daily meditations, visualisations (letting the tumour shrink and dealing with the fear of the diagnosis) and tried to go out for one-hour walks as often as possible. I also took MMS (Miracle Mineral Solution, an unfortunate name for a very effective remedy). I took MMS for over a year as suggested, first orally and for several months in combination with DMSO (dimethyl sulphoxide) topically.

On this diet I lost about 5kg over a span of two months. So did my husband who supported me on the diet, a good indication for me that I hadn't lost weight because of the cancer but because of my change in diet. It was a reassuring observation as advancing cancer is accompanied by weight loss.

Meanwhile, I tried to find a medical practitioner who would support me in my endeavour to heal the cancer with natural methods. I found a former GP who now works as an acupuncturist and nutritional therapist in Devon, UK.

It was clear from the start that he had many suggestions and insights regarding my condition but he couldn't take me on as a patient (law in the UK [Cancer Act, 1939] forbids anybody from claiming to heal cancer by any other means than chemotherapy, radiation or surgery). However I felt it was a step in the right direction.

After seeing him I slightly altered my diet, started to take supplements, dropped the regular colonics and introduced daily coffee enemas instead.

Phase 2

Diet

From my initial detoxifying diet I switched to a kind of building up or strengthening diet. Essentially it was the same as before but I added a few of the so called 'super foods' like bee pollen, goji berries, freshly ground-up flax and hempseeds, flaxseed and hempseed oils in my breakfast porridge, and augmented my usual lunches and suppers with fish, organic chicken or lamb's liver twice a week.

Supplements

As far as supplements went, I started to take iodine, krill oil, zinc, selenium, magnesium, a multi-vitamin, I ate apricot kernels and drank Essiac tea.

Naturopathic approaches

I also added the following naturopathic techniques to my daily routine: coffee enemas as mentioned earlier, castor oil packs over the liver, dry brushing, hot and cold showers, occasional Epsom salt bath, continued with my one-hour walks several times a week and tried to get into the sun without sun protection for 20 minutes a day to top up on the spirit-raising sun's health-bringing vitamin D stimulus.

Working with the mind

I carried on with my daily meditations and visualisations, as I understood the importance of working with the mind. I needed to have each and every aspect of my life supporting my longing for health. I listened to the 'Teaching of Abraham' These are teachings channelled by Esther Hicks. I know it sounds batty, but in fact they have been very important for me, as have lectures by the writer Eckart Tolle.

Mental attitude

During all this time I tried to stay clear of talking about trying to 'fight the cancer'. Ultimately my body had created the illness and I saw it more as a wake-up call that somewhere along the line I had gone against my own truth. I wanted to be kind to my body. I felt that was my way forward in all areas of my life. I wanted to learn again to go with the flow without compromising my own truth. At the same time I wanted to stay open to learn new things and change my approach along the way if needed. As long as it benefited my general health and wellbeing.

Electromagnetic radiation

During this time I also came to realise how health damaging electromagnetic radiation is. So we stopped using wireless broadband and went back to using cables, exchanged our cordless phone for an old fashioned hand held phone and I tried to use my mobile phone as little as possible (if I had to, I used an ear piece).

Creativity

On my quest for health I also wanted dedicate time to pottery again. I had started years before but had given it up when I got too busy with work. Now seemed the perfect time to start. So I enrolled on a course again. Two years on and I am still doing it. I really love to have my hands in wet clay and forming objects out of it. Mostly I do objects I can use around the house. My pots are getting better and looking less wonky, the glazes become more predictable, and they crack less.

This year for the first time I will exhibit some of my 'masterpieces' together with other friend's art in Cornwall. For me it is not so much about making perfect pieces of art, it's more about expressing an important part of myself.

Toxicity in cosmetics and cleaning products

The other important area of possible toxin burden that needed to be addressed was cleaning products, toiletries and cosmetics.

We basically switched them all to environmentally friendly products that were free of petrolatum, mineral oils, sodium lauryl/laureth sulfate, parabens, lanolin, and that hadn't been tested on animals, didn't contain any animal by-products and were biodegradable.

High quality water

On top of all that we installed a reverse osmosis filter for our so-important daily water consumption. This filters out the good and the bad, so we added extra mineral drops to our drinking water. We also installed a filter in our shower head that cleans out fluorides and other damaging ingredients.

Monitoring my progress

When I was first diagnosed and I wanted to go onto my alternative health regime, one big issue for me was how to monitor my progress.

The oncologist couldn't offer me any on-going tests other than invasive PET scans that they normally do every six months. As I was considered opting for 'no treatment' in the eyes of conventional medicine I wasn't given this test.

However, as I mentioned before, these tests are taxing on the body and I was rather looking for a test that was less invasive. We eventually came across the 'Navarro Test', which quite few people do when approaching cancer in a natural way.

Initially the test seemed to be very complicated to do and sounded a bit 'cowboy'-like. However, we overcame all obstacles and I did the test every three months. Besides feeling good in my body, the test became an important indicator of how I was doing on a less obvious level. After doing the test a few times it wasn't all that complicated as it initially seemed.

Success

After 18 months on this regime the lump in my breast had dissolved. Where there used to be a bulge that was as big as a chestnut, there was now nothing. At this point I felt that my body was strong enough to do another PET scan.

A reluctant oncologist eventually agreed to do the test. It showed that I had no cancer in my body anymore and I was declared as being 'in complete remission'. The oncologist was very surprised.

What now?

After the result of the PET scan, I had a big celebration with friends who had supported me through my healing journey. Everybody asked me if I would go on with my strict diet.

Well, there were a few things in my mind that I wanted to eat again. I tried them out but I can't really say that it was the big 'wow' experience that I was expecting.

For one thing, I have now completely lost my appetite for alcohol. It makes me feel strange and I don't like it any longer. Croissants with butter, strawberry jam and a coffee used to be my ultimate fantasy while I was on my regime. Even that has lost its appeal. However, I still love my daily crunchy organic veggie salads, the occasional bit of chicken and fish here and there.

My healthy diet has become a way of life. I still have the odd bits that I regard as not that healthy but I easily find my way back.

One thing that I find important for me is not to become too obsessed with food. I still like to go out for a meal every so often and eat what feels right for me without being too concerned, and then I go home and carry on with my daily green juice, the salads and steamed veggies and plenty of good quality water.

As a result of my healing journey I have enrolled in a nutritional healing course. That course teaches more or less the approach that has helped me immensely.

Over the last two years I feel as if I have done a crash course in healthy living. The nutrition course gives me the time and the support to go over everything I have done to get better and to come to a deeper understanding. I hope that with my own experience and the help of this course I will be able to inspire people to try out the gentle way of healing cancer.

Summary

Initially I was trying to find the 'right' healing method. Everything I read felt very overwhelming, confusing and at times was contradictory. Initially, when I came across these contradictions they felt like a major obstacle and a big worry on my journey. But now I feel much more relaxed about them. Gradually, all the reading I did and the information I had accumulated fell into place. I developed a sense of when to incorporate another healing method, and which one I wanted to incorporate. I needed to stick to something that felt right to me before I understood all other methods.

I am sure I could have done it in a different way, but the methods I chose felt right to me at the time. What I want to express here is the fact that there is not only one right method of healing. Finding my own inner voice and my own intuition was pivotal.

Although initially it was a very scary situation, it eventually became a very empowering process. I was, and I am, still amazed by the way my body reacted to positive, loving, caring and gentle attention. It felt that there was this part in me that wanted to be heard and acknowledged. Once I had tuned in, it was delighted to support my healing process on every conceivable level. The illness was a true blessing in disguise for me.

Having said all that, I don't feel I have reached a place from where I can simply go back to my life how it used to be. On a physical level my healing is complete for now but emotionally I feel like a work in progress.

Nevertheless I felt that I had a story that might help others so I contacted *The Guardian* newspaper Health Editor to offer her my story. This was the reply I got back: 'I'm sorry—it's good to hear you are well, but we are a very science-based, evidence-based newspaper and would not run stories based on one person's experience, which may well not be typical.'

If that's their attitude, how is anyone going to learn that it is possible, as I have proved for myself, that you can cure cancer by natural means?

If anyone wishes to know more I can be contacted at nuro@insafehands.co.uk.

Appendices

The rich can afford the very best medicine

When it comes to cancer, I feel sorry for the rich. They can afford the very best treatments that money can buy. And they must be the best treatments—right?—because they are the treatments proposed by the most eminent doctors to whom only the very rich have access.

Often these treatments are the very latest, most cutting-edge. The more you can pay, the more you are going to suffer. But since these oncologists don't have the cure for most cancers and are not going to have that cure for the conceivable future—(read oncologist Siddhartha Mukherjee's best-selling book, *The Emperor of All Maladies*, if you don't believe me)—then all this money spent on painful treatments is just buying the pain. The more money you have the more pain you can afford.

But if we can't put our hopes on these latest, cutting-edge treatments what can we do? Well, there are so many options that I could suggest, that I don't know where to start. That's why I wrote the *Cancer Survivor's Bible* (see www.fightingcancer.com). That's where you will find the answers that suit you.

But let's return to the issue of wealth, fame and cancer. Recently we have had two famous pancreatic cancers: Steve Jobs' and Patrick Swayze's and a long time ago we had Steve McQueen's mesothelioma. Both of these cancers—pancreatic and mesothelioma—are considered to be pretty much untreatable (by conventional means). But that doesn't mean they won't treat you anyway. Doctors will often treat you just to stop you becoming so depressed that you'll do something crazy like go to the alternative treatments (I'm not joking. This is policy in some quarters. They treat you until you're so far along that there's little anyone can do for you).

Swayze and Jobs both went the conventional route. Although Jobs did also follow an alternative regime to start with, and very possibly continued doing some through his conventional treatments (certainly he survived much longer than most people diagnosed with pancreatic cancer), Swayze was only interested in following the conventional route. He died 18 months after diagnosis. Felicity Corbin-Wheeler, whose story I tell in this section is today alive and cancer free, having recovered from the same cancer using the much derided alternative, Laetrile. If you get pancreatic cancer, which do you think is the best model to follow?

And then there was Steve McQueen who famously, having exhausted his conventional options, chose to work with the alternative cancer therapist, William Kelley, then after a year with him allowed himself to be operated on—and died on the operating table. Who gets the praise and who the blame?

Dr Nicholas Gonzalez, who has continued William Kelley's work (for details of Kelley's approach see Section 3: *Cancer Research and Politics*—Kelley, too, cured himself of terminal stage pancreatic cancer), has complained about the way the media responds differently to conventional doctors on the one hand and alternative therapists on the other:

'You see, when a conventional oncologist loses a celebrity patient, they [the media] portray him as a hero fighting this terrible disease against enormous odds; working late into the night trying to keep the celebrity alive. But when an alternative practitioner loses a patient, they consider him a sleazy quack getting money from unsuspecting cancer victims.'

The Steve McQueen case has been used particularly to stigmatise alternative approaches, but Gonzales has responded robustly to the suggestion that Kelley killed McQueen:

'He [Steve McQueen] was terminal when he came to Dr Kelley. He had failed radiation, failed immunotherapy. He had been misdiagnosed for a year. The reason he ended up with Stage 4 mesothelioma is because he was misdiagnosed by his fancy conventional doctors in Southern California. Then they gave him radiation—there's not a study in the history of the world showing that radiation helps in mesothelioma; they gave it anyway. Then they gave him immunotherapy. There's not a study in the history of the world saying that immunotherapy helps in mesothelioma. They did it anyway. Then he was dying and he went to see Kelley. He died, and Kelley got all the blame. Not the doctors who misdiagnosed him! In fact when you read the newspaper articles, there are still articles about how Dr Kelley killed McQueen. No! Cancer killed McQueen. You see, an oncologist at Sloan-Kettering can do a bone marrow transplant on celebrity patients. They die, and he's written up like a hero .... Kelley tries to help after conventional doctors failed miserably and misdiagnosed him, and McQueen lived longer than he should. (He was a half-compliant patient—he continued to smoke, drink, and eat ice cream.) .... About two or three years ago, there was an op-ed piece in the Wall Street Journal attacking unconventional cancer therapy. They talked about McQueen, and how Kelley killed him. ... Conventional oncologists lose patients every day, and no-one says they're murdering anybody. Instead they're considered heroes for trying so hard.'

So there it is. Two morals to this article. First, money may or may not buy happiness but, when it comes to cancer, it doesn't necessarily buy a longer, healthier life. Second, don't believe everything you read in the national press when they criticise alternative medicine.

Letter to oncologists

For decades you have been seeking to cure cancer—first through surgery, attempting, at first, to achieve your aims by increasingly disfiguring and life-threatening operations until sanity came to the rescue and you realised (I do hope you have realised) that surgery only works at a very early stage of a cancer's growth, and therefore a lumpectomy is as much as needs be done—but of course if the cancer has spread to other parts of the body, then even this is useless—possibly even worse than useless, as the healing process may incidentally provoke a more rapid growth of distant metastases.

Then came radiation, which is still with us, which has the same limitations as surgery—and more besides. You realised eventually that only a systemic approach could work. So you turned your focus on chemotherapy. But despite repeated attempts to cure cancer with multiple, highly toxic, drug regimes, this approach too has sadly failed. You now recognise it only works in about five to six per cent of cancers (for the 'benefit' ultimately of maybe three per cent). This benefit, sadly, comes with it an extraordinary range of qualifications—early onset of new cancers, slowing down of brain functions, and so on. But you know all this. Patients generally don't, but you do. Oncologist Siddhartha Mukherjee has admitted as much in his wide-ranging, best-selling book, *The Emperor of All Maladies*, but this fact has been known for a very long time. The problem is in persuading you oncologists to be straight with us on this. Now it seems there is a move in this direction.

Currently, you are placing all your hopes on smart drugs that attack proteins and enzymes specific to each of the 2,000 (or some say 20,000) different cancer types you have discovered. But even this approach you understand will not work. The closer you get to the bio-chemistry of these 'evil' cells the greater their complexity. And of course, cancer changes genetically very fast and each drug ceases to be effective equally rapidly. The cure for cancer has simply disappeared over the horizon. But you have not told people that. You go along with the press releases from drug companies that announce each supposed advance. You allow the press to laud these developments. You remain satisfied with the small incremental improvements in mortality measure, decade on decade. But you know that the pain and failure of conventional cancer treatments will go on and on—perhaps forever, because you cannot see any alternative. And yet the alternative is there in plain sight. You even call it 'alternative medicine'.

For the most part you have given up on the hope of cure and are now moving to a philosophy of palliative medicine. It is your hope that if you cannot cure cancer you can at least help cancer patients live longer. It is here that the horizons of the alternative movement converge on your own sphere.

If you allowed yourself to embrace alternative medicine—and why should you not? There is no research to show that a regime of diet, supplements, herbs and other health supporting does not also substantially extend life, and quality of life. And as the stories in this section demonstrate clearly, some people cure themselves of cancers that conventional doctors have given up on. Yes 'cure' is the word we can use when someone remains free of cancer for 30 years, as Beata Bishop has done.

So here is a suggestion, one first suggested to me by Ian Clements The suggestion is this. All cancer patients should be seen long-term on an outpatient basis. They should be given regular blood tests to determine not only the progress of various cancer markers but also to monitor other key indicators of overall health. Then they should be encouraged to follow whatever therapies and treatments they may deem to be appropriate—alternative as well as conventional—all the time maintaining a beady eye on changes to these markers for cancer and health. Offer everyone this book so that they can see the full range of the options that may be beneficial. And of course keep testing, keep evaluating the results, keep being prepared to fiddle with the regime.

I can assure you, you will be amazed. Suddenly, people you expected to die will recover. Perhaps not everyone but certainly more than do so currently. Others—the vast majority, I suspect, of those who take the job of getting well again seriously—will go on living far longer than predicted.

It is really that simple. So the question I put to you now is this: Why have you not already done this?

You see, cancer is not just a problem for doctors, it is—more pressingly—a problem for the patients, the people with the cancer. Cancer patients need to learn to begin to take responsibility for their own cancers (and their own health overall) and doctors need to help them. Indeed, more and more patients are seeing for themselves the benefits of complementary and alternative treatments. People are already moving towards CAM treatments for their cancer—and they are not telling their doctors because of the weight of disapproval. It's a secret move away from orthodox medicine, and this movement is getting bigger and bigger all the time. (Ask yourself this: if people believed doctors had a good cure for cancer there wouldn't be a need for alternative therapies. So if more and more people are using CAM: complementary and alternative medicine—what does that indicate?)

Here's what University of Toronto cancer researcher Heather Boon discovered in 2005: '… more than 80 per cent of all women with breast cancer report using CAM (41 per cent in a specific attempt to manage their breast cancer), *CAM use can no longer be regarded as an "alternative" or unusual approach to managing breast cancer.*' (my emphasis). According to her, younger, more educated women, in particular, are more likely to have a high commitment to CAM therapies.

Cristiane Spadacio, another cancer researcher, says: '… there has been an exponential growth in interest in—and use of—complementary and alternative medicine (CAM), especially in developed western countries …. *Studies show that the number of patients who use some form of alternative therapy after the diagnosis of cancer is high … [and they experience] high levels of satisfaction with alternative therapies.*' (my emphasis).

At present, the situation is this: if patients decline to undergo surgery, radiation or chemotherapy—or any of the other treatments on the conventional menu—then you oncologists wash your hands of them. 'We offered them treatment and they refused, what can we do?' You tell yourselves.

Well, what you can do is this: continue to see them on an outpatient basis, offering your access to blood tests, scans and so on, so that these patients can monitor their own bodies. That's what you can do, and indeed should be doing. Otherwise you are monopolising certain services to the detriment of the health of people who wish to work out their own solutions to their cancers—and they have every right to do this because it is they, ultimately, who are going to suffer the consequences.

So, please, please, can you set aside your prejudices and help them.

Jonathan Chamberlain
www.fightingcancer.com

Cancer: a systemic disease demands a systemic response

What causes cancer? Is it A or B or C? Is it bad diet, depression, chemicals in the atmosphere or what? This is the way most people approach the question of causation. This approach is reductionist: if there is a problem there must be a chain of causation. A causes B and that makes C happen and the result of that is cancer.

This is the way all medical research approaches the problems they study. They look for linear chains of cause and effect. 'The problem with this approach is that it has trouble explaining dynamic complexity,' David Brooks (*The Social Animal*, Short Books 2011, p.131). But it seems so obvious a way of thinking, that to imagine there is another way of looking at a problem is at first difficult to conceive. But there is another way.

'Emergent systems' describes situations where there is a complex dynamic context underlying a phenomenon, but where no specific element of the dynamic context is causative by itself.

Let's take the example of poverty and IQ . Poverty has the effect of reducing IQ—but how? Is it a question of genes? Parental relationships? Bad diet? Poor living conditions? Living in crime-ridden neighbourhoods? Well, it appears that none of the above single conditions on its own causes lower IQs. Lower IQs occur when they—and other factors—are all present together. It is the combination of factors that causes the negative cascade, one of the results of which is a lower IQ.

What is interesting about this way of looking at the problem, is that it leads us to a different way of trying to solve the problem. Instead of tinkering (by, say, improving diet or trying to add special remedial classes etc.) the only way to change the result is to change the entire underlying context—change everything all at once.

If we apply this idea to cancer, that is if we see cancer as being an emergent system, then if we are to reverse the situation, we need to change everything at once: habits, diet, relationships, activities, attitudes, goals, biochemical terrain—everything. The more factors we can change in a positive direction, the more likely we are to induce a new emergent system—one that will initiate a positive cascade of results.

That leads to a very interesting conclusion: the more things you do to improve your health in relation to cancer, the more likely you are to live longer, the more likely you are to recover.

Summing up

Taken individually, each of these stories can be, and generally has been, dismissed by doctors as inexplicable. In each case the doctor might say that the recovery was unexpected but 'it is unlikely that alternative therapies have had any real impact'. However, taken collectively, the case they make for the potential of a wide variety of alternative therapies from diet, herbs, supplements and so on becomes increasingly hard to reject.

Many doctors will claim that they know of sad cases where ill-advised patients have taken to the alternative route and died shortly thereafter, But they don't mention the cases where patients have undergone painful and damaging conventional treatments and who have, like my wife did, died shortly after.

Of the dead we cannot speak. Undoubtedly, many people going the alternative route do die—perhaps because they have not done enough of the right things or they have stuck to one thing, or who knows what other reason (but undoubtedly they will have saved themselves a great deal of pain and very likely will have lived longer than expected). But what these stories do tell us, is that many people following alternative approaches have cured their cancers, or are continuing their battle against cancer, never allowing themselves to think they have defeated it but that, for the time being, they are winning. And let us remind ourselves of the extraordinary range of cancers represented by these stories—breast cancer, prostate cancer, melanoma, sarcoma, cancers of the colon, kidney, bladder, pancreas and anus, brain tumours, lymphoma and myeloma. Whatever is working is working across the whole spectrum of cancer.

How many times do you need to press a light switch to know—with 100 per cent certainty—that there is a causal relationship between pressing the switch and the light coming on. Two? Three times at most. How many cases do you need to read of people recovering from cancer using alternative means before you can accept that maybe there is something to the alternative approaches to cancer?

It is my hope that you will see that the promise of freedom from cancer by means of health-enhancing (not health-damaging) therapies is real. As one contributor to my blog said recently: 'It was very early on in my journey that I began to question the conventional methods of treatment. I was sitting in the break room at work one morning, and I posed a question to a co-worker: 'Why would God want to use radioactive poison to heal me? Why would He want to kill all that is right and good to kill that which is not?' The 'logic' in that has never computed in my mind and is something I cannot get around. The answer that came to me was that He wouldn't. That question became the driving force behind my decision to find a natural remedy for my cancer.'

It is by asking these simple innocent questions that we discover the nakedness of the Emperor of Conventional Medicine. Cancer comes from nature—the answer too must be available in nature.

Respect for me is a word that has enormous power. If we respected each other, if we respected our environment, if we respected ourselves more fully, then the world would be a very different place. But we don't respect this planet we are all travelling on enough. We don't respect other people—people who are different from us—enough. And we don't respect our bodies enough. If we did, we wouldn't allow them to be attacked with such toxic chemicals or with such toxic and damaging radiation (see Section 2: *Cancer: Diagnosis and Conventional Treatments: The Pros and Cons of Cancer Tests, Surgery, Radiation and Chemotherapy* for a full discussion of this topic).

It is my hope that this book will be helpful to you in extending the length and the quality of your life, the lives of your family members, and the lives of your friends, neighbours, colleagues and even casual acquaintances.

Tell others

If you have found this book useful, then tell all your family and friends. Cancer is part of all our lives—either the cancers we are harbouring in our own bodies, or the cancers that are affecting the lives of loved ones, friends, neighbours, colleagues and so on.

The better we are prepared, the better our outcome is likely to be. If we build into our lives strategies that can 'cure' cancer, then by adopting them in advance we will be doing a great deal to prevent that cancer in the first place.

As a cancer patient wrote after reading one of my books: 'I wish I'd read this book before I was diagnosed. My doctor and the cancer charities didn't tell me any of this.' If you found one of the sections of this book particularly useful, you may be interested to know that each section is published as a separate book in the *Cancer: The Complete Recovery Guide* series of eight books (available from all Internet bookshops).

Help your family and friends avoid the pain and suffering that goes along with cancer. You could save someone's life.

Testimonials

Cancer: The Complete Recovery Guide

'Mr Chamberlain has a voice that is at once humble and powerful. I like writers that cut to the chase, and then do not skimp on the practical details … and I really like his attitude. He speaks from the heart, but clearly wants you to use your head. Good combination.'—*Andrew Saul PhD, in the Doctor Yourself Newsletter*

'This book tells me everything I want to know. Why didn't my doctor tell me this?'—*Rev Bill Newbern*

'First of all let me say: Congratulations on your superb book! I have a vast experience in this field of alternative cancer treatment going back to 1999. I have attended dozens of alternative, complementary, and integrative cancer conferences and workshops (I attend every such event that I hear about); have had discussions with hundreds of holistic cancer practitioners and thousands of cancer patients; am active on all the alternative cancer email discussion groups; and have read or am familiar with almost every book written on alternative cancer treatment (and have compiled an annotated bibliography of them). Let me say immediately that your book is authoritative, reputable, and much more comprehensive and better balanced than the vast majority of other books on the topic. Also, it has much valuable material that I don't recall seeing in any other book. The book would strongly appeal to cancer patients and their families. The tone is perhaps a bit too strong for conventional medical practitioners, but the book isn't written for them. But it is very suited towards the general public and certainly to cancer patients for whom it was clearly written. In fact the tone is engaging and lively and will appeal to anyone sympathetic to alternative approaches to cancer. You have succeeded in making a complicated subject accessible.'—*Leonard S Rosenbaum MA, Board of Directors, International Association of Cancer Victors and Friends (IACVF; www.cancervictors.net)*

'An excellent, up-to-date resource.'—*Patty Feist*

'Having just been through surgery myself to remove a breast cancer lump and facing follow-up treatments such as chemotherapy, radiotherapy and hormone therapy, I am so glad I was tipped off to read this book …. This book helps to put things in perspective and was invaluable to me in making my decisions about follow-up treatment.'—*Lucy W (Amazon review)*

'I recently bought your book because I have become very involved in the life of an old friend, and the challenges she faces with a diagnosis of secondary liver cancer. We were both comforted and somewhat inspired by the broad sweep of your book.'—*Ron Crennel*

'Over the last six years or so, I've had a sporadic correspondence with Jonathan Chamberlain. I knew we shared a passion to get the word out about gentle, non-toxic ways to heal cancer and that he had written several books on the subject. But I was not prepared for the experience I got when I read his new book he sent me a couple of weeks ago. This is an incredibly informative and useful book. Every one of you needs it in your library.'—*Bill Henderson, author of* Cancer-Free

'The section on conventional treatment was riveting. For someone like me, who's chosen the alternative route right from the start, that section is actually very comforting! Leaves you in no doubt that there is no alternative to the alternatives!'—*Ann Napier, Publisher, Cygnus Book Club*

'Well done, I do think you have made a good job of covering such a wide variance in subjects and keeping it readable. I particularly like your writing style, factual and calm about what is frankly the ridiculous state of relationships between orthodox and alternative approaches.'—*Patricia Peat, Cancer Options (cancer consultancy)*

Cancer Recovery Guide: 15 Alternative and Complementary Strategies for Restoring Health

'Jonathan Chamberlain's *Cancer Recovery Guide* is loaded with practical ways to beat cancer now. If you have been told that your only options are surgery, radiation, and chemotherapy, then this is the book for you. In my 33 years as a health educator, I have seen very few books on cancer that are so upbeat and so well written.'—*Andrew W Saul, Assistant Editor,* Journal of Orthomolecular Medicine

'For a book shorter than 200 pages, with big print, Chamberlain's *Cancer Recovery Guide* [the little book] packs a lot of discussion on theory and treatment into what may be the best read on alternative therapies for cancer.'—*Jonathan Collin MD, Editor-in-chief,* Townsend Letter for Doctors

'This book is just SUPERB!!!!'—*'Feemeister' (Amazon review)*

Testimonials for both books

'Jonathan, I bought both of your books …. They are excellent and should be on every list of recommended cancer resources. Thank you for the excellent research and writing you did to create them.'—*Phil Zachary*

'These two books should be on the shelves of every medical practitioner who counsels or treats cancer patients, as well as cancer patients and their families.'—*Positive Health Magazine*

Other testimonials can be found at www.fightingcancer.com

Index

About the author

Jonathan Chamberlain was brought up in Ireland and Hong Kong but now lives in the UK. He describes himself as a novelist who got hijacked by life.

When his daughter was born with Down's Syndrome and later became profoundly disabled when a heart operation went wrong, he went on to found two charities for families with disabled children, one in Hong Kong and one in China. He has written about this time in his memoir: *Wordjazz for Stevie*, described by one newspaper as 'Maybe the most moving story you will ever read'.

When Bernadette, his wife, got cancer he started the research that led to a series of cancer books resulting in *The Cancer Survivor's Bible*. In addition he has written these titles:

Fiction

Dreams of Gold

The Alphabet of Vietnam

Whitebait & Tofu

Non-fiction

King Hui: The man who owned all the opium in Hong Kong

Chinese Gods

Wordjazz for Stevie

Cancer

Cancer: The Complete Recovery Guide (2008 Edition)

Cancer Recovery Guide: 15 Alternative and Complementary Strategies for Restoring Health

Cancer: The Complete Recovery Guides Books 1-8 (2012 Edition)

Other books by Jonathan Chamberlain

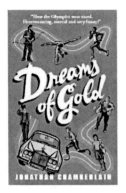

Dreams of Gold

A wild, zany—and very funny—romp as a motley crew of athletes save the London 2012 Olympics from the bizarre machinations of a crazed dictator. P G Wodehouse meets Tom Sharpe—with a dash of Spike Milligan!

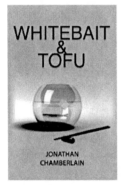

Whitebait & Tofu

American noir. Sam, British photographer living in an urban sprawl on the American Pacific coast gets caught up in a conspiracy. Who is Tulip, the beautiful Japanese woman who moves into his life? Where does she fit in and what does she really want of him? Crisp as haiku tale of love and sex and death.

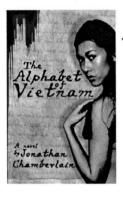

Alphabet of Vietnam

When men come back from war they bring the war back with them.

'I loved this book. An extraordinary page-turner. Intricately plotted, with astute observations that capture the fingernails-on-a-blackboard atmosphere of Vietnam, then and now. Reminiscent of Joseph Conrad and Graham Greene. It's up there with the best.'—Colin Leinster, former Vietnam correspondent, LIFE magazine.

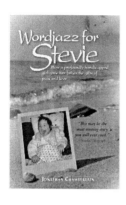

Wordjazz for Stevie

Deeply moving memoir of living with a profoundly disabled daughter and the gift of pain and love that she bequeaths her father.

'May be the most moving story you will ever read'—*Sunday Telegraph*

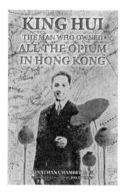

King Hui: The man who owned all the opium in Hong Kong

Kung fu fighter, gambler, playboy, collaborator with the Japanese, CIA spy, associate of triads—Hui was many things. His story is the living story of Hong Kong.

'This is a true story but it reads like a novel. It is a cracking read.'—Sir David Tang

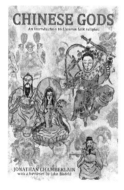

Chinese Gods: An introduction to Chinese folk religion

An introduction to the folk religion of the Chinese people—the belief system that informs the thinking of over one billion people.

'Even for the casual reader, this is a hugely satisfying book.'—Nick Walker, *Bangkok Post*

CPSIA information can be obtained at www.ICGtesting.com
Printed in the USA
BVOW041859300413

319525BV00006B/313/P